CURRENT PSYCHOTHERAPIES

CURRENT PSYCHOTHERAPIES
TENTH EDITION

Editors

Danny Wedding
Raymond J. Corsini

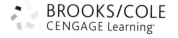
BROOKS/COLE
CENGAGE Learning·

Australia • Brazil • Japan • Korea • Mexico • Singapore • Spain • United Kingdom • United States

BROOKS/COLE
CENGAGE Learning

Current Psychotherapies, Tenth Edition
Editors: Danny Wedding, Raymond J. Corsini

Publisher: Jon-David Hague

Editorial Assistant: Amelia Blevins

Media Editor: Elizabeth Momb

Brand Manager: Elisabeth Rhoden

Market Development Manager: Kara Kindstrom

Manufacturing Planner: Judy Inouye

Rights Acquisitions Specialist: Roberta Broyer

Text Researcher: PreMedia Global

Production Management and Composition: Teresa Christie, MPS Limited

Copy Editor: S.M. Summerlight

Art and Design Direction: Carolyn Deacy, MPS Limited

Cover Designer: Kathleen Cunningham

Cover Image: Bendy Poppies, 1995 (colour photo) © Norman Hollands / Private Collection / The Bridgeman Art Library

For product information and technology assistance, contact us at
Cengage Learning Customer & Sales Support, 1-800-354-9706
For permission to use material from this text or product,
submit all requests online at **www.cengage.com/permissions**
Further permissions questions can be e-mailed to
permissionrequest@cengage.com

Library of Congress Control Number: 2012955798

Student Edition:

ISBN-13: 978-1-285-08371-1
ISBN-10: 1-285-08371-7

Loose-leaf Edition:

ISBN-13: 978-1-285-41905-3
ISBN-10: 1-285-41905-7

Brooks/Cole
20 Davis Drive
Belmont, CA 94002-3098
USA

Cengage Learning is a leading provider of customized learning solutions with office locations around the globe, including Singapore, the United Kingdom, Australia, Mexico, Brazil, and Japan. Locate your local office at **www.cengage.com/global**

Cengage Learning products are represented in Canada by Nelson Education, Ltd.

To learn more about Brooks/Cole, visit **www.cengage.com/Brooks/Cole**

Purchase any of our products at your local college store or at our preferred online store **www.CengageBrain.com**

Printed in the United States of America
1 2 3 4 5 6 7 17 16 15 14 13

In memory of Raymond J. Corsini (1914–2008)

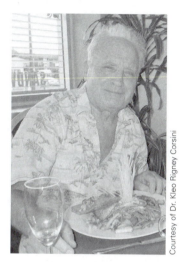

Dedication

To Pamela Susan Tarzian Broadman
*Who taught me how profoundly one human being
can love another*

CORE STRUCTURE

CONTENTS

CONTRIBUTORS

Martin M. Antony
Martin M. Antony, PhD, is Professor of Psychology at Ryerson University, Toronto, Canada, where he conducts research on the nature and treatment of anxiety disorders and perfectionism. An author of more than 200 scholarly publications, Dr. Antony has coauthored or edited 28 books, including *Behavior Therapy and the Oxford Handbook of Anxiety and Related Disorders*. Dr. Antony has received many career awards for his contributions to research and training, and he also has served as president of the Canadian Psychological Association.

Aaron T. Beck
Aaron T. Beck, MD, founded Cognitive Therapy. He currently directs the Psychopathology Research Unit in the Department of Psychiatry at the University of Pennsylvania, where he is an emeritus professor. Dr. Beck is the recipient of numerous awards, including the 2006 Albert Lasker Clinical Medical Research Award for developing Cognitive Therapy.

Larry E. Beutler
Larry E. Beutler, PhD, is Professor Emeritus at the University of California Santa Barbara and at Palo Alto University. He is past editor of the *Journal of Consulting and Clinical Psychology* and of the *Journal of Clinical Psychology*. He is past president of two APA divisions (the Society of Clinical Psychology and the APA Division of Psychotherapy) and author or coauthor of 29 books and more than 450 scholarly papers on psychotherapy and assessment.

Lillian Comas-Díaz
Lillian Comas-Díaz, PhD, is a clinical psychologist in full-time private practice and a Clinical Professor at the George Washington University Department of Psychiatry and Behavioral Sciences. Lillian has published extensively in psychology, serves on several editorial boards, and currently is an Associate Editor for the *American Psychologist*. Her most recent book is *Multicultural Care: A Clinician's Guide to Cultural Competence*.

Frank Dumont
Frank Dumont, EdD, Professor Emeritus, McGill University, was Director of the PhD program in counseling psychology at McGill, where he served as a chair of his department. He published widely on inferential processes in psychotherapy, collaborated with Raymond Corsini on *The Dictionary of Psychology*, and most recently authored *A History of Personality Psychology*.

Albert Ellis (1913–2007)
Albert Ellis, PhD, wrote more than 80 books and more than 800 articles, but he is best known for developing and championing Rational Emotive Behavior Therapy (REBT). He was consistently ranked as one of the most influential psychologists of the 20th century. In addition to his writing, Al trained and supervised practitioners, and he helped thousands of clients in his clinical practice. Dr. Ellis was posthumously awarded the 2013 Award for Outstanding Lifetime Contributions to Psychology by the American Psychological Association.

Debbie Joffe Ellis
Debbie Joffe Ellis, MDAM, is a licensed psychologist and mental health counselor, author, and presenter who conducted public and professional workshops with her husband, Albert Ellis, until his death in 2007. Debbie currently maintains a

clinical practice and travels around the world presenting on Rational Emotive Behavior Therapy.

Irene Goldenberg

Irene Goldenberg, EdD, is a Professor Emerita in the Department of Psychiatry, University of California Los Angeles. She has trained generations of psychiatrists and psychologists in family therapy, and she coauthored *Family Therapy: An Overview*, now in its eighth edition. Currently, Irene is in independent practice in Los Angeles, California.

Herbert Goldenberg (1927–2009)

Herbert Goldenberg, PhD, was a Professor Emeritus at California State Los Angeles, where he taught for 40 years. His books on clinical and abnormal psychology and family therapy were widely adopted. He was honored along with his wife, Irene Goldenberg, with the Lifetime Achievement Award by the American Family Therapy Academy in 2007.

Lynne Jacobs

Lynne Jacobs, PhD, cofounded the Pacific Gestalt Institute in Los Angeles, where she continues to practice. She is also a training and supervising analyst at the Institute of Contemporary Psychoanalysis, and she maintains a private practice in Los Angeles. Lynne has numerous publications and teaches Gestalt therapists internationally.

Ruthellen Josselson

Ruthellen Josselson, PhD, is a professor of clinical psychology at the Fielding Graduate University and a practicing psychotherapist. She is author of many books and articles, including *Playing Pygmalion: How People Create One Another* and *The Space Between Us*. She is codirector of the Yalom Institute of Psychotherapy, and she has received both the Henry A. Murray and Theodore R. Sarbin Awards from the American Psychological Association.

Alexander Kriss

Alexander Kriss, MA, is a doctoral candidate in clinical psychology and a writer. He currently trains at The New School for Social Research in New York City and is a former editor of *The New School Psychology Bulletin*. Alexander's plays have been performed in New York and London, and his e-books have been published for Amazon.

Michael P. Maniacci

Michael P. Maniacci, PsyD, is a licensed clinical psychologist in private practice in Chicago and Naperville, Illinois. He teaches at numerous institutions and consults with several organizations, and he has written more than 40 articles or book chapters and authored, coauthored, or edited 5 textbooks.

Harold H. Mosak

Harold H, Mosak, PhD, received his doctorate in clinical psychology from the University of Chicago in 1950. In 1952, he cofounded, with Bernard H. Shulman and Rudolf Dreikurs, the Adler School of Professional Psychology, where he currently holds the rank of Distinguished Service Professor.

John C. Norcross

John C. Norcross, PhD, ABPP, is Professor of Psychology and Distinguished University Fellow at the University of Scranton and a clinical psychologist in part-time practice. Author of more than 300 scholarly publications, Dr. Norcross has cowritten or edited 20 books, including *Psychotherapy Relationships That Work, Handbook of Psychotherapy Integration, Insider's Guide to Graduate Programs in Clinical and Counseling Psychology,* and *Self-Help That Works*. John also has served as president of the APA Society of Clinical Psychology and the APA Division of Psychotherapy.

Erica Goldenberg Pelavin

Erica Pelavin, LCSW, PhD, is a family psychologist specializing in bullying prevention, relational aggression, digital drama, cybersafety, and conflict resolution. In addition to her counseling work with adolescents, she teaches seminars in media literacy and 21st-century learning skills.

Kenneth S. Pope

Kenneth S. Pope, PhD, is a licensed psychologist and diplomate in clinical psychology whose works include more than 100 articles and chapters. The most recent of Ken's 12 books is *Ethics in Psychotherapy and Counseling: A Practical Guide* (4th ed.) (coauthored with Melba J. T. Vasquez). A Fellow of the Association for Psychological Science (APS), Ken provides free psychology resources at kspope.com and free disability resources at kpope.com.

Tayyab Rashid

Tayyab Rashid, PhD, provides psychological services for the Health & Wellness Centre, University of Toronto Scarborough, Canada. Dr. Rashid completed his pre- and postdoctoral clinical training at the University of Pennsylvania under the mentorship of Dr. Martin Seligman, with whom he developed and empirically validated Positive Psychotherapy (PPT). Dr. Rashid guest edited the 2009 *Journal of Clinical Psychology* special issue on Positive Interventions.

Nathaniel J. Raskin (1921–2010)

Nathaniel J. Raskin, PhD, has been called a "quiet giant" of the client-centered approach. He was a student of Carl Rogers, later a colleague and close friend, and a Professor of Clinical Psychology at Northwestern University Medical School. Everyone who experienced Nat in small groups, in classes, or as clients, recalls his decency, generosity, and profound embodiment of unconditional positive regard, empathic understanding, and genuineness.

Carl Rogers (1902–1987)

Carl Ransom Rogers, PhD, pioneer of the client-centered and person-centered approach, is regarded as one of the most influential and revolutionary psychologists of the 20th century. He was a master therapist whose emancipatory theory and practice, not only of therapy but also of interpersonal relationships, is widely studied. His later work included large group encounters between parties to international conflicts in Northern Ireland and Central America.

Laurie Sackett-Maniacci

Laurie Sackett-Maniacci, PsyD, is a licensed clinical psychologist and an adjunct faculty member and clinical supervisor at the Adler School of Professional Psychology in Chicago, Illinois, where she teaches Adlerian theory and Adlerian treatment approaches. Laurie maintains a private practice in Naperville and is a consultant to the Rush Copley Heart Institute Rehabilitation Center.

Jeremy D. Safran

Jeremy D. Safran, PhD, is Professor of Psychology at The New School for Social Research, Clinical Professor at the New York University Postdoctoral Program in Psychotherapy and Psychoanalysis, and past president of the International Association for Relational Psychoanalysis and Psychotherapy. He is the author of numerous books, including *Psychoanalysis and Psychoanalytic Therapies*.

Martin E. P. Seligman

Martin Seligman, PhD, is the Zellerbach Family Professor of Psychology and Director of the Positive Psychology Center at the University of Pennsylvania. Seligman cofounded the field of positive psychology in 1998 and since then has devoted his career to furthering the study of positive emotion, positive character traits, and positive institutions. Seligman's earlier work focused on learned helplessness and depression. Seligman is an often-cited authority in Positive Psychology and a best-selling author.

Helen Verdeli

Helen Verdeli, PhD, is an Associate Professor of Clinical Psychology at Teachers College, Columbia University. Her teaching and research focuses on treatment and prevention of mood disorders with a focus on underresourced regions around the world. She serves on advisory committees for the World Health Organization, United Nations nongovernmental organizations, and many other international organizations.

Roger Walsh

Roger Walsh MD, PhD, DHL, is professor of psychiatry, philosophy, and anthropology and a professor in the religious studies program at the University of California at Irvine. He is a long-term student, teacher, and researcher of contemplative practices, and his relevant publications include *Paths Beyond Ego, The World of Shamanism*, and *Essential Spirituality: The Seven Central Practices*, as well as an American Psychological Association psychotherapy video, *Positive and Transpersonal Approaches to Therapy*.

Danny Wedding

Danny Wedding, PhD, MPH, is the Associate Dean for Management and International Programs at the California School of Professional Psychology, Alliant International University. Although based in San Francisco, he oversees psychology training programs in Tokyo, Hong Kong, and Mexico City. Danny has published widely in psychology and is the current and longtime editor of the journal *PsycCRITIQUES: Contemporary Psychology—APA Review of Books*.

Marjorie E. Weishaar

Marjorie E. Weishaar, PhD, is a Clinical Professor of Psychiatry and Human Behavior at the Alpert Medical School of Brown University. She teaches cognitive therapy to psychology and psychiatry residents. She has widely published in cognitive therapy and has received several teaching awards.

Myrna M. Weissman

Myrna Weissman, PhD, is a Professor of Epidemiology and Psychiatry at the College of Physicians and Surgeons and the Mailman School of Public Health, Columbia University. She is also Chief of Epidemiology at the New York State Psychiatric Institute. Myrna has won numerous awards for her research on depression, and she has been elected to the Institute of Medicine of the National Academy of Science.

Marjorie C. Witty

Marjorie C. Witty, PhD, is Professor and University Fellow at the Illinois School of Professional Psychology, Argosy University, Chicago. She has taught and practiced client-centered therapy since 1974. She has published articles on the subject of social influence and nondirectiveness in client-centered therapy and served on the editorial boards of *The Person-Centered Journal* and the *Person-Centered and Experiential Psychotherapies* journal.

Irvin Yalom

Irvin Yalom, MD, is Emeritus Professor of Psychiatry at Stanford University and currently in private practice in Palo Alto and San Francisco. He has published widely, including textbooks (*The Theory and Practice of Group Psychotherapy* and *Existential Psychotherapy*) and collections of psychotherapy tales (*Love's Executioner* and *Momma and the Meaning of Life*) as well as several psychotherapy teaching novels (*When Nietzsche Wept, Lying on the Couch, The Schopenhauer Cure*, and, most recently, *The Spinoza Problem*).

Gary Yontef

Gary Yontef, PhD, ABPP, is a cofounder of the Pacific Gestalt Institute, past president of the Gestalt Therapy Institute of Los Angeles, and an Associate Editor of Gestalt Review. He formerly taught at UCLA but is now in private practice in Los Angeles. Gary teaches and consults internationally, and his publications about the theory and practice of relational gestalt therapy include the book *Awareness, Dialogue, and Process: Essays on Gestalt Therapy*.

ACKNOWLEDGMENTS

Every book is shaped and improved by the comments of those readers who take time to provide feedback. This book is no different, and we have benefited from the suggestions of literally hundreds of our students, colleagues, and friends. We have been particularly vigilant about getting feedback from those professors who use *Current Psychotherapies* as a text, and their comments help shape each new edition. I also benefited from numerous suggestions from colleagues in the Society of Clinical Psychology (Division 12 of the American Psychological Association).

The faculty and staff of the California School of Professional Psychology, Alliant International University, have been supportive and helpful during the preparation of the 10th edition of *Current Psychotherapies*, and they were always there for me when I needed advice and encouragement. I especially appreciate the support of President Geoff Cox, Provost Russ Newman, and CSPP Dean Morgan Sammons. Dalia Ducker, Ron Duran, Jennifer Kulbeck, Pamela Broadman, Robyn Moyer, Connie Horn and Karen Harrington also helped in a variety of ways, as did my friend Shelia Henderson, who served as a sounding board for many of the decisions made as I worked on this new edition. Chris Pearce and Christoph Zepeda helped with the day-to-day management of *PsycCRITIQUES: Contemporary Psychology—APA Review of Books* while I focused on editing *Current Psychotherapies*, and Ryan Niemiec did most of the heavy lifting in updating our book *Positive Psychology at the Movies*. I am more grateful than any of them will ever know.

PREFACE

This new edition of *Current Psychotherapies* reflects a commitment to maintaining the currency alluded to in the book's title, and the text in its entirety provides a comprehensive overview of the state of the art of psychotherapy. The book was first published in 1973, and since that time it has been used by more than a million students and translated in more than a dozen languages. One reviewer referred to the text as "venerable."

Ray Corsini originally recruited me to work with him in 1976 while I was a graduate student at the University of Hawaii, and recruiting the best possible authors and maintaining the quality of the book has been a consuming passion for the past 40 years. I'm now the age Ray Corsini was when he brought me on as a coeditor for *Current Psychotherapies* and *Case Studies in Psychotherapy*, and I have recruited Barbara Cubic, a cherished colleague, to work with me as coeditor for all future editions of both books.

New chapters on Interpersonal Psychotherapy and Multicultural Psychotherapy were added to the 9th edition, and the 10th edition includes a new chapter on Positive Psychotherapy written by Tayyab Rashid and Martin Seligman. I was simply delighted to be able to recruit authors of their stature. In addition, the 10th edition includes a new chapter on Psychoanalytic Psychotherapies written by Jeremy Safran and Alexander Kriss, and the chapters on Adlerian Psychotherapy and Behavior Therapy have both been totally rewritten.

I reluctantly dropped the chapter on Analytical Psychotherapy for this edition. This was done primarily to keep the size of the book manageable for those students who will be reading the book within the limits of a 16-week semester. Any professor who wants to continue to include Jung in his or her course will have easy access to the chapter on Analytical Psychotherapy from the 9th edition on the Cengage Website, **CengageBrain.com**.

All other chapters retained for this edition have been updated to include the most current relevant research findings. Each chapter describing a particular approach to psychotherapy examines the evidence base supporting that particular theory, and I have asked each contributor to share his or her ideas about the importance—and limitations—of evidence-based practice. In addition, all of the core chapters now address the very important topic of multiculturalism.

In a preface to an earlier edition, Raymond J. Corsini described six features of *Current Psychotherapies* that have helped ensure the book's utility and popularity. These core principles have guided the development of each new edition.

1. *The chapters in this book describe the most important systems in the current practice of psychotherapy.* Because psychotherapy is constantly evolving, deciding what to put into new editions and what to take out demands a great deal of research. The opinions of professors were central in shaping the changes we have made.

2. *The most competent available authors are recruited.* Newly established systems are described by their founders; older systems are covered by those best qualified to describe them.

3. *This book is highly disciplined.* Each author follows an outline in which the various sections are limited in length and structure. The purpose of this feature is to make it as convenient as possible to compare the systems by reading the book "horizontally"

(from section to section across the various systems), as well as in the usual "vertical" manner (from chapter to chapter). The major sections of each chapter include an overview of the system being described, its history, a discussion of the theory of personality that shaped the therapy, a detailed discussion of how psychotherapy using the system is actually practiced, and an explanation of the various applications of the approach being described. In addition, each described therapy is accompanied by a case study illustrating the techniques and methods associated with the therapy. Students interested in more detailed case examples can read this book's companion volume, *Case Studies in Psychotherapy* (Wedding & Corsini, 2013). Those students who want to understand psychotherapy in depth will benefit from reading both *Current Psychotherapies* and *Case Studies in Psychotherapy.*

4. *Current Psychotherapies is carefully edited.* Every section is examined to make certain that its contents are appropriate and clear. In the long history of this text, only one chapter was ever accepted in its first draft. Some chapters have been returned to their original authors as many as four times before finally being accepted.

5. *Chapters are as concise as they can possibly be and still cover the systems completely.* We have received consistent feedback that the chapters in *Current Psychotherapies* need to be clear, succinct, and direct. We have taken this feedback seriously, and every sentence in each new edition is carefully edited to ensure that the information provided is not redundant or superfluous.

6. *The glossary for each new edition is updated and expanded.* One way for students to begin any chapter would be to read the relevant entries in the glossary, thereby generating a mind-set that will facilitate understanding the various systems. Personality theorists tend to invent new words when no existing word suffices. This clarifies their ideas, but it also makes understanding their chapter more difficult. A careful study of the glossary will reward the reader.

Ray Corsini died on November 8, 2008. He was a master Adlerian therapist, the best of my teachers, and a cherished friend. I will always be grateful for his friendship, his support of my career, and everything I learned from him during the many years we worked together.

Danny Wedding
San Francisco
dwedding@alliant.edu

1 | INTRODUCTION TO 21ST-CENTURY PSYCHOTHERAPIES

Frank Dumont

> *Other men are lenses through which we read our own minds.*
> Ralph Waldo Emerson (1850)

> *Psychotherapy, as far as it leads to substantial behavior change, appears to achieve its effect through changes in gene expression at the neuronal level.*
> Eric Kandel (1996)

EVOLUTION OF THIS SCIENCE AND PROFESSION

This book surveys a diverse set of effective psychotherapies. Each represents a vision of the Human as well as a set of distinct treatment procedures for addressing the emotional distress and the accompanying behavioral and cognitive problems that drive people to seek help. As one reviews the evolution of this textbook through 10 editions, and the theories of personality development that underpin each therapeutic modality treated within it, it's evident that these modalities have an increasingly short half-life. Entire schools of psychotherapy have undergone dramatic change, some more rapidly than others—and some have virtually disappeared (e.g., Transactional Analysis). New and increasingly integrative approaches to mental health have been presented. Although built on strong historical foundations, these recent modalities would strike even psychotherapists of the 1960s and 1970s as novel if not strange.

Several contemporary psychotherapies have their roots in the early 20th century, but they evolved dramatically over the past century and have been seamlessly woven into the warp and weft of many disparate approaches to improving mental health. They continue to merit description in some early chapters of this textbook. Advances in personality psychology, developmental psychology, relationship science, and neuroscience are, where appropriate, reflected in the evolving psychotherapies presented in this book. The structure of these therapies and their interdisciplinary and clinical effectiveness have continued to improve. I must note in this context that a new chapter titled *Psychodynamic Psychotherapies* has been added encompassing the Freudian and Jungian schemas, which have provided a prolific matrix for Kleinian and other *analytical* relational therapies. In this introductory chapter, other modifications of this 10th edition will be noted.

To understand where our profession is heading, we need to know where psychotherapy historically started in the West and how it has been transformed by the ongoing global integration of scientific and cultural perspectives on behavior and cognition. This issue is briefly addressed in the following section.

Historical Foundations of Psychotherapy

From the origins of recorded history, humans have sought means to remedy the mental disorders that have afflicted them. Some of these remedies, such as the ceremonial healing rituals found in shamanistic societies, were and continue to be patently unscientific—though not necessarily ineffective for that reason. Pre-Christian, temple-like *asklepeia* and other retreat centers of the eastern Mediterranean region, using religio-philosophical lectures, meditation, and simple rest, competed with secular medicine to assuage if not remedy psychological disorders. The secularistic stream of psychophysiological treatment, in which Hippocrates worked, was surprisingly scientific.

Hellenist physicians understood by their empirical investigations that the brain was not only the seat of knowledge and learning but also the source of depression, delirium, and madness. Indeed, Hippocrates wrote, "Men ought to know that from nothing else but the brain come joys, delights, laughter and sports, and sorrows, griefs, despondency, and lamentations . . . and by the same organ we become mad and delirious, and fears and terrors assail us . . . all things we endure from the brain when it is not healthy" (fifth century B.C.E., quoted by Stanley Finger, 2001, p. 13). Hippocrates himself insisted that his students address illnesses by natural means. He repudiated the popular notion that such illnesses as seizures were "divine" and should be treated by supplicating or appeasing a deity. Although the Hippocratic tradition endured uninterruptedly to the time of his renowned disciple Galen who lived six centuries later, psychotherapy as a domain of science in its modern sense did not clearly emerge until the 18th century.

The Unconscious

A Primordial Construct

The reader will find that the construct *unconscious* plays a salient role in certain chapters of this volume. Although it was examined and debated by Hellenists thousands of years ago, the unconscious was also a key construct in the psychotherapies that emerged in the West in the 19th century. The *scientific* study of the unconscious is commonly thought to have started with renowned polymath Gottfried Wilhelm Leibniz (1646–1716).

Leibniz studied the role of subliminal perceptions in our daily life (and, incidentally, coined the term *dynamic* to describe the forces operative in unconscious mentation). His investigations of the unconscious were continued by Johann Friedrich Herbart (1776–1841), who attempted to mathematicize the dynamics describing the passage of memories to and from the conscious and the unconscious. Herbart suggested that tacit ideas struggle with one another for access to consciousness as dissonant ideas repel and depress one another. Associated ideas help draw each other into consciousness (or drag each other into unconscious realms). Leibniz and Herbart are salient examples of 17th- and 18th-century scientists who attributed significance to an understanding of the unconscious in their work (Whyte, 1960).

Mesmer and Schopenhauer

Two of the most influential and creative thinkers in the early 19th century were Franz Anton Mesmer (1734–1815) and Arthur Schopenhauer (1788–1860). Their impact can be seen in the psychiatric literature that evolved into the full-fledged systems of Pierre Janet, Sigmund Freud, Alfred Adler, and Carl Gustav Jung. An example is Nobel laureate Thomas Mann's observation that, in reading Freud, he had an eerie feeling that he was actually reading Schopenhauer translated into a later idiom (Ellenberger, 1970, p. 209). Analogous statements could be made about many of the other system builders.

Mesmer and his disciples, regarded as the pioneers of hypnotherapy, effectively discredited the exorcist tradition that had dominated pre-Enlightenment Europe (Leahey, 2000, pp. 216–218). That there are many quaint and unsubstantiated hypotheses in the Mesmerian system does not diminish the fact that one can trace to Mesmer the principle that rapport between therapist and patient is important in therapy. He also stressed the influence of the unconscious in shaping behavior, and he clearly demonstrated the influence of the personal qualities of the therapist; the spontaneous remission of disorders; hypnotic somnambulism; the selective, inferential function of memories of which we have no conscious awareness (reaffirmed later by Helmholtz in 1861); the importance of patients' confidence in treatment procedures; and other common factors in our current therapeutics armory.

Three distinct streams of investigation into how the mind works emerged in the 19th century. The contributors to these streams were (1) systematic, lab-bench empiricists; (2) philosophers of nature; and (3) clinician–researchers. A multitude of psychotherapies were spun off from these investigations.

PSYCHOTHERAPY-RELATED SCIENCE IN THE 19TH CENTURY

The Natural Science Empiricists

Some of the greatest scientists of the 19th century such as Gustav T. Fechner (1801–1887) and Herman von Helmholtz (1821–1894) conducted seminal research in the area of cognitive science. Fechner's work tapped into and overlapped with the investigations of Herbart. Fechner began with the distinction between the theaters of the waking and sleeping states—and especially the dream state. That the unconscious exists as a realm of the mind was evident even to the untutored farm laborer. Anyone who had ever struggled to recall a memory—and succeeded—knew that he or she retained knowledge that was not always readily accessible. This knowledge had to reside somewhere. In the late 1850s in his psychophysics experiments, Fechner attempted to measure the intensity of psychic stimulation needed for ideas to cross the threshold from the unconscious to full awareness—what is referred to today as *working memory*—as well as the intensity of the resultant perception. Fechner's studies reverberated throughout Europe, and the reader may unknowingly resonate to his findings not only in Freud's writings (Freud quoted him in several of his works) and the chapters of this book but also in those of myriad other contemporary theorists and practitioners, most notably the Gestaltists and (Milton H.) Ericksonians.

In 1861 Helmholtz, another experimentalist, "discovered the phenomenon of 'unconscious inference,'" which he perceived "as a kind of instantaneous and unconscious reconstruction of what our past taught us about the object" (Ellenberger, 1970, p. 313). This idea has been given modern trappings in a popular and influential book by Daniel Kahneman (2011), *Thinking, Fast and Slow*. Wilhelm Griesinger, Joannes von Müller, and many other such experimentalists and brain scientists dominated the academic scene of Vienna, Berlin, Heidelberg, Tübingen, Leipzig, and other German-language universities and institutes in the 19th century, making many contributions that infused the work of later psychodynamicists.

The spirit and approach of these lab-based scientists resounded throughout Europe and in large part constituted what became known there as the *organicist* tradition. Several of Freud's mentors, including Ernst Brücke (1819–1892) and Theodor Meynert (1833–1892), were organicists. Although the organicists worked feverishly throughout the century to find solutions to psychiatric disorders, Emil Kraepelin on the cusp of the 20th century finally conceded defeat, admitting that 50 years of hard bench work had given medicine few tools for curing psychiatric disorders (Shorter, 1997, pp. 103, 328). Kraepelin turned his attention to classifying diseases, meticulously describing them, schematizing their course, and establishing benchmarks for ongoing prognoses—thus generating as a by-product a paradigm for the contemporary *Diagnostic and Statistical Manual* (DSM). Kraepelin's views provided an opportunity for those so inclined to argue that only a psychological approach to mental illness would prove effective. Thereafter, the work of all the brass-instrument methodologists and empiricist dream scholars of the second half of the 19th century paled in significance by comparison with the influence of the psycho-philosophical clinicians.

The Psychologist–Philosophers

The philosophers of nature had a much greater long-term influence on the development of the psychotherapies described in the following chapters of this book than did laboratory-based scientists. These philosophers can be historically situated in the same school of thought that nurtured Schiller and Goethe. They were Romantics in the philosophical sense, firmly rooted in nature, beauty, homeland, sentiment, the life of the mind, and, of course, the mind at its most enigmatic: the unconscious. Arthur Schopenhauer, Carl Gustav Carus, and Eduard von Hartmann were among the most notable of this group.

Schopenhauer published *The World as Will and Idea* in 1819. This masterpiece of the Western canon, once it caught on, provided ideational grist for generations of psychological researchers. This book especially inspired those psychologists who were imbued with the 19th-century historical school *Philosophy of Nature*. They had embraced (or resigned themselves to) nonbiological methods for curing the fashionable disorders of the day—even those that today would be classified as DSM axis I disorders. Schopenhauer's book was in large part a treatise on human sexuality and the realm of the unconscious. His principal argument was that we know things that we are unaware that we know and that we are largely driven by blind, irrational forces. His irrationalist and pansexual view of human behavior and mentation was deterministic and also pessimistic (see Ellenberger's 1970 analysis, pp. 208–210). Schopenhauer's thoughts influenced the psychology of many later thinkers, not least Friedrich Nietzsche and Sigmund Freud.

Carl Gustav Carus (1789–1869), a contemporary of Schopenhauer, is largely unread today. However, he can justifiably be singled out in a book on psychotherapy because he developed an early and sophisticated schema for the unconscious (see Ellenberger, 1970, pp. 202–210). Carus speculated that there are several levels to the unconscious. Humans interacting among themselves do so simultaneously at various reaches of their unconscious as well as conscious minds. In the clinic, as patient and therapist are at work, the conscious of each speaks to the unconscious as well as to the conscious of the other. But further, the unconscious of each speaks to the conscious as well as the unconscious of the dyadic other. Both are communicating with each other simultaneously in paravocal, nonverbal, organic, and affective modes of which both participants are not fully aware. Thus, *both* the therapist and the patient, willfully or not, engage in transference and countertransference (see Dumont & Fitzpatrick, 2001). Nonlinear messages systemically and simultaneously radiate in all directions. Therapist transference, Carus taught us, occurs at an unconscious level even as therapist and patient greet each other for the first time. Pillow talk and huge rallies unconsciously evoke such deep-seated emotional resonances. So does the clinical psychotherapeutic relationship.

The tracts of Schopenhauer and Carus set the epistemological stage for von Hartmann's and Nietzsche's influential writings on our tacit cognitions, which they believed drove the daily, unreflective behavior of people. Nietzsche affirmed that what we are consciously thinking is "a more or less fantastic commentary on an unconscious, perhaps unknowable, but felt text" (cited in Ellenberger, 1970, p. 273). He developed notions of self-deception, sublimation, repression, conscience, and "neurotic" guilt. In his view, humans lie to themselves even more than they lie to each other. Cynic par excellence, Nietzsche averred that every complaint is an accusation and every admission of a behavioral fault or characterological flaw is a subterfuge to conceal more serious personal failures. In brief, he unmasked many of the defense mechanisms that humans employ to embellish their persona and self-image. In his unsystematic and aphoristic way, Nietzsche cast a long shadow over the personology and psychotherapies of the 20th century.

The Clinician–Researchers

In the nascent clinical psychology of the 19th century, a great number of gifted clinicians made discoveries and innovations in their clinical practices that had implications for the development of theories of personality as well as for psychotherapy. Some were humble practitioners such as the celebrated hypnotherapist Ambroise Liébault. Others were great scholars such as Moritz Benedikt (1835–1920), whose work in criminology, psychiatry, and neurology won the admiration of Jean-Martin Charcot. Benedikt developed the useful concept of seeking out and clinically purging *pathogenic secrets*, a practice that Jung later made an essential element of his analytic psychotherapy. Théodore Flournoy, Josef Breuer, Auguste Forel, Eugen Bleuler, Paul Dubois (greatly admired by Raymond Corsini), Sigmund Freud, Pierre Janet, Adolf Meyer, Carl Gustav Jung, and Alfred Adler all made signal contributions to the science of psychotherapy. Though many of their contributions have outlived their usefulness, the numerous offshoots of their findings and systems can be traced in current clinical psychotherapy and in other psychological disciplines.

Although psychotherapies are in constant evolution, clinicians often continue to use the strategies, techniques, and guiding principles they learned in their graduate professional programs, dated though they may have become. Under the pressures of private clinical practice, they may feel unable to develop new procedures and apply novel principles that their professional practice and a diligent reading of the literature could afford them. Remaining at a fixed stage of one's continually evolving profession is not a desirable outcome of training. To paraphrase an aphorism from sport psychology, practice makes permanent but not necessarily perfect. Improving our performance of an outdated or largely flawed technique is not a clinical desideratum.

Chapters 2 through 15 of this volume represent scientifically recognized advances over the theories and practices that preceded them. Like all current and major psychotherapies, each has emerged to a greater or lesser degree from the historical matrix previously described. Although the contemplative therapies described in Chapter 12 have their roots in the ancient traditions of the Far East and Middle East, some derive from those of the Near East and the asklepeia of Hellenic Greece.

THE IMPACT OF THE BIOLOGICAL SCIENCES ON PSYCHOTHERAPY

When patients[1] learn new ideas, whether true, false, or simply biased, whether in the clinic or in the course of daily life, concomitant alterations of the brain occur (see, e.g., LeDoux's *Synaptic Self*, 2002). Every encounter with our environment causes changes within us and especially in our neural functioning. Once skills and ideas are truly learned and lodged in permanent storage, it is difficult if not impossible to unlearn them. Education implies permanence. Given the solution to a puzzle or taught procedural skills such as cracking a safe or riding a bicycle, one cannot unlearn that knowledge. Neuronal decay and lesions can, of course, undo memory and occur to a certain extent in normal aging and catastrophically in strokes, illness, or violent accidents. The task of the therapist in most cases is to help the patient fashion *alternative* and "future memories" supported by newly adopted motivational schemas.

In his important book *Neuropsychotherapy: How the Neurosciences Inform Effective Psychotherapy* (2007), Klaus Grawe noted, "Psychotherapy, as far as it leads to substantial behavior change, appears to achieve its effect through changes in gene expression at the neuronal level" (p. 3, citing Kandel, 1996, p. 711). Further neuronal embedding of patients in their dysfunctional past by prodding them to ruminate about that past does not erase their painful memories nor their penchant for dwelling on these memories. Nor does it teach them more adaptive patterns of behavior. Effective therapists teach patients how to avoid dysfunctional ruminations, harmful behavioral routines, and maladaptive habits. They also help their clients develop social, interpersonal, self-disciplinary, and technical skills that will advance their well-being and that of others with whom they interact. The neurosciences have demonstrated that neuronal restructuring, which occurs in all learning processes, enables the adaptive changes in behavior, affect, and mentation that are the core objectives of psychotherapy (see, e.g., Dumont, 2009, 2010a, 2010b).

The plasticity of the human organism, and especially its central nervous system, provide us the affordances of redemption and improved well-being. Much of the plasticity in our neuro-emotional systems is achieved through *epigenetic changes*. External events (as well as those of the "internal milieu") can turn genes on or off by enabling the synthesis of proteins that act, in the moment, on the genome in cell nuclei. Introducing even minor novelties in clients' lives can have enormous impact on the way they perceive and experience themselves. We now know that effective therapists and their

---

[1] Throughout this chapter, I have used the term *patient*, which etymologically implies *suffering* and characterizes most people who seek therapy. It is a derivative of a Latin verb that means to endure a painful situation. In the eighth edition of this book, Raymond Corsini noted the discipline-specific connotations of patient and *client*; Ray believed the former term was appropriate for medical contexts, but he used the latter term in his private practice.

clients can optimize desirable outcomes using neural circuit-altering, placebo-laden talk, and by epigenetically triggering the expression of dormant genes through exposure to nurturant social events (see, e.g., Güntürkün, 2006; LeDoux, 2002, pp. 260–300). This ancillary neurological perspective on psychotherapy allows the creative exploration of the cognitive and emotional variables at play in clients' lives that are central to their improvement.

Culture generally—and one's immediate family specifically—function as genetic enablers. As Merleau-Ponty (Bourgeois, 2003, p.370) reminds us, culture is sedimented in the body and pervades our central nervous system. Epigenetic effects can operate for better or for worse, depending on the richness and benignancy of one's culture—and one's access to what it can provide. In brief, it is the complex biocultural matrix of the organic *and* the environmental that co-construct our way of being in the world and our potential for growth (Baltes, Reuter-Lorenz, & Rösler, 2006). The therapeutic procedures explained in the chapters of this textbook derive from this matrix.

Organicists and Dynamicists: Clashing Standpoints

Readers will immediately recognize the potential for cultural confrontations in these propositions. However, confrontation is neither necessary nor useful. A recent book integrating evolutionary, neuroscience, and sociocultural approaches to understanding close relationships among humans (Gillath, Adams, & Kunkel, 2012) provides a good model for uniting disparate approaches to the study of human nature. The ancient tensions between environmentalists and organicists, psychopharmacologists and psychodynamicists, behavioral geneticists and cognitive-behaviorists can be resolved through a systemic integration of the many variables that are at play at any moment. Indeed, such integration is necessary because to ignore organic *or* environmental variables in the treatment of one's clients is to neglect essential aspects of the whole person. And it is an ancient error to treat all affective disorders as if there were no organicity in the causal skein of variables that brought them about.

One example of this error is ignoring patients' medication histories. Kenneth Pope and Danny Wedding (2012) discuss in the final chapter of this book the danger inherent in neglecting to monitor patients who are taking psychotropic medication. Patients need to be pharmacologically guided and their experiences between sessions closely followed. Medicating patients for psychological purposes requires preset clinical objectives and conscientious ongoing assessment of progress. Grawe (2007) stated:

> From a neuroscientific perspective, psychopharmacological therapy that is not coordinated with a simultaneous, targeted alteration of the person's experiences cannot be justified. The widespread practice of prescribing psychoactive medication without assuming responsibility for the patient's concurrent experience is, from a neuroscientific view, equally irresponsible. . . . The use of pharmacotherapy alone—in the absence of the professional and competent structuring of the treated patient's life experience—is not justifiable. . . . (pp. 5–6)

Nurture is profoundly shaped by nature. Indeed, as Robert Plomin and Avshalom Caspi (1999) suggest, we may be genetically driven to seek the very environments that presumably shape us. As Nestler (2011) reminds us, even "[mouse] pups raised by a relaxed and nurturing mother" are more resistant to stress than pups deprived of such nurturance. Nurturance melts away inhibitory methyl groups and "leaves the animals calmer" (p. 82). He concludes that scientists have learned that "exposure to the environment and to different experiences (including random occurrences) throughout development and adulthood can modify the activities of our genes and, hence, the ways these traits manifest themselves" (p. 83). Thus, aspects of our nature get epigenetically expressed for better or for worse. In other words, genes get chemically tagged by the kinds of experiences to which we are subjected throughout our lives and can subsequently be turned on (or off). Like matryoshka dolls, genetic tags may hide inside *perceived* environmental cues. Therapists, to the extent that they can guide the experiences of their clients, become responsible to some degree for *both* nurturant *and* natural components of their patients' lives.

Evolutionary Biology and Behavioral Genetics

Neuroscience is not the sole biological research domain whose findings will have implications for psychotherapy. Evolutionary psychology is closely related to the field of behavioral genetics and will further clarify many of the temperamental traits that therapists need to understand. This discipline will have an impact on the therapeutic modalities that clinicians of the future will assuredly develop. Further, it will shine a focused light on the human genome and the lawfulness that governs its complex transcriptions into the biopsychosocial regularities that occur in the course of one's life. Anthropologists have discovered that there are at least 400 universal behavioral traits—products of our evolved monomorphic genes. This is more than we have traditionally imagined (see Brown, 1991), and it places some constraints on the cultural relativism that nevertheless justifiably qualifies all our therapies.

Steven Pinker (2002) has further documented the principle that all humans share a unique human nature. If we exclude anomalous genetic mutations, the normative stance of all clinicians treating a patient is that they are dealing with an organism struck from the same genetic template as themselves. Remaining cognizant of these human regularities, clinicians will still need to uncover those traits influenced by patients' personal life events. In that holistic context, therapists can cast light on client strengths, treat the dysfunctions that patients reveal to them, and monitor the situational variables and events that can contribute to the remediation of their condition. Those environmental variables, and their influence on thought, speech, and behavior, are described in the cutting-edge chapters on behavior therapy (Chapter 6, newly authored by Martin Antony and cognitive therapy (Chapter 7, written by Aaron Beck and Marjorie Weishaar)—therapies that are distinct enough to deserve separate chapters but are still tightly intermeshed in certain aspects of their assessment and treatment procedures.

Finally, the related fields of molecular genetic analysis, cognitive neuropsychology, and social cognitive neuroscience, which are all advancing at impressive rates, will inevitably infiltrate our porous integrationist models of helping. Various psychotherapies influence each other and thus are converging, and they all depend on various human sciences whose advances *promote* that very convergence.

CULTURAL FACTORS AND PSYCHOTHERAPY

Demographics

In the ninth edition of *Current Psychotherapies,* a new chapter was devoted to current approaches to multicultural psychotherapy. This change reflected the self-evident importance of cultural factors in psychotherapy; however, it also acknowledged the changing demographic character of the planet, the human tides that are swirling about the previously distant continents of the globe, and the tightening communication networks that result when masses of people engage in commerce, armed conflict, research, diplomacy, higher education, or professional psychological counseling. Although existential psychotherapy (Chapter 8), and most notably contemplative psychotherapies

(Chapter 12), have dealt heretofore with the ethnocultural variables implicated in the treatment of diverse ethnic populations, Chapter 15 is dedicated exclusively to this approach.

Multicultural Psychotherapy

The complexities involved in multicultural counseling are incomparably greater than those involved in conducting therapy in a homogeneous culture in which each member of the therapeutic dyad springs from the same ethnocultural background. When the patient and the therapist are solidly grounded in different traditional cultures, it *matters* if the "authority" figure is a member, say, of a minority, nondominant culture or the dominant, majority culture. In marital counseling, the difficulties multiply like fractals if the couple seeking help is biracial or bicultural. In this case, the matrix of interactive variables becomes even more complex should the therapist or counselor *unknowingly* identify with one spouse rather than the other—which is not unlikely. Gender-by-culture permutations add another layer of systemic interactions. And, of course, it is not enough to simply acknowledge one's differentness. Counselors are never fully aware of how different they are from the clients sitting across from or beside them for the simple reason that they are never fully conscious of the dynamics driving their own reactions to the client's socially conditioned sensitivities. Much of therapists' mentation operates beyond awareness, for their own cognitive and affective structures are intermeshed in the invisible, bottomless depths of their unconscious.

Cantonese speakers counseling Cantonese speakers in Hong Kong face different challenges than Hispanic counselors in San Diego counseling other Hispanics. The philosophical and socioeconomic differences that characterize members of the same society will determine the suitability of nonindigenous psychotherapies that are more or less congenial to both of them. But within homogeneous non-Caucasian populations, there is the same constellation of contingencies that confront Euro-American peoples. Job stresses, finances, physical illness, personal history, family dynamics, personological variables of genetic and environmental origin, and even the weather and season will all affect what happens between a therapist and a client.

Language and Metaphor

Language, behavioral mannerisms, local and national poetry, myth, and metaphor are the instruments that shape the structures of our mind (see, for example, Lakoff & Johnson, 1980). Popular metaphors permeate all aspects of human thought. They ultimately shape a nation's culture and collective "personality." Those who are not familiar with these elements of their clients' culture will find it difficult to enter the labyrinthine recesses where their ancestral and self-made demons (some benevolent, some hurtful) reside.

All therapists can tell clinical stories of mistakes they have made by the innocent use of a metaphor, a careless juxtaposing of questions, a refusal of a courtesy, or an insensitivity to a taboo of their client's culture. Painfully, their former patients and friends have left, often never to return, and with hardly a word of explanation. For this reason, it has often been proposed that psychotherapies need to be indigenized. Rather than exporting Euro-American psychotherapies, say, to China, some would encourage Chinese healers to develop psychotherapies that reflect *their* philosophies, values, social objectives, and religious convictions. Yang (1997, 1999), for example, has suggested that Chinese counselors can more easily help resolve the paradoxes and dilemmas that characterize Chinese village, family, and personal life than non-Chinese can. Likewise, Hoshmand (2005, p. 3) avers that "indigenous culture provides native ways of knowing what is salient and congruent with the local ethos and what are credible ways of addressing human problems," a view supported by Marsella and Yamada (2000). Similarly, Cross and Markus (1999) note that "the articulation of a truly universal understanding of human nature and personality . . . requires the development of theories of behavior *originating* in the indigenous psychologies of Asian, Latin American, African, and other non-Western societies" (p. 381).

Even within the same society, the intergenerational differences in culture are as striking and important as the cross-national. These differences are apparent in attitudes to single-member households, premarital sex, marriage and divorce, family structure, religious practices and beliefs, sexual preferences, modesty and skin exposure in dress, use of soft drugs, and myriad other lifestyle choices. The complex challenges these issues present to mental-health service providers will be more fully addressed in Chapter 15.

NEGOTIATING FAULT LINES IN THE EBT TERRAIN

Psychotherapy: An Art or a Science?

Division 12 of the American Psychological Association (APA) established a Task Force on Promotion and Dissemination of Psychological Procedures (1995) to grapple with the issues of empirically based treatments (EBTs). A flood of research has since followed to demonstrate the scientific validity of those therapies their partisans espouse. As in earlier editions of *Current Psychotherapies,* the contributors to this book have wrestled with this issue. Many serious fault lines in the terrain define this debate, and although they have all been addressed by the professions serving the mental-health needs of society, they still constitute threats to clinical credibility.

Patients typically work in session with one therapist for 50 minutes a week but are exposed for the rest of the week to innumerable contingencies outside the clinic that can confound fine-tuned plans and firm resolve. Many of these contingencies are unforeseen and beyond their control. Paul Meehl (1978) called these random events *context-dependent stochastologicals* (p. 812). They are a tangle of variables internal and external to the person that intertwine with job stresses, financial concerns, troubled children, angry spouses or in-laws, difficult colleagues, bad weather, life-threatening illness, contested insurance claims, and the forgotten baggage of personal history and past defeats. All patients have a unique set of such variables, but to make the situation even more complicated, they are often afflicted by a number of distinct disorders—some overlapping. This comorbidity complicates the diagnostic coding of disorders and patients for purposes of validating therapy for them (Beutler & Baker, 1998). For many practitioners and onlookers, the science of prognosticating outcomes in psychotherapy inspires as much confidence as predictions of stock-market fluctuations. There is simply too much opacity in the universe of variables, known and unknown, to make confident prognoses.

Spontaneity and Intuition: "Throw-Ins"

Readers of the chapters of this book will be faced with clients who present complex puzzles to them, each client manifesting varying degrees of anxiety, coping skills, and emotional stability—and often with no clear idea what their treatment will consist of or how effective this expensive service will be. Long before clinical interns enter this arena, they will need to have made some multilayered existential choices: whether (or not) to become artisanal therapists, manual-based "craftsmen," or complex humanistic variants between these two extremes. Yalom (1980) wrote about a group course in cooking he once took with an Armenian chef. As she spoke, the students learned by watching, like so many Inuit children. Besides noting the main ingredients, Yalom observed that as the pots and skillets were shuffled from counter to stove, a variety of spices were tossed in—a pinch of this and a pinch of that. "I am convinced," he wrote, "those surreptitious throw-ins made all the difference" (p. 3). He likened this process to psychotherapy. Often unknown to therapists, it's their unscripted "throw-ins" that can make all the difference.

I include at this point a slightly redacted excerpt written by Ray Corsini that appeared in previous editions of this book. It is reminiscent of the throw-ins that Yalom wrote about—less a traditional version of psychotherapy than a conversational but therapeutic throw-in. It demonstrates how a verbal intervention, even in a nonclinical setting, can alter a person's life—in this case, for the better. This anecdote has implications for our daily social lives.

AN UNUSUAL EXAMPLE OF PSYCHOTHERAPY

A Corsini Throw-In

About 50 years ago, when I was working as a psychologist at Auburn Prison in New York, I participated in what I believe was the most successful and elegant psychotherapy I have ever done. One day an inmate, who had made an appointment, came into my office. He was a fairly attractive man in his early 30s. I pointed to a chair, he sat down, and I waited to find out what he wanted. The conversation went something like this (P = prisoner; C = Corsini):

P: I'm leaving on parole Thursday.
C: Yes?
P: I didn't want to leave until I thanked you for what you had done for me.
C: What was that?
P: When I left your office about two years ago, I felt like I was walking on air. When I went into the prison yard, everything looked different, even the air smelled different. I was a new person. Instead of going over to the group I usually hung out with—they were a bunch of thieves—I went over to another group of square Johns [prison jargon for noncriminal types]. I changed from a cushy job in the kitchen to the machine shop, where I could learn a trade. I started going to the prison high school and I now have a high school diploma. I took a correspondence course in drafting and I have a drafting job when I leave Thursday. I started back to church even though I had given up my religion many years ago. I started writing to my family and they have come up to see me and they remember you in their prayers. I now have hope. I know who and what I am. I know I will succeed in life. I plan to go to college. You have freed me. I used to think you bug doctors [prison slang for psychologists and psychiatrists] were for the birds, but now I know better. Thanks for changing my life.

I listened to this tale in wonderment, because to the best of my knowledge I had never spoken with him. I looked at his folder and the only notation there was that I had given him an IQ test about two years before. "Are you sure it was me?" I finally said. "I'm not a psychotherapist, and I have no memory of ever having spoken to you. What you are reporting is the sort of personality and behavior change that takes many years to accomplish—and I certainly haven't done anything of the kind."

"It was you, all right," he replied with great conviction, "and I will never forget what you said to me. It changed my life."

"What was that?" I asked.

"You told me I had a high IQ," he replied.

With one brief sentence I had (inadvertently) changed this person's life.

(continued)

(continued)

Let us try to understand this event. If you are clever enough to understand why this man changed so drastically as a result of hearing these five words, "You have a high IQ," my guess is that you have the capacity to be a good therapist.

I asked him why this sentence about his IQ had such a profound effect, and I learned that up to the time that he heard these five words, he had always thought of himself as "stupid" and "crazy"—terms that had been applied to him many times by his family, teachers, and friends. In school, he had always received poor grades, which confirmed his belief in his mental subnormality. His friends did not approve of the way he thought and called him crazy. And so he was convinced that he was both an ament (low intelligence) and a dement (insane). But when I said, "You have a high IQ," he had an "aha!" experience that explained everything. In a flash, he understood why he could solve crossword puzzles better than any of his friends. He now knew why he read long novels rather than comic books, why he preferred to play chess rather than checkers, why he liked symphonies as well as jazz. With great and sudden intensity he realized through my five words that he was really normal and bright and not crazy or stupid. He had experienced an abreaction that ordinarily would take months. No wonder he had felt as if he were walking on air when he left my office two years before!

His interpretation of my five words generated a complete change of self-concept—and consequently a change in both his behavior and his feelings about himself and others.

In short, I had performed psychotherapy in a completely innocent and informal way. Even though there was no agreement between us, no theory, and no intention of changing him—the five-word comment had a most pronounced effect, and so it was psychotherapy.

MANUALIZATION OF TREATMENT

Spontaneous, unplanned throw-ins are hardly a basis for a *science* of psychotherapy. Doing psychotherapy in this manner makes it more like a craft or at its pinnacle—as Yalom and Josselson do it—an art. Even repeatedly demonstrating that one can improve client well-being and achieve therapeutic objectives by a manualized series of interventions does not explain *how* the variables have caused the outcome. Intensive research has been conducted in the last decade precisely to identify the mechanisms that are bringing about change. Although ambitious programs of process research, as distinguished from outcome research, are being conducted (e.g., see Norcross & Goldfried, 2005), the identity of the causal links and their nature are not yet fully understood. Such understanding will only surface when we have a mature neurobiology that can describe the organism's interaction with its environment. This, of course, will further facilitate the integration of psychologists as professional coequals in medical primary care facilities. These challenges are obviated for those who are only seeking manualized approaches to therapy, that is, sets of sequential, algorithmized steps for proceeding through phases of therapy (see Prochaska, Norcross, & DiClemente, 1995, for one cogent model).

There are several practical advantages to manualized psychotherapy. Engineering therapy in the guise of an architecture of stages or building blocks makes sense pedagogically. One proceeds from the known to the unknown and untried in a methodical, stepwise fashion, clearly specifying layered objectives and mobilizing the personal, social, and institutional resources that are so useful—and so often necessary. These processes through which the patient can be guided are amenable to various configurations.

The chapters of this book (2 through 15) have been structured in such a way that the enterprising student can design a manual for each, using the elements as they are presented.

OBSTACLES TO A SCIENCE OF PSYCHOTHERAPY

The sheer number of potent situational, somatic, and psychological variables that must be considered when computing the outcome variances of diverse therapies for a client dwarfs considerations of procedural variables. Moreover, citing numerous studies, Michael Mahoney wrote in 1991 "the *person* of the therapist is at least eight times more influential than his or her theoretical orientation and/or use of specific therapeutic techniques" (p. 346). Norcross and Beutler (2008) stated that there are "tens of thousands of potential permutations and combinations of patient, therapist, treatment, and setting variables that could contribute" to improving treatment decisions (p. 491). They noted the earlier studies of Beutler and colleagues who conducted analyses of these numerous variables with a sample of depressed patients. They reduced "tens of thousands" to a manageable number, trusting that the loss of specificity in their constructs would not overshadow the utility of their generic approach. This is analogous to the task undertaken by Allport and Odbert (1936) and several generations of trait psychologists who followed them, who reduced 18,000 personality descriptors to a handful of core personality factors using the factor analytic techniques largely developed by Raymond B. Cattell.

The immensity of the task weighs on us when we consider the hundreds of other disorders cataloged in the DSM and *International Classification of Diseases* (ICD) that call for varied treatments on the one hand and evoke Meehl's innumerable random events on the other. But proposing many therapies that are disorder specific is as vexing a proposition as proposing one therapy that can purportedly remedy all axis II disorders as defined, say, in the DSM. Nevertheless, the complex and changing context of our patients' daily lives is like a headwind that keeps pushing us back toward Yalom's kitchen and pulling us outside the comfortable conceptual boxes in which we have been trained.

SOURCES OF HOPE

The pursuit of *what* works in psychotherapy is more important to a pragmatic species such as *Homo sapiens* than the pursuit of *why* it works. This is especially true in applied and very practical disciplines. But like wave and particle theories in the physics of light, art and science in psychotherapy are not incompatible paradigms. Both are valid, and elements of both appear in every clinical session. As unanticipated material comes to light, all clinicians to one degree or another rely on intuitive inspiration and creative imagination in deciding what to do next.

Some therapies, such as behavior therapy and cognitive therapy, are more amenable to manualization than others such as existential psychotherapy, but they ought not to be preferred simply for that reason. On the other hand, the manualization of therapies must not be caricatured simply as a cookbook approach to treating disorders. The variables and the random events that frequently pop up in a patient's life and complicate therapists' best-thought-out plans require adjustment and compromise. Therapeutic judgment and creativity are always called into play. Pursuing the mirage of a blueprint that unfolds seamlessly from start to finish entails a loss of therapists' time and effectiveness and drains patients' emotional and financial resources. There is room in evidence-based therapies and manualized therapies for the poetry, spirituality, spontaneity, sentiment, free will, and even the mystery and romance of human self-discovery and growth that both patients and humanistically inclined therapists crave. There should be no tension between getting better and *feeling* better. In fact, like butter in the batter, affect and reason are as inseparable here as elsewhere.

INDUSTRIALIZING PSYCHOTHERAPY

Although pastoral counseling and faith-based therapeutic procedures are widely practiced not only in North America but also globally, secular, science-based approaches to treating mental disorders have become normative. As psychotherapy has gained recognition as a health discipline, a growing chorus of advocates (of both patients and professionals engaged in mental-health services) has clamored for insurance companies to reimburse mental-health costs. The growth in number of managed health-care units is partly a business issue and perhaps of little interest to students who have a laserlike focus on simply developing effective therapeutic skills, but the reality is that clinical and counseling psychologists, social workers, psychiatric nurses, psychoeducators, school psychologists, psychiatrists, sports psychologists, and occupational therapists will increasingly be working in teams with medical professionals (see Cummings & Cummings, 2013, for advances in integrated health care). A primary advantage of integrated health-care teams is that they provide readily accessible colleagues who can serve as our intellectual prostheses. Nevertheless, even those who choose to work independently will still need to become part of a local professional network—and, further, ensure that they have the skills to run a solvent enterprise. Like it or not, therapists are quickly drawn into a web of institutional requirements that will secure not only the safety of the public they serve but also their own livelihood.

The industrialization of all health professions has "been the linchpin of the development and use of empirically based clinical practice guidelines" (Hayes, 1998, p. 27). Readers may recoil from these institutional realities, but they are well advised to generate their personal therapeutic, professional, and business models during their studies and training such that they meet the demands of the accreditation, licensure, insurance, and medical organizations that will facilitate the growth and solvency of their practice.

WHO CAN DO PSYCHOTHERAPY?

Psychotherapy is a generic term that encompasses a large number of clinical procedures intended to improve clients' well-being. The practice of professional psychotherapy is not "owned" by one profession or another. Adequately educated, trained, and certified professionals can typically practice psychotherapy whether they are, say, clinical psychologists, psychiatrists, counseling psychologists, social workers, psychiatric nurses, school psychologists, or occupational therapists. However, *whatever the mental-health profession* in which they have received training, therapists must, in the public interest, be able to demonstrate their competence to treat their *particular* patients in accordance with currently accepted standards of the larger mental-health services community and the discipline in which they work. The principal caveat that all therapists must take seriously is that they should never overstep the limits of their competencies, whether it be, say, in the administration and interpretation of diagnostic and assessment tools or the use of a procedure in which they have not been adequately trained.

Positive Psychology

The momentum toward fashioning psychologies that are increasingly *positive* has accelerated in the 21st century, most notably (in North America) through the work of Martin Seligman and Mihaly Csikszentmihalyi. This trend has inevitably affected the practice of a range of psychotherapies. This recent emphasis is not a novelty—there have been precursors—and the whole approach is built on solid historical foundations. Alfred Adler was a positive psychologist who gave luster to the idea of *self-actualization*, the overriding—arguably the only—innate drive he acknowledged in his personality psychology. Abraham Maslow was also a positive psychologist whose seminal book *Toward a Psychology of Being* (1962; see also Maslow, 1954) was a beacon for those who were fleeing the psychiatric illness models of the previous century (see the chapter titled "From Illness to Wellness Models of Human Nature," Dumont, 2010b). These scholars were joined by other influential therapists such as Carl Rogers and Milton H. Erickson who insisted that the potential for personal well-being and creative solutions to personal problems on which therapists should focus resided in every human. In recognition of the growing importance of positivity in the mental-health professions, a new chapter titled "Positive Psychotherapy" has been added to this book (Chapter 13). The author, Tayyab Rashid, has analyzed, among other facets of positive therapy, the usefulness of film and other art media in furthering this approach.

CONCLUSION

Efficacy, Therapist aptitudes, and Diagnostic Coding

This chapter closes with a passage that Ray Corsini wrote in this introductory chapter some years ago. He insisted that one should choose to develop expertise in therapeutic approaches that suit one's personality. He concluded his introductory chapter with the following thoughts.

> I believe that if one is to go into the fields of counseling and psychotherapy, then the best theory and methodology to use must be one's own. The reader will not be either successful or happy using a method not suited to her or his own personality. Truly successful therapists adopt or develop a theory and methodology congruent with their own personality. . . . In reading these accounts, in addition to attempting to determine which school of psychotherapy seems most sensible, the reader should also attempt to find one that fits his or her philosophy of life, one whose theoretical underpinnings seem most valid, and one with a method of operation that appears most appealing in use. (2008, p. 13)

Valid as this statement appears, it raises three critical issues: (1) treatment efficacy, (2) therapist aptitudes, and (3) diagnosis and diagnostic coding.

First, relative to efficacy, some disorders appear to be most aptly treated by a specific modality irrespective of what suits the therapist's personality, just as there are certain cancers, say, that are best treated by a specific intervention, irrespective of the satisfaction an oncologist might get by using a different treatment. Choosing a therapy that is less well-validated for treatment of a specific disorder simply because one finds it personologically more congenial should not be encouraged. Intrinsic treatment efficacy should normally override the congeniality factor—albeit therapists' personality can powerfully enhance efficacy. In contrast, some eminent researchers in this domain affirm that factors common to all therapies, including the personality of the therapist, swamp the effects that flow from the specific procedures that are used.

Second, relative to therapists' aptitudes, some studies (e.g., Kraus, Castonguay, Boswell, Nordberg, & Hayes, 2011) suggest that certain therapists achieve clinical success superior to others when they treat one kind of disorder but inferior to others when they treat a different disorder. In general one can't be certain whether this is a function of therapists' comfort or discomfort in the face of the client's specific dysfunctions, their negative transference toward the client they have yet to meet in person, or the perhaps less-suitable but preferred modality they use for specifically different disorders. These process issues have still to be fully resolved. While studying this textbook students and trainees have an early opportunity to select a domain of competence and a demographic sector in which to work where these conflictual issues can be minimized.

A variety of personological (and random) reasons can motivate students' choices of therapies in which they wish to achieve expertise. Career choices also need to be made among the kinds of disorders to which students wish to devote their professional lives. It's unlikely they can be equally successful working with all mental-health disorders. One will need to assess the level of one's discomfort in the face of serious dysfunctions and specific clienteles. This will involve acknowledging the potential for negative subliminal and conscious transference to future clients with certain dysfunctions—for example, pedophilia or sadism. Because of this, all trainees must understand that their personalities and competencies limit the spectrum of clientele they can treat. This book presents an array of some of the most esteemed and well-validated psychotherapies of the 21st century in which students may wish to be trained—and for the disorders they feel inclined to treat. However, the treatments explicated in this textbook must be personalized and attuned to the psychological needs of the patient. Every human being presents with complex and unique problems.

Third, relative to diagnosis and diagnostic coding, if choosing the most efficacious therapy for the disorder a client presents is imperative, then the need for an accurate diagnosis is obvious. This will also necessitate learning the diagnostic skills and mastering whatever assessment tools exist that will allow therapists to match procedures to problems. One doesn't want to treat a nonexistent problem that has been erroneously inferred from misinterpreted data. That would risk creating another problem in addition to the one the client presented. A practical corollary to this is that students need to become proficient in the use of the most current DSM. Soon many will need to transition to the *International Classification of Diseases* (ICD-10-CM). Beginning October 1, 2014, U.S. practitioners will be obliged to use it. Learning this system is all the more urgent because insurers will require the ICD coding of diseases for reimbursement. Finally, Corsini added:

> A value of this book lies in the greater self-understanding that may be gained by close reading. This book about psychotherapies may be psychotherapeutic for the reader. Close reading vertically (chapter by chapter) and then horizontally (section by section) may well lead to personal growth as well as to better understanding of current psychotherapies. (p. 13)

This advice from a great therapist and scholar[2] is a fitting conclusion to this chapter.

---

[2] Raymond Corsini died November 8, 2008, in Honolulu at age 94. He was a creative, loyal, challenging, and inspiring colleague. All of us who had the privilege of working with Ray over the years acknowledge our debt to him.

REFERENCES

Allport, G. W., & Odbert, H. S. (1936). Trait-names: A psycho-lexical study. *Psychological Monographs, 47,* (1, whole no. 211).

Baltes, P. B., Reuter-Lorenz, P. A., & Rösler, F. (2006). Prologue: Biocultural co-constructivism as a theoretical metascript. In P. B. Baltes, P. A. Reuter-Lorenz, & F. Rösler (Eds.), *Lifespan development and the brain: The perspective of biocultural co-constructivism* (pp. 3–39). Cambridge, UK: Cambridge University Press.

Beutler, L. E., & Baker, M. (1998). The movement toward empirical validation: At what level should we analyze, and who are the consumers? In K. S. Dobson & K. D. Craig (Eds.), *Empirically supported therapies: Best practice in professional psychology* (pp. 43–65). Thousand Oaks, CA: Sage.

Bourgeois, P. (2003). Maurice Merleau-Ponty: Philosophy as phenomenology. In A.-T. Tymieniecka (Ed.), *Phenomenology world wide: Foundations–dynamics–life engagements* (pp. 343–383). Dordrecht, Netherlands: Kluwer Academic.

Brown, D. E. (1991). *Human universals.* New York: McGraw-Hill.

Corsini, R. J. (2008). Introduction. In R. J. Corsini & D. Wedding (Eds.), *Current psychotherapies* (8th ed., pp. 1–14). Belmont, CA: Thomson/Brooks/Cole.

Cross, S. E., & Markus, H. R. (1999). The cultural constitution of personality. In L. A. Pervin & O. P. John (Eds.), *Handbook of personality* (pp. 378–396). New York: Guilford.

Cummings, N. A. & Cummings, J. L. (2013). *Refocused psychotherapy as the first line intervention in behavioral health.* New York: Routledge.

Dumont, F. (2009). Rehearsal, confession, and confabulation: Psychotherapy and the synaptic self. *Journal of Contemporary Psychotherapy, 39*(1), 33–40.

Dumont, F. (2010a). *A history of personality psychology: Theory, science, and research from Hellenism to the twenty-first century.* Cambridge, UK: Cambridge University Press.

Dumont, F. (2010b). From illness to wellness models of human nature. In F. Dumont, *A history of personality psychology: Theory, science, and research from Hellenism to the twenty-first century* (pp. 35–74). Cambridge, UK: Cambridge University Press.

Dumont, F., & Fitzpatrick, M. (2001). The real relationship: Schemas, stereotypes, and personal history. *Psychotherapy: Theory, Practice, Research, and Training, 38,* 12–20.

Ellenberger, H. F. (1970). *The discovery of the unconscious: The history and evolution of dynamic psychiatry.* New York: Basic Books.

Finger, S. (2001). *Origins of neuroscience: A history of explorations into brain function.* Oxford, UK: Oxford University Press.

Gillath, O., Adams, G., & Kunkel, A. (2012). *Relationship science: Integrating evolutionary, neuroscience, and sociocultural approaches.* Washington, DC: American Psychological Association.

Grawe, K. (2007). *Neuropsychotherapy: How the neurosciences inform effective psychotherapy.* Mahwah, NJ: Erlbaum.

Güntürkün, O. (2006). Letters on nature and nurture. In P. B. Baltes, P. A. Reuter-Lorenz, & F. Rösler (Eds.), *Lifespan development and the brain: The perspective of biocultural co-constructivism* (pp. 379–397). Cambridge, UK: Cambridge University Press.

Hayes, S. C. (1998). Scientific practice guidelines in a political, economic, and professional context. In K. S. Dobson & K. D. Craig (Eds.), *Empirically supported therapies: Best practice in professional psychology* (pp. 26–42). Thousand Oaks, CA: Sage.

Hoshmand, L. T. (2005). Thinking through culture. In L. T. Hoshmand (Ed.), *Culture, psychotherapy, and counseling: Critical and integrative perspectives* (pp. 1–24). Thousand Oaks, CA: Sage.

Kahneman, D. (2011). *Thinking, fast and slow.* New York: Doubleday

Kraus, D. R., Castonguay, L. G., Boswell, J. F., Nordberg, S. S., & Hayes, J. A. (2011). Therapist effectiveness: Implications for accountability and patient care. *Psychotherapy Research, 21,* 267–276.

Lakoff, G., & Johnson, M. (1980). *Metaphors we live by.* Chicago: University of Chicago Press.

Leahey, T. H. (2000). *A history of psychology: Main currents in psychological thought* (5th ed.). Upper Saddle River, NJ: Prentice Hall.

LeDoux, J. (2002). *Synaptic self: How our brains become who we are.* New York: Viking/Penguin.

Mahoney, M. (1991). *Human change processes: The scientific foundations of psychotherapy.* New York: Basic Books.

Marsella, A. J., & Yamada, A. M. (2000). Culture and mental health: An introduction and overview of foundations, concepts, and issues. In I. Cuellar & F. A. Paniagua (Eds.), *Handbook of multicultural mental health: Assessment and treatment of culturally diverse populations* (pp. 3–24). New York: Academic Press.

Maslow, A. H. 1954. *Motivation and personality.* New York: Harper.

Maslow, A. H. 1962. *Toward a psychology of being.* Princeton, NJ: Van Nostrand.

Meehl, P. (1978). Theoretical risks and tabular asterisks: Sir Karl, Sir Ronald, and the slow progress of soft psychology. *Journal of Consulting and Clinical Psychology, 46,* 806–834.

Nestler, E. J. (2011). Hidden switches in the mind. *Scientific American, 304*(6), 77–83.

Norcross, J. C., & Beutler, L. E. (2008). Integrative psychotherapies. In R. J. Corsini & D. Wedding, *Current psychotherapies* (pp. 481–511). Belmont, CA: Thomson/Brooks Cole.

Norcross, J. C., & Goldfried, M. R. (Eds.) (2005). *Handbook of psychotherapy integration* (2nd ed.). New York: Oxford University Press.

Pinker, S. (2002). *The blank slate: The modern denial of human nature.* New York: Viking.

Plomin, R., & Caspi, A. (1999). Behavioral genetics and personality. In L. A. Pervin and O. P. John (Eds.), *Handbook of personality: Theory and research* (2nd ed., pp. 251–276). New York: Guilford Press.

Pope, K. S., & Wedding, D. (2012). Contemporary challenges and controversies. In R. J. Corsini & D. Wedding (Eds.), *Current psychotherapies* (9th ed., pp. 568–603). Belmont, CA: Brooks/Cole, Cengage Learning.

Prochaska, J. O., Norcross, J. C., & DiClemente, C. C. (1995). Stages of change: Prescriptive guidelines. In G. P. Koocher, J. C. Norcross, & S. S. Hill (Eds.), *Psychologists' desk reference* (pp. 226–231). New York: Oxford University Press.

Schopenhauer, A. (1819/1969). *The world as will and representation* (Trans. E. F. J. Payne). Toronto: General Publishing.

Shorter, E. (1997). *A history of psychiatry: From the era of the asylum to the age of Prozac.* New York: Wiley.

Task Force on Promotion and Dissemination of Psychological Procedures. (1995). Training in and dissemination of empirically validated psychological treatments. *Clinical Psychologist, 48,* 3–23.

Whyte, L. L. (1960). *The unconscious before Freud.* New York: Basic Books.

Yalom, I. D. (1980). *Existential psychotherapy.* New York: Basic Books.

Yang, K. S. (1997). Indigenizing Westernized Chinese psychology. In M. H. Bond (Ed.), *Working at the interface of cultures: Eighteen lies in social science* (pp. 62–76). New York: Routledge.

Yang, K. S. (1999). Towards an indigenous Chinese psychology: A selective review of methodological, theoretical, and empirical accomplishments. *Chinese Journal of Psychology, 41*(2), 181–211.

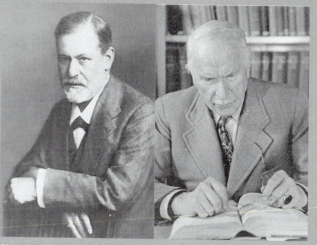

Sigmund Freud (1856–1939)
© Bettmann/CORBIS

Carl Jung (1875–1961)
Interfoto/Alamy

2 | PSYCHOANALYTIC PSYCHOTHERAPIES

Jeremy D. Safran and Alexander Kriss

OVERVIEW

Psychoanalysis is a distinctive form of psychological treatment and a model of psychological functioning, human development, and psychopathology. Sigmund Freud (1856–1939) was a Viennese neurologist who became known as the founding father of psychoanalysis. Psychoanalysis, however, is not synonymous with Freudian theory. There is no one psychoanalytic theory of personality or treatment but a host of different theories and treatment models that have developed over more than a century through the writings of theorists and practitioners from many different countries. The massive body of psychoanalytic theory that evolved over the course of Freud's lifetime was developed by Freud in conversation and collaboration with numerous colleagues, including Wilhelm Stekel, Alfred Adler, Karl Abraham, Otto Rank, Paul Federn, Sandor Ferenczi, Carl Jung, Eugene Bleuler, Max Eitingon, Hans Sacks, and Ernest Jones. Subsequent elaborations of psychoanalytic theory and the emergence of diverse psychoanalytic traditions were inspired by the work of key theorists such as Anna Freud, Melanie Kein, Ronald Fairbairn, Donald Winnicott, Heinz Hartmann, Heinz Kohut, Wilfred Bion, Charles Brenner, Jacques Lacan, Harry Stack Sullivan, and Stephen Mitchell. Although there are important similarities between all of these traditions, there are also important differences. Despite this lack of a unified perspective, it is possible to speak in general terms about certain basic principles that tend to cut across different psychoanalytic perspectives. These include:

1. an assumption that that all human beings are motivated in part by wishes, fantasies, or tacit knowledge that is outside of awareness (this is referred to as *unconscious motivation*);

2. an interest in facilitating awareness of unconscious motivations, thereby increasing choice;

3. an emphasis on exploring the ways in which we avoid painful or threatening feelings, fantasies, and thoughts;

4. an assumption that we are ambivalent about changing and an emphasis on the importance of exploring this ambivalence;

5. an emphasis on using the therapeutic relationship as an arena for exploring clients' self-defeating psychological processes and actions (both conscious and unconscious);

6. an emphasis on using the therapeutic relationship as an important vehicle of change; and

7. an emphasis on helping clients to understand the way in which their own construction of their past and present plays a role in perpetuating their self-defeating patterns.

The purpose of this chapter is to introduce psychoanalytic theory as a framework for conceptualizing human behavior and conducting psychotherapy. We seek to emphasize not only those concepts that are universally upheld, but also the controversies, unique perspectives, and ongoing dialectics between and within different schools of thought that have been a part of psychoanalysis since its beginning.

Basic Concepts

The Unconscious

One of Freud's most important insights was that "we are not masters of our own houses." By this, he meant that rational understanding of the factors motivating our actions often proves inadequate. Freud understood the *unconscious* as an area of psychic functioning in which impulses and wishes, as well as certain memories, are split off from awareness. This occurs either because the associated affects are too threatening or because the content of the impulses and wishes themselves are learned by the individual to be unacceptable through cultural conditioning.

Many contemporary psychoanalysts no longer conceptualize the unconscious in precisely the same way that Freud did. Some still contend (as did Freud) that there is a hypothetical psychic agency (i.e., the *ego*) that keeps aspects of experience deriving from the more primitive, instinctually based aspect of the psyche (referred to as the *id*) out of awareness. Others, however, argue that it is problematic to speculate about the nature of hypothetical psychic agencies such as the ego and the id. For example, Brenner (2002) argued that it is more useful to simply conceptualize any experience or action as reflecting a particular type of compromise between an underlying wish versus a fear of the consequences of achieving it. Other theorists find it useful to think of the unconscious as the dissociation of experience because of the failure of attention and narrative construction (e.g., Bromberg, 1998, 2006; Davies, 1996, 1998; Mitchell, 1993; Pizer, 1998; Stern, 1997, 2010). Notwithstanding theoretical differences of this type, however, common threads running through the differing perspectives are the premises that (1) our experience and actions are influenced by psychological processes that are not part of our conscious awareness and (2) these unconscious processes are kept out of awareness in order to avoid psychological pain.

Fantasy

Psychoanalytic theory holds that people's fantasies play an important role in their psychic functioning and the way in which they relate to external experience, especially their relationships with other people. These fantasies vary in the extent to which they are part of conscious awareness, ranging from daydreams and fleeting fantasies on the edge of awareness to deeply unconscious fantasies that trigger psychological defenses. In Freud's early thinking, these fantasies were linked to instinctually derived wishes involving sexuality or aggression, and they served the function of a type of imaginary wish fulfillment. Over time, Freud and other analysts developed a more elaborate view of the nature of fantasy and became convinced that fantasy served a number of psychic functions, including the need for the regulation of self-esteem, the need for a feeling of safety, the need for regulating affect, and the need to master trauma. Because fantasies are viewed as motivating our behavior and shaping our experience—and yet for the most part operate outside of focal awareness—exploring and interpreting clients' fantasies is viewed as an important part of the psychoanalytic process.

Primary and Secondary Processes

Primary process is a raw or primitive form of psychic functioning that begins at birth and continues to operate unconsciously throughout the lifetime. In primary process, there is no distinction between past, present, and future. Different feelings and experiences can be condensed together into one image or symbol, feelings can be expressed metaphorically, and the identities of different people can be merged. Infants are considered to operate in this mode as part of normal development. Primary process can be seen operating throughout childhood and adulthood in dreams and fantasy, as well as more consistently in individuals suffering from acute psychosis.

By contrast, *secondary process* is the style of psychic functioning associated with consciousness. It is logical, sequential and orderly, and the foundation for rational, reflective thinking.

Defenses

A *defense* is viewed as an intrapsychic process that functions to avoid emotional pain by pushing thoughts, wishes, feelings, or fantasies out of awareness. In the heyday of ego psychology, a systematic attempt was made to conceptualize and categorize the various defenses that people employ (e.g., Freud, 1937), such as *intellectualization* (in which an individual talks about something threatening while keeping an emotional distance from the feelings associated with it), *projection* (in which a person attributes a threatening feeling or motive he is experiencing to another person), and *reaction formation* (in which someone denies a threatening feeling and proclaims she feels the opposite).

Another defense which is particularly important to Kleinian theory is called *splitting*. When an individual attempts to avoid his or her perception of the other as good from being contaminated by negative feelings, he or she may split the representation of the other into two different images. Melanie Klein (1975) believed that this defense is commonly used by infants so that they are able to feel safe with their mothers. Rather than developing a complex representation of the mother that entails both her desirable and undesirable qualities, two separate representation of the mother are established: one that is all good and another that is all bad. According to Klein, the ability to integrate the good and bad representations of the mother is a developmental achievement that requires the ability to tolerate ambivalent feelings about the mother.

Clients who have more severe psychological disturbances never achieve this ability as adults and as a result are more likely to use splitting as a defense than healthy individuals. Splitting tends to have a more serious impact on the individual's everyday functioning than other defenses because the individual who commonly employs it experiences dramatic fluctuations in his or her perception of and feelings toward others. These fluctuations make it very difficult to maintain stable relationships with others, including therapists, who are often experienced as evil, persecutory, and completely untrustworthy.

Transference

Though *transference* has been defined and emphasized differentially throughout the development of psychoanalysis, it is a fundamental concept that played an important role in Freud's evolution of thought. Freud began to observe that it was not uncommon for his clients to view him and relate to him in ways that were reminiscent of the way they viewed and related to significant figures in their childhoods—especially their parents. He thus began to speculate that they were "transferring" a template from the past onto the present situation. For example, a client with a tyrannical father might begin to see the therapist as tyrannical. A client with an overly vulnerable father or mother who needed protecting might begin to relate to the therapist in the same way that she had related to her parents.

At first, Freud believed transference was an impediment to treatment (Freud, 1912). He speculated that transference was a form of resistance to remembering traumatic experiences, and he thought clients would act out previous relationships in the therapeutic setting rather than remember them. Over time, however, Freud came to see the development of transference as an indispensable part of the psychoanalytic process (e.g., Freud, 1917). In a sense, by reliving the past in the analytic relationship, the client provided the therapist with an opportunity to help him develop an understanding of how past relationships were influencing the experience of the present in an emotionally immediate way.

One- Versus Two-Person Psychologies

An important development that has taken place across a range of different psychoanalytic schools has been a shift from a *one-person psychology* to a *two-person psychology*. Many psychoanalysts have replaced Freud's view of the therapist as an objective and neutral observer who could serve as a blank screen onto whom the client projects his transference with a perspective in which therapist and client are viewed as coparticipants who engage in an ongoing process of mutual influence at both conscious and unconscious levels. This conceptual shift has important implications for the evolution of many of the concepts we will discuss later (e.g., resistance, transference, countertransference) as well as for psychoanalytic technique because it implies that the therapist cannot develop an accurate understanding of the client without developing some awareness of his own ongoing contribution to the interaction. Although the therapist's goal still remains one of ultimately understanding and helping the client, this cannot be accomplished without an ongoing process of self-exploration on the therapist's part.

This is especially the case with difficult or more disturbed clients who tend to evoke complex feelings and reactions in others, and therapists may not always be aware of these responses. But the process of exploring one's own contributions to the therapeutic relationship often illuminates subtle aspects of psychic functioning and interpersonal style in less-disturbed clients as well.

Shifting focus toward a two-person psychology has permitted helpful reconceptualizations of several of the aforementioned basic concepts of psychoanalysis. For instance, a two-person psychology emphasizes that the therapist often plays an important role in the emergence of resistance. Working through a client's resistance in modern psychoanalysis thus often involves an exploration of the therapist's contribution to it (Benjamin, 1990; Safran & Muran, 2000).

Other Systems

Psychoanalysis is the first modern Western system of psychotherapy, and most other forms of therapy that evolved out of it were strongly influenced by it or developed partially in reaction to it. Two founding fathers of cognitive therapy, Aaron Beck and Albert Ellis, were originally trained as psychoanalysts, and the seeds of many cognitive behavioral ideas can be found in psychoanalysis. Some of the early emphases of cognitive therapy (e.g., not focusing on the past, deemphasizing the therapeutic relationship) can be understood as attempts to discard aspects of psychoanalysis that were seen as problematic, but some cognitive therapists are reintroducing these concepts.

One difficulty in comparing psychoanalysis to other systems of psychotherapy is that psychoanalysis is not just form of therapy—it is a worldview. As such, it has had a profound effect on the development of Western culture. Although Freud initially began developing psychoanalysis as a treatment for clients presenting with symptoms that other physicians were unable to treat, his ambitions and the ambitions of subsequent psychoanalysts ultimately came to extend beyond the realm of therapy into social theory and cultural critique.

There are many reasons for the declining fortunes of psychoanalysis. One factor has been the tendency for psychiatry to become increasingly biological. Another is the rise of the cognitive-behavioral tradition and growing emphasis on evidence-based treatment. Another factor influencing the decreasing popularity of psychoanalysis has been a negative public reaction to an attitude of arrogance, insularity, and elitism that came to be associated with the psychoanalytic tradition. Psychoanalysts have also been guilty of a lack of receptiveness to valid criticism and empirical research. Many of these problems emerged as a result of various historical, cultural, and social-political forces that shaped the development of psychoanalysis but are not intrinsic to it. For example, for many years psychoanalysis in North America was a subspecialty of psychiatry and dominated the mental-health system. Psychiatrists who had completed the intensive process of formal psychoanalytic training were seen as the elite within their discipline. Psychoanalysis became a lucrative, prestigious, and socially conservative profession, attracting candidates who often had an interest in becoming respected members of the establishment rather than challenging it.

This development was in many respects ironic. The early psychoanalysts in Europe tended to be members of a liberal and progressive intelligentsia. Freud and many of his closest colleagues came from Jewish backgrounds and were accustomed to being members of a socially oppressed and marginalized group. Many of these early analysts were progressive social activists committed to political critiques and social justice. They viewed themselves as brokers of social change and saw psychoanalysis as a challenge to traditional societal and political norms (Danto, 2005; Jacoby, 1983; Safran, 2012).

Many of these problematic features of psychoanalysis have diminished in the last two decades as a result of internal reforms and modifications that have taken place within the psychoanalytic tradition—reforms that are partially the result of generational changes among the leading figures in psychoanalysis. Many of today's leading psychoanalytic theorists came of age during the 1960s during the anti–Vietnam War protests, and the emergence of a youth counterculture that was characterized by a rejection of conventional social norms (Safran, 2012). Unfortunately, many people in the broader mental-health field and the general public are unaware of these changes within mainstream psychoanalysis and are responding to a caricatured understanding of the tradition based on aspects of psychoanalytic theory, practice, and attitude that are no longer characteristic of psychoanalysis. In addition, a partial or somewhat distorted understanding of what older traditions of psychoanalysis were trying to do has contributed to this lack of awareness by the broader mental-health profession.

The current marginalization of psychoanalysis is attributable not only to valid criticism but also to unhealthy contemporary cultural biases, especially in the United States. These biases include an emphasis on speed, pragmatism, instrumentality, and an intolerance of ambiguity (Cushman, 1995; Hoffman, 2009; Safran, 2012). Notwithstanding growing political cynicism in the United States, U.S. culture is traditionally optimistic. Although this optimism certainly has its value, it can also lead to a type of naïveté that tends to underestimate the complexity of human nature and the difficulty of the change process. American culture traditionally tends to gloss over the more tragic dimensions of life, espouse the belief that we can all be happy if we try hard enough, and be biased toward a "quick fix mentality." The massive increase of the number of people taking antidepressants is one symptom of this mentality. Psychoanalysis originated in continental Europe and in a culture that had experienced centuries of poverty, oppression of the masses by the aristocracy, ongoing religious conflict and oppression, and generations of warfare that culminated in two world wars that were unprecedented in scale and tragedy.

Because of these cultural differences, American psychoanalysis is more optimistic than its European counterpart, but it still retains many of the traditional psychoanalytic values such as the appreciation of human complexity, a recognition that contentment or the "good life" are not necessarily the same as a two-dimensional version of "happiness," and an appreciation that change is not always easy or fast. A greater understanding of what contemporary psychoanalysis is about and a deeper appreciation of the more valuable dimensions of psychoanalytic theory and practice can enrich our understanding of how best to help people and serve as a corrective to some of our cultural biases (Safran, 2012).

HISTORY

Precursors

Freud's development of psychoanalytic theory and practice was influenced by a number of cultural and intellectual trends and scientific models that dominated European circles in the late 19th and early 20th centuries. It was also influenced through Freud's ongoing engagement with the thinking of numerous mentors, colleagues, and critics whose ideas he built on, critiqued, assimilated, and transformed.

One formative influence on Freud's early thinking was his exposure to developments in French neurology and psychiatry that explored the role that the splitting of consciousness played in psychopathology—in particular, the work of the renowned French neurologist Jean-Martin Charcot, who had established an international reputation through his use of hypnosis with hysterics. *Hysterics* were clients who presented with a variety of dramatic physical problems—such as paralysis of the limbs, blindness, and convulsions—that could not be accounted for on an organic basis. Today this particular pattern of symptom presentation and the associated diagnosis is far less common. Charcot's theory was that hysterical symptoms emerged as a result of a type of splitting off of aspects of consciousness as a result of an organic weakness; hypnosis could both induce and intensify hysterical symptoms as well as lead to their improvement.

In 1886, Freud began collaborating with an older colleague, Josef Breuer, who had earned high respect in his own right as a practicing physician working with a wide range of problems, including syndromes without an obvious organic basis. He told Freud about a female patient who presented with severe hysterical symptoms: Breuer treated her using an innovative technique that involved experimenting with different therapeutic approaches and modifying what he was doing in response to her feedback. Rather than treating her exclusively through somatic means (as was common at the time), Breuer made the assumption that the patient's symptoms had a psychological meaning. Over time, he found that the young woman would experience relief from her symptoms after talking freely about painful and traumatic experiences and recovering painful memories that had been dissociated. The young woman—who was given the pseudonym Anna O. in the case report that Breuer and Freud ultimately published collaboratively—referred to Breuer's approach as "the talking cure."

Partially influenced by Charcot's thinking about the role of dissociation in hysteria, Freud and Breuer came to believe that hysterical symptoms were the result of suppressed emotions that had been cut off at the time of the trauma, and that these emotions expressed themselves in the form of physical symptoms. Freud felt that hypnosis could help clients recover memories of the trauma and experience the associated affect, eventually resulting in a cure. In contrast to Charcot, Freud came to believe that the origins of the problem were not the result of an organic weakness but were, in fact, entirely psychological. In 1895, Breuer and Freud published *Studies in Hysteria* (Breuer & Freud, 1995), which consisted of a number of case histories and a theoretical section outlining their beliefs about the psychological origins of hysteria (Makari, 2008).

Beginnings

Although Freud's early forays into psychoanalysis used hypnosis to help clients recover lost memories and associated emotions, over time he found this technique to be unreliable. Although some clients were good candidates for hypnosis, many were simply not sufficiently suggestible. Instead of hypnotizing his clients, Freud began to encourage them to "say everything that comes to mind without censoring." This was the origin of the psychoanalytic principle of *free association*, a technique in which clients are encouraged to attempt to suspend their self-critical function and verbalize thoughts, images, associations, and feelings that are on the edge of awareness (Makari, 2008).

Another factor influencing the theoretical emphasis on clearly distinguishing psychoanalysis from hypnosis and suggestibility was the evolving conception of the goals of psychoanalysis. Freud was highly invested in establishing psychoanalysis as a rigorous scientific discipline, and he therefore saw the need to differentiate it from methods that were increasingly viewed as quackery by the scientific community and public alike. There was also a growing sense that one of the important goals of psychoanalysis involved the pursuit of truth. Hypnosis helped people through suggestion, whereas in contrast psychoanalysis was supposed to help people become more skeptical and face uncomfortable truths about themselves (Safran, 2012). Psychoanalysis came to be seen as a kind of counterindoctrination (to social and cultural brainwashing) rather than as a form of indoctrination (Reiff, 1966).

From Seduction Theory to Drive Theory

Another critical stage in the evolution of Freud's thinking was a shift in his belief that sexual trauma always lies at the root of psychological problems, which had been dubbed *seduction theory,* toward an emphasis on the role of fantasy and instinctual drive. Over time, he abandoned his theory that all of his clients had been sexually abused as children and instead began to focus on the role that sexual instincts play in the developmental process. He theorized that rudimentary sexual feelings are present even during early infancy and give rise to sexually related wishes and fantasies that are pushed out of consciousness because they were experienced as too threatening. Freud speculated that often the recovered memories of sexual trauma were actually the product of reconstructed fantasies rather than real sexual trauma. Although he never discounted the impact of real sexual abuse or trauma, he did come to place less emphasis on these experiences, and he no longer saw them as the ubiquitous core of all neurotic problems. Freud began to abandon a model of simple, mechanical linear causation and instead moved toward a view of memory as constructive. At the same time, Freud's growing emphasis on unconscious fantasy opened the way to a deeper appreciation of the complex nature of psychic life that was not always obvious to the everyday observer. Freud's evolving perspective involved tracing the chain of the client's association in order to help formulate hypotheses about childhood fantasies and wishes that had been covered over and disguised.

By the early 1900s, Freud had come to believe that all thinking and action were fueled by a type of psychic energy that is linked in a complex way to sexuality. Building on contemporary developments in a variety of scientific disciplines (e.g., neurology, biology, evolutionary theory, psychophysics), Freud developed a motivational model that held that psychic energy (which he termed *libido*) could be activated by both external and internal stimuli, which in turn produces an organismic sense of tension or "unpleasure." Consistent with early 20th-century thinking in neurology, Freud theorized that maintaining psychic energy at a constant level was a biological imperative. Thus, once psychic energy became activated it needed to be discharged, which restored psychic equilibrium and was experienced as pleasure. This discharge of psychic energy could take place in a variety of ways (e.g., the expression of affect, the satisfaction of a sexual urge, or the repetition of an experience that has become associated with tension reduction through experience). For example, during the process of nursing, a type of presexual feeling in the infant's mouth is elicited by oral stimulation and satisfied by sucking the mother's breast. The mother's breast thus becomes an object that is invested with psychic energy through its association with previous experiences of tension reduction. This psychobiological push to repeat experiences that have become associated with tension reduction is known as the *pleasure principle,* and the general model of motivation is known as *drive theory.*

Freud theorized that the process of psychological development was linked to the biological process of sexual development from infancy to adolescence. Freud's emphasis on instinctual sexuality as the cornerstone of his entire theoretical edifice (what is referred to as his *psychosexual theory*) was controversial from the beginning. There has been much speculation as to why psychosexual theory became so central to Freud's thinking, and it is likely that multiple factors played a role. One factor may have been that the puritanical Victorian culture of Freud's era exacerbated the role of sexual conflicts in many of the hysterical patients that he initially treated. In addition, Freud was influenced by a growing interest in the study of human sexuality among academic psychiatrists. Another factor may have been Freud's desire to ground psychoanalysis in biology and Darwinian theory. Freud reasoned that because of its link to reproduction and survival of the species, sexuality was likely to play a particularly prominent role in human psychology. It is important to note, however, that although there was a time when Freud's drive theory was widely adopted by the mainstream psychoanalytic community, the trend within today's psychoanalysis is to replace it with a model of motivation that is more consistent with contemporary developments in emotion theory and research and the affective neurosciences.

Jung, Bleuler, and the Zurich Psychoanalytic Society

The first psychoanalysts were for the most part Viennese physicians who met in Freud's home every Wednesday evening to discuss evolving psychoanalytic ideas and explore their relevance to clinical practice. The publication of Freud's *The Interpretation of Dreams* in 1900 began to attract attention from a wider professional audience. A development that was to become particularly important for the future of psychoanalysis was the growing interest in Freud's work by Eugene Bleuler, a prominent Swiss psychiatrist. Bleuler, the director of the prestigious Burgholzli Psychiatric Clinic in Zurich, had become interested in the use of methods borrowed form experimental psychology to investigate the thought processes of psychiatric patients. In 1900, he hired a young medical graduate named Carl Jung to work in the clinic and help him with his research. With Bleuler's encouragement, Jung began to use a type of word-association test to investigate the response time latencies to emotionally charged words in different groups of psychiatric patients. Bleuler and Jung began to account for their findings using Freud's theories about the nature of unconscious processes. Jung argued that delayed response times to emotionally charged words reflect the unconscious functioning of what he termed emotional *complexes*—that is, affectively charged ideas that are repressed because they are emotionally threatening. Jung's published articles on the topic were well received by the mainstream psychiatric community, and his reputation began to grow.

Bleuler and Jung began corresponding with Freud, keeping him abreast of their work and asking for clinical advice. At the same time, a number of the psychiatrists at the Burgholzli clinic began to experiment with the use of treatment methods that they had gleaned from Freud's writings. The growing interest in Freud's work by staff members at the Burgholzli played an important role in spreading Freud's thinking in the medical community. Unlike Freud and his Viennese associates, who worked primarily in private practice settings without important institutional affiliations, Jung, Bleuler, and other staff members at the Burgholzli worked in a psychiatric setting considered to be on the cutting edge of teaching and research. It was common for psychiatrists from across Europe to spend time there in order to learn about the latest developments in psychiatric treatment. In this manner, a growing number of physicians and psychiatrists from around the world became familiar with Freud's work, and many of them were ultimately to become some of the more prominent members of the psychoanalytic community and contributors to the development of psychoanalytic theory and practice.

In 1907, Jung traveled to Vienna to meet with Freud personally. After this visit, Jung's alliance with Freud and the growing psychoanalytic movement became increasingly stronger, and Freud began to see Jung and his colleagues in Zurich as indispensable to the future development of psychoanalysis. The psychiatrists working with Jung and Bleuler established the Zurich Psychoanalytic Society, and Jung organized the First International Psychoanalytic Congress in 1908. Freud hoped that Jung, who was

20 years younger, would ultimately become his successor as the leader of the psychoanalytic movement, and for a period of time there was a general understanding that Jung would fulfill this expectation. There were, however, from the beginning, both theoretical and personal tensions between Freud and Jung that grew over time and ultimately led to the end of their collaboration. At a theoretical level, Jung believed that Freud was mistaken in viewing sexuality as the most important motivational principle. He also believed that Freud's view of the unconscious was one-sided in nature and that Freud failed to recognize the more creative and growth oriented aspects of unconscious processes. And, finally, Jung felt that Freud failed to recognize the importance of the spiritual and transpersonal aspects of the human psyche.

At a personal level, both Freud and Jung were highly ambitious men with intense needs for promoting their own unique worldviews and establishing their respective legacies. Freud viewed Jung as a brilliant protégé who would help to further establish and consolidate the psychoanalytic perspective that Freud had pioneered. And although Jung deeply appreciated and benefited from Freud's mentorship and support, his own needs for individuation and creative aspirations ultimately made it impossible to remain in Freud's shadow. By 1912, the strains between Jung and Freud had become insurmountable, and their relationship came to a mutually bitter and emotionally painful end. Jung subsequently went on to develop his own unique and highly influential school of psychotherapy known as *analytical* or *Jungian psychology*.

The Development of Structural Theory and Ego Psychology

In 1923, Freud published *The Ego and the Id* (Freud, 1923) and laid out the foundations for what subsequently became known as his *structural theory*. In this paper, he distinguished three different psychic agencies—the id, the ego, and the superego—and described how they interact to deal with the demands of reality versus the pleasure principle. The *id* is the aspect of the psyche that is instinctually based and present from birth. The *ego* gradually emerges out of the id and functions to represent the concerns of reality. Although the id presses for immediate sexual gratification, the ego evaluates the suitability of the situation for satisfying one's instinctual desires, and it allows the individual to delay instinctual gratification or find other ways of channeling instinctual needs in a socially acceptable fashion.

The *superego* is the psychic agency that emerges through the internalization of social values and norms. Although some aspects of the superego can be conscious, other aspects are not. One important function of the ego is to mediate between the demands of the id and the superego. For a variety of reasons, the superego often becomes overly harsh and demanding and can lead to self-destructive feelings of guilt and a rejecting stance toward one's own instinctual needs and wishes. One goal of analysis traditionally has been to help individuals become more aware of the overly harsh nature of their superegos so that they become less self-punitive.

The Development of Object Relations Theory in Britain

A second major psychoanalytic tradition emerging out of some of Freud's more mature thinking came to be known as *object relations theory*, which is particularly concerned with the way in which we develop internal representations of our relationships with significant others. Object relations theory developed primarily in Britain, stemming from the work of Melanie Klein and those she influenced. Klein, originally a practitioner of child analysis who pioneered the technique of play therapy, was particularly interested in understanding the early relationship between the mother and the infant, and she developed a line of theory that laid the groundwork for understanding the way in which psychological maturation involves a process of developing internal representations of our relationships with significant others. Throughout the 1940s and 1950s, some of the more innovative theoretical and technical advances in psychoanalysis emerged out of the work of Klein (e.g., 1975) and her followers, who became particularly interested in working with difficult, treatment-resistant cases.

At the same time, another group of psychoanalytic theorists started to appear, consisting of those who were influenced by both Freudian and Kleinian ideas but were unwilling to align themselves politically with either tradition. These analysts, who became known as the *British Independents* or the *Middle Group*, consisted of theorists such as Ronald Fairbairn (1952, 1994), Michael Balint (1968), Donald Winnicott (1956, 1958, 1960), and John Bowlby (1969, 1973, 1980). Some of the key qualities associated with the work of these analysts were an emphasis on the importance of spontaneity, creativity, therapist flexibility, and the value of providing clients with a supportive and nurturing environment. Many developments coming out of the Kleinian and Middle Group traditions have subsequently been assimilated into more recent developments in American psychoanalysis. Winnicott, in particular, has become an important inspiration to many contemporary North American psychoanalysts who emphasize creativity, spontaneity, and authenticity. Bowlby's work has given rise to the extremely fertile area of attachment theory and research.

Current Status

Toward Psychoanalytic Pluralism in North America

Unlike the British system, which formally institutionalized the existence of three different psychoanalytic traditions (Freudian, Kleinian, and the Independent or Middle Group), the United States formally recognized the existence of only one psychoanalytic tradition. Ego psychology centered firmly around Freud's structural theory and refinements of it developed by Anna Freud (Freud's daughter), colleagues in Britain, and émigré American analysts such as Heinz Hartmann, Ernst Kris, Rudolph Loewenstein, Edith Jacobson, and Erik Erickson and subsequently American-born analysts such as Charles Brenner and Jacob Arlow.

American ego psychology gradually consolidated into an orthodoxy that is sometimes referred to as *classical psychoanalysis*. Classical psychoanalysis was characterized by an adherence to certain core theoretical premises as well as specific technical guidelines. The core theoretical premises included an adherence to Freud's drive theory of motivation and to his psychosexual model of development. Following Freud, classical psychoanalysis viewed transference as a projection of the client's unconscious dynamics, and they believed that therapists who had mastered their own unconscious conflicts as a result of undergoing their own personal analyses could function as blank screens onto which clients would project their transferences. In classical psychoanalytic thinking, the key mechanism of change was theorized to involve the process of gaining insight into one's own unconscious conflicts.

Important technical guidelines (derived from six essays that Freud published between 1911 and 1915) specified that therapists should strive to maintain anonymity (in order to function as a blank screen that would not contaminate the client's transference), attempt to remain neutral (by refraining from giving the client direct advice or letting the therapist's own biases influence the client), and avoid gratifying the client's immediate wishes (e.g., requests for personal information about the therapist's life, requests for direct guidance or advice, requests for active interventions or help with problem solving) because such wishes were viewed as derivatives of unconscious wishes and fantasies that need to be explored and understood rather than acted on.

Practitioners of American ego psychology were by and large unfamiliar with British object relations theory, and theorists diverging too far from mainstream ego psychology tended to become marginalized; in some cases, they started their own schools of thought. One of the more notable mavericks was Harry Stack Sullivan (1953), an iconoclastic American-born psychiatrist who had never received any formal psychoanalytic training. Sullivan developed his own model of psychoanalytically oriented psychiatry that was strongly influenced by a type of field theory emerging out of American sociology as well as the American philosophical school of pragmatism. Unlike ego psychologists, Sullivan theorized that the need for human relatedness is the most fundamental human motivation, and he deprivileged the motivational role of sexuality. He also believed that it is impossible to understand the individual apart from the context of relationships with others. In the context of psychotherapy, he argued that everything transpiring in the therapeutic relationship needed to be understood in terms of both the client's and therapist's ongoing contributions rather than exclusively in terms of the client's psychology or the transference. In collaboration with Clara Thompson and Erich Fromm, Sullivan founded the tradition of *interpersonal psychoanalysis*.

Another figure who came to play an important role in the movement toward a more pluralistic perspective in North American psychoanalysis was Heinz Kohut (1984), a European émigré who for many years was a well-respected mainstream ego psychologist. As his thinking and clinical work evolved, however, he became particularly interested in the treatment of narcissism, and over time his theoretical formulations diverged increasingly from mainstream psychoanalytic ideas. Kohut became particularly interested in understanding the processes through which the individual develops a cohesive sense of self, an experience of inner vitality, and a capacity for self-esteem. He placed an increasing emphasis on the role that the therapist's empathic stance plays as a mechanism of change in and of itself and in the centrality of this process in repairing ruptures in the therapeutic relationship when they occur as a result of the therapist's inevitable lapses in empathy.

The development of *relational psychoanalysis* was another important stage in the ultimate fragmentation of the monolithic psychoanalytic perspective that had dominated American psychoanalysis in the 1950s and early 1960s. In particular, Greenberg and Mitchell's *Object Relations in Psychoanalysis* (1983) helped to crystallize developments that were already taking place and catalyze the emergence of a new paradigm. The book established a legitimate role for the tradition of American interpersonal psychoanalysis within the mainstream psychoanalytic tradition by drawing parallels between what Sullivan was trying to accomplish theoretically and what other more "legitimate" mainstream psychoanalysts were attempting to achieve. The book also introduced the seminal works of British object relations theorists such as Klein, Fairbairn, and Winnicott to an audience of ego psychologists that had been largely unfamiliar with them.

Subsequently, Stephen Mitchell (1988, 1997) published several highly influential books articulating many of the key principles of the emerging relational paradigm in psychoanalysis. Over the next two decades, several creative psychoanalytic theorists emerged as leading voices in the relational tradition. These included Lewis Aron, Philip Bromberg, Emmanuel Ghent, Adrienne Harris, Jessica Benjamin, Muriel Dimen, Irwin Hoffman, Neil Altman, Jody Davies, and Donnel Stern.

An important thrust of the early relational thinking involved critiquing aspects of classical psychoanalytic theory that were viewed as problematic. Various threads of the relational critique had already been articulated by diverse psychoanalytic theorists who had been marginalized by classical psychoanalysis (e.g., Carl Jung, Sandor Ferenczi, Otto Rank, Melanie Klein, Ronald Fairbairn, Donald Winnicott, Harry Stack Sullivan, Erich Fromm, and Heinz Kohut). But the relational critique and the systematic articulation of alternative theoretical ideas and technical prescriptions emerged at a time when changes already taking place in the broader culture created a particularly fertile climate for changes within the psychoanalytic world.

Examples of relevant cultural changes included the rise of humanistic and existential alternatives to psychoanalysis in the 1960s, the emergence of the cognitive-behavioral tradition, the growing marginalization of psychoanalysis within psychiatry, and the rise of feminist and postmodern thinking. Relational theorists rejected Freud's drive theory of motivation and placed greater emphasis on the instinctual need for human relatedness. They argued that it is impossible for the therapist to function as a blank screen for transference projection because anything he or she does reveals elements of his or her unique subjectivity. They further argued that the relationship between the therapist and client is one of mutual influence and that it is impossible for the therapist to step completely outside of the emergent relational field and observe the client objectively. Relational thinking emphasized the inevitable fallibility of the therapist and maintained that no matter how well-analyzed she is, she can never be fully transparent to herself. And they argued that the therapeutic relationship in and of itself is a critical ingredient of the change process and emphasized the importance of the authentic human encounter between therapist and patient.

What does the current scene in American psychoanalysis look like? The dominant paradigm of American ego psychology has given way to the emergence of a variety of different traditions. Contemporary ego psychology has evolved into what is called *modern conflict theory*. Conflict theory emphasizes the centrality in human experience and the action of ongoing conflict between unconscious wishes and defenses against them. Many of the more abstract and speculative ideas about the structure of the human psyche, the relationship between the psychological and biological and the nature of human motivation, are deemphasized in modern conflict theory. There is a more pragmatic emphasis on principles of technique and practice, and efforts to develop an overarching model of the human psyche tend to have been replaced by less-ambitious attempts at theory construction. Although it would be an overstatement to say that relational tradition has emerged as the dominant paradigm in American psychoanalysis, there is little doubt that it has significantly influenced the mainstream.

Kleinian and Lacanian Traditions in Europe and Latin America

Two additional developments have been remarkably influential in other parts of the world and are increasingly coming to have an impact on American psychoanalysis. The first development can be designated as the Kleinian and post-Kleinian thinking of various innovative theorists, one of the most notable being Wilfred Bion, a British psychoanalyst who trained with Klein. Bion's concept of *containment* has proven especially popular in contemporary analytic thinking, and it is described later in this chapter.

A final major psychoanalytic tradition is Lacanian and post-Lacanian theory. French psychoanalyst Jacques Lacan (1988a, 1988b) was extremely critical of the American tradition of ego psychology, which he viewed as emphasizing conventionality and societal conformity, as well as betraying Freud's most radical and important insights about the centrality of unconscious processes. In contrast to American ego psychologists, who emphasized the adaptive aspects of the ego, Lacan argued that the ego—that is, one's sense of "I"—is an illusion. According to Lacan, our identity or sense of "I-ness" is forged out of a misidentification of ourselves with the desire of the other. Unlike theorists such as Winnicott, however, Lacan does not believe that there is a *true self* waiting to be discovered. Rather, there is emptiness or what Lacan refers to as a *lack*—a fundamental sense of alienation from the self. This lack stems in part from the fact that our experience cannot be communicated without the medium of language. The very process of symbolizing our experience through language, however, results in a distortion of this experience.

Lacanian psychoanalysis played an important role in breaking up the hegemony of the traditional psychoanalytic institutes in Latin America in the same way that traditions such as self psychology and relational psychoanalysis did in the United States. Lacanian concepts are beginning to make their way into American clinical psychoanalysis as well.

PERSONALITY

There is no one psychoanalytic theory of personality. Rather, psychoanalysis provides a kaleidoscopic lens, informed by different schools of thought, through which one can view human experience and development. Although space constraints do not allow for a comprehensive review of psychoanalytic perspectives on personality development, we will briefly outline a few of the most influential psychoanalytic theories of personality.

Theory of Personality

Conflict Theory

Beginning with Freud and his colleagues, *intrapsychic conflict* has been viewed as playing a central role in the development of the individual's specific personality. From the perspective of conflict theory, different personality or character styles can be understood as resulting from the compromise between specific underlying core wishes and characteristic styles of defense that are used to manage these wishes. For example, the obsessional individual is typically involved in a conflict between obedience and defiance. Intellectualization is the key defense used to manage underlying emotions that are threatening; words and details are used to obscure underlying feelings. The hysterical personality style has an underlying wish for emotional intimacy that is defended against by superficial or dramatic emotionality and seductiveness. The phobic style involves displacing intrapsychic conflicts onto external situations. Conflicts around underlying sexual feelings are defended against by displacing anxiety onto public situations. Common defenses are displacement, projection, and behavioral avoidance. Unacceptable feelings of anger are transformed into the experience of panic. The narcissistic style involves defending against underlying wishes for dependency and fear of abandonment by surface feelings of grandiosity and self-aggrandizing behaviors.

Object Relations Theory

Object relations perspectives on personality theorize that internal representations (referred to as *internal objects* or *internal object relations*) influence the way in which people perceive others, choose particular types of people with whom to establish relationships, and shape their relationships in an ongoing fashion through their own perceptions and actions (e.g., Meissner, 1981; Schafer, 1968). This basic perspective has influenced a wide range of specific theories of personality and development. Much of the writing about internal objects or internal object relations, while clinically rich, can be conceptually ambiguous. Different theorists have developed different understandings of what an internal object is and different models of how internal objects become established (a process referred to as *internalization*).

In recent years, there has been a growing interest in John Bowlby's (1969, 1973, 1980) model of object relations known as *attachment theory*. According to Bowlby, humans have an instinctively based need (a motivational system referred to as the *attachment system*) to maintain proximity to their primary caregivers (referred to as *attachment figures*). The attachment system serves an adaptive function, in that it increases the possibility that the infant will be able to obtain the caretaking and protection that are essential for its survival. To maintain proximity to the attachment figure, infants develop representations of their interactions with their attachment figures that allow them to predict what type of actions will increase the possibility of maintaining proximity versus what type of actions will threaten the relationship. Bowlby referred to these representations as *internal working models*. When an infant learns that certain ways of being jeopardize the relationship with attachment figures, they develop a propensity for dissociating experiences and feelings—such as aggression, anger, and vulnerability—linked to these ways of beings.

One major difference between the conceptualization of internalization emerging out of attachment theory and mother–infant developmental research (e.g., Bowlby, 1973, 1980; Main, 1991; Stern, 1985) and the thinking of objects theorists is that models deriving from attachment theory and developmental research tend to assume that internal working models are based on the representation of actual interactions that have taken place between the infant and significant others. In contrast, *object relations theory* assumes that internal models are shaped by a combination of these real experiences with unconscious wishes and fantasies and other intrapsychic processes that are not reality based. Different object relations theories, such as those of Melanie Klein and Ronald Fairbairn, emphasize the role of different types of unconscious fantasies.

Klein (1975) theorized that people are born with instinctual passions related to both love and aggression that are linked to unconscious fantasies and images about relationships with others. These unconscious fantasies exist before any actual encounter with other human beings and serve as the scaffolding for the perception of others. In Klein's thinking, instinctual aggression played a particularly important role. She believed that infants experience their own aggression as intolerable, and therefore they need to fantasize that this aggression originates in the other (typically, the mother in Klein's writing) rather than themselves. Klein uses the term *projective identification* to designate the intrapsychic process through which feelings that originate internally are experienced as originating from the other. These unconscious fantasies of aggressive, persecuting others, referred to as *internal objects* by Klein, become part of the infant's psychic world and color his or her perception of significant others who are seen as dangerous and persecuting.

To retain some perception of the other as potentially good and nondangerous, infants unconsciously split the image of the other or the internal object into good and bad aspects. The good aspect is thus able to remain uncontaminated by the bad aspect. Over time, as a result of both cognitive and emotional maturation and ongoing encounters with real significant others, the child is able to begin integrating the good and bad objects into one whole and to reclaim aggression as emerging from the self.

Klein's thinking, while clinically rich, lacks systematic consistency and can be difficult to grasp conceptually. Much of her writing suggests she is trying to put into words intuitions gleaned from years of clinical experience that don't lend themselves easily to explicit articulation. Reading Klein is hard work, typically accompanied by the experience of confusion and befuddlement interspersed with moments of new clarity and deep insights into what she is trying to say about human experience and clinical work.

In contrast to Klein, Fairbairn's thinking is more systematic in nature. At the same time, his writing can have a hermetic or self-referential quality to it that can make it difficult to fully grasp. Fairbairn (1952, 1994) theorizes that internal objects are established when the individual withdraws from external reality because the caregiver is unavailable, frustrating, or traumatizing, and individuals instead create a type of internal reality as a substitute. These fantasized relationships become important building blocks for one's experience of the self because the self is always experienced in relationship to others, whether in fantasy or reality. The problem is that these defensive attempts to control significant others by developing fantasized relationships with them, rather than real ones, are only partially successful. The reason for this is that the depriving or traumatizing aspects of the significant other that provide the raw material for the unconscious fantasy or internal object inevitably end up becoming part of the internal structure or enduring psychic organization that is developed.

In important respects, the concept of internal object relations serves the same function in object relations theory as the concept of internal working model does for Bowlby. (This should come as no surprise because Bowlby was strongly influenced by Melanie Klein and was an object relations theorist himself). Both the concepts of internal object relations and internal working models provide ways of thinking about the way in which our internal representations of relationships with others shape our ongoing relationships. Some of the implications of object relations theory are identical to those of attachment theory (e.g., we tend to dissociate experience that would have threatened our relationship with our primary caregivers). Other implications cannot be derived as easily from attachment theory.

Klein has a unique ability to touch on some of the more disturbing unspeakable terrors of psychic life, especially in more severe forms of psychological disturbance. She also provides brilliant clinical insights into human destructiveness toward both self and others. Her thinking has helped to establish a foundation for working clinically with clients who can seem untreatable to many clinicians. Fairbairn's thinking can provide tremendous clinical insights into working with clients who are "addicted" to romantic relationships that are self-destructive. For example, according to Fairbairn, as adults we seek out others (e.g., romantic partners) who resemble our parents in certain respects as a type of loyalty to our internal objects. Or we project our internal objects onto others, thereby increasing the possibility that we will see them in predictable ways (e.g., hostile and abusive) and react in predictable ways to our projections (e.g., hostility in response to perceived abuse). Or we act in a way that will elicit responses from others that resemble the way our parents would have responded because at some level this is what feels most comfortable or natural to us. From Fairbairn's perspective, in a sense people are addicted to these pathological modes of relating because they are the only form of relating they know. The abusive relationship becomes the template for love. To give up this model of relating would mean to give up all hope of relating to others.

Developmental Arrest Models

Developmental arrest models such as Winnicott's developmental theory or Kohut's *self psychology* theorize that psychological problems emerge as a result of the failure of caregivers to provide a "good enough" or optimal environment. As a result of this failure, the normal developmental process becomes arrested. According to Winnicott (1956, 1958, 1960), the infant begins in a state of subjective omnipotence, believing that his or her wishes make things happen and that the mother will satisfy all of his or her needs. Over time, it is inevitable that the mother will fail the infant in various ways, and the infant begins to lose his or her experience of omnipotence and to experience a distinction between his or her fantasies and reality. If the mother is too unresponsive or her needs impinge too much on the infant's, then the infant will become overadapted to the needs of the other and develop a *false self*. This allows the infant to maintain relatedness with the other as well as protect himself. However, this arrangement comes at a price. By defining himself in regard to the needs and desires of others, the infant may grow up to feel alienated from himself, resulting in the subjective experience of a lack of inner vitality.

If, on the other hand, the process by which the infant's sense of omnipotence is frustrated takes place in a sufficiently gradual fashion, then the infant can come to accept the limitations of the other without being traumatized. This process of *optimal disillusionment* is an important mechanism in therapy as well.

Kohut (1984) theorizes that, to develop a cohesive sense of self, the developing child requires caregivers who are able to provide adequate mirroring or attunement to his or her needs. In addition, he theorizes that failures in attunement or empathy are inevitable and that the experience of working through these empathic failures with the parents is also critical to the development of a cohesive sense of self. Both Winnicott and Kohut theorize that change in treatment requires a new kind of relationship with the therapist that remobilizes the natural developmental process that has been arrested.

PSYCHOTHERAPY

Theory of Psychotherapy

What Is Psychoanalytic Therapy?

Traditionally, psychoanalysts have made a clear distinction between *psychoanalysis* versus what is referred to as *psychoanalytic* or *psychodynamic therapy*. The term *psychoanalysis* has been reserved for a form of treatment with certain defining characteristics or parameters. The term *psychodynamic therapy* has been used to refer to forms of treatment that are based on psychoanalytic theory but lack some of the defining characteristics of psychoanalysis. Over the years, there has been some controversy over which parameters of psychoanalysis are and are not defining criteria.

A common stance has been that psychoanalysis (as opposed to psychoanalytic therapy) is long term (e.g., four years or more), intensive (e.g., four or more sessions per week), and open ended (no fixed termination date or number of sessions). In addition, psychoanalysis is characterized by a specific therapeutic stance that involves (1) an emphasis on helping clients to become aware of their unconscious motivation, (2) refraining from giving the client advice or being overly directive, (3) attempting to avoid influencing the client by introducing one's own belief and values, (4) maintaining a certain degree of anonymity by reducing the amount of information one provides about one's personal life or one's feeling and reactions in the session, (5) attempting to maintain the stance of the neutral and objective observer rather than a fully engaged participant in the process, and (6) a seating arrangement in which the client reclines on a couch and the therapist sits upright and out of view of the client.

Many psychoanalysts no longer make such rigid distinctions. The differences between psychoanalysis and psychoanalytic treatment have more to do with the politics of the discipline and professional elitism than any theoretically justifiable criteria, but at the same time it is a mistake to assume that all of the parameters associated with traditional psychoanalysis are of no value. For example, although some clients benefit from short-term treatment, many people require longer term treatment, and the tendency to pathologize the practice of long-term psychoanalytic treatment reflects an overemphasis in our culture on the value of individualism and a devaluation of the interdependency more characteristic of traditional cultures. Similar arguments can be made not only for the benefits of one versus multiple sessions per week but also the use of the couch. Psychoanalysts are increasingly coming to develop a more pluralistic perspective on both theory and practice - there is no one theory that has a unique purchase on truth, and no single "right" way to do psychoanalytic therapy.

The Therapeutic Alliance

The concept of the *therapeutic alliance* originated in early psychoanalytic theory (Sterba, 1934; Zetzel, 1956). Although Freud did not use the term explicitly, he did emphasize the importance of establishing a good collaborative relationship with the client. Ralph Greenson's (1965, 1971) formulation of the alliance was particularly influential in North America. Greenson spoke about the importance of distinguishing between the transferential aspects of the therapeutic relationship (which are distorted), and the alliance, which is based on the client's rational, undistorted perception of the therapist, and on a feeling of genuine linking, trust, and respect. Greenson emphasized that the caring, human aspects of the therapeutic relationship play a critical role in allowing the client to benefit from psychoanalysis.

Edward Bordin's (1979) conceptualization of the alliance, which was strongly influenced by Greenson's thinking, has become particularly influential among psychotherapy researchers. According to Bordin, the strength of the alliance depends on how much the client and therapist agree about the tasks and goals of therapy and on the quality of the relational bond between them. The tasks of therapy consist of the specific activities (either overt or covert) that the client must engage in to benefit from treatment (e.g., exploring dreams and exploring transference). The goals of therapy are general objectives toward which the treatment is directed (e.g., symptom reduction and personality change). The bond element of the alliance refers to the degree of trust the client has in the therapist and the extent to which he or she feels understood by the therapist. Bond, task, and goal components of the alliance are always influencing one another.

Transference

Like most psychoanalytic concepts, the notion of *transference* has evolved considerably since Freud first developed it in 1905. Transference refers to the client's tendency to view the therapist in terms that are shaped by his or her experiences with important caregivers and other significant figures who played important roles during the developmental process. Thus, early experiences establish templates or schemas that shape the perception of people in the present. Although this tendency is true for all new relationships, the role of the therapist tends to be imbued with a particular set of expectations by virtue of the fact that he or she is in the role of the helper. The client is thus particularly likely to be in a dependent role vis-à-vis the therapist, and the therapist has a greater likelihood of functioning as a stand-in for a larger than life parental or authority figure than another person selected at random.

The therapeutic relationship therefore provides an opportunity for the client, in a sense, to bring the memory of the relationship with the parent or other significant figure from the past (aspects of which are often unconscious) to life through the relationship with the therapist. This provides the therapist with an opportunity to help clients gain insight into how their experiences with significant figures in the past have resulted in unresolved conflicts that influence their current relationships. Because transference involves a type of reliving of clients' early relationships in the present, the therapist's observations and feedback can help them to see, understand, and appreciate their own contribution to the situation. The resulting insight will have an experiential quality to it that will lead to change rather than a purely intellectual understanding that has no ultimate impact on the client.

Countertransference

The therapist's *countertransference* is his or her counterpart to the client's transference. Freud conceptualized the therapist's countertransference as his or her feelings and reactions to the client's transference that are a function of his or her own unresolved conflicts. From Freud's perspective, these reactions were an obstacle to therapy, and the therapist's task was to analyze or work thorough countertransference in personal supervision, in therapy, or through self-analysis.

These days *countertransference* tends to be defined more broadly as the totality of the therapist's reactions to the client (including feeling, associations, fantasies, and fleeting images). Beginning in the 1950s, analysts in different parts of the world began to talk about countertransference as a potentially valuable source of information for the therapist (e.g., Bollas, 1987; Heimann, 1950, 1960; Jacobs, 1991; Ogden, 1994; Racker, 1953, 1957). Although this view can be extremely useful therapeutically, it is not without its own potential dangers. There is a tendency in some psychoanalytic writing to assume that countertransference experience provides an infallible source of information about the client's unconscious experience and a tendency to underemphasize the therapist's own unique contribution to the countertransference.

Both sides of the coin must be considered before one's countertransference can provide any real clinical value. Take, for example, the following dramatic illustration. Imagine a situation in which a therapist has just found out that one of his children has developed a chronic illness. It is highly likely that this knowledge is going to have an important impact on the type of experience he will have with any client he sees. And yet the particular form and shading of the experience will also be influenced by the client with whom he is working. With one client he may be more aware of feeling helpless and sad. With another his feelings may tend toward rage at the cosmic injustice of the situation. The interaction of two subjective perspectives (client and therapist) results in a unique *transference–countertransference matrix* for each therapeutic dyad.

Resistance

Resistance is conceptualized as the tendency for an individual to resist change or act in a way that undermines the therapeutic process. It is often considered alongside the aforementioned concept of *defense* because resistance is the way in which defensive processes manifest in the therapy session and interfere with the therapist's goals or agenda. For example, the client's inability to think of anything to say while in the session may be understood as a form of resistance. The tendency to consistently come late for sessions or to forget about sessions can be thought of as a form of resistance. In both examples, a primary motivating factor may be the unconscious wish to avoid emotional pain (e.g., the pain associated with exploring threatening feelings or the fear of changing). This tendency to avoid pain or fear manifests in a behavior that thwarts or impedes the therapist's agenda and the process of treatment.

The concept of resistance, although valuable both theoretically and clinically, can also be problematic. It can be used by the clinician in a pejorative or blaming fashion by implying that the client is doing something wrong in not "cooperating" with the therapist in the therapeutic process. Over time, an important shift in analytic theory and technique took place in which resistance came to be seen not as an obstacle but as an intrinsic mode of the client's psychic functioning or as an aspect of his or her character that needs to be illuminated and understood rather than bypassed. Moreover, greater emphasis has been placed on the self-protective aspects of resistance. There has thus been an important shift toward conceptualizing the notion of resistance in empathic and affirmative terms (Safran & Muran, 2000).

Intersubjectivity

As the two-person psychology perspective grows in influence, some analytic thinkers find that conceptualizing the psychotherapy situation in terms of the client's perspective (including transference distortions) and the therapist's perspective (including countertransference reactions) is incomplete. Rather, the meeting of two minds is thought to produce a new, emergent product—the analytic dyad—and understanding in psychotherapy derives out of the dialogue between therapist and client through which meaning is constructed. This perspective is a radical departure from the classical psychoanalytic idea that the therapist works from a position of authority to uncover the "truth" of the client's reality.

Stephen Mitchell (1993) goes so far as to say that this process of intersubjective negotiation is actually at the heart of the therapeutic process because it allows the client to gradually learn that human relationships are flexible, and that it is possible to recognize the potential validity of the other person's perspective without feeling demolished or invalidated. Stuart Pizer (1998) describes the therapy session as an ongoing negotiation about the meaning and substance of reality. What is traditionally conceptualized as transference can be understood as the client's initial bid at defining reality. For example, the client who views the therapist as critical and withholding is defining reality in one possible way. The therapist can accept this claim and acknowledge these qualities in himself, or he can reject them and interpret them as the client's transference (e.g., "You see me as cold and withholding because I remind you of your father."). The client in turn can accept the therapist's bid at redefining reality or respond with a counterbid (e.g., "Maybe I have a tendency to view others as cold and withholding because of my past, but for all that I still believe that you are acting in a cold and withholding way, or that you have cold and withholding characteristics."). The therapist in turn can reject the client's counterbid or begin to shift his perspective (e.g., "Perhaps you're right. . . . I didn't see it before, but there is a way in which I'm acting more cold and withholding than I realized.").

In this fashion, what is traditionally conceptualized as transference–countertransference can instead be understood in terms of an ongoing implicit and explicit negotiation about what is taking place in the therapeutic relationship, who is doing what to whom, and what both the client and therapist are really experiencing. Jessica Benjamin (1990) argues that this process plays an important role in helping the client to develop the capacity for *intersubjectivity*—that is, the ability to hold onto one's own experience while at the same time beginning to experience the other as an independent center of subjectivity.

Enactment

Enactment has become a central concept in contemporary psychoanalytic thinking, once again reflecting a general shift toward a two-person psychology (Chused, 1991, 2003; Jacobs, 1991; Sandler, 1978). Because client and therapist are always influencing one another at both conscious and unconscious levels, they inevitably end up playing complementary roles in relational scenarios of which neither is fully aware. Both the client's and the therapist's working models or relational schemas will inevitably influence these scenarios. The process of collaborating in the exploration of how each of them is contributing to these scenarios provides clients with an opportunity to see how their own relational schemas contribute to the enactment, and it provides an opportunity for playing out new scenarios with other important human beings in their lives, thereby contributing to a modification of their current relational schemas.

The traditional psychoanalytic wisdom was that the therapist should avoid participating in these enactments and instead try to maintain a neutral position from which he or she could interpret the client's transference toward the therapist, thereby helping the client see how the present is being shaped in maladaptive ways by his or her own unconscious assumptions, projections, and previous developmental experiences. A common position in contemporary psychoanalytic thinking, however, is that the therapist cannot avoid participating in these enactments no matter how psychologically healthy or mature she is because (1) we are inevitably influenced by complex nonverbal communications from others that are difficult to decode, and (2) therapists, like other human beings, are never fully transparent to themselves (Chused, 2003).

Furthermore, even if it were possible to avoid participating in enactments with our clients, the ability to do so would deprive us of participating in our clients' relational worlds and developing a lived experience of what those worlds feels like. Participation in enactments thus allows us, in Philip Bromberg's words, to know our clients "from outside in" (Bromberg, 1998). Those things that our clients cannot express to us verbally are communicated through nonverbal behavior and action, and the only way we can come to know important dissociated aspects of the client's internal experience is to play a complementary role in their relational scenarios and experience the feeling of playing this role.

Process of Psychotherapy

Empathy

From a contemporary psychoanalytic perspective, the most fundamental intervention is empathy (Kohut, 1984; McWilliams, 2004; Safran, 2012). The ability to identify with our clients and immerse ourselves in their experience is critical in the process of establishing an alliance. In addition, this capacity to identify ourselves with our clients and communicate our empathic experience to them is a central mechanism of change in and of itself. The topic of empathy was traditionally neglected in psychoanalytic writing, where the emphasis was placed on the importance of making "accurate" interpretations. With Heinz Kohut and the development of self psychology, however, the topic of empathy was placed in the foreground. Kohut argued that it is not enough for an interpretation to be "accurate"—it also has to be experienced as empathic by the client.

Psychoanalytically oriented therapists also help clients make sense of their experience by making empathic conjectures. For example, "I think if I were in your shoes in the situation you're describing, I might be feeling patronized" or "I think I might be feeling genuinely happy for your sister's good fortune, but at the same time maybe a little envious." Well-timed questions can also serve a clarifying function. For example, "Do you have any sense of what it was about the situation that you found troubling?" or "Can you put your experience into words at all?"

Interpretation

Historically, one of the most important interventions at the psychoanalytic therapist's disposal has been what is called an *interpretation*. An interpretation has traditionally been conceptualized as the therapist's attempt to help clients become aware of aspects of their intrapsychic experience and relational patterns that are unconscious. Although empathic reflection is the therapist's attempt to articulate meaning that is implicit in what the client is saying, interpretation is the therapist's attempt to convey information that is outside of the client's awareness.

A distinction has often been made between the *accuracy* of an interpretation (in the sense of the extent to which an interpretation corresponds to a "real" aspect of the client's unconscious functioning) versus the *quality* or *usefulness* of an interpretation (in the sense that the client can make use of the interpretation as part of the change process). In theory, an interpretation can be accurate without being useful. The dimension of quality is spoken about in a variety of ways such as *timing* (Is the context right? Is the client ready to hear it?), *depth* (To what extent is the interpretation focused on deeply unconscious material versus material that is closer to awareness?), and *empathic quality* (To what extent is the interpretation sensitive to the impact it has on the client's self-esteem and how does it contribute to the client's experience of being deeply and genuinely understood?).

To the extent that a strong therapeutic alliance exists, an interpretation that is potentially threatening can be experienced in a more benign way because it is being delivered by somebody the client trusts. It is important to bear in mind that the immediate relational context colors the meaning of anything the therapist says (Mitchell, 1993). Interpretations with exactly the same words can be experienced as critical or caring, depending on whether or not the client feels respected and cared for by the therapist.

Clarification, Support, and Advice

Despite the traditional psychoanalytic emphasis on refraining from providing excessive reassurance or advice, many contemporary psychoanalytic therapists find that support, reassurance, and advice can play vitally important roles in the change process. Although ideally we wish to promote our clients' ability to trust in themselves, we also recognize that in many circumstances a genuine word of reassurance can be vitally important for a client who is struggling with a difficult situation or feeling anxious. Similarly, a word of well-timed advice to a client who is feeling genuinely overwhelmed or confused or who is in a state of crisis can be an extremely important intervention. A traditional psychoanalytic concern has been that when therapists give advice or share their opinions with clients, this places undue influence on them and risks compromising their autonomy. Critics such as Owen Renik (2006), however, argue that the practice of withholding one's opinions as a therapist is disingenuous, because our beliefs implicitly influence the message we convey to our clients without giving them a chance to fully reflect on our position and disagree with us if they wish. A willingness on the therapist's part to give advice, especially when asked for it, is consistent with reducing the power imbalance because we are "playing our cards straight up" with our clients rather than engaging in a process of mystification.

Termination

Termination is considered to be one of the most important phases of treatment. A well-handled termination can play a vital role in helping clients consolidate any gains that have been made. On the other hand, poorly handled terminations can negatively affect the treatment process. In a non–time-limited treatment, the topic of termination can be initiated by either client or therapist. Often clients who are contemplating termination will have difficultly bringing it up directly, and it is important for the therapist to be attuned to cues that the client may be considering ending treatment.

Ideally, the decision to terminate is made collaboratively by client and therapist and marks the end of a treatment that has been helpful and satisfying. In real life, termination in open-ended treatment is often somewhat messy and often the result of extraneous factors (e.g., the client moves to another city, the therapist moves to another city, or the therapist-in-training changes externship placements). In other situations, termination takes place when the client becomes frustrated with what he or she perceives as a lack of progress and decides to take a break or seek another therapist.

There is a stereotype about the psychoanalytic therapist's difficulty in accepting the client's reasons for wanting to leave treatment at face value or for probing incessantly for negative feelings that the client either doesn't have or is unable to disclose in the moment. In one respect, this is not surprising: An important thread to analytic work involves looking beneath the surface explanation to find deeper meaning or unconscious motivation. If the therapist explores the client's reasons for initiating termination in a sensitive and respectful manner, then in some circumstances it can lead to the exploration of feelings of resentment, mistrust, or disappointment on the client's part, which in turn can strengthen the therapeutic relationship and lead to the client's recommitment to therapy. Alternatively, the client may wish to leave treatment because he or she is feeling too intimate, vulnerable, or dependent on the therapist.

When, however, the therapist fails to accept the client's stated reasons for wanting to leave at face value and repeatedly attempts to badger her into admitting feelings or motivations she either doesn't experience or is unaware of, the client can feel undermined, coerced, or pathologized. The therapist thus needs to strike a balance between on one hand trying too hard to hold on to a client who wants to terminate and, on the other, failing to adequately explore the client's underlying motivations for terminating.

When the process of exploring the client's desire to leave treatment does lead to a final decision to terminate, it is useful to establish a contract to meet for a certain number of final sessions and thus provide an opportunity to terminate in a constructive fashion. This involves several different principles such as reviewing the changes that have taken place in treatment, constructing a shared understanding of the factors that have led to change, helping the client to recognize her own role in the change process, and creating a space that allows the client to express a range of positive and negative feelings about the termination and the treatment (Safran, 2012).

Mechanisms of Psychotherapy

Making the Unconscious Conscious

Psychoanalytic theory postulates a host of different change mechanisms, and a multitude of new ways of conceptualizing the change process continue to emerge as psychoanalytic theories themselves continue to evolve and proliferate. At the most basic level, there is an understanding that change often involves making the unconscious conscious or, in Freud's oft-cited axiom, "Where id has been there shall ego be" (Freud, 1932). Central to Freud's mature thinking was the idea that change involves becoming aware of our instinctual impulses and related unconscious wishes and then learning to deal with them in a rational or reflective fashion. For Freud, we typically delude ourselves as to reasons for doing things, and this self-deception limits our choice. By becoming aware of our unconscious wishes and our defenses against them, we increase the degree of choice available to us. We then decrease the degree to which we are driven by unconscious factors and assume a greater degree of agency.

Emotional Insight

There has been a tendency to privilege the role of conceptual understanding in psychoanalytic change. A central notion has been that psychoanalysis works by making the unconscious conscious and that the primary vehicle for doing this is through the use of verbal interpretations that give the client *insight* into the unconscious factors that are shaping his or her experience and actions. Although the psychoanalytic process of interpretation and insight has been criticized as intellectualized and detached, there has always been an emphasis on the importance of *emotional insight*—that is, combining the conceptual with the affective so that the client's new understanding has an emotionally immediate quality to it and is not relegated to the realm of intellectual understanding that has no impact on his or her daily functioning. It has long been held that one of the key ways of increasing the possibility that the insight will be emotional is through the use of *transference interpretations* (Strachey, 1934) that lead the client to reflect on his or her immediate experience of the therapeutic relationship rather than construct an abstract formulation. In other words, by directly observing the way in which he or she is construing things and acting in the here and now, the client is able to develop an experience of himself as an agent in the construction and creation of his own experience.

Creating Meaning and Historical Reconstruction

People often come to therapy with varying degrees of difficulty in the construction of meaningful narratives about their lives. These failures of meaning can include both the absence of narratives that make sense of important aspects of their experience or their lives in general, as well as the existence of maladaptive narratives they have constructed to make sense of their experience.

As sociologist Philip Reiff (1966) argued, in premodern cultures, traditional systems of healing (e.g., shamanic practices, religious beliefs) helped people in psychological pain by giving some sense of meaning to their suffering in culturally normative terms (e.g., spiritual possession) and by reintegrating the alienated individual back into the community. Contemporary psychoanalytic practice performs a similar function by providing culturally normative psychological or psychoanalytic explanations for symptoms and emotional pain. Because we live in a more individualistic culture, however, psychoanalytic practice adds an additional dimension of creating meaning through a process of co-constructing an idiosyncratic narrative that is tailored to the client's unique history and psychology.

The process of constructing a viable narrative account of the role that one's childhood experiences played in contributing to one's problems can also decrease the experience of self-blame that typically complicates and exacerbates emotional problems. By coming to understand one's emotional problems as arising from psychological coping strategies that were adaptive and made sense in the context of a dysfunctional childhood situation—but are maladaptive in the present context—the client can become more tolerant and accepting toward him- or herself and begin the process of developing coping strategies that are adaptive in the current context.

Often the problems that clients bring to therapy extend beyond a concern with specific symptoms to a more pervasive sense of meaninglessness and existential despair. When this is the case, the process of exploring and clarifying one's own values and engaging in a meaningful dialogue with the therapist can help clients reorient themselves and develop a more refined sense of what is meaningful to them. This process of meaning construction often involves becoming more aware of and articulating the nuances of one's emotional experience in the context of the relationship with the therapist so that the client can begin to get a sense of feeling more vitally alive and in touch with his or her inner experience.

Increasing and Appreciating the Limits of Agency

Clients often begin treatment with a diminished sense of personal agency. They experience themselves to be at the mercy of their symptoms or to be victims of misfortune or of other people's ill intent or neglect. They often fail to see the relationship between their symptoms and their own internal and interpersonal conflicts. They also commonly do not recognize their own roles and contributions to the conflictual patterns they repeat in their lives. As clients gain a greater appreciation of the connections between their symptoms, their ways of being, and their own contributions to conflictual patterns, they come to experience a greater degree of choice in their lives and experience themselves as agents rather than as victims. This growing awareness or understanding of one's personal agency must be experientially based rather than purely conceptual. Coming to experience a sense of agency is, however, only half the battle. The other half involves coming to appreciate and accept the limits of agency. In a culture such as ours that promotes the myth that we can "have it all" if only we drink the right beer or drive the right car, it is easy to feel that something is missing or that somehow we are being left behind. Although American psychoanalysts tend to have a more romantic sensibility than many European analysts, there is still recognition that the freedom we experience is freedom within the constraints of our character structures, environmental realities, and the uncontrollable contingencies of life (Safran, 1993, 1999, 2012).

Containment

One of the most important skills for therapists to develop is not technical in nature but personal and internal. This skill involves attending to our own emotions when working with clients and cultivating the ability to tolerate and process painful or disturbing feelings in a nondefensive fashion. How do we help our clients hold on to some sense of faith that things will work out when we are beginning to feel hopeless? How do we work with our own feelings when we begin to feel the same sense of despair that our client feels?

British psychoanalyst Wilfred Bion referred to this process as *containment*. According to Bion (e.g., 1970), as part of the normal developmental process children defend against feelings that are too threatening or toxic for them to experience by projecting them onto the parent. Bion argues that children (and clients) not only imagine that unacceptable feelings belong to the caregiver or therapist but that they also exert subtle pressures that evoke the dissociated feeling in the other. So, for example, the client who experiences nameless feelings of dread and terror dissociates these feelings and in subtle ways evokes these feelings in the therapist. The client who experiences rage that he or she finds unbearable, dissociates these feelings and evokes them in the therapist. Bion also theorizes that children need their parents to help them process raw emotional experience and learn to tolerate, symbolize, and make sense of this experience.

How do children or clients evoke powerful and sometimes dissociated feelings in parents or therapists? Although Bion did not elaborate on the precise mechanisms, contemporary emotion theory and research suggest that (1) it is not uncommon for people to experience the nonverbal aspects of emotion in the absence of conscious awareness and (2) people are remarkably good at reading and responding to other people's emotion displays without conscious awareness (e.g., Ekman & Davidson, 1994; Greenberg & Safran, 1987; Safran & Muran, 2000). The process of containment is conceptual and affective in nature. Helping the child or client to put feelings into words is certainly one component of it. The more challenging component involves processing and managing powerful feelings that are evoked in us as parents or as therapists so that our own affective responses can help to regulate the others emotions rather than further deregulate them (Safran, 2012).

Rupture and Repair

Tronick (2007) and colleagues have demonstrated that in normal mother–infant face-to-face interactions, affective coordination between the two occurs less than 30% of the time. Transitions from coordinated to miscoordinated states and back occur about once every 3 to 5 seconds. Tronick and colleagues hypothesize that this ongoing process of interactive disruption and repair plays an important role in the normal developmental process by helping the infant develop a form of implicit relational knowing that represents both the self and other as capable of repairing disruptions in relatedness. This paradigm provides a useful model for understanding an important nonverbal mechanism through which the process of working through the inevitable misunderstandings and disruptions in relatedness that take place between client and therapist contribute to a change in the client's implicit relational knowing.

The principle of relationship *rupture and repair* has come to assume a central role in the thinking of many psychoanalytic theorists as an important element of the change process (e.g., Kohut, 1984; Safran, Crocker, McMain, & Murray, 1990; Safran & Muran, 1996, 2000, 2006). It has a long history in psychoanalytic thinking, dating back to Sandor Ferenczi (1931), who came to believe that it is inevitable that the therapist will ultimately fail the client by not being adequately attuned to his or her needs; when this happens, a retraumatization will occur for the client. The process of working through this retraumatization in a constructive fashion allows the client to begin to bring split-off parts of the self into the therapeutic relationship. From this perspective, the therapist's inevitable failures provide opportunities for *working through* in a way that helps the client to begin to bring him- or herself into the relationship in a way that is experienced as real.

APPLICATIONS

Who Can We Help?

No treatment is effective for all individuals, and psychoanalytically oriented treatments are no exception to this rule. This is especially true when it comes to the use of certain specific psychoanalytic interventions. For example, because of intellectual, psychological, or emotional factors, some clients have a limited capacity for self-reflection, and interventions designed to promote reflective capacity such as interpretation are simply not helpful. Some clients find any attempt to explore the transference or the therapeutic relationship too threatening. Clients who are too psychologically disorganized or disturbed may find any attempt to explore defenses or unconscious wishes equally threatening. Clients who are in a state of crisis may find any insight-oriented treatments meaningless because they have an immediate need for guidance, structure, and support. Interventions that involve the use of therapist self-disclosure of their own countertransference may be experienced as threatening or intrusive by some clients. The psychoanalytic emphasis on underlying psychodynamic issues and character changes rather than immediate symptom relief may be of little use for a client who is currently in intense emotional distress and does not have the luxury of or interest in focusing on underlying issues.

Similarly, when it comes to parameters related to treatment length or session frequency, many clients may not have the interest, time, or financial resources to be in long-term treatment. And many clients may not have the interest, time, or psychological resources to be in treatment more than once a week—or even once a week. For all of these reasons, "psychoanalysis" when defined in a rigid or purist fashion is most appropriate for clients who are neurotic (as opposed to borderline or psychotic), who have a relatively high level of ego strength and cohesiveness, and the capacity for self-reflection.

If, however, psychoanalysis is conceptualized in a more flexible fashion as a broadly based theoretical framework, then it can be useful for a wide range of clients (Safran, 2012). This requires an understanding of the diversity of change mechanisms that can be involved in the treatment process and an openness to the incorporation of different treatment interventions (e.g., empathy, interpretation, guidance, advice giving, and collaborative problem solving). Although there will always be theoretical purists who cling to a more rigid definition of psychoanalysis, there is a growing trend in the direction of a more pluralistic and flexible perspective in North America and many other parts of the world. In turn, a growing number of individuals suffering from problems mild and severe, acute and chronic, are able to benefit in therapy from the psychoanalytic orientation without being burdened by the dogmatic elements that were once prominent in North American psychoanalysis.

Treatment

As psychoanalysis is not a specific treatment modality but a philosophical framework, its theories and techniques can be applied in a range of settings and integrated with the theories and techniques of other approaches. Although the prominence of psychoanalysis within the health-care professions has declined, it is important to recognize that many of our shared cultural assumptions have, in fact, been shaped by the psychoanalytic tradition (e.g., the role of the unconscious, the idea that people can act defensively, the idea that people's psychiatric symptoms can be understood in psychological terms, and so on). There is thus an important sense in which we live within a psychoanalytic culture. The concepts inherent in psychoanalytic therapies are therefore appropriate for and practiced regularly in hospitals, clinics, and private practices within individual, group, and family contexts.

Evidence

Despite a common misconception that little or no empirical research supports the efficacy of psychoanalytic therapy, numerous studies actually document the value of the psychoanalytic approach. The most rigorous evidence comes from *randomized clinical trials* (RCTs) examining the efficacy of *short-term dynamic psychotherapy* (STDP) relative to various types of control groups. Recent meta-analyses have found substantial effect sizes for short-term dynamic psychotherapies that are as large as or larger than those commonly found for short-term cognitive therapies (see Shedler, 2010, for an excellent review).

For example, a meta-analysis by Abbass and colleagues included 23 randomized clinical trials that collectively analyzed data for 1,431 clients (Abbass, Hancock, Henderson, & Kisely, 2006). All treatments included in the studies lasted less than 40 sessions and compared different types of STDP treatment to control groups (wait-list, minimal treatment, or "treatment as usual"). The meta-analysis yielded an overall effect size of 0.97 for general symptom improvement. Particularly striking was that the effect sizes actually increased substantially at long-term follow-up. The effect size increased to 1.51 when clients were assessed at a 9-month or longer interval after treatment concluded.

A meta-analysis of RCTs conducted by Leichsenring and Rabung (2008) provides one of the more compelling current sources of evidence that longer-term psychoanalytic therapy is a particularly effective treatment for complex mental disorders such as personality disorders, chronic mental disorders (defined as lasting at least a year), multiple mental disorders or complex depression, and anxiety disorders. The authors reviewed 23 studies conducted between 1960 and 2008 involving a total of 1,053 clients. The studies compared long-term psychoanalytically oriented treatments to a range of different short-term treatments, including cognitive behavior therapy, dialectical behavior therapy, family therapy, and STPD therapy. The results showed that long-term psychoanalytic therapy was more effective than these shorter-term treatments with regard to overall outcome, target problems, and personality functioning. Long-term psychoanalytic therapy produced large and stable effect sizes, and these effect sizes increased significantly between the end of therapy and follow-up.

Many practical and logistical problems make it difficult to conduct RCTs of long-term psychoanalytic treatment as it is typically practiced in the real world. Because of these constraints, most studies evaluating the effectiveness of long-term psychoanalysis tend to be of a more naturalistic nature. For instance, Leichsenring and colleagues have reported the results of a naturalistic study of the effectiveness of psychoanalytic therapy for 36 clients seeking treatment for chronic psychiatric problems (e.g., depression, anxiety, obsessive–compulsive disorder, and nonorganic sexual dysfunction), with the majority of clients presenting with co-morbid diagnoses (Leichsenring, Biskup, Kreisch, &

Staats, 2005). Although there was no control group, the effect size of a control group from another study was used as a point of reference. The average duration of treatment was 37.4 months, and an average of 253 sessions were conducted. In general, effect sizes were large for changes in symptoms, interpersonal problems, quality of life, well-being, and the target problem formulated by the clients at the beginning of treatment. These changes were stable at follow-up one year later, and in some areas they actually increased.

An extremely ambitious naturalistic outcome study conducted in Sweden by Sandell and colleagues (2000, 2001, 2002) evaluated the outcome of over 400 clients who received either psychoanalysis or psychoanalytic therapy. The mean duration of treatment in psychoanalysis was 51 months, and the mean frequency was 3.5 sessions per week. The mean length of treatment in psychoanalytic therapy was 40 months, and the mean frequency of sessions was 1.4 times per week. In general, both treatments were found to be effective, but three conclusions were clear: (1) At the 3-year follow-up, clients in psychoanalysis achieved better outcomes on a number of dimensions than clients in psychotherapy, (2) more experienced psychoanalysts achieved better outcome than therapists with less psychoanalytic training and experience, and (3) the variables of frequency and duration interacted to moderate outcome in a positive direction.

In summary, a growing body of empirical evidence supports the efficacy of psychoanalytic therapies for a range of disorders. Note that the extant research suggests that the impact of psychoanalytic therapy continues to increase after termination—a finding that is not emerging to the same extent in the case of cognitive-behavioral interventions. At this time, the evidence for the effectiveness of intensive, long-term psychoanalysis is garnered from naturalistic studies rather than RCTs, and logistical realities make it highly unlikely that there are going to be many RCTs evaluating the efficacy of long-term intensive psychoanalysis in the near future. However, absence of evidence is not the same thing as evidence of absence.

Moreover, the results of the many naturalistic studies supporting the effectiveness of long-term psychoanalysis should not be dismissed out of hand. As psychology students learn in introductory research methods classes, empirical research inevitably purchases internal validity (the ability to infer causation and rule out alternative hypotheses) at the expense of external validity (generalizability to real-life situations). If the results of psychotherapy are to be of any real value, then we must adopt a pluralistic perspective on research that weighs the evidence yielded by a range of different methodologies in light of an understanding of the strengths and weaknesses of any given methodology (Seligman, 1995).

Psychotherapy in a Multicultural World

Psychoanalysis was originally developed as a form of treatment by and for educated, middle-class Western Europeans suffering from "neurotic" problems in living. As psychoanalysis became the dominant theoretical influence within the public health-care system, a paradoxical process took place. On one hand, therapists influenced by psychoanalytic thinking were placed in the position of treating a broad range of clients from different cultures and social classes. On the other hand, psychoanalytic therapists were simultaneously being guided by theoretical premises and treatment interventions that were ill equipped to fit the diversity of clients being treated.

As a society, we are officially committed to the ideal of tolerance of diversity, and psychoanalytic theorists and researchers share this focus on the importance of learning about racial and cultural differences and of adapting treatments in a culturally responsive fashion. The psychoanalytic perspective's unique contribution to this area, however, is its emphasis on the role that unconscious biases and prejudices about race, culture, and class play in shaping our daily interactions. We inevitably internalize societal prejudices, and these unconscious internalized attitudes influence the way in which we relate to others and ourselves. When we treat someone coming from a different cultural background or race in therapy, internalized cultural attitudes play out unconsciously in the transference–countertransference matrix for both client and therapist.

Clinical psychology students trained with a bias toward therapies that use self-reflection and are insight oriented can often feel powerless when working in the public sector, where many clients do not come from a culture that privileges self-reflection and where the daily aspects of their existence (e.g. poverty, social instability, physical illness, lack of control over their living environment) are so overwhelming that such an approach can seem irrelevant. This can lead to a defensive stance on the part of the therapist that contributes to devaluing clients. Therapists may tend to disown experiences and qualities in themselves such as aggression, sexuality, criminality, or exploitativeness and feel particularly critical of such qualities in working-class clients. Or they may underestimate the influence of class and social conditions on an individual's life and feel critical of clients coming from an unstable and economically disadvantaged background who are not able to "pull themselves up by their bootstraps" and choose better life options for themselves (Altman, 1995; Gutwill & Hollander, 2006). This kind of attitude can mirror larger societal attitudes that equate poverty with moral depravity, thereby condoning a social system that privileges the wealthy and the middle class.

As discussed throughout this chapter, a contemporary psychoanalytic perspective does not privilege insight as the sole or even primary mechanism of change, but it instead emphasizes the role of a host of different change mechanisms, including empathy, new relational experience, and containment. From this perspective, it is the relational meaning of the intervention that is critical. Students of psychoanalytic therapy therefore must remember that treatment can consist of a range of different interventions such as exploring internal experience, providing guidance or advice, negotiating a common goal or task with a client, or simply attempting one's best to be there for the client in a reliable fashion. At the same time, they must reflect internally on the possible relational meaning of a given interaction, becoming aware of and modulating their own affective experiences, and learning about the way unconscious prejudices influence one's work.

CASE EXAMPLE

The case of Ruth (previously described in Safran, 2002) provides a good example of a patient treated with a contemporary, shorter-term psychoanalytic approach. Ruth contracted to receive 30 sessions of treatment from me (JDS) as part of an ongoing brief psychotherapy program. She was an attractive, young-looking 52-year-old woman who had been divorced for 16 years. Since her divorce, she had had a series of short-term affairs with men, which typically would end because of her dissatisfaction with her partners. As she grew older, she became increasingly concerned about the possibility of spending the rest of her life alone. She hoped psychotherapy would help her understand her pattern of pursuing relationships that ultimately left her feeling dissatisfied and unfulfilled.

Although I initially felt very sympathetic toward Ruth, a pattern developed fairly rapidly in which I had difficulty maintaining a sense of emotional engagement with her and found myself biding time until the sessions ended. I became aware of a tendency on Ruth's part to tell long stories with obsessional detail and to do so in an unemotional, droning fashion that left me feeling distant and unengaged. In an attempt to understand what was being enacted between us, I tried to tactfully communicate my sense of emotional disengagement, hoping to clarify potential links between my experience, Ruth's characteristic style of presentation, and the intrapsychic processes underlying it. Ruth seemed responsive to my feedback and a dialogue ensued that, over time, shed some light on the nature of the enactment. Ruth was able to articulate an underlying fear of abandonment that led her to defend against vulnerable feelings by controlling her style of presentation. She was also able to articulate a semiconscious perception of my disengagement and a tendency to intensify her deadening monologue as a way of dealing with feelings evoked by this perception.

Following these explorations, Ruth began, for the first time, to complain more directly about what she felt she was not getting from me in treatment. Whereas the first phase of treatment had been marked by an emotional flatness, by session 20 Ruth's frustration, anger, and disappointment felt more tangible. She began the session by indicating that she was aware that the treatment was more than halfway through, and she asked for my evaluation of how things were going so far and for a plan for the rest of the treatment. With my encouragement, Ruth was eventually able to tell me that she needed more emotional engagement from me, and that she did not want to try to be a more interesting person in order to keep my interest. Her ability to express these needs helped me to empathize more fully with her experience of not feeling accepted and validated. In this and subsequent sessions, Ruth was also able to contact sad and painful feelings of being hurt by my failure to accept and prize her.

The experience of directly challenging me and seeing that our relationship was able to survive enabled Ruth to bring her underlying feelings of despair, vulnerability, and dependency into the therapy. She began session 21 by saying that, although she had left the previous session "all fired up" and ready to make changes in her life, she found herself sinking back into an apathetic inertia. She then made a passing allusion to feeling that she needed someone to help her out of her inertia. When I asked her if she felt as though she needed help from me right now, Ruth began to cry slightly and to speak about her feelings of disappointment and loss in life in general. Her downward glance was particularly salient for me, and I mentioned it to Ruth and asked her if she was aware of it. Ruth acknowledged that she was aware of looking away and that she felt that she wanted to push her feelings back inside, because she felt she was being self-pitying. Further exploration led her to articulate a fear of "blubbering and not even being able to talk," her anticipation of consequent embarrassment, and a desire to be by herself. At this point, I conveyed to her my own sense of being "kept outside," and my remark led to an exploration of the way in which Ruth was pulling away from me in her pain and sadness. This helped Ruth articulate a fear of being abandoned by me, accompanied by deep and heartfelt sobbing. There followed a tearful exploration of how Ruth had spent so much of her life depriving herself of real contact and support from people because of her difficulty in acknowledging to herself how deeply she wanted to be nurtured and cared for. She then expressed her relief at being able to share her painful feelings and longings with me, mixed with sadness and feelings of loss in the acknowledgment of having spent so many years without receiving the contact and support she needed.

In subsequent sessions, we explored Ruth's fears and sadness about imminent abandonment by me, as well as her anger. She began session 23 by talking about her fears of abandonment in general.

Ruth: I have this fear of being abandoned and disappointed. And so I guess I just shut down and cut people out of my life.

Jeremy: In the back of my mind I'm thinking that we only have six or seven more sessions, and so I'm wondering about this whole issue of opening up and being abandoned in this context.

Ruth: Well, it does make me sort of scared when I start thinking about the ending. And I guess that's true of me in general. I guess I'm reluctant to really involve myself deeply in relationships . . . but the desire is still there.

Jeremy: Uh-huh . . . I have a sense of a real yearning inside of you. [Patient begins to cry and then stops herself.] What's happening for you?

Ruth: Well, it starts to hurt, and then I think, intellectually, "It's so inappropriate for me to be upset about therapy ending."

Jeremy: It doesn't seem inappropriate to me. We've worked together for a while now and really started to develop a relationship, and my sense is that you're beginning to open up and trust. And we're ending soon . . . and that's got to be painful.

Ruth: Well, and I guess part of it is the finiteness of it. I leave with whatever feelings I have, and for you, it's like, "Good. That was a tough one. That's over." And then you go on with something else.

We began to discuss the inequity of the situation and Ruth's anger at me. She also spontaneously drew a parallel between the asymmetry of our investment in the relationship and a general tendency for the men she felt deeply about to not reciprocate the depth of her feelings. In the following session, the theme of inequity emerged once again. Ruth returned to the concern that I would be glad when things were over because (she believed) I found her frustrating and difficult to work with. Although it was true that I had felt frustrated, bored, and disengaged from Ruth, especially in the earlier part of the treatment, I was now experiencing our sessions as vitally alive and engaging, and I had a growing feeling of empathy for her dilemma and a sense of real caring for her. I struggled with the question of whether or not to say anything to Ruth about the change in my feelings toward her. I tentatively resolved not to say anything, trusting that Ruth would be able to experience the change at an affective level and fearing that verbal reassurances would be experienced as hollow.

Further exploration helped Ruth to flesh out her concerns about my feelings toward her and to articulate her desire that I really care about her. Putting this yearning into words led not only to more sadness but also to a feeling of satisfaction about her ability to take the risk of revealing her desires. The session ended with Ruth returning to her feelings of hurt and anger about the fact that I had not volunteered to meet beyond the preestablished termination session. I empathized with Ruth's feelings and told her that I believed it was legitimate for her to feel both hurt and angry with me.

In session 28, Ruth spoke about her difficulty trusting that men care about her unless they go overboard in their attempts to woo her. She also indicated that her experience had been that ironically the kind of man who was likely to go overboard in an effort to woo her, inevitably turned out to be (in her words) a "player" or charmer who ultimately turned out to be particularly untrustworthy. Given this long-standing pattern, therefore, Ruth said it felt good that she was starting to feel okay about our relationship, despite my not having actively reassured her. In other words, Ruth felt good about beginning to trust her instincts about our relationship rather than my words.

The final two sessions were devoted to summing up and consolidation. Ruth's feeling was that the seed of a new way of being in relationships was beginning to grow in her. She was able to acknowledge her sadness about separating from me and her anxiety about the future—in addition, she spoke of a growing optimism and belief that things could be different in her life. Various strands in the therapeutic work were never completely tied together, and certain issues were touched on but not explored in depth. Though this was partly the result of the short-term nature of the treatment, my experience has been that a lack of total closure exists in any therapy. Termination in a time-limited context, however, tends to intensify a process that we therapists must inevitably undergo of grappling with the ultimate frustration of the type of grandiose ambitions that are common for less experienced therapists, and of coming to terms with the intrinsic ambiguities of life and the limits of our understanding and control.

SUMMARY

Psychoanalysis originated more than 100 years ago, and it has evolved dramatically over time. It has become more flexible, less authoritarian, more practical, and more responsive to the needs of a wider range of clients from diverse racial, cultural, and social class backgrounds. There is a growing cohort of dedicated and rigorous psychoanalytic researchers, and there is a growing body of empirical evidence that supports the effectiveness of psychoanalytic treatments.

For many years psychoanalysis had a dominant role in our health-care system. By the mid to late 1960s, however, psychoanalysis was under siege: on one side by the behavioral tradition, and on the other by the "third force"—the tradition of humanistic psychology. Although the behavioral tradition critiqued psychoanalysis for its lack of scientific legitimacy, the humanistic tradition faulted psychoanalysis for its mechanistic and reductionist tendencies and its failure to appreciate the more noble aspects of human nature and the fundamental dignity of human experience.

To the behavioral criticism that psychoanalysis lacks scientific rigor, the current resurgence of interest in empirical research among psychoanalysts is all for the good. Nevertheless, it would be a mistake to disregard or devalue those dimensions of psychoanalysis that fall outside of the natural sciences—those aspects of psychoanalysis that are more accurately conceptualized as a hermeneutic discipline, a philosophy of life, a critical theory, or a craft.

The humanistic critique of psychoanalysis for its failure to appreciate and affirm the fundamental nobility and dignity of human nature is also valuable. Many people have had traumatic experiences with psychoanalytic therapy, particularly during the heyday of dogmatic American ego psychology, and they have left treatment feeling fragmented, objectified, and pathologized rather than appreciated, understood, and whole. Contemporary psychoanalysis has in many respects assimilated some of the more positive, creative, and affirmative qualities of the humanistic psychology of the 1960s. This has largely been a positive development that benefits clients, therapists, and students alike.

However, it will be important for the future of psychoanalysis not to discard what many have described as Freud's tragic sensibility: his belief that there is an inherent conflict between instinct and civilization; his emphasis on the importance of acknowledging and accepting the hardships, cruelties, and indignities of life without the consolation of illusory beliefs. Freud saw the goal of psychoanalysis as one of "transforming neurotic misery into ordinary human unhappiness." Although this view runs counter to the typical American sensibility of optimism, opportunity, and the pursuit of happiness, it directs our attention toward the ways in which some of our cultural values can lead to an insidious type of oppression that marginalizes and silences those who are suffering and judges them as failures or as morally inferior.

There is a well-known anecdote that when Freud was crossing the Atlantic with Jung and Ferenczi to deliver his 1909 lecture series at Clark University, (an event which was subsequently to become a turning point in North America's receptiveness to psychoanalysis), Jung spoke excitedly and enthusiastically about the growing interest in psychoanalysis by Americans. Freud was much more measured in his reaction and is reputed to have replied, "Little do they realize we are bringing the plague" (Fairfield, Layton & Stack, 2002, p. 1). Looking toward the future, it is important for us not to discard those aspects of psychoanalysis that do not easily assimilate to mainstream American culture. Although American psychoanalysis was remarkably influential in its heyday, this success came at a cost: It became an elitist, insular, and culturally conservative force. The contemporary marginalization of psychoanalysis provides us with the opportunity to recover and build on some of the revolutionary and culturally progressive qualities that were present at the beginning.

 Counseling CourseMate Website:
See this text's Counseling CourseMate website at www.cengagebrain.com for learning tools such as chapter quizzing, videos, glossary flashcards, and more.

ANNOTATED BIBLIOGRAPHY

Mitchell, S. A., & Black, M. J. (1995). *Freud and beyond: A history of modern psychoanalytic thought.* New York: Basic Books.
This is a wonderful introduction and survey of the theories of many of the key historical and contemporary thinkers whose ideas shaped the development of psychoanalytic theory and practice. The authors find the perfect balance between depth and accessibility and are able to convey complex theoretical ideas with great clarity. Although this is not a hands-on book about clinical practice, anyone interested in developing a grasp of the remarkable panorama of the psychoanalytic landscape will find it a rewarding read and a valuable reference book.

McWilliams, N. (2004). *Psychoanalytic psychotherapy: A practitioner's guide.* New York: Guilford Press.
This is an excellent primer on psychoanalytically oriented treatment written for beginning clinicians. McWilliams covers key theoretical and technical principles in a jargon-free fashion. She also provides clear guidelines for dealing with the nuts and bolts of clinical practice and for handling common clinical challenges and dilemmas. In addition, McWilliams offers valuable advice regarding important topics such as therapist self-care, professional development, and personal therapy for the clinician.

Safran, J. D. (2012). *Psychoanalysis and psychoanalytic therapies.* Washington, DC: American Psychological Association.
Psychoanalysis and Psychoanalytic Therapies examines the origins of psychoanalysis in the work of Freud and his colleagues at the turn of the century, and it charts the major turning points in the development of psychoanalytic theory and practice over time. It also introduces the reader to cutting-edge developments in theory, practice, and research. Key theoretical concepts are examined, and principles of intervention are clearly spelled out. Central theoretical controversies in the field are discussed, and the treatment process is illustrated with detailed case examples. A valuable feature of the book is that it is linked with a DVD illustration of six sessions of psychoanalytic treatment (available from the American Psychological Association). Another unique feature of the book is the way in which it contextualizes the origins and evolution of psychoanalytic theory and practice in cultural, historical, and political terms.

Safran, J. D. (2008). *Psychoanalytic therapy over time.* www.apa.org/pubs/videos/4310864.aspx

Part of the *Psychotherapy in Six Sessions Video Series*

Format: DVD (closed caption)
In *Psychoanalytic Therapy Over Time*, Jeremy D. Safran demonstrates the relational psychoanalytic approach. Over the course of the six sessions on this DVD, Dr. Safran works with a young woman with a history of serious depression, substance abuse, and a pattern of romantic involvement with abusive men. Through a process of exploring tensions and relational patterns emerging in the therapeutic relationship, Safran helps the client begin to recognize her own needs and strengths and to feel more optimistic about the future. Over the course of therapy, the client progresses from a stance of wary and resentful compliance to one of growing trust and healthy self-assertion. The case is also described in Safran (2012).

CASE READINGS

The case of "Sophie." In S. A. Mitchell (1993), *Hope and dread in psychoanalysis.* New York: Basic Books.
Stephen Mitchell describes the case of "Sophie," an architectural graduate student in her early 30s who began treatment with a characterological depression and a history of problematic relationships with men. Mitchell's discussion of Sophie's case is used to illustrate important principles from a relational psychoanalytic perspective. One key principle is that the psychoanalytic process involves an ongoing negotiation between the subjectivities

of the patient and the analyst, in which the analyst finds his own particular way of way of confirming and participating in the patient's experience yet, over time, establishes his own presence and perspective in a way that the patient can find enriching rather than demolishing.

The case of "Alec." In P. M. Bromberg (2000). Potholes on the royal road: Or is it an abyss. *Contemporary Psychoanalysis, 36,* 5–28.

In the case of "Alec," Philip Bromberg cogently illustrates the process of working through a transference–countertransference enactment that allows both therapist and patient to make authentic contact with one another. The case is an excellent example of how the therapeutic dyad can openly explore and work with each member's respective experiences, including undisclosed anger toward one another and mutual feelings of masked shame.

The case of "Simone." In J. D. Safran (2012). *Psychoanalysis and psychoanalytic therapies.* Washington, DC: American Psychological Association. [Reprinted in D. Wedding & R. J. Corsini (2013), *Case studies in psychotherapy* (7th ed.). Belmont, CA: Brooks/Cole.]

"Simone" was a 26-year-old African American woman who began psychoanalytically oriented treatment complaining of a "general feeling of emptiness" as well as a moderate problem with bulimia. She had been involved in a few very short-lived romantic relationships, which she had always ended abruptly when she started to feel that her partners were "too needy." Over the course of treatment, Simone and her therapist, Jeremy Safran, spent considerable time exploring the factors contributing to her feelings of emptiness as well as her binging behavior. She fluctuated dramatically (both within sessions and at various stages of the treatment) in her ability to look at her own feelings and actions in a self-reflective fashion. Over time, part of the work involved exploring the way in which Simone's skittishness about commitment to the treatment were related to her fears of abandonment, and she gradually became more trusting of her therapist and more committed to the therapeutic relationship.

The case of Simone provides a good example of the way in which the exploration of transference–countertransference enactments can help a client become more aware of the link between her dynamic conflicts and problematic relational patterns, and also the way in which the therapeutic relationship can play a vital role in providing a new relational experience that challenges the client's internalized representation of self–other relationships.

REFERENCES

Abbass, A. A., Hancock, J. T., Henderson, J., & Kisely, S. (2006). Short-term psychodynamic psychotherapies for common mental disorders. *The Cochrane Database of Systematic Reviews, 4,* CD004687.

Altman, N. (1995). *The analyst in the inner city: Race, class, and culture through a psychoanalytic lens.* Hillsdale, NJ: The Analytic Press.

Balint, M. (1968). *Basic fault: Therapeutic aspects of regression.* Evanston, IL: Northwestern University Press.

Benjamin, J. (1990). An outline of intersubjectivity: The development of recognition. *Psychoanalytic Psychology, 7,* 33–46.

Bion, W. R. (1970). *Attention and interpretation.* London: Routledge.

Bollas, C. (1987). *The shadow of the object: Psychoanalysis of the unthought known.* New York: Columbia University Press.

Bordin, E. (1979). The generalizability of the psychoanalytic concept of the working alliance. *Psychotherapy: Theory, Research and Practice, 16,* 252–260.

Bowlby, J. (1969). *Attachment and loss: Vol. 1. Attachment.* New York: Basic Books.

Bowlby, J. (1973). *Attachment and loss: Vol. 2. Separation, anxiety, and anger.* New York: Basic Books.

Bowlby, J. (1980). *Attachment and loss: Vol. 3. Sadness and depression.* New York: Basic Books.

Brenner, C. (2002). Conflict, compromise formation, and structural theory. *The Psychoanalytic Quarterly, 71,* 397–414.

Breuer, J., & Freud, S. (1893–1895/1995). *The standard edition of the complete psychological works of Sigmund Freud.* (Vol. 2). London: Hogarth Press.

Bromberg, P. M. (1998). *Standing in the spaces: Essays on clinical process, trauma, and dissociation.* Hillsdale, NJ: Analytic Press.

Bromberg, P. M. (2000). Potholes on the royal road: Or is it an abyss. *Contemporary Psychoanalysis, 36,* 5–28.

Bromberg, P. M. (2006). *Awakening the dreamer: Clinical journeys.* Mahwah, NJ: Analytic Press.

Chused, J. F. (1991) The evocative power of enactments. *Journal of the American Psychoanalytic Association, 39,* 615–639.

Chused, J. F. (2003). The role of enactment. *Psychoanalytic Dialogues, 13,* 677–687.

Cushman, P. (1995). *Constructing the self, constructing America.* Reading, MA: Addison-Wesley.

Danto, E. (2005). *Freud's free clinics.* New York. Columbia University Press.

Davies, J. M. (1996). Linking the "pre-analytic" with the post-classical: Integration, dissociation, and the multiplicity of unconscious process. *Contemporary Psychoanalysis, 32,* 553–576.

Davies, J. M. (1998). Multiple Perspectives on Multiplicity. *Psychoanalytic Dialogues, 8,* 195–206.

Ekman, P., & Davidson, R. J. E. (Eds.). (1994). *The nature of emotions: Fundamental questions.* New York: Oxford University Press.

Fairbairn, W. R. D. (1952). *Psychoanalytic studies of the personality.* London: Tavistock/Routledge & Kegan Paul.

Fairbairn, W. R. D. (1994). *Psychoanalytic studies of the personality.* New York: Routledge/Taylor & Francis.

Fairfield, S., Layton, L., & Stack, C. (Eds.). (2002). *Bringing the plague: Toward a postmodern psychoanalysis.* New York: Other Press.

Ferenczi, S. (1931/1980). Child analysis in the analysis of adults. (E. Mosbacher, Trans.). In M. Balint (Ed.), *Final Contributions to the problems and methods of psychoanalysis.* (pp. 126–142). London: Karnac Books.

Freud, A. (1937). *The ego and the mechanisms of defense.* Honolulu: Hogarth Press.

Freud, S. (1912/1958). *The dynamics of transference.* (Standard Edition ed. Vol. 12). London: Hogarth Press.

Freud, S. (1917/1963). *Mourning and melancholia.* (Standard Edition ed. Vol. 14). London: Hogarth Press.

Freud, S. (1923/1961). *The ego and the id.* (Standard Edition ed. Vol. 19). London: Hogarth Press.

Freud, S. (1932). *Introductory lectures on psychoanalysis.* (Standard Edition ed. Vols. 15–16). London: Hogarth Press.

Greenberg, J., & Mitchell, S. A. (1983). *Object relations in psychoanalytic theory.* Cambridge, MA: Harvard University Press.

Greenberg, L.S., & Safran, J.D. (1987). *Emotions in psychotherapy: Affect, cognition, and process of change.* New York: Guilford Press.

Greenson, R. (1965). The working alliance and the transference neurosis. *Psychoanalysis Quarterly, 343,* 155–181.

Greenson, R. (1971). The real relationship between patient and the psychoanalyst. In M. Kanzer (Ed.), *The unconscious today* (pp. 213–232). New York: International Universities Press.

Gutwill, S., & Hollander, N. C. (2006). Class and splitting in the clinical setting: The ideological dance in the transference and countertransference. In L. Layton, N. C. Hollander, & S. Gutwill (Eds.), *Psychoanalysis, class, and politics: Encounters in the clinical setting.* New York: Routledge, Taylor & Francis Group.

Heimann, P. (1950). On countertransference. *International Journal of Psychoanalysis, 31,* 81–84.

Heimann, P. (1960). On counter-transference. *British Journal of Medical Psychology, 33,* 9–15.

Hoffman, I. (2009). Doublethinking our way to "scientific" legitimacy: The desiccation of human experience. *Journal of the American Psychoanalytic Association, 57*(5), 1043–1070.

Jacobs, T. (1991). *The use of the self: Countertransference and communication in the analytic setting.* Madison, CT: International Universities Press.

Jacoby, R. (1983). *The repression of psychoanalysis: Otto Fenichel and the political Freudians.* Hillsdale, NJ: The Analytic Press.

Klein, M. (1975). *"Envy and gratitude" and other works, 1946–1973.* New York: Delacorte.

Kohut, H. (1984). *How does analysis cure?* Chicago: University of Chicago Press.

Lacan, J. (1988a). *The seminar of Jacques Lacan: Book 1. Freud's papers on technique, 1953–1954* (J. Miller, Ed., & J. Forrester, Trans.). New York: Norton. (Original work published 1975)

Lacan, J. (1988b). *The seminar of Jacques Lacan: Book 2. The ego in Freud's theory and in the technique of psychoanalysis, 1953–1954* (J. Miller, Ed., & S. Tomaselli, Trans.). New York: Norton. (Original work published 1978)

Leichsenring, F., Biskup, J., Kreisch, R., & Staats, H. (2005). The Göttingen study of psychoanalytic therapy: First results. *The International Journal of Psychoanalysis, 86,* 433–455.

Leichsenring, F., & Rabung, S. (2008). Effectiveness of long-term psychodynamic psychotherapy: A meta-analysis. *Journal of the American Medical Association, 300,* 1551–1565.

Main, M. (1991). Metacognitive knowledge, metacognitive monitoring, and singular (coherent) vs. multiple (incoherent) model of attachment: Findings and directions for future research. In C. M. Parkes, J. Stevenson-Hinde, & P. Marris (Eds.), *Attachment across the life cycle* (pp. 127–159). New York: Tavistock/Routledge.

Makari, G. (2008). *Revolution in mind: The creation of psychoanalysis.* New York: Harper Collins.

McWilliams, N. (2004). *Psychoanalytic psychotherapy: A practitioner's guide.* New York: Guilford Press.

Meissner, W. W. (1981). *Internalization in psychoanalysis.* New York: International Universities Press.

Mitchell, S. A. (1988). *Relational concepts in psychoanalysis.* Cambridge, MA: Harvard University Press.

Mitchell, S. A. (1993). *Hope and dread in psychoanalysis.* New York: Basic Books.

Mitchell, S. A. (1997). *Influence and autonomy in psychoanalysis.* Hillsdale, NJ: Analytic Press.

Mitchell, S. A., & Black, M. J. (1995). *Freud and beyond: A history of modern psychoanalytic thought.* New York: Basic Books.

Ogden, T. (1994). *Subjects of analysis.* Northvale, NJ: Aronson.

Pizer, S. A. (1998). *Building bridges: The negotiation paradox in psychoanalysis.* Hillsdale, NJ: Analytic Press.

Racker, H. (1953). A contribution to the problem of countertransference. *International Journal of psychoanalysis, 34,* 313–324.

Racker, H. (1957). The meanings and uses of countertransference. *Psychoanalytic Quarterly, 26,* 303–357.

Reiff, P. (1966). *The triumph of the therapeutic: Uses of faith after Freud.* Chicago: University of Chicago Press.

Renik, O. (2006). *Practical psychoanalysis for therapists and patients.* New York: Other Press.

Safran, J. D. (1993). The therapeutic alliance rupture as a transtheoretical phenomenon: Definitional and conceptual issues. *Journal of Psychotherapy Integration, 3,* 33–49.

Safran, J. D. (1999). Faith, despair, will, and the paradox of acceptance. *Contemporary Psychoanalysis, 35*, 5–24.

Safran, J. D. (2002). Brief relational psychoanalytic treatment. *Psychoanalytic Dialogues, 12*, 171–195.

Safran, J. D. (2012). *Psychoanalysis and psychoanalytic therapies.* Washington, DC: American Psychological Association.

Safran, J. D., Crocker, P., McMain, S., & Murray, P. (1990). Therapeutic alliance rupture as a therapy event for empirical investigation. *Psychotherapy: Theory, Research, Practice, Training, 27*, 154–165.

Safran, J. D., & Muran, J. C. (1996). The resolution of ruptures in the therapeutic alliance. *Journal of Consulting and Clinical Psychology, 64*, 447–458.

Safran, J. D., & Muran, J. C. (2000). *Negotiating the therapeutic alliance: A relational treatment guide.* New York: Guilford Press.

Safran, J. D., & Muran, J. C. (2006). Has the concept of the alliance outlived its usefulness. *Psychotherapy, 43*, 286–291.

Sandell, R. (2001). Can psychoanalysis become empirically supported? *International Forum of Psychoanalysis, 10*, 184–190.

Sandell, R., Blomberg, J., & Lazar, A. (2002). Time matters: On temporal interactions in long-term follow-up of long-term psychotherapies. *Psychotherapy Research, 12*, 39–58.

Sandell, R., Blomberg, J., Lazar, A., Carlsson, J., Broberg, J., & Schubert, J. (2000). Varieties of long-term outcome among patients in psychoanalysis and long-term psychotherapy: A review of findings in the Stockholm Outcome of Psychoanalysis and Psychotherapy Project (STOPP). *The International Journal of Psychoanalysis, 81*, 921–942.

Sandler, J. (1978). Counter-transference and role-responsiveness. *The International Review of Psychoanalysis, 3*, 43–47. Reprinted in J. Sandler (1998), *Internal objects revisited* (pp. 47–56). London: Karnac.

Schafer, R. (1968). *Aspects of internalization.* Madison, CT: International Universities Press.

Seligman, M. (1995). The effectiveness of psychotherapy. *American Psychologist, 50*, 965–974.

Shedler, J. (2010). The efficacy of psychodynamic psychotherapy. *American Psychologist, 65*, 98–109.

Sterba, R. (1934). The fate of the ego in analytic therapy. *International Journal of Psycho-Analysis, 15*, 117–126.

Stern, D. B. (1997). *Unformulated experience.* Hillsdale, NJ: Analytic Press.

Stern, D. B. (2010). *Partners in thought: Working with unformulated experience, dissociation, and enactment.* New York: Routledge/Taylor & Francis Group.

Stern, D. N. (1985). *The interpersonal world of the infant: A view from psychoanalysis and developmental psychology.* New York: Basic Books.

Strachey, J. (1934). The nature of the therapeutic action of psychoanalysis. *International Journal of Psycho-Analysis, 15*, 127–159.

Sullivan, H. S. (1953). *The interpersonal theory of psychiatry.* New York: Norton.

Tronick, E. (2007). *The neurobehavioral and social-emotional development of infants and children.* New York: W.W. Norton.

Winnicott, D. W. (1956). Primary maternal preoccupation. *Through paediatrics to psychoanalysis.* (pp. 300–305). New York: Basic Books.

Winnicott, D. W. (1958). The capacity to be alone. *The maturational process and the facilitating environment.* (pp. 29–36). New York: International Universities Press.

Winnicott, D. W. (1960). Ego distortion in terms of true and false self. *The maturational process and the facilitating environment.* (pp. 140–152). New York: International Universities Press.

Zetzel, E. (1956). Current concepts of transference. *International Journal of Psychoanalysis. 37*, 369–375.

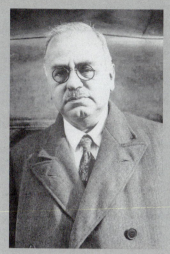

Alfred Adler (1870–1937)
© Bettmann/CORBIS

3 | ADLERIAN PSYCHOTHERAPY

Michael P. Maniacci, Laurie Sackett–Maniacci, and Harold H. Mosak

OVERVIEW

Adlerian psychotherapy was first developed by Alfred Adler. His original name for his system was Individual Psychology, and he viewed human nature from a holistic, teleological, phenomenological, social, and constructivist perspective. He saw people as active co-creators of their worlds, and he believed that prosocial adaptation was a requirement for healthy living. Feelings of inferiority, self-centeredness, hostile competition and competitiveness, certain biological predispositions, and discouragement all lead to psychopathology. Psychotherapists needed to work cooperatively, flexibly, and actively with their clients to help them develop better self-esteem, a more egalitarian view of others, and a more proactive and constructive view of life and other people.

Basic Concepts

Adlerian psychotherapy was originally developed when Adler was a co-worker with Sigmund Freud (Hoffman, 1994). Although Freud's influence was crucial, as Adler (1931/1964b) himself wrote, Adler soon introduced his own concepts and assumptions, which differed greatly from Freud's. The basic assumptions of Adlerian psychology can be summarized in the following 12 key principles (Mosak & Maniacci, 1999).

1. *Holism.* Adler believed that people should not be broken into parts. Emotional versus intellectual processes, conscious versus unconscious, individual versus group, and so forth are all artificial dichotomies. Adlerians prefer to look primarily at people and not to break them into parts (e.g., "My anger overwhelmed me!"). Just as Adlerians approach individuals holistically, so they approach interpersonal dynamics. People need to be considered in their social contexts. To examine an emotion in isolation from the total person is as unproductive as it is to examine a person without examining that person's social context. The field of study is the whole person in the person's social network.

2. *Teleology.* Adlerian psychology is concerned with purposes. As Aristotle (1941) first outlined in 350 B.C.E., to understand a thing, it must be analyzed according to the following four causes.

   Material: What is it made of?

   Efficient: What caused it to be?

   Formal: What shape does it take?

   Final: What purpose does it serve?

   Although many systems of psychotherapy emphasize the first three causes (which Adlerians acknowledge), Adlerians emphasize the fourth. For example, anxiety can be viewed in the following ways.

   Material cause: Rapid heart beat, sweaty palms, shortness of breath, perspiration.

   Efficient cause: Exposure to fearful childhood situations, predisposition to a disturbance of the neurotransmitter GABA.

   Formal cause: An anxiety disorder diagnosis, such as panic disorder, or a generalized anxiety disorder.

   Final cause: A signal to self and others to take charge and stay in control.

   Although many systems would agree with the first three causes and write extensively about them, Adlerians are relatively unique in adding the fourth—to be in control. The purpose of anxiety is to take charge, to be in control of something or someone (including oneself). Emotions, for example, can be viewed much the same way. The final cause of love is to move toward something. The final cause of apathy is to gain power (if someone does not care about anything, it is tough to control him or her). The final cause of hate is to move away from something.

3. *Creativity.* People are viewed as actors, not merely as reactors. As stated already, they are viewed as co-creators of the worlds. Parents affect children, that much is well understood, but what is often overlooked is that children affect parents too. A new baby influences family dynamics as much as family dynamics influence a baby. People are all too aware of how other people affect them, but seldom are they aware of how they affect other people; however, all relationships are bidirectional (see holism presented previously). Although heredity and environment are crucial to development, so too is the child's perception of the internal and external worlds he or she experiences. As Adlerians are fond of writing, no two children ever grow up in the same family: With the birth of each child, the family dynamic changes forever. No other child will ever know what it is like to be the oldest child, but neither will anybody else know what it is like to be the youngest.

4. *Phenomenology.* Although it is important to understand what children are born with material and efficient causes, it is equally (and oftentimes more) important to know how the children perceive what they were born with. By understanding

children's perceptions of their situations, a key insight is gained into the children's worlds. Many children who appear to have (by external standards) a "gift" perceive it as a "curse." One young client with whom one of the authors worked (MPM) stated that being a gifted athlete with a strong, superb physique was no blessing because he could never "coast" in sports or physical activities. He always felt the pressure was on him to perform well, to lead. Anything less than "first" or "top" was considered a disappointment. Adlerians do want to know the objective situation, but the subjective situation is quite often far more helpful.

5. *Soft Determinism.* Adlerians advocate for soft determinism. Hard determinism states unequivocally that "A leads to B." Nondeterminism states that there are no causes, and everything is a matter of free will. Adlerians tend to split the difference: "A most often leads to B, if that is of use to the person and that is how the person perceived the situation." Soft determinism stresses influences, not causes. It speaks of probabilities, not certainties. As has been pointed out in other works (e.g., Mosak & Maniacci, 1999), choosing does not always mean wanting. People may choose an alternative without necessarily wanting it. For instance, if the building is on fire, I may choose to jump out the window, but that does not mean I wanted to jump out the window. Next, freedom to choose does not always mean freedom of choice. Life does impose limits, and we are rarely free to choose from an unlimited menu. Life has limits, and given those limits, we still have some choice (even if those choices are not great). Finally, choice, responsibility, and blame need to be clarified. When all is said and done, people are responsible for their choices, though they are not necessarily to blame. The fact that people may not be aware of their choices does not mean they have not made them. Given the assumptions detailed previously, it is very understandable why certain people make certain choices. Instead of blaming them, Adlerian point out those choices—educate them about their choices—and then reeducate them, teach them new choices, and provide them with new skills and learning opportunities, both in and out of session.

6. *Social Field Theory.* As noted in the assumption about holism, Adlerians tend to closely examine the social field in which behavior takes place. It is not enough to know that someone is "crying." Where does that person cry? With whom? Who is the first to know when the person cries? Who is the last? Who never knows the person cries? Who is most affected by the person's crying? These types of questions elucidate the field in which the crying takes place. The person cries only partially because of "being sad" (an efficient cause) but also because crying can be used to produce an effect on others (final cause). What effect might that crying have?

    Adler (1956) wrote that there were three main tasks of life, and other Adlerians have elaborated on his original formulation (e.g., Manaster & Corsini, 1982; Mosak & Maniacci, 1999). For Adler, the three main tasks of life were work, community, and love. All psychopathology was designed to avoid or evade one or more of life's tasks. By looking at how clients meet—or do not meet—the tasks of life, psychotherapists can better understand clients.

7. *Motivation as Striving.* The most common way of expressing this concept in Adlerian psychology is to state that people are motivated to move from a perceived minus situation to a perceived plus situation. What the "minus situation" is and what the "plus situation" is varies from person to person and situation to situation. One person's minus situation may be "weak" and the plus "strong." Another's may be "fat" and "thin." Yet another may be "poor" and then "rich"—or "hated" and then "loved." Throughout Adler's career, he used different

phrases for each position (Adler, 1956; Ansbacher, 1964, 1978). The minus situation was variously labeled:

inferior

weak

hated

neglected

inadequate to the task

the plus situation was variously labeled:

superior

a real man

power

security

self-esteem

perfection

overcoming

completion

Early in Adler's writings, he believed that the feeling of a minus situation came first—that is, that children felt inferior and then strove to become superior (Adler, 1912/2002; Ansbacher, 1964). As his thinking and experience grew, he reversed the order. By the end of his life, Adler thought that children all strive to achieve some goal first; only when frustrated do they feel inferior or inadequate (Adler, 1935/2012b). It was an important change—and far more than terminological in nature. Adler's original position was a variant of Freud's tension reduction model: People felt a tension they had to reduce, only instead of the tension being caused by blocked libido, Adler felt it resulted from feeling inferior. Adler shifted to a growth model of human nature—tension reduction was not the principle objective, striving was, and only secondarily was tension produced when the person could not achieve his or her goals (Ansbacher, 1964, 1977, 1978).

8. *Idiographic Orientation.* Adlerians emphasize the *idiographic* rather than the *nomothetic* nature of people. The specifics of the case are more important than the generalities. Saying people have a major depressive disorder is nomothetic in nature. How do they manifest their particular depression? With whom? Where and when? Are they more sad or more irritable? Lonely and isolated or social and needy when down? Given the assumptions of phenomenology, creativity, holism, social field theory, striving, and so forth, far more specific data are required. Mary's major depressive disorder only seems to "arise" when she's alone and when her children go back to school in the fall. Jane's major depressive disorder only seems to "flare up" when her husband is around and trying to control her. Both may meet the diagnostic criteria for major depressive disorder, but the idiographic nature is crucial to their treatment.

9. *Psychology of Use.* This concept is an outgrowth of the aforementioned concepts. Although it is important to know what a person "has," it is often far more important to know what "use" a person makes of what he or she has. As opposed to the language of a psychology of possession, the language of a psychology of use is far more active, directive, and complex. "Bill has quite a temper!" reflects the psychology of possession in that he "has" a temper. Adlerians would phrase it (and conceptualize it) differently (McKay & Dinkmeyer, 1994; Rasmussen, 2010): "Bill uses his temper to control others," or to "get out of stuff he dislikes," and so forth. Hence, certain psychological processes are reframed in rather interesting ways such as emotions,

memory, or cognition. Adlerians are not as interested in the specific emotions a person has as much as they are in how those emotions are used. Similarly, what a person remembers is important, but it is far more interesting to know for what purpose the person has held onto that memory (see how Adlerians assess personality in the "Process of Psychotherapy" section later in the chapter). Many people may be intelligent, but how are they using their intelligence, for what purposes?

10. *Acting "As If."* People form maps of their worlds. They then act "as if" those maps were accurate representations of reality. The extent to which they cling to their maps is what is of interest to Adlerians. No map ever can be more important than the terrain itself, or survival is at risk. If Jack believes that people are always safe and to be trusted, then most times that may be quite useful. There may be times when such an assumption would put him as risk of being harmed, however, and if he too rigidly clings to his belief and too often acts as if it were true, then he is avoiding reality. Life will not yield to Jack's map. Jack must yield or face the consequences of such an overgeneralization. Adlerians tend to analyze how useful people's maps are given the particulars of their lives. What Adler referred to as the "style of life," which contemporary Adlerians call the "lifestyle," provides clues to the maps individuals act on. The lifestyle can be summarized as having four main components (Mosak & Maniacci, 1999; Shulman & Mosak, 1988):

Self-Concept—all the instructions about who I am or am not,

Self-Ideal—all the instructions about who I should be or should not be,

Worldview—all the instructions about people, life, and the world, and

Ethical Convictions—all the instructions about what is right or wrong, good or bad.

Psychopathology can be conceptualized (in part) as a matter of "goodness of fit" between the terrain and the map. The better the fit, the less likely behavior will appear as maladaptive.

11. *Self-Fulfilling Prophecy.* When people act "as if" their maps were "real," "true," or "correct," they tend to actively shape the feedback they receive. The feedback they receive is really partially a by-product of the feed-forward mechanisms they have sent out. If they act as if people are hostile, then quite often they will get back hostile responses, which then seem to justify their beliefs. As Adlerians have written, "believing is seeing" (Mosak & Maniacci, 1998, p. 4).

12. *Optimism.* Adler (1956) was quite emphatic about human nature being neutral, contrary to what is often stated. He did not believe that people were fundamentally good, nor did he (like Freud) believe that they were fundamentally bad. They could be either, depending on many factors (such as those already described). It is human nature's neutrality that leads to the psychotherapeutic stance of optimism. Everybody can be better than he or she is at any given point, no matter how discouraged or dysfunctional he or she may appear to be. Education, encouragement, teaching new choices, empathy, understanding, helping to usefully compensate for organic inferiorities, insight, and the acquisition of new skills can all help people to feel better, do better, and be better. Again, given the idiographic nature of Adlerian psychology, what "better" means varies from person to person and from situation to situation. Hope, faith, and compassion are crucial to optimism. If therapists do not use them and model them for clients, then clients often cannot find them for themselves.

Other Systems

Adlerian theory offers a comprehensive framework for understanding people as well as a method for creating direction in helping those whom Adlerian clinicians serve. The relationship between Adlerian theory and other theories can be described in a twofold manner. First, the theoretical underpinnings of various theories share many of the same assumptions that Adlerian theory embraces. Second, many of the therapeutic approaches that are utilized by other theories, regardless of whether they have sprung from similar assumptions, are consonant with those utilized by Adlerians. This twofold explanation lends itself to a considerable amount of overlap between Adlerian theory and other theories. Moreover, it speaks to (1) the ability of clinicians who practice from a different theoretical orientation to broaden their repertoire of methods in helping clients and (2) the notion that Adlerian psychology offers a comprehensive theory that can be seen as truly integrated. The following is a description of the many ways in which Adlerian theory compares to a variety of other approaches.

Adlerian psychology is a phenomenological, holistic, teleological, optimistic, and socially embedded theory that is predicated on a variety of basic assumptions. These assumptions can be seen as a common thread woven into various other theories, and they provide a good basis of comparison between Adlerian theory and other theories including cognitive-behavioral and newer cognitive-behavioral theories, solution-focused theory, positive psychology, attachment theory, and multicultural theory.

Cognitive-Behavior Therapy

Adler was the first phenomenological, cognitive therapist (Mosak & Maniacci, 1999). Like Adlerian theory, cognitive-behavioral theory emphasizes a relationship between people's belief systems and their emotions and behavior (Watts, 2003). Adlerians seek to understand the clients' lifestyle convictions, a task consonant with cognitive-behavior theory. Cognitive therapists seek to identify distortions in a client's thinking such as "should" statements that represent unrealistic expectations that the client holds. These "should" statements would be analogous to unrealistic self-ideal beliefs that Adlerians seek to identify. Cognitive theory also emphasizes not only what a person thinks but also how the person thinks. For example, the key cognitive therapy concept of *dichotomous thinking* (a tendency to view things in terms of mutually exclusive categories) is similar to Adler's notion of *antithetical modes of apperception*, where the client mistakenly evaluates and dichotomizes impression in terms of above–below, masculine–feminine, or all or nothing (Adler, 1912/2002).

The therapeutic approach in both of these theories share similarities as well. Both cognitive-behavior theory and Adlerian theory emphasize the importance of the therapeutic relationship. One of the primary ways in which Adler diverged from the traditional psychoanalytic approach was in his emphasis on establishing a strong therapeutic relationship in general and a collaborative, egalitarian, respectful rapport in particular. Cognitive therapists also place considerable emphasis on establishing a strong therapeutic alliance. Both theoretical orientations approach treatment as an educational endeavor (Watts, 2003).

Newer Cognitive-Behavioral Approaches: Mindfulness and Acceptance and Commitment Therapy

Mindfulness and acceptance and commitment therapies are new cognitive theories that have grown in use over the past decade or so (Hayes, Follette, & Linehan, 2004). Both of these theories have similar underpinnings and share some similarities with Adlerian theory and can be used within an Adlerian framework. Given that they are both cognitive in nature, they share with Adlerian thinking that what and how people think affects their behavior and well-being. Mindfulness and acceptance approaches seek to have clients become aware of internal and external stimuli—and accept rather than judge these stimuli. So even though the Adlerian therapist has traditionally sought to identify and help modify negative beliefs and thought patterns, mindfulness and acceptance therapy helps clients accept their current thought patterns as "just thoughts" without modifying them. Although these two approaches may be somewhat divergent on this point, both seek to help clients increase their well-being, learn to be their own best friend, and become more accepting of anxiety and feelings of inferiority.

The commitment aspect of acceptance and commitment therapy (Hayes, Follette, & Linehan, 2004) also shares a similar approach to Adlerian therapy. Commitment therapy seeks to help a client articulate what he or she wants life to mean. From this articulation, the therapist helps a client create a life plan and move toward his or her goals. This forward-thinking, goal-oriented approach is consonant with the Adlerian approach. More specifically, the Adlerian therapist collaborates with clients to help define what they would like to change with respect to the tasks of life (i.e., work, love, social, spiritual, and self tasks).

Solution-Focused Therapy

For many reasons, psychotherapy has moved to a brief-therapy model. Solution-focused therapy and Adlerian therapy are both models that lend themselves well to a brief-therapy approach (de Shazer, 1988). Moreover, these two theories share other similarities as well. Both theories are goal oriented. In this way, they both work toward identifying client goals via a collaborative relationship. The emphasis is on helping the client move forward. Inherent in Adlerian theory is the emphasis on teleology and investigating the purpose of symptoms and behaviors. Indeed, Adlerians have used "The Question" as a means of identifying the potential purpose of symptoms for some time (Mosak & Maniacci, 1998). Solution-focused therapists have employed the "The Miracle Question" (de Shazer, 1988, p. 5). Adler is not cited by de Shazer, but the use of the tactic is virtually identical.

In addition to the goal-oriented focus of both Adlerian therapy and solution-focused therapy, there are other areas of overlap. Both therapies embrace an optimistic view of people, both focus on identifying and building on the strengths of the clients, and both focus on the importance of establishing a solid therapeutic alliance. Lastly, solution-focused brief therapy focuses on the future. Adlerian therapy shares this focus as well, although Adlerian therapists will also focus on the present and the past. Adlerians will occasionally "glimpse" into the clients' past as a means for understanding how they got to where they are now as well as how they parlay those past experiences into their current motivation and goals.

Attachment Theory

Adlerian theory considers the role of attachment in development, whereas attachment theory (Wallin, 2007) explores it in detail. Via early experiences, children develop working models of self and others principally through interactions with caretakers. Attachment theory identifies common attachment styles, and each style seems to be differentiated by the views and expectations that are commonly concluded in certain situations. Although attachment theory may at times be a little too deterministic and lack the acknowledgment of the creative power of the individual, it can augment the investigation of a client's lifestyle. Attachment theory shares with Adlerian theory an emphasis on the importance of the social field. In their research, Peluso, Peluso, Buckner, Kern, and Curlette (2009) found attachment style and lifestyle to be similar constructs.

Positive Psychology

Over the past decade or so, positive psychology has emerged as a new, optimistic, and strength-focused psychology that stands in contrast to many earlier systems of psychology that embraced the medical model (Carlson, Watts, & Maniacci, 2006; Seligman, 2011). Positive psychology focuses on those aspects related to well-being versus those that make us "ill." Elements such as positive emotions, engagement in life, having a sense of meaning, and interpersonal relationships have been identified as important elements that promote a sense of well-being (Seligman, 2011). The focus on strengths of the individual as well as those elements related to well-being share a considerable amount of overlap with Adlerian psychology. Despite this overlap, the positive psychology literature almost never mentions Adler's ideas. Indeed, Adler's focus on what is good with the individual, the emphasis on encouragement of the individual, and the notion of expanding social interest (i.e., a feeling of belonging to and participating with others) in the individual are all consonant with those elements outlined in positive psychology.

HISTORY

Precursors

Adler is often described as a man ahead of his time (e.g., Ellenberger, 1970), and his assumptions were often out of step with the prevailing medical and scientific tenor of his time (Maniacci, 2012). Several reasons for this have been detailed by many authors in another work (Carlson & Maniacci, 2012), but they can be summarized here.

Adler was a scientist. He earned a degree in medicine and was a practicing physician. He initially wrote about and conceptualized cases from a materialistic, relatively hard deterministic perspective. Such a perspective won him the recognition and attention of several people in his home town of Vienna, most notably Sigmund Freud. Such a hard deterministic stance was most evident in his first major publication on organ inferiority in 1907, when he was still an active member of the original inner circle of Freud and his colleagues (Adler, 1907/1917). This perspective did not suit Adler for long, however.

Adler read widely—and more than medical and psychiatric journals and publications. Soon after his initial publication on organ inferiority, Adler began making references to nonscientific authors. He was dissatisfied with the logic and assumptions of the materialistic perspective so prevalent at the time. In fact, in one publication, Adler wrote that among the greatest influences on his system of psychology were "the Bible, Shakespeare, and Goethe" (Adler, 1956, p. 329). Two of his most frequent referenced authors in his first main psychological text published in 1912 were philosophers Friedrich Nietzsche and Hans Vaihinger (Adler, 1912/2002; Maniacci, 2012). Adler was struggling for a new way of describing personality and psychology, and the prevailing scientists of his day were not providing him with a conceptual foundation for his thinking, so he looked elsewhere.

From Aristotle, Adler borrowed many concepts such as the notions of humans being social animals. He also borrowed the notions of common sense, practical wisdom, and the final cause. From Immanuel Kant and one of his disciples, Vaihinger (1911/1965), Adler found more reinforcement for the notion of common sense and the idea of cognitive maps. From Nietzsche (1901/1967), he borrowed the notions of the will to power, "illness" or "sickness" as a potential means of gaining power and influencing people, and the notion of the creative use of memory to serve a purpose and as justification for one's actions.

Adler also learned a great deal from Shakespeare (Maniacci, 2012). He cited Shakespeare's characters in several places, and he praised the playwright for his astute understanding of human nature. He cited Shakespeare as one of the main resources for his notion of compensation and overcompensation of organic inferiorities (see his references to the character of Richard III in Adler, 1956, p. 168). Also from Shakespeare he learned that what leads people to trouble was a mismatch between their characters and the demands of the situation. Shakespeare often portrayed characters of great moral and intellectual virtues who nonetheless had flaws that were frequently outgrowths of their very strengths. For example, Othello was a man of honor, honesty, and loyalty, but he was either tragically too trusting of others or devastatingly not trusting enough. When he ran into a situation for which he was unprepared—that is, a deceitful comrade—he did not handle it well, and it led to his downfall. It was the combination of character and situation that led to trouble, not one or the other.

Finally, Adler (1931/1964b) borrowed several concepts from Freud, even in his last years writing that he was indebted to Freud for the concepts of unconscious processes, dream interpretation, guessing, the crucial role of childhood in personality formation, and the importance of developing a "talking cure" for what until then had been primarily a somatic attempt to cure psychiatric disturbances.

Beginnings

Adler was born in Vienna on February 7, 1870, and died while lecturing in Aberdeen, Scotland, on May 27, 1937. He graduated from the University of Vienna in 1895 with a degree in ophthalmology. He was crucially aware of how disturbances in the way people see their worlds could affect their health. He soon switched to general medicine and then neurology. He served as an Austrian army physician during World War I and had been very politically active before that. He marched in women's liberation parades, wrote on social medicine and the health of the working class, and advocated for the handicapped and poor and established clinics for the underserved across Austria. He consulted with prisons, hospitals, and sanitariums. He gave public lectures, worked in schools, trained guidance counselors and pubic school teachers to intervene with students, and set up marriage clinics.

Sometime in 1902, Adler received a written invitation to meet with Sigmund Freud on a Wednesday evening to discuss matters relating to psychology and medical practice (Hoffman, 1994; Orgler, 1939/1963). How Freud knew of Adler has never been fully clarified, though there is some evidence that Freud had sent some patients to Adler for evaluation and that Adler may have even treated one of Freud's relatives, though whether the treatment was primarily medical or psychiatric is unclear (if it happened at all). Nonetheless, they met, and Freud was impressed. Within a short time, Adler was elected president of the Wednesday Psychological Society (before the group took the name of Vienna Psychoanalytic Society) and Adler was coeditor (with Freud) of their journal.

The two men worked together for nine years. They seemed to have been friendly but not quite friends. Adler was the only member of the original society not to have been psychoanalyzed by Freud. Why he never underwent a "training analysis" has never been explained, but it may have been a crucial factor in their eventual split. Adler was very different in style and temperament from his senior colleague, and he practiced "psychoanalysis" very differently. He invited patients to sit up and talk freely about real-life challenges they faced, as opposed to reclining on a couch and free associating as the analyst sat behind and took notes. He advocated asking questions and structuring the interviews, especially early in treatment, something Freud found risky because of the potential "contamination of the data" that might ensue if the analyst were too directive. Adler saw couples, children, and families, and he worked with the physically impaired in clinics, prisons, schools, and in front of other professionals to demonstrate his methods. Freud never demonstrated his work to anyone, even on invitation. Freud would only work with a very specific population in individual treatment in private, as opposed to Adler, who treated anyone, from neurotics to psychotics and criminals. If the patients did not meet Freud's criteria for treatment, then he would not treat them. Adler would modify his methods until he found what worked with any particular individual (Maniacci, 1999).

In 1911, their differences came to a head (Adler, 1956; Ansbacher, 1978). Adler's papers and lectures were becoming more and more divergent from Freud's work, and a meeting was held. At issue were several key points, two of which became irreconcilable. First, Freud presented his views; a week or so later, Adler presented his. Freud felt that women were biologically inferior to men, and their lack of a penis determined that they could not go through the oedipal stage of development as men did, and therefore they were destined to be psychologically inferior for the rest of their lives and should not be trusted with positions of leadership and authority (e.g., Freud 1933/1965, p. 119). Adler, married to a very educated, politically active woman who made sure her first two daughters received doctorates (in philosophy and medicine, respectively), would not agree (Hoffman, 1994). He felt that women used psychiatric services more because of social inferiorities rather than constitutional inferiorities: They were denied access to equal rights and respect, and given their status as social inferiors, they developed psychiatric symptoms to rebalance the power in their social situations. It was only through symptoms that they could exercise some degree of power and control. Freud felt that was an unacceptable position.

Second, Freud felt that repression was a necessary function of humanity, that only through repression could people ever hope to survive together. Fundamentally, people were animals who, without repression, would kill each other. Adler disagreed. He felt repression was only needed because people refused to accept the logic of social living and failed to use their "drives" to work cooperatively with others. People did not have to be in conflict with themselves or others if they attached the right meaning to life and were educated to be well adjusted, cooperative, and compassionate. It was not that people were animals, it was that they were poorly educated and did not see things clearly enough. If they were treated warmly, respectfully, and fairly, they would grow up and be cooperative, useful members of society, and society would be all the better for it.

The society held a vote, and Adler lost. It was declared that his position was incompatible with Freud's, and Adler resigned his presidency and editorial position. After some heated debate, Adler's followers were informed that their vote for his positions made them also unwelcome, and that to hold membership with Adler's new group (which was being formed) made it impossible for them to be in Freud's. The rift was formalized.

Adler and his colleagues formed their own group and searched for a name. Personality Psychology was chosen but soon dropped because somebody else had claimed that title. Holistic Psychology was tried, but a new group had already claimed the word *holism* (in German, they were known as the *Gestalt* psychologists). Adler and his group called themselves the Society for Free Psychoanalytic Research, though no one is quite clear what "Free" meant (it has been alluded to by people who were there at the time that it meant "Free from Freud"). Again, that title was objected to by none other than Freud, who wanted the word *psychoanalysis* to be the exclusive property of his group. Adler (perhaps for the last time) yielded and called his group Individual Psychology, from the Latin word *individuum*, indivisible, a synonym for holism. Unfortunately, it was frequently misunderstood as meaning "individual," exactly the opposite of Adler's original intention. Still, it stood (Maniacci, 2012).

Adler continued the work he began before Freud. He was socially aware and active, lectured extensively, published often, and opened training centers throughout the world. Adler and his followers established clinics and advocated group therapy, child guidance, family therapy, couples therapy, and the writing of self-help books for the general public so that psychological information could be used preventatively and reach as many people as early as possible.

Current Status

The current status of Adlerian psychology reflects vibrancy, innovation, and forward movement and can be seen in the recent work of many Adlerians. These undertakings include opportunities for training and continuing education and the inclusion of Adlerian theory in counseling and therapy and other areas such as wellness.

Currently, Adlerian schools are located in Chicago, Minnesota, Washington, and San Francisco, all of them offering advanced degrees and postdoctoral training in Adlerian theory. The North American Society of Adlerian Psychology (NASAP) is an organization that provides ongoing training opportunities, clinician collaboration, and camaraderie via conferences and newsletters. It also publishes the quarterly Adlerian journal, the *Journal of Individual Psychology*, a peer-reviewed journal that includes research and articles related to the use of Adlerian principles and techniques in clinical work and education. A variety of other Adlerian training materials exist as well, such as the *Collected Clinical Works of Alfred Adler*, edited by Henry Stein, and a library of training videos produced by Jon Carlson and distributed by the American Psychological Association (see Carlson, Watts, & Maniacci, 2006, p. 280, for a complete list of videos). Mozdzierz, Peluso, and Lisiecki (2009) and Rasmussen (2010) have written recent books that link Adlerian theory and therapy with current research in the field. Both are highly recommended.

Wellness is another pertinent area in which Adlerians have written and continue to work. Wellness—an interest in the physical, mental, and social well-being of individuals—continues to be a motivating force in helping others. Adlerians such as Thomas Sweeney (2009, pp. 36–43) have developed the WEL and 5F-Wel assessment instruments to measure a person's degree of wellness. These assessment instruments have been derived from Adlerian psychology and cross-disciplinary studies that identify areas of health, quality of life, and longevity. Laurie Sackett-Maniacci continues to run semi-structured groups for cardiovascular patients out of Rush-Copley Heart Institute near Chicago. The groups focus on issues of wellness, adjustment to illness, modifying maladaptive health behaviors, and increasing stress-management skills. This is a continuation of her work with medical patients she first researched at the Diamond Headache Clinic in Chicago (Sackett-Maniacci, 1999). This research examined lifestyle factors of chronic migraine headache sufferers and has served as a guide for targeted areas of treatment.

PERSONALITY

Theory of Personality

Adlerian psychology describes personality from the perspective of the style of life, or as it is more commonly called, the *lifestyle* (Ansbacher, 1977). First, some clarifications are in order.

Temperament refers to the inborn characteristics children have, which are primarily genetic. Experts have debated how many temperaments there are, but the fact that humans are born with certain predisposition seems clear. Those temperaments are quickly modified via learning and socialization.

Personality can be defined as a collection of traits and characteristics children develop through the process of socialization. Given their temperamental predispositions and early childhood experiences, personality develops.

Lifestyle (as the Adlerians define it) is the *use* of the personality, traits, temperament, and psychological and biological processes in order to find a place in the social matrix of life. As alluded to previously, someone may *have* a shy temperament, but how that person comes to *perceive* and *use* it in either a socially useful or useless manner is what is of greatest interest to Adlerians. The link between lifestyle and attachment theory is important (Peluso et al., 2009). Children come to believe, and therefore act "as if," they can only belong if they do certain things they perceive are required for them to find their place (Dreikurs & Soltz, 1964). For example, Karl may believe that to find his place, he has to be the boss. He uses his large size, imposing voice, and aggressive nature to find his place by being in charge. If he is encouraged, he could be a leader; if discouraged, he might be a bully. The bully and the leader both may have similar biological predispositions, traits, and characteristics, but one uses them in a socially constructive way whereas the other does not.

There are many factors that influence the development of the lifestyle (Mosak & Maniacci, 1993, 1999; Powers & Griffith, 1987; Shulman & Mosak, 1988). A brief overview will detail some of them.

1. *Degree of Activity*. Adler (1927/1957, 1956) referred to *degree of activity* and alluded to the fact that it is partially learned and partially a product of temperament (possibly endocrine functions, or so he believed in 1927). Some children are just more active then others. How this matches the caretakers' degree of activity is crucial. A mismatch can be trouble: A parent who has a low degree of activity paired with a child who has a high degree of activity may not be the best possible match. The degree of activity children display in childhood often becomes the amount of energy adults have in solving problems later on in life.

2. *Organ Inferiority*. Some children have constitutionally inferior organ systems. The law of compensation will then begin along three dimensions (Dreikurs, 1967; Maniacci, 1996b):

Somatic: One organ system will take over, such as one kidney becoming overactive to compensate for the weaker one.

Sympathetic: The body may change the way it moves, sits, reclines in order to unconsciously protect the weaker body part. A limp that may develop to accommodate a weaker leg is one such example.

Psychic: The brain or mind may develop a belief system that over- or underemphasizes certain bodily functions. A person with poor eyesight may become overly preoccupied with visual stimuli and become a painter. A man with a club foot may become a world class athlete (as did the English poet and nobleman, George Gordon, Lord Byron).

An organ inferiority can influence the development of the lifestyle. It can shape the process directly, for example, through the law of compensation (Adler, 1956) or indirectly such as through the perceptions and attitudes of the parents, siblings, caretakers, and others. They may treat the child specially, and that can influence the lifestyle.

3. *Birth Order and Sibling Relationships*. Adler (1920/2012a) discussed the birth order of children. He identified five positions: only, oldest, second, middle, and youngest. He also described the characteristic attributes for each position—for example,

only children tend to be perfectionists, oldest borns become leaders, second borns become rebels, middle children become pleasers, and youngest borns become attention seekers. Many authors, including some Adlerians, have written best-selling books describing birth-order roles (Forer & Still, 1976; Leman, 1985). The utility of the concept of birth order in Adlerian psychology has been debated, and differing opinions exist even among Adlerians (Shulman & Mosak, 1977). Nonetheless, sibling relationships are crucial, even when they do not fit neatly into the traditionally defined birth-order roles. Parents are crucial to the development of the lifestyle, but siblings are as well—and sometimes even more important. Why? It is not so mysterious. Children will often spend more time with siblings than parents, and that extra time can influence many of the choices children make. Sibling relationships and the role children carve out for themselves in childhood often manifest later in life as the stance adults take toward socialization across many different contexts and roles.

4. *Family Values.* The values families hold influence the lifestyle (Powers & Griffith, 1987; Shulman & Mosak, 1988). Typically, though not exclusively, values come in three varieties: maternal, paternal, and family.

    Maternal values are held by the mother or mother figure. Paternal are held by the father or father figure. Although both are important, neither is necessarily binding. What does that mean? If mother values education and father does not, the children usually have some sense of freedom about accepting the value. If they do, they can fit in with mother; if they do not, they still have father to bond with. A family value is held by both. That is binding. To accept the value therefore becomes synonymous with fitting in with the key authority figures in the family; to reject allows no ally and no bonding with either key figure. That can be tantamount to not fitting in at all. Family values children accept or reject in childhood often become what are now referred to as *psychosocial stressors* in adulthood.

5. *Family Atmosphere.* There is an emotional tone that characterizes every family (Dewey, 1971). Families that are more emotionally sensitive and intelligent have different atmospheres than do families that are more emotionally cold, distant, or hostile. Children's reactions to the prevailing atmosphere often helps set their moods as adults (Powers & Griffith, 1987). Although adult mood may be a by-product of temperament, genetics, and overall health and nutrition, it is also very often a response to what was the perceived family atmosphere in childhood. For example, a hostile, unpredictable family atmosphere in childhood may lead children to develop an anxious, inhibited mood as adults if they come to believe that that is the best way to prepare themselves for the future.

6. *Parenting Style.* Adlerians have long written about parenting dynamics. Autocratic, democratic, and permissive styles (to only name a few) and their possible effects on children's lifestyles have been documented for decades. In general, Adlerians have long advocated for a democratic style of parenting children, believing that it best influences the characteristics of belonging, cooperation, and useful bonding that Adlerians see as crucial to society (Dreikurs, 1971; Dreikurs & Soltz, 1964).

Other features are also important such as school, religion, economics, peers, and culture. When Adlerians assess a lifestyle, all of these factors and others are inquired about during what is known as a *lifestyle interview*. Once these factors are assessed, the core structures of the lifestyle can be formulated in collaboration with the client. The client's self-concept, self-ideal, worldview and ethical convictions can be expressed, sometimes in a shorthand manner that can be summarized in this example:

I am small and weak (self-concept).

I should be big and strong (self-ideal).

The world is a tough place where only real men survive (worldview).

It is better to be the top dog than to be eaten by the other dogs (ethical convictions).

Such a lifestyle has been described as a "superiority seeker" in the Adlerian literature (Mosak & Maniacci, 1999).

When the self-concept falls short of the self-ideal, feelings of inferiority result. When the self-concept falls short of the worldview, feelings of inadequacy typically ensue. When the self-concept falls short of the ethical convictions, guilt feelings emerge. Historically, these are described as "feelings," but in actuality they are merely the results of discrepancies in convictions. The lack of congruence between convictions feels like a pain, a subjective sense of anguish or a discomfort of some sort. How the person does or does not compensate for such discrepancies is crucial (Mosak & Maniacci, 1999).

The more encouraged a person is, the greater the chances that he or she will handle the discomfort prosocially. The more discouraged the person is, the greater the chances he or she will develop symptoms of psychopathology. This is a crucial point, often misunderstood even in Adlerian circles. Everybody has some incongruence in lifestyle convictions; that is normal. Nobody ever lives up to his or her expectations all the time. When he or she falls short, how is that handled? That is the critical question.

People want to belong, to bond. We are social creatures. Attachment is synonymous with survival. Children may perceive, or misperceive, how they should attach or belong. As long as they are encouraged, they have a place regardless of their sense of inferiority, and they will typically adapt to life's challenges in a healthy, productive manner.

Variety of Concepts

Adlerians tend to favor simple language and concepts. Adlerian psychology is not a "depth" psychology; it favors a "breath" perspective (Powers & Griffith, 1987 p. 5). It does not dig deeply into any one idea or stage of development but rather chooses to look across situations and processes to detect patterns and themes. The lifestyle provides the blueprint for the recurring patterns people experience in life. This is reflected in the concepts discussed in Adlerian psychology.

Common Sense and Private Logic

Thinking can be divided into two categories. Common sense reflects the thinking shared by the community, the consensual thinking shared by others. It is learned by interaction and communion. Private logic entails thinking that is unique to the person. It is unshared, except by a small group, which is most often (but not always) the family of origin. Common sense is almost always verbal and linguistically based, and private logic can be linguistic but is most often attitudinal, personal, and "felt." When Adler (1956) declared that people know more than they understand, he was referring to private logic. People know they are mortal, that bad things can and do happen to people—in their common sense. For many, in their private logic, they believe they are special and immune, hence they can take risks. In his early formulations, Adler (1912/2002) emphasized the degree of common sense a person had as a barometer of overall mental health. The greater the amount of common sense, the better the overall adaptation. The cognitive map matched the terrain. More was needed, however, as Adler learned all too well.

Community feeling is an important concept (Ansbacher, 1992b). Sometimes referred to as *social interest*, it refers to the feeling of being a part of the community, the group, in a cooperative, egalitarian manner (Mosak & Maniacci, 1999). People who display community feeling feel at home in the world, as if they belong. They treat others with respect and fairness. They realize that their way of belonging should not interfere with others finding their place, and they find a way to coexist. As Adler observed, common sense could be corrupted. What appeared as common sense to a community could be grossly inadequate (as he observed in Germany's preparation for World War II). Community feeling and social interest served his theory as a check on the potential corruption of common sense. Whereas common sense led to adaptation in the here and now, community feeling was intended to lead to a greater good for all people at all times. This concept embodies the idea that what is good cannot be defined to any particular culture or time but rather for the species as a whole.

Reason is a fascinating concept in Adlerian psychology. Intelligence is the ability to solve problems, and Adler accepted that definition. He felt that intelligence that included the human element, the concern for others and their well-being, was reason (Adler, 1928/1964a). Many people can be intelligent but not reasonable. Their intelligence is not used in service of the greater good; it lacks community feeling.

Life tasks are the main theaters of operation for people (Adler, 1956). Individuals must work, socialize, and love in order to find their place. Typically, in Western culture, work is the easiest of the original life tasks to meet. It requires the least community feeling. Socialization, or the social task, requires more. Love and intimacy require the most. People who get into psychological difficulties often first show those difficulties in the love task.

Safeguarding operations are those mechanisms people use to evade life tasks (Adler, 1956; Mosak & Maniacci, 1999). Because of an erroneous conception of life, self, and the interaction between them, people may attempt to act "as if" the life tasks can only be met in a particular manner. Gerry may believe that she only belongs and can function if she is right. As long as people tell she is right, all is well. When they do not, problems may arise. She may develop excuses, symptoms, evasions, fears, and all sorts of difficulties in order to attempt to rearrange life to meet her requirements rather than the other way around. Psychoanalysts have traditionally defined safeguarding operations as *defense mechanisms*.

Stress can be conceptualized as a person doubting his or her place in the world (Mosak & Maniacci, 1999). People can be tired for simply physiological reasons. Stress, on the other hand, happens when people's lifestyles do not seem to match the terrain: Their maps are not adequate to the territory.

Unconscious is used more as a verb than a noun in Adlerian psychology. Given the holistic hypothesis, Adlerians do not see a discrepancy between conscious and unconscious processes. People may be unconscious of what they are doing, but there is no "unconscious place" where ideas or impulses exist. Typically, they are unconscious of what they are doing because they have never had it explained to them. The eye can see everything but itself, the saying goes, and people learn their lifestyle convictions mostly nonverbally. Seldom is a lifestyle formed out of one traumatic experience; most often, it is learned through thousands of little transactions, experiences, and interactions over a long period of time. No one incident is typically recalled as being worthy of significance, yet the total accumulation of life's events and interactions leads to patterns and maps.

Movement is a term Adlerians use frequently. It implies behavior, but it is more than that. The best indicator of a person's intentions is what he or she does, but movement also means intention. Adlerians focus on thinking, feeling, and behaving, but Adlerian psychotherapy is primarily interested in motivation modification, not simple behavior modification or changes in feelings and emotions (Manaster & Corsini, 1982).

PSYCHOTHERAPY

Theory of Psychotherapy

Adlerian theory is consistent and unified. Over the course of its existence, little has changed in the basic assumptions of Adlerian psychology. The postulates derived from the basic assumptions may change, but that is normal. For example, the basic assumption about the relevance of a social field theory has not changed, and it has received considerable support across disciplines. However, what the concept of a social field *means* has changed. In Adler's day, homosexuality was considered psychopathological (Adler, 1978; Ansbacher, 1978). Adlerians today realize it is not (Chandler, 1995). So even though Adlerians' views about homosexuality have changed, the underlying assumption about the necessity of understanding the social field and treating those in it in an encouraging, egalitarian manner has not. Gay or straight, understanding how people treat each other and teaching them to treat each other cooperatively, fairly, compassionately, and encouragingly is as relevant today as it was in Adler's time.

Although the basic assumptions have not changed and are consistent and clearly delineated, the process of therapy continues to evolve (Carlson, Watts, & Maniacci, 2006; Kopp, 1995; Mozdzierz, Peluso, & Lisiecki, 2009; Oberst & Stewart, 2003; Sperry, 1989, 1995; Sweeney, 2009). What Adlerians do and how they do it continues to adapt and change as people and situations evolve in a culture across time. This was a point of contention between Freud and Adler as far back as 1911. Because Freud tied his theory to the science of the day (i.e., the steam engine and Newtonian physics), as the science changed so has psychoanalytic theory. His technique, however, has not. Classical psychoanalysis is still the same. If the patients do not fit the system, they cannot be in classical psychoanalysis. Adler's theory was not tied to the science of the day, so his system has not had to change its metaphors or concepts (Kopp, 1995; Maniacci, 2012). He would adapt his theory to the needs of his patients, and much the same is true today. Outlining Adlerian psychotherapy is difficult because it is so tied to the particulars of the case (the idiographic nature of the theory). Still, six common factors can be outlined as goals of Adlerian psychotherapy (Mosak & Maniacci, 2011):

1. fostering community feeling;
2. decreasing feelings of inferiority, and therefore, psychological symptoms;
3. modifying the lifestyle to make it more adaptive, flexible, and prosocial;
4. changing faulty motivation and destructive values;
5. encouraging equality and acceptance of self and others; and
6. helping the person to be a contributing member of the world community.

Diagnosis, as in the medical model, is typically not relevant to the therapy itself. Adlerians are not opposed to multiaxial systems like the one that was previously used in the *Diagnostic and Statistical Manual of Mental Disorders* (DSM-IV; American Psychiatric Association, 2000), and have even written extensively about how a unification can be achieved between traditional psychiatric case conceptualizations and Adlerian case formulations (Maniacci, 1999, 2002; Maniacci & Sackett-Maniacci, 2002; Sperry, 2002).

The five axes of the DSM-IV were previously defined as:

Axis I—Clinical Syndromes and Disorders,

Axis II—Personality Disorders,

Axis III—Medical Conditions,

Axis IV—Psychosocial Stressors, and

Axis V—Global Assessment of Functioning Scale.

On axis I, a typical diagnosis might have been dysthymic disorder, a form of chronic, low- to midlevel depression. On axis II, it might be listed a dependent personality disorder. On axis III, the person might have a broken leg that limits his or her motility. On axis IV, it could be listed the psychosocial stressor of a recent divorce that has precipitated the onset of the dysthymic disorder diagnosis. Axis V used the Global Assessment of Functioning (GAF) scale, which quantifies a person's overall functioning in the areas of working and socializing on a scale from 1 (extremely low) to 100 (extremely high). A typical diagnostic work up might have looked like this:

Axis I—Dysthymic Disorder;

Axis II—Dependent Personality Disorder;

Axis III—Fracture of the left tibia; diabetes (per physician diagnosis);

Axis IV—Recent Divorce; and

Axis V—Current GAF 45 (serious impairment).

In contrast, an Adlerian case formulation would be done this way:

Axis I—The Arrangement,

Axis II—The Lifestyle,

Axis III—Organ Inferiority (organ jargon),

Axis IV—The Shock, and

Axis V—A Barometer of the Life Tasks.

The case formulation might be this. A person, Hillary, believes that in order to belong she needs others (axis II). This was learned in her family of origin and also from having childhood onset diabetes. Without help and support from others in getting her needs met, she might die (axis III). She has run into a situation for which she is unprepared, what Adler (1956) referred to as a shock: Her husband has left her for another woman (axis IV). In attempting a home repair without him, she fell and broke her leg (axis III). This only served to reinforce her sense of needing someone in order to survive (axis II). Unconsciously she is furious and is having a silent temper tantrum (axis I). To be openly mad might drive her ex-husband and others even farther away, so she must bite her tongue and rage quietly. It serves its purpose: Her dysthymia "arranges" her adult children to come near her and makes her ex-husband look bad. She attains the support she needs and makes him look bad—and she hopes that if he feels bad enough, he might come back. Her functioning in the life tasks has decreased dramatically (axis V): She cannot work, she has stopped socializing unless people come to her, and she has given up on men.

Such a case formulation allows Adlerians to communicate with professionals of different disciplines and theories. Although far from perfect, the DSM language and multiaxial system can allow for greater communication and teamwork (Maniacci, 2002). In addition, treatment planning can be facilitated. Adlerians can plan what to do using both their theory and the diagnostic system. A comprehensive treatment plan would look like this (Carlson, Watts, & Maniacci, 2006; Maniacci, 1999):

1. crisis stabilization,

2. medical and somatic interventions,

3. short-term goals,

4. long-term goals, and

5. ancillary services.

Level 1 interventions are directed to dealing with whatever crisis is most critical—for example, homicidal or suicidal ideation. These level 1 interventions are typically designed to address whatever major issues exist on axis I. Level 2 interventions are directed at axes I and III. Any underlying medical or somatic interventions may have to be dealt with by physicians or other health-care providers. Level 3 interventions are typically short term in nature and directed at providing immediate relief from the pain and discomfort typically experienced by clients. The most effective way of achieving this is to address the axis IV dynamics. As clients learn to deal more effectively with their stressors (shocks), the need for the axis I arrangement to cope with the stressor fades. Level 4 interventions entail long-term goals that typically are directed at modifying the key lifestyle issues found on axis II. This can take awhile, and if clinicians attempt to deal with these issues without attempting at least some symptomatic relief (via interventions aimed at axis IV), then the chances increase that clients will be lost to treatment dropout or discouragement. More traditional interventions of analysis, insight, and interpretation are commonly used here. Level 5 interventions are called *ancillary services* because they involve processes that may be additional to the services provided in traditionally defined psychotherapy such as tutoring for academic problems, consultations with clergy for spiritual issues, 12-step support groups for substance abuse issues, and psychological, vocational, or neuropsychological testing. All of these are aimed at further improving functioning on axis V, the tasks of life, and therefore better preparing clients for future shocks.

Process of Psychotherapy

Adlerian psychotherapy has been characterized as having four stages (Dreikurs, 1967). In reality, these are not stages, but really processes that roughly appear in the following order, but can occur anytime. The four stages are *relationship* building; *investigating* and uncovering the dynamics of the clients, typically via the collection of lifestyle material; *interpretation* of the lifestyle so as to gain insight and reeducation as to the meaning clients have attached to life, themselves, and others; and *reorientation*, the process of teaching new skills and attitudes to encourage community feeling and social interest.

Adlerians believe *relationship* involves mutual respect between equals. The psychotherapist may be an expert in psychology, but the client is an expert about him- or herself. Both need to work collaboratively in order to achieve the desired outcome. Goals for treatment are mutually decided on whenever possible. If either the client or the therapist unilaterally impose treatment goals, therapy is likely to fail. Resistance is defined as a misalignment of goals between two equals.

Therapy can be conceptualized as a meeting of two worlds (Mahoney, 1980). Ideally, the psychotherapist represents common sense and community feeling. The client represents a misunderstanding of such things, and private logic is dominating his or her thinking. The client's world is nonconsensual about some key issue or issues. At one time, in the family of origin, it might have worked, but it does not now, and the client is suffering and stubbornly trying to impose his or her way on life and it is not working. The therapist must first join the client's world and see life from the client's perspective. As the client feels understood and warmly accepted, the therapist gradually begins to shift perspective and encourage the client to see life from another, more common-sense, perspective. If the relationship is strong, the client will follow and see things in a new light. The process of change has begun.

Investigation typically entails a lifestyle assessment but also begins in the initial interview. After a one- or two-session initial interview, if the client feels understood and can see the utility of the process, then typically one or two sessions are spent gathering the relevant historical material needed to formulate the lifestyle. The aforementioned Adlerian case formulation using the DSM is referred to as the *general diagnosis* by Adler and Adlerians (Adler, 1956; Carlson, Watts & Maniacci, 2006; Powers & Griffith, 1987).

The clients are described in somewhat nomothetic terms because they have been initially interviewed cross-sectionally, so to speak. They are interviewed in five key areas (Maniacci, 1999):

1. identifying information,
2. presenting problem,
3. relevant recent history of the problem,
4. current functioning, and
5. treatment expectations.

These five key areas (generally) answer these questions:

1. *Identifying information*: Who are you? Where do you live and work? How much education do you have? Are you in a relationship? Are you medically ill and on medications or receiving treatment of any kind?

2. *Presenting problem*: What brings you here? Why now? When did it start? What else was happening in your life when it began? Who is the first to notice when it happens? Who is most affected by your having this problem?

3. *Relevant recent history of the problem*: How far back have you had such a problem? How did you get along with peers as a kid? What made you choose certain people to be your friends? With teachers? What teachers did you learn best from? What teachers did you learn the least from? Have you ever had treatment for this problem before and with whom? What worked and did not work in that treatment? What was helpful and what was not?

4. *Current functioning*: Where do you work? How do you spend your time if you do not work? What kind of job do you like? What is your social life like? Who are your friends? Why them? What is your love life like? Are you satisfied? Why or why not? What makes someone attractive or unattractive to you?

5. *Treatment expectations*: What would be different in your life if you did not have this problem? Why do you think it is happening? What would you like us to do about it? How long will it take? How will we know when we are finished? Should anyone else be involved? Who is the most famous person of all time and why?

There are more questions, but initial interview questionnaires have been published and detailed elsewhere in Adlerian literature (Adler, 1956; Carlson, Watts, & Maniacci, 2006; Dreikurs, 1967; Maniacci, 1999; Powers & Griffith, 1987). These questions provide an overview and help formulate the general diagnosis.

The next part, the lifestyle assessment, Adler called the *special diagnosis* (Adler, 1956; Carlson, Watts, & Maniacci, 2006; Maniacci, 1999; Powers & Griffith, 1987). It is here where the specifics of the case, the particular idiographic nature of the process, shines through. Clients are given a semistructured interview that asks about their early childhood experiences. They typically are interviewed in the following key areas (Dreikurs, 1967; Shulman & Mosak, 1988):

sibling relationships and birth-order dynamics;

sibling ratings on a list of traits;

physical development;

school experiences;

sexual development;

social development;

religious or spiritual development, including meanings given to life;

> parental or caretaker descriptions;
>
> marriage or relationship description of the parental figures;
>
> cultural and economic dynamics of the community; and
>
> other role models and adults in the children's lives.

After these areas are assessed, the clients' *earliest memories* are elicited. Early recollections are those memories from before age 10 that can be visualized and have a clear narration to them (Shulman & Mosak, 1988). They must have a "one time this happened" quality to them (as opposed to a general description such as "we used to go to the beach all the time"). After the detailed narration is gathered, clients are asked to locate the most vivid moment of the memory and describe the relevant feeling or feelings associated with the memory. Typically, 7 to 10 memories are collected, but fewer may be all that are needed in many circumstances. The early memories are interpreted as a projective technique, and patterns are elicited that strikingly reveal the client's lifestyle (Clark, 2002; Mosak & DiPietro, 2006). An example of an early recollection is the following: "I was six years old. When I walked outside, I found a twenty dollar bill in the street. I thought wow, how awesome! The most vivid part: Finding the bill. Feeling: Happy."

This recollection might be indicative of someone with a low degree of activity who values getting great things with little effort. If such a theme persists throughout the other recollections, then a central theme (Mosak, 1977) would be identified that can reveal the core elements of the lifestyle.

Interpretation begins when the general diagnosis is initially presented via the case formulation and later when the lifestyle material is discussed and summarized for the client. The classical lifestyle summary has four parts to it (Shulman & Mosak, 1988):

1. a summary of the family constellation;

2. a summary of the early recollections;

3. a list of the client's faulty premises, which serve as a basis for his or her private logic (variously termed "errors," "basic mistakes," "interfering attitudes, beliefs behaviors," "interfering ideas," or "growth impeding convictions" in the literature; see Adler, 1956; Dreikurs, 1967; Powers & Griffith, 1987; Shulman & Mosak, 1988); and

4. a list of the client's assets and strengths.

Referring back the aforementioned case of Hillary, her lifestyle assessment revealed the following:

Summary of Family Constellation

Hillary is the youngest of four and only girl who was looked after by her siblings and mother. Her diabetes frightened all of them, and they overprotected her to the point of suffocating her. Hillary complied and even used their attentiveness to elicit attention and service, but it did not work as well with father. He was more stern and demanding. Hillary never quite knew how to handle him. She did figure out how to handle her brothers and her teachers at school, however, further proving to her how powerful being ill or fragile could be.

Summary of Early Recollections

I am a little lost soul. I need others to protect me from the dangers of life. People are a help to me when they care for me, but not when they criticize me. Life is unpredictable when I am alone, but safe in the care of others.

INTERFERING ATTITUDES, BELIEFS, BEHAVIORS

1. Hillary believes that life is dangerous.
2. She assumes she has to have others to make life safe. She cannot do it on her own.
3. She wants help but abhors criticism.

ASSETS AND STRENGTHS

1. She will accept help.
2. She cares and is a genuinely kind person.
3. Hillary loves sharing and giving.

The lifestyle assessment is presented to the client, and her feedback is elicited. Should she have any questions or objections, they are taken seriously and discussed; if needed, the summaries are amended until she feels comfortable.

Reorientation begins once the client accepts the lifestyle summary. Work begins on modifying the basic mistakes and encouraging the assets. Many tactics are available to Adlerian psychotherapists that help modify the lifestyle convictions that are troublesome (K. A. Adler, 1967; Carlson & Slavik, 1997; McKay & Dinkmeyer, 1994; Mosak & Maniacci, 1993, 1998; Nikelly, 1971; Rasmussen, 2010; Sherman & Fredman, 1986; Sperry, 1989, 1995; Starr, 1977; Watts & Carlson, 1999).

Mechanisms of Psychotherapy

Modeling

Adler (1956) felt that, for many people, the first good human relationship in their lives occurred in psychotherapy; hence, it was important for the therapist to model proper behavior. Ideally, the psychotherapeutic relationship should be between equals who are working together on a common task. Through empathy, goal alignment, and mutual discovery and encouragement, the clients begin to see things differently. The psychotherapist's next goal is to spread that to others outside of therapy.

Guessing

This may seem obvious to some and foolhardy to others, but Adlerians guess. They offer hypotheses to clients, typically but not always in the form of "Could it be that . . .?" or "Maybe you do that because. . ." Guessing does several things. First, it speeds up treatment. All therapists form hypotheses, but not many share them. By guessing, and sharing those guesses, Adlerians receive helpful feedback from clients. Second, guessing demonstrates *the courage to be imperfect*. Adlerians will simply look for a recognition response from the client, and if it is not there, say, "I am wrong. Let's try again." Seldom will clients be put off by such a stance. Often they will join in and help. Third, it facilitates the relationship. Clients often feel understood and appreciate the feedback, frequently reporting that it is better than when other therapists simply sit there silently. Fourth, it leads to faster problem solving and exploration. Until everyone agrees on what is going on, it is tough to move forward with treatment.

Pattern Recognition

Once they feel accepted, clients need to recognize their patterns and see the coherence in their choices and goals. By seeing the connections throughout life tasks, understanding the consistency from childhood into adulthood via the lifestyle assessment, and catching themselves enacting their lifestyles in session, clients gain a useful sense of control over their lives. It is difficult to accept their choices and make new ones when they are not even aware of their choices to begin with.

Task Setting

In sessions, clients are given something to do. They are encouraged to practice social skills, write letters, role play, draw, or simply think differently. As they feel more comfortable practicing in session, these tasks are assigned as homework in order to generalize the learning that occurs in therapy to real-world situations.

Encouragement

Encouragement is a technical term in Adlerian psychology. Courage has been defined as the willingness to risk even when the outcome is uncertain (Mosak, 1995). To *encourage* means to instill courage in clients. Adlerians believe that a key dynamic that leads to psychopathology is discouragement—a lack of faith in themselves and others. Reflecting feelings, offering gentle prompts to try again, showing faith in their abilities, accepting clients with their flaws and still demonstrating respect for them, and showing concern and interest— all of these help to encourage.

Early Recollections

Early recollections are most often used for assessment to help clients detect their patterns and see their goals (Mosak, 1977; Mosak & DiPietro, 2006). They can also be used to foster change. One way is to point out the similarity between what clients are currently doing and their early recollections. It can be quite startling when they realize the "rhythm of reoccurrence" (Dreikurs, 1933/1950, p. 44) in their lives. Another use of early recollections is to ask clients to take a painful memory from childhood and retell it, this time reworking it to have it "turn out any way you would want it to." They are instructed that they "are in complete control" and can have it "redone." This is often a clear depiction of the limits of their reasoning ability. Even the most intelligent clients are amazed at how difficult it can be to see how to restructure the recollection in a socially useful manner (Maniacci, 1996a). An example is this memory from an adult male client:

> Age 7. I was riding my bike and I cut the corner too closely. I fell off and tore up my arm. It hurt like heck, but I was too embarrassed to go home and show my parents, so I tried wiping it off in the grass and waiting to see if it stopped bleeding. It didn't and now it was dirty. Most vivid part: Wiping my arm in the grass. Feeling: Hurt and shame.

The therapist's original interpretation follows:

> He cuts things too closely. He takes risks and then tries to cover them up for fear of looking bad. His cover up is often worse than his original offense. He does not trust people to help him. When asked to restructure the memory, he produced the following:
>
> Age 7. I was riding my bike and I cut the corner too closely. I fell off and cut my arm, but not too badly. I was able to clean it up at a water fountain in the park and cover it up, so no one could see it.

The limits of his private logic are evident. He did change some aspects of the memory, but the crucial issue is unchanged. He still is a risk taker who cuts things too closely, and he still tries to cover up his mistakes. It took *four* additional attempts at restructuring before he even realized and could visualize the change of being more careful and deliberate and not taking such a chance to being with; even then, he still was too hesitant to trust people.

Dream Interpretation

Adlerians use dream interpretation. Even near the end of his life, more than 30 years after his initial meetings with Freud, Adler (1931/1964b) gave him credit and spoke well of Freud's attempt to understand dreams. Although he did not agree with Freud's view of dreams, he nonetheless valued the effort. Adlerians tend to see dreams as ways of preparing for the future (Adler, 1956; Gold, 1981; Shulman, 1973) and as rehearsals for future courses of action. One of their main functions is to be a factory of emotions in that they generate a feeling or mood that persists into the waking state and therefore spurs action in a particular direction. Unlike early recollections, which are about long-standing, lifestyle-based issues, dreams reflect the more recent concerns of the clients. Recurring dreams most likely represent more long-standing dynamics, but generally speaking dreams are attempts to solve current issues. Here is a dream from an adult female client: "I woke up, in bed, and I was alone. I felt something funny in my mouth and when I checked, I had no teeth. Most vivid part: Having no teeth. Feeling: Kind of happy."

Unlike early recollections, the key imagery in dreams requires associations and definitions in order to understand the references the clients are making. Her key associations were as follows: bed = a place to relax, be herself; alone = free; teeth = power; no teeth = I'm old. The dream was confusing until a connection was made: Her husband was missing from the bed. When asked about this, she grinned widely and said, "Hooray! I outlived the bastard!" Needless to say, couples counseling was offered. She declined.

Questioning

Adlerians are very proficient at asking questions and leading clients to find answers. An outline of some of the questions asked during the initial interview was presented previously. The significance of some of the questions can be detailed now.

"What would be different if you did not have your symptoms?" This has been referred to as "The Question." Adlerians have been using it for decades (Mosak & Maniacci, 1998). It serves two principle purposes. First, the answer to it often reveals what the client is avoiding. A client presents with symptoms of panic. She is asked The Question and responds that without her panic she would be able to work harder and spend more time with her kids. From an Adlerian perspective, this implies that she is using her panic to avoid the work and love tasks. Second, The Question can be used to aid in differential diagnosis. If the client said, "I'd be able to catch my breath and not feel my heart about to explode," a whole different meaning is assumed. There is no apparent social purpose implied in her answer. The chances are pretty high that her "panic" is not anxiety. There probably is some somatic pathology occurring. Another response could be, "I'd be able to catch my breath and not feel my heart about to explode, and I'd work harder and spend more time with the kids." This is clearly a blend between the two types of answers and implies that both psychosocial and somatic issues are occurring. She might be using genuine organic pathology for a social purpose. Both issues need to be addressed.

"Who is most affected by your symptoms?" This question typically elicits the target of the symptoms (Dreikurs, 1967). Many clients will (initially) respond that they are the most affected by their symptoms. Clinicians can be supportive, empathize, and then query further. "I know, it is tough. But after you, then who is most affected?" Often the client will then acknowledge, "Oh, my wife." This suggests the symptom is being used to alter or rebalance something with the client's wife. That needs to be explored.

"When did your symptoms start? What else was going on in your life at that time?" This is examining axis IV, psychosocial stressors, or what Adlerians refer to as the *shock* or *exogenous factor*. This frequently reveals what situation arose that the client was unprepared to handle (Dreikurs, 1967; Maniacci, 2002).

"Who is the most famous person of all time and why?" This question typically reveals a key organizing value for the client (Lombardi, 1973). As important as the answer itself is, the response to the query "why?" is even more crucial. A common answer is, "Jesus Christ." The answers to why can be quite varied. "Because he died for our sins" is a far cry from "Because his name is known everywhere." In the first instance, helping and sacrifice may be key values. In the second, attention and acknowledgment may be important.

Family Sculpting

This action-oriented technique is designed to reveal family dynamics and expectations (Sherman & Fredman, 1986). It is most easily done in family or group counseling, but it can be done in individual treatment as well. Clients are asked to stand up and, using other people or playing roles themselves, are then asked to sculpt the members of their family (either their current family or family of origin). They can put family members in any part of the room, in any pose, that would symbolize how they see them. After they have sculpted the cast of characters, they are asked to redo the sculpture to have the group be in an ideal pose, the way they would really want them to be. The two sculptures are compared.

It is fascinating to note who is sculpted first. Most times, that is the key member of the family the clients are most focused on. Next, the clients are taught that their symptoms are most often designed to move the people depicted from the first sculpture to the ideal sculpture. They do not realize it, but it is very often the case.

Confrontation

Adlerians are not shy about confrontation (Mosak & Maniacci, 1998; Shulman, 1973). However, although clients are often confronted, this never occurs in a hostile or demeaning manner. A confrontation is different from an interpretation. An interpretation does not require a response. It is offered by the therapist as a statement. The confrontation is designed to provoke a response and thereby increase discomfort. "So when do you plan on telling her?" is a confrontation as opposed to "You are afraid to tell her," which is an interpretation. Questions such as "When?" or "If you keep doing that how will you feel two hours from now?" are used to have the clients accept some accountability for their choices and engage the therapist in a meaningful dialogue.

Spitting in the Soup

Adler (1956) borrowed this unpleasant image but very helpful tactic from Charles Dickens' *Oliver Twist*. In the orphanage, children were starving. Typically, they were given bowls of thin soup as their main meal. It was not enough, so the children would run down the isles of the hall and spit in some inattentive child's bowl. The child would be so disgusted he or she would give up the soup, and the spitting child would get double the portion. Should the child choose to still eat the soup, it would taste horrible. Adler would use an interpretation to reframe the clients' symptoms in such a way that they would give them up—or if they still used them, they would be "spoiled." For example, a very proud client who was obsessive about hand washing was told that his symptom was really a declaration of disdain for others. "Cleanliness is next to Godliness, and you must be god-like in your desire to not touch what the rest of use and accept as normal." This explanation left a rather bad taste in his mouth, and sharply decreased the hand washing.

APPLICATIONS

Who Can We Help?

Adler himself and Adlerians in general work with a wide array of clients. As previously noted, Adler worked with all sorts of clients across diverse settings. Because the psychotherapy is so client based (as opposed to theory based), modifying tactics is easy as long as the basic assumptions of Adlerian psychology are not violated.

Non-Adlerian therapists often ask, "Are there any clients for whom Adlerian therapy does not work?" The surprising answer is, "No." Adlerians are flexible and rather eclectic in their styles. It is hard to find a tactic or approach that could not be used effectively. Some clients are not open to psychotherapy, and nothing works with them if they will not cooperate.

Adlerians have worked with and continue to help people with neuroses, psychotic symptoms, personality disorders, medical conditions, adjustment disorders, interpersonal problems, vocational problems, career-counseling issues, business consultations, and school problems. Adlerians consult and work with businesses, schools, clinics, hospitals, prisons, churches, and temples.

Adlerians have long been involved in parent and couple educational programs as well. Adler (1927/1957); Dreikurs (Dreikurs & Soltz, 1964); Dinkmeyer, McKay, and Dinkmeyer (1997); Popkin (1987); Nelsen (1996); West (1986); Main (1986); and Leman (1995) have all written best-selling parenting and couple education programs that are still in print.

In addition, authors such as Beecher and Beecher (1966/1986), Dreikurs (1946), Newman and Berkowitz with Owen (1971), Forer (Forer & Still, 1976), Leman (1985), McKay and Dinkmeyer (1994), and Dinkmeyer and Carlson (1984, 1989) have written top-selling self-help books for the general public. This goes back to a tradition Adler (1927/1957) himself started in 1927 with his best seller *Understanding Human Nature*.

Treatment

Adlerians engage in practically every type of treatment. As with most all of the founding members of psychotherapy, individual one-on-one therapy was the gold standard for years. Adler himself and other Adlerians have expanded the scope of practice ever since (Ansbacher 1992a).

The literature on couples and marriage treatment continues to grow (Carlson & Sperry, 1998, 1999; Dinkmeyer & Carlson, 1984, 1989; Evans & Dinkmeyer, 1993; Huber & Baruth, 1981; Kern, Hawes, & Christensen, 1989; Sperry & Carlson, 1991). Considering the social field theory assumption of Adlerian psychology, this is a natural progression. Couples counseling from the Adlerian point of view can be unique. The lifestyle-assessment process that is routinely conducted with individuals also has been used with couples. The tactic is called *lifestyle matching*. Each person's lifestyle is assessed, and then both parties are brought together with their lifestyles in hand. Typically, the two summaries are matched along the following dimensions:

psychological vantage point,

gender expectations,

family atmosphere,

family values, and

current approaches to life.

Psychological vantage point refers to how both partners saw their sibling relationships. Were both the oldest born who found their places by leading, taking charge? Was one a youngest and the other a middle? What did these roles mean? How did they learn to relate to others, and what did they expect others to do in response to them?

Gender expectations explores what the partners think about issues of masculinity and femininity. Were there traditional roles assigned in their respective families? Who did what and how? Do they have unique perspectives on gender that may not match each other's expectations?

Family atmosphere is next to be examined. Did each partner grow up with similar family atmospheres? If not, how did they differ? As already noted, the adult correlate of the childhood family atmosphere is frequently seen as the adult's prevailing mood. Is there a mismatch in mood and emotional tone?

Family values are discussed and matched next. As discussed, the dominant family values can find their adult correlate as stressors. "These issues are important to me." "I care and get worked up about these issues." Are the couple's values congruent? Do they discuss and negotiate them or "sweep them under the rug"?

Current approaches to life are examined by looking at the central themes in the early recollections of each partner. Is there any overlap? Do they radically differ? Is one person mostly a risk taker and the other a homebody? Do they both have competitive attitudes, or are they peacemakers?

Adlerians are quite involved in family treatment (Bitter & Main, 2011; Carlson, Sperry, & Lewis, 1997, 2005; Christensen & Schramski, 1983; Dagley, 2000; Grunwald & McAbee, 1999; Kottman, 1995; Maniacci & Carlson, 1991; Mosak & Maniacci, 1993; Sherman, 1999; Sherman & Dinkmeyer, 1987; Sherman & Fredman, 1986). Family treatment has typically been delineated along two dimensions in Adlerian psychology: family counseling and family therapy.

Family counseling can often be done in a public setting (though it is regularly done in private as well) and frequently is the cornerstone of family education centers that Adlerians establish in communities. This tradition goes back to Adler and Dreikurs and continues to this day. Families are screened and invited to participate in two ways: as the demonstration family on stage and in the audience watching. Those in the audience can be invited on stage in the future. The families are counseled about typical family issues such as bedtimes, chores, mild family fights, sibling rivalry, and general lack of cooperation. The recommendations are direct and encouraging, and they usually follow the ones discussed in popular Adlerian-based self-help parenting manuals (e.g., Nelsen, 1996).

Family therapy is done in private. The issues may be quite the same as in family counseling, but they also can be rather different. More personal and more demanding issues are addressed such as delinquency, substance abuse, issues of neglect, and high-conflict fighting, as well as extreme disrespect and defiance. Although many of the typical Adlerian parent recommendations are still applied, the core lifestyle dynamics of the individual members often become the focus as well.

Adlerians are enthusiastic about group therapy (e.g., Corsini, 1971; Shulman, 1973). Similar to the distinction between family counseling and family therapy, groups can be found along a spectrum.

Group counseling is mostly psychoeducational in nature. Many times, the groups can be content specific such as a couples group, a parenting group, or a cardiac survivors group. Books can be read and discussed, and minilectures can be provided (e.g., Dinkmeyer, McKay, & Dinkmeyer, 1997).

Group therapy has many of the same dynamics as family therapy. Oftentimes, more complex and involved issues are addressed, and the structure is less didactic and more exploratory and interactive.

Multiple psychotherapy has been used by Adlerians for a long time (Dreikurs, Shulman, & Mosak, 1984). Many Adlerians prefer to work in a practice with other Adlerians. It is common to have a second therapist occasionally sit in on sessions and offer feedback. This facilitates training; the handling of challenging clients, families, and groups; and keeping cases from going "too far off course" because of a therapist's blind spots. The therapists can model cooperation, disagreement while maintaining mutual respect, and "good cop–bad cop" dynamics, to mention but a few of the possibilities. Unique to the Adlerian approach to multiple psychotherapy is the use of two therapists to assess the lifestyle. In the classical approach, one therapist spends two or three sessions gathering the data, and another comes in for the interpretation and composes the summaries and lists the basic mistakes and assets (see Powers & Griffith, 1987, for actual transcripts of such sessions).

Adlerians also routinely use art therapy (Dreikurs, 1986), movement therapy, psychodrama (Starr, 1977), and role playing (Corsini, 1966). Some have recently branched out into mindfulness, meditation, biofeedback, neurofeedback, and relaxation training as part of their work.

The Setting

Although Adlerians operate in many settings, private practice, hospitals, clinics, schools, prisons, businesses, and family education centers are the most common settings. There is no distinctly Adlerian way to set up an office other than personal preference and taste. The common thread would most likely be a sense of warmth, equality, and comfort.

Testing

Because Adlerian psychotherapy is mostly a psychoeducational model of treatment, physical examinations are often recommended to rule out clear-cut organic pathology and assess the need for somatic interventions. Depending on a number of factors, including the response to "The Question," physical examinations can be required before any further psychotherapy is tried.

Adlerians often use psychological testing, and some have written about it (e.g., Carlson, Watts, & Maniacci, 2006; Sperry, 1995). The most common psychological tests Adlerians use are intelligence tests, projective tests (most often the Rorschach inkblot test, and the Thematic Apperception Test, or TAT), drawings (Draw-a-Person Test, House-Tree-Person Test), and objective personality inventories (Minnesota Multiphasic Personality Inventory).

Two standardized and normed tests have been published. The Basic Adlerian Scales for Interpersonal Success (BASIS-A) inventory has been used extensively in research and practice over the past several years. It is a 65-item test grounded in Adlerian theory. It measures individuals along five dimensions: belonging–social interest, going along, taking charge, wanting recognition, and being cautious. In addition, there are five supporting scales that round out the personality profile: harshness, entitlement, liked by all, striving for perfection, and softness. The other test on the market is the Children's Apperceptive Storytelling Test (CAST). It is similar to the TAT in that it has a standard series of cards depicting social scenarios. Clients are prompted to tell stories that are coded and scored along several dimensions derived from Adlerian principles.

The Therapist

Adlerians typically do not practice as anonymous therapists, and they seldom simply withdraw and observe. They interact, challenge, question, and debate but always in a respectful, egalitarian manner. Of course they make mistakes—all people do—but they see these mistakes as an opportunity to model the courage to be imperfect. Because Adlerians tend to guess, they "put themselves out there." Therapy goes faster that way, because all therapists guess, but at least Adlerians tend to share those guess with clients and receive feedback sooner than later.

Patient Problems

Adlerian therapists will deliberately avoid the most challenging situations. The three most common problems Adlerians face are probably true for all therapies: disliking clients, sexual feelings for and from clients, and suicide.

The first two issues are not unique to Adlerians and are handled much the same way as in other therapies. It is hard to work collaboratively with clients therapists do not like. Can it be done? Probably. Should it be done? That is more complex, and there is no clear answer. Supervision and consultation are strongly recommended in such cases, and multiple therapy can help as well. Referral to another therapist is often appropriate in these cases. Sexual intimacy with a client is never acceptable and should never happen, and neither are any other forms of dual relationships, with one possible exception. Adlerians will frequently move between treatment formats, for example, from family to individual therapy and back again. As long as the limits of confidentiality are clearly spelled out and maintained, and clients are clear about communications, boundaries, and expectations, the flow is fairly natural and generally not difficult.

Suicide is another matter, and suicide threats are always taken seriously. Once again, Adlerians mostly handle these situations as others do—with contracts, phone calls to relevant caretakers, and hospitalization if needed. Unique to the Adlerian perspective is the "spitting in the soup" tactic described previously. Once the situation is contained and safe, clients can be confronted with the purposes of their suicidal ideation, threats, plans, and actions. Evasion, revenge and retaliation, and hopelessness are common purposes and should be processed and explored (K. A. Adler, 1961, 1967) .

Evidence

The field of psychology has moved toward an evidence-based approach to provide the best treatment for clients. Adlerians have both encountered challenges to this movement and have stepped up to this challenge by engaging in and providing a growing body of research that validates many Adlerian constructs and techniques. The challenges that Adlerians have faced have been twofold: (1) Adlerians focus on understanding and treating the idiographic aspects of the individual and (2) clients present with complex problems and concerns that often don't fit the simple research paradigms sometimes associated with the emphasis on evidence-based therapies.

Adlerians have long emphasized the idiographic aspects of the clients they serve. They are interested in knowing the client's self-created goals and belief systems, as well as the role of symptoms. In this way, the Adlerian seeks to "treat the person" rather than "treat the symptoms." The assessment of the client's experience, goals and belief system, and role of symptoms yields a unique picture from one client to the next. The study of this process therefore lends itself to a case-study approach versus the randomized controlled trial method. Moreover, because Adlerians utilize a wide range of techniques that varies from client to client based on the client's idiographic presentation, a manualized approach to treating symptoms, such as seen with cognitive-behavioral therapy, becomes difficult. A final distinction to be made that illustrates the difficulties in fully moving toward evidence-based practice is in the differences inherent in the quantitative versus qualitative approaches to research. Although Adlerians have conducted quantitative research, as will be presented later, Adlerian psychology lends itself especially well to qualitative and case-study research approaches.

A second challenge in the evidence-based model involves the complex presentation of many if not all clients who come to therapy and counseling. Of course, this is a challenge for other systems as well. Clients typically come to therapy with a variety of symptoms rather than "just" depression or "just" anxiety, and these symptoms often compound one another, making it difficult to only target one set of symptoms. Moreover, clients do not live in a vacuum, and their lives are complex and changing, which also compounds the symptom pattern as well as the area of focus in the therapy. Although the Adlerian emphasis on understanding each individual's lifestyle and how it relates to current challenges is unique, it does not provide a "prescription" of treatment of symptoms that cuts across the board for all clients. Research on Adlerian therapy may be difficult, but research on Adlerian theory is plentiful.

Despite these challenges, Adlerian theory has undergone a good deal of research. For example, considerable research has looked at some of the nomothetic constructs of Adlerian theory, such as that seen in the research on birth order (Eckstein et al., 2010). Much research has also been undertaken that confirms the validity and reliability of techniques such as early recollections (Mosak & Di Pietro, 2006) and the use of "The Question" (Sackett-Maniacci, 1999). There also is a substantial body of evidence, more quantitative in nature, that measures lifestyle themes. This can be seen by the use of the BASIS-A in research (Kern, Gormley, & Curlette, 2008).

Birth order has been widely studied and has been shown to be a valid construct of personality development. Eckstein and colleagues (2010) provided a meta-analysis of birth-order research and found several lifestyle (personality) factors associated with birth order. For example, a tendency toward success and achievement were seen in first-born children, middle children were shown to demonstrate a tendency toward high sociability, and only children were found to also be high in achievement motivation. Although there has been some controversy related to the evidence of birth order and its relationship to personality, research has demonstrated support for differences in birth-order characteristics according to psychological birth-order position.

The concept of lifestyle is hallmark to Adlerian theory. Lifestyle assessment has a goal to glean a comprehensive picture of the client's subjective experience and as such is a highly subjective tool that can make objective measurement a challenge. However, attempts have been made to measure lifestyle from a more objective framework that offers the ability to measure lifestyle themes. The BASIS-A inventory was designed with that purpose in mind. To date, the BASIS-A has been widely used in many research studies. In a review of these studies, Kern, Gormley, and Curlette (2008) demonstrate the validity of the BASIS-A inventory and its use with a variety of populations, including substance abusers, incarcerated sexual offenders, chronic migraine headache sufferers, eating disorders, and others. The BASIS-A has also been used to determine the similarity of the construct of lifestyle with the construct of attachment styles described in attachment theory (Peluso et al., 2009).

According to Mozdzierz, Peluso, and Lisiecki (2009), research has revealed four crucial elements that appear to be present in effective therapy: warmth, empathy, acceptance, and encouragement of risk taking. Adlerians seek to establish a warm, collaborative relationship based on mutual respect, and much has been written about techniques that can be used to encourage, motivate, and demonstrate concern for the client (Mosak & Maniacci, 1998). Early recollections have also been used not only as a method of understanding and empathizing with the client but also as a means of deciding how to work with the clients based on their beliefs surrounding seeking help (Kern, Stoltz, Gottlieb-Low, & Frost, 2009). Early recollections also enhance the therapeutic alliance because therapists can adjust their style and interventions according to clients' preferred methods of help seeking.

There is also research that has been conducted outside of the Adlerian theory that validates many Adlerian constructs. Two particularly excellent examples are the works of Roy Baumeister and Brene Brown. Baumeister and Leary (1995) validated the construct of the need to belong. The need to belong is part and parcel of Adler's thinking with respect to his notion of social interest. In her qualitative research on shame and resilience, Brown (2007) finds support for Adler's ideas that people are motivated to strive from a feeling of *less than* (i.e., inferior, inadequate) to a feeling of *more than* (i.e., perfection, superiority). Similarly, the works of Jeffery Binder (2004) and John Gottman (1999) have provided empirical validation for many Adlerian constructs.

Psychotherapy in a Multicultural World

Psychotherapy is an interpersonal process. Adlerians especially see it as a meeting of two worlds: the client's and the therapist's. This interface requires both tact and respect.

In a multicultural world, psychotherapy can be perceived as intrusive. This occurs especially when clinicians fail to appreciate the worldviews of clients. The Adlerian use of the lifestyle assessment addresses this problem to a large extent. Through the process of inquiry about early childhood situations; parenting styles and values; religious, economic, and cultural themes; and educational and social situations, Adlerians rapidly become educated about the dynamics of many cultures and races. Guessing and providing feedback helps as well, so clients can correct and amend any preconceptions clinicians have. The authors have conducted detailed lifestyle assessments over the years with numerous clients. The list of countries includes China, Ghana, Israel, Ireland, Iraq, Iran, South Africa, Belize, Thailand, Vietnam, Korea, Japan, France, England, Canada, Italy, Columbia, Turkey, and Germany. Several lifestyles have been done on Native Americans as well. The lifestyle assessment process has helped clients teach us about the world as well as themselves. Never have they found it intrusive or problematic, and we have benefited greatly from hearing their stories. Working with clients from diverse cultures is much like taking a personal tutorial in multiculturalism with each new client.

CASE EXAMPLE

Kate presented for psychotherapy reluctantly. She was "sent in" by two of her friends, both of whom had previously seen one of the authors (MPM) for brief psychotherapy. She was uncomfortable but willing to give it a try—"once or twice." After a few awkward silences, she began her story.

Identifying Information

Kate was 48 years old and in her second marriage of 16 years after having been previously married for 13 years. She had a stepson from her husband's previous marriage and three of her children from her first marriage, all adults (one female, two males). She had a master's degree, worked as an elementary school librarian, and was not religious, though her parents came from a "mixed marriage" of a Polish-Catholic father and a Native American (Cherokee) mother. She was on no medication but reported a very long history of anxiety and social withdrawal.

Presenting Problem

"I think about dying, all the time," she stated matter of factly. "I never acted on it—except at age 16, when I overdosed." She called a friend, passed out, and paramedics were called. "I can't take my mother and my kids emotionally blackmail me," she forcefully stated. She reported being anxious "all my life," and she could not pinpoint a time when she was not anxious. Her children and mother would be most hurt if she acted her suicidal thoughts, but she had not formulated any concrete plans—"yet." Her favorite youngest child was marrying in a few weeks, and because of pressure from their father and her two other children, he had informed Kate she was not invited to his wedding.

Relevant Recent History

She was the youngest of five, with a sister 12 years older, a brother 11 years older, a brother 10 years older, and a third brother 5 years older. She was "never right and never could do anything right." "I was an afterthought." She always suspected her eldest sister was, secretly, her mother, but no one would talk about it or deny it when Kate pressed for an answer. She left her first husband because he beat her and threatened on three separate occasions to kill her and the children with a shotgun if she did not leave. She did, after much "agony," and left the kids with him. The children never forgave her, and she never forgave herself. She had "a little bit of counseling with the divorce, but it went nowhere."

Current Functioning

She loved her career and the kids she worked with, and she acknowledged being "very closed, private" at work but well respected and loved by students. "I just refuse to share anything with anybody." Everybody ended up disappointing her after "great starts," she declared.

She sees her friends frequently but maintains a distance, keeping her "true self" to herself. For fun, they ride motorcycles. Her best friend, Gail, had a "similar background" and does not let people get close to her either. "We're close in our silence." Gail had been a client of one of the authors (MPM), and said, "You can trust him, he's different." That was enough for Kate. Her friendships always started out strong, then fizzled after she got "tired of them and they wound up disappointing and hurting me."

Her marriage was "wonderful." "I'm a spoiled rotten brat—Finally!" Her husband cooked for her, filled her car with fuel, and loved her deeply. "I'm waiting for the rug to be pulled out," she added. "How can it last?" It was "just a matter of time until he leaves," and she secretly tested him by acting tempestuously to see if he would stay. He always did, much to her surprise.

Treatment Expectations

When asked what would be different in her life if she was not so chronically suicidal, she replied, "I can't imagine. I always have been." She then paused before adding, "I'd relax and let go. I wouldn't have to work so hard at staying alive." She did not know why she was so suicidal in her thoughts. She wanted therapy to tell her why the thoughts were always there because she no longer trusted herself. She wanted no one else in treatment with her because her husband "wouldn't understand" and her kids "wouldn't care." She had two responses to who she thought the most famous person of all time was: Her first response was "No one," then after a few minutes added, "Jesus" because "if you're going to die, go out for a cause."

General Diagnosis

Kate was a survivor, someone who has gone through life believing that she was better off alone. She could take care of others, but she did not expect others to take care of her. She was both happy and pessimistic about her husband's attention and believed it was not going to last. It was explained to her she did not appear to be suicidal but rather seemed to be testing herself to see how strong she really was. Given the fact that she was "too comfortable" with all of the pampering from her husband, she needed to regularly prove she was strong (on her own) by regularly *not killing herself!* Each time she did not act on it, she felt a triumph, a victory, and accomplished. *She was strong enough to survive all on her own without any help from him or anyone else!*

Axis I: Anxiety disorder not otherwise specified.

Axis II: Avoidant personality disorder (with borderline features).

Axis III: None reported.

Axis IV: Conflict with her children; too comfortable with husband.

Axis V: GAF: 65 currently; 65 highest past year (long-standing moderate impairment).

Kate was presented with a (verbal) summary of the diagnosis and was "blown away." She had never thought of it like that before. She broke out in tears. "I need to think," she added, and she scheduled the next appointment before wanting to leave. She was offered a brief therapy contract of 10 sessions. She thought 10 was "a bit much," yet she agreed and hurried out.

Session 2. Her son's wedding was approaching, and Kate wanted one session to discuss how to handle it. He had called, and she was invited. This was worst than before. At least, when she was not invited, she could avoid the tension. Now what? She was taught some deep breathing and relaxation techniques, and given this directive: At the wedding, instead of having a low degree of activity and waiting for others to approach her, she would "take charge, assert herself, and greet people warmly." With a higher degree of activity, she might feel more in charge and therefore, less anxious. She loved the thought, but did not know if she could "pull it off." As the session ended, she added warmly that for the first time in her memory, she had gone a whole week without a suicidal thought. She could not explain why, but felt it could have "something to do with that last comment about proving how strong" she was.

Sessions 3–5: Special Diagnosis. Her lifestyle was collected during two sessions and summarized back to her during the third session. She had an alcoholic, physically abusive father who beat her mother and the children regularly. All of the children scattered. Mother, a Cherokee, was ridiculed by her own people in their small home town for marrying a "white man" and was also rejected by the "whites." Not welcomed in school, shunned by all but one peer, and sent away to a private "Indian" school, she withdrew into herself and her books. Kate's earliest recollections follow:

1. Age 6. Bill, James, and I were playing in the backyard with Rich. He said let's go to the garage, and the next thing I know it burned down. Most vivid part: The fire. Feeling: Fun, then dread.

2. Age 6. Sitting in the sandbox. Everybody started yelling my name, hoping I'd run away. Mom's (female) best friend grabbed hold of me and took me home and dad yelled, furious at me. Most vivid part: Laughing, I didn't understand what all the fuss was about. Feeling: Fun.

3. Age 8. My (male) dog died. I came home from school and mom said "Your damn dog died." Most vivid part: Sad and trying to get away because if you cried in front of her, you'd be in trouble. Feeling: Sad.

4. Age 9. The (male) principal and some lady walked into my classroom and said come to the office. I asked what was wrong and they said "You're Indian." Most vivid part: Mom was there, crying. Feeling: Sadness, I just got kicked out of school for being Indian.

5. Age 7. I went out the backdoor and when I came back, it was locked. I went over to a girlfriend's house, but her mom said I couldn't come in because they were having a party. I went to another house, and they weren't home. I sat and cried. Most vivid part: Looking for somewhere to go and realizing no one was there. Feeling: Sadness and a sense of being lost.

6. Age 7. Sitting on the porch with Grandfather. It was stormy and mom was going crazy trying to get us into the basement. Grandfather said "If God's going to get you, he'll get you here or there." People were ridiculous, screaming like little girls, running down the street, and a tornado came right by us. Most vivid part: The excitement and the tornado. Feeling: Excited.

7. Age 6. Riding my bike into the porch. My brother had hold of the seat and let go without telling me. I didn't know how to brake, went over the handlebars, and into my other brother's lap. Most vivid part: Dave teaching me. Feeling: I guess happy—anything with my brother Dave made me happy, even if I got hurt.

8. Age 5. I went to the wrong school bus stop. Big brother, who was a crossing guard, wasn't there and I went too far. I cried and some guy in a white van took me home. Mom yelled at him when we got there. Most vivid part: Mom yelling at him for driving me home. Feeling: Happy to be home but confused—why was she so mad at him?

Summary of Family Constellation

Kate is the fifth of five children and psychologically an only child who grew up with an older sister and three older brothers who mostly had nothing to do with each other, making this a 2–1–1–1 family constellation. This was a family dominated by father's tyrannical behavior. He couldn't resist showing his superiority, which usually meant showing others their inferiority. Mother was defeated by him when she was with him, but when he left (as he often did for days at a time), she blossomed. At those times, the home changed, and people were allowed to shine for themselves. Kate valued and even cherished such moments. She wanted to be kind, hardworking, and giving—as mother was when father was gone—but it couldn't last. Whether from father's ignorance or the town's bigotry, Kate felt rejected and humiliated. She decided to fight for herself, unlike mother, and not let the bastards get away with it. Her stance only worked to a point. Her friend's father, her mother (at times), and her idolized brother (when he was around) all served to keep her from becoming totally hopeless. Add to that her positive experience at the Indian school, where, despite her hardened exterior, she decided to keep a soft underbelly. When she couldn't fight, she opted for withdrawal into fantasy, mostly through books and reading. She vowed, mostly to herself, never to be dependent on anyone again, and to fight before she would be taken down; yet inside she still hoped for that special place, and she also hoped that special someone would help her find hope and love—and eventually acceptance.

Summary of Early Recollections

Nothing good lasts. I had better prepare myself for the worst and not get upset and scream like a "little girl." I refuse to panic, even when I am upset (inside). I sometimes don't see how things go so bad, but they will. I want to count on a man to back me up and help me achieve, but if I do, and he lets go, I'll be hurt because I fell head over heels for him.

INTERFERING ATTITUDES, BELIEFS, BEHAVIORS

1. Kate is so busy preparing for the worst she misses the best.
2. She confuses being emotional with being weak.
3. She wants support and is hurt when she doesn't get it, but she doesn't tell people about it or her fears.
4. Unconsciously, Kate sets herself up to "burn things down" without knowing she does it. She is so busy focusing on the negative that she might precipitate what she fears.
5. She doesn't give herself enough credit for her strength and all she has survived.

ASSETS AND STRENGTHS

1. She cares.
2. She is brave.
3. Kate will accept help.
4. She knows how to have fun and enjoy herself.
5. She is an excellent student.
6. Once she gives her heart and loyalty to someone, she is faithful to the extreme. (She may even believe more in others than in herself.)

Kate was stunned. She said, "Wow, you nailed it. That's me! I swear it's just like you grew up with me." She took the prepared copy of her lifestyle assessment and went home to think and reflect.

Session 6. Kate reported a change. She went to the wedding, warmly greeted everybody, and didn't even attend to some of the "dirty looks" she got. She felt different, as if she somehow "wasn't so alone." She couldn't explain why. She thought she felt understood and that she realized she wasn't a little girl anymore.

Sessions 7–10. The next four sessions went very smoothly. She asked a lot of questions about her assessment. These sessions focused on her misunderstanding of her role in life. She thought she had to prove her worth, but that was tough because she had to do it anonymously. If she stood out too much, she might be singled out, and like the recollection about school, the reward for being singled out (even as great) might be rejection. She was "trying to chase two rabbits at once" (Beecher & Beecher, 1966/1986, p. 73). If she was too outstanding, she would bring attention to herself, and that could lead to trouble. So she was quiet, but then she felt she was not earning her keep, and people would not find her worthwhile and would abandon her. She was damned if she did, and damned if she didn't. In session, she practiced countering her negative thinking and anticipating rejection if she spoke up. At the 10th session, she warmly asked if she could "stay a little longer, just a bit." Six more sessions were negotiated.

Sessions 11–16. Kate wanted to examine interfering attitude number four—that she unconsciously might be setting herself up for trouble. She wanted to learn how to expect more from life and accept the good. It was pointed out to her that she regularly believed that, like mother, the only truly good times were to be had when father was out of town on business and that maybe she felt that the only time she could really relax and enjoy herself was when she was alone—and the possible implications that had for her marriage. Tearfully, she admitted she secretly longed for alone time, and that as much as she loved her husband, it was somehow wrong to enjoy having him at home. She worked to change that. Her sessions ended with no more suicidal ideation, no anxiety, and much more self-acceptance. The gains lasted at three- and six-month follow-up calls.

Sessions 17–18. Seven months after the last session (i.e., one month after the six-month follow-up call), Kate called and requested two additional sessions. Something "truly frightening yet eye opening" had happened, and she didn't want to talk about it over the phone. Kate, her husband, and some friends took a cross-country motorcycle ride. In the Northwest, at the side of a mountain, she wandered over to take a picture. Despite warnings from her husband and friends, she went to the edge of a cliff. The ground gave way and she fell. She dropped the camera, grabbed a vine, and held on for "dear life." She frantically managed to claw her way up, her husband and friends dove to the ground, formed a chain, and pulled her back. She cried for almost an hour. At the moment she grabbed the vine and began clawing, she reported two things flashed through her mind. First, the initial interview "guess" vividly came back to mind—she really did not want to die. Second, she caught herself in interfering attitude number four—she was a person who unconsciously set herself up for the negative. She would never do that again.

Kate is doing well. Follow up at one year, two years, and three years (via phone) found no symptoms. She recently sent a letter with an enclosed check for the one last session she owed with the following explanation:

> Dr. Mike:
>
> OK by now I bet you thought I forgot to pay you. Well no—it's just hard to explain. Actually now you can take the check and throw the letter away or you could read on for one of my crazy thoughts!
>
> I thought about writing this letter and sending out the check almost on a daily basis but every time I started I felt like I was completely saying good bye to a friend. So in a weird sort of way my mind was saying if you don't pay him then you will always have a connection without closure. OK here's where you are saying that you will always be a phone call away, right? But to me putting closure on how you helped me change is a very sad thing. I find myself hearing your explanations when life throws something at me. I hear you sighing and rolling your eyes when I try to control something I can't control. I even see your hand tapping your knee telling me that I'm ok and everything else comes after that. So how do I put closure on that? Why would I want to? I have changed so much because of you helping me put things in perspective that I can only say that I procrastinated sending you a check because now I'm ok and everyone else can ****ing wait. ☺
>
> Hope you have a Merry Christmas and a great new year!
>
> Thanks again,
>
> Kate

SUMMARY

Adlerian theory is alive and well. Its holistic, teleological, phenomenological, interpersonal, motivational, and cognitive aspects are now mainstream, and many other systems keep rediscovering its basic tenets and principles. Ellenberger (1970) noted, "It would not be easy to find another author from which so much has been borrowed from all sides without acknowledgment than Adler" (p. 645). Adler himself wrote in 1933,

> Individual Psychology, which is essentially a child of this age, will have a permanent influence on the thought, poetry, and dreams of humanity. It will attract many

enlightened disciples, and many more who will hardly know the names of its pioneers. It will be understood by some, but the numbers of those who misunderstand it will be greater. It will have many adherents, and still more enemies. Because of its simplicity many will think it too easy, whereas those who know it will recognize how difficult it is. (Adler, 1933/1950, p. vii)

After understanding Adlerian psychotherapy, clinicians find it easy to integrate the diverse systems and findings of many other schools. It communicates well to clients, and it serves as a comfortable bridge for treatment planning, case formulation, and integrating contemporary diagnostic language.

 Counseling CourseMate Website:

See this text's Counseling CourseMate website at www.cengagebrain.com for learning tools such as chapter quizzing, videos, glossary flashcards, and more.

ANNOTATED BIBLIOGRAPHY

Adler, A. (1956). *The Individual Psychology of Alfred Adler: A systematic presentation in selections from his writings* (H. L. Ansbacher & R. R. Ansbacher, Eds.). New York: Basic Books.
This has been the main reference to Adler's key writings for decades. It is still required reading for anyone wishing a detailed introduction to Adler's original writings.

Adler, A. (2002–2006). *The collected clinical works of Alfred Adler*: Volumes 1–12 (H. Stein, Ed.). San Francisco: Classical Adlerian Translation Project. (Original works published 1898–1937)
The clinical works of Alfred Adler have been newly translated and edited and are available online, in print, and via Kindle. The new translations reflect masterful work by all concerned.

Carlson, J., & Maniacci, M. P. (Eds.). (2012). *Alfred Adler revisited*. New York: Routledge.
The editors assembled 23 of Adler's original articles and requested comments from 21st-century experts in various fields. The new introductions by those experts, along with the articles themselves, prove refreshing and stimulating. The articles cover everything from early recollections to dream analysis, birth order, psychoanalysis, education, and therapy—plus more.

Carlson, J., Watts, R. E., & Maniacci, M. P. (2006). *Adlerian therapy: Theory and practice*. Washington, DC: American Psychiatric Association.
This is the latest textbook on Adlerian therapy. Individual, couple, group, and family therapies are covered in detail with updated references, resources, and a list of videos that demonstrate Adlerian therapy in different formats.

Hoffman, E. (1994). *The drive for self: Alfred Adler and the founding of Individual Psychology*. New York: Addison-Wesley.
This is the best biography of Adler. Painstakingly researched, it includes many details previously unknown to scholars. The section on Adler's work with Abraham Maslow is especially fascinating.

Manaster, G. J., & Corsini, R. J. (1982). *Individual Psychology: Theory and practice*. Itasca, IL: F. E. Peacock.
This is the first textbook written in English by two students of Rudolf Dreikurs. It remains a classic in the Adlerian field and one of the best written works in Adlerian psychology.

Mosak, H. H., & Maniacci, M. P. (1998). *Tactics in counseling and psychotherapy*. Itasca, IL: F. E. Peacock.
This textbook covers more than 100 tactics used in Adlerian psychotherapy and presented from the perspective of "What do I do when . . . ?"

Mosak, H. H., & Maniacci, M. P. (1999). *A primer of Adlerian psychology: The analytic- cognitive-behavioral psychology of Alfred Adler*. Philadelphia: Brunner/Mazel.
This book examines the basic assumptions of Adlerian theory and detail such topics as personality development, lifestyle, psychopathology, and interventions.

Mozdzierz, G. J., Peluso, P. R., & Lisiecki, J. (2009). *Principles of counseling and psychotherapy: Learning the essential domains and nonlinear thinking of master practitioners*. New York: Routledge.
This is an excellent text for both novice and experienced clinicians who want to learn the skills necessary for all aspects of effective treatment and the development of core competencies in counseling and therapy. This book speaks to both Adlerians and non-Adlerians as it breaks down the complex process of psychotherapy.

Rasmussen, P. R. (2010). *The quest to feel good*. New York: Routledge.
In this excellent new perspective on Adlerian theory and therapy, the author integrates the works of Alfred Adler with Theodore Millon and produces a rare book that is good for both clinicians and clients. His integration of the latest research on emotions with Adlerian theory is excellent.

CASE READINGS

Adler, A. (1929). *The case of Miss R. : The interpretation of a life story* (E. Jenson & F. Jenson, Trans.). New York: Greenberg.

> This classic by Adler is a verbatim transcript of his interpreting the case history of a patient he did not treat as the case was presented to him. This is a complex case that demonstrates many of basic Adlerian principles.

Adler, A. (1964). The case of Mrs. A. In A. Adler, *Superiority and social interest: A collection of later writings* (H. L. Ansbacher & R. R. Ansbacher, Eds.) (pp. 159– 190). Evanston, IL: Northwestern University Press. (Original work published 1931)

> Similar to *The case of Miss R.,* Adler does a line-by-line interpretation of a case for an audience of professionals. This presents another very challenging case but a much shorter presentation.

Dreikurs, R. (1997). Family counseling: A demonstration. In J. Carlson & S. Slavik (Eds.), *Techniques in Adlerian psychology* (pp. 466–484). Washington, DC: Accelerated Development. (Original work published 1972)

> This is a classic example of how "Dr. D" would do family counseling, an actual transcript of the session conducted before an audience of professionals.

Manaster, G. J., & Corsini, R. J. (1982). *Individual Psychology: Theory and practice.* Itasca, IL: F. E. Peacock.

> Chapter 17 offers a verbatim transcript of a client who keeps getting into trouble when he is only trying to help. This is an especially useful teaching case.

Maniacci, M. P. (1998). The psychotic couple. In J. Carlson & L. Sperry (Eds.), *The disordered couple* (pp. 57–81). Bristol, PA: Brunner/Mazel.

> In 15 sessions, a psychotic man was provided couples therapy from an Adlerian perspective. Follow-ups at 1 month, 3 months, 6 months, 1 year and 4 years, found him to be free from psychosis, off all medications, and stable.

Maniacci, M. P. (1999). Clinical therapy. In R. E. Watts & J. Carlson (Eds.), *Interventions and strategies in counseling and psychotherapy* (pp. 59–85). Philadelphia: Accelerated Development.

> Clinical therapy is defined as the psychotherapy of complex cases. This is a detailed case history involving 94 sessions over a 4-year period with several years of follow-up. This case demonstrates an integration of the DSM-IV diagnostic system with an Adlerian case formulation from general diagnosis through special diagnosis and long-term treatment. Psychological testing and individual and family therapies were used to treat this challenging but hardworking woman with multiple diagnoses.

Maniacci, M. P., & Sackett-Maniacci, L. (2002). The use of the DSM-IV in treatment planning: An Adlerian view. *Journal of Individual Psychology, 58,* 388–397.

> This is another case that demonstrates the integration of a DSM diagnostic formulation with an Adlerian case conceptualization. This case involved a man with multiple hospitalizations for treatment-resistant migraine headaches who was underwent outpatient Adlerian psychotherapy. This is a clear example of the concepts of holism and psychology of use.

Mosak, H. H. (1997). Life style assessment: A demonstration focused on family constellation. In J. Carlson & S. Slavik (Eds.), *Techniques in Adlerian psychology* (pp. 39–55). Washington, DC: Accelerated Development.

> This book presents transcripts of a live demonstration of a lifestyle assessment. Mosak has a short time to help a troubled teen understand herself and her strained relationship with her family.

Mosak. H. H., & Maniacci, M. P. (2013). The case of Roger. In D. Wedding & R. J. Corsini (Eds.), *Case studies in psychotherapy* (7th ed.). Belmont, CA: Brooks/Cole.

> In nine audio-recorded sessions before a class, Mosak helps a very anxious agoraphobic man overcome his fears and become more at peace with himself and the world. This is a detailed study of how Adlerians do therapy.

REFERENCES

Adler, A. (1917). *Study of organ inferiority and its psychical compensation: A contribution to clinical medicine* (S. E. Jelliffe, Trans.). New York: Nervous and Mental Diseases Company. (Original work published 1907)

Adler, A. (1950). Forward. In R. Dreikurs, *Fundamentals of Adlerian psychology* (p. vii). New York: Greenberg. (Original work published 1933)

Adler, A. (1956). *The Individual Psychology of Alfred Adler: A systematic presentation in selections from his writings* (H. L. Ansbacher & R. R. Ansbacher, Eds.). New York: Basic Books.

Adler, A. (1957). *Understanding human nature* (W. B. Wolfe, Trans.). Greenwich, CT: Premier Books. (Original work published 1927)

Adler, A. (1964a). Brief comments upon reason, intelligence and feeble-mindedness. In A. Adler, *Superiority and social interest: A collection of later writings* (H. L. Ansbacher & R. R. Ansbacher, Eds.) (pp. 41–49). Evanston, IL: Northwestern University Press. (Original work published 1928)

Adler, A. (1964b). The differences between Individual Psychology and psychoanalysis. In A. Adler, *Superiority and social interest: A collection of later writings* (H. L. Ansbacher & R. R. Ansbacher, Eds.) (pp. 205–218). Evanston, IL: Northwestern University Press. (Original work published 1931)

Adler, A. (1978). *Cooperation between the sexes: Writings on women, love and marriage, sexuality and its disorders*

(H. L. Ansbacher & R. R. Ansbacher, Eds.). New York: Jason Aronson.

Adler, A. (2002). *The neurotic character: Fundamentals of Individual Psychology and psychotherapy* (C. Koen, Trans., & H. Stein, Ed.). San Francisco: Classical Adlerian Translation Project. (Original work published 1912)

Adler, A. (2012a). Individual psychological education. In J. Carlson & M. P. Maniacci (Eds.), *Alfred Adler revisited* (pp. 129–137). New York: Routledge. (Original work published 1920)

Adler, A. (2012b). The fundamental views of Individual Psychology. In J. Carlson & M. P. Maniacci (Eds.), *Alfred Adler revisited* (pp. 11–18). New York: Routledge. (Original work published 1935)

Adler, K. A. (1961). Depression in the light of Individual Psychology. *Journal of Individual Psychology, 17,* 56–67.

Adler, K. A. (1967). Adler's Individual Psychology. In B. B. Wolman (Ed.), *Psychoanalytic techniques: A handbook for the practicing psychoanalyst* (pp. 299–337). New York: Basic Books.

American Psychiatric Association. (2000). *Diagnostic and statistical manual of mental disorders* (4th ed., text rev.). Washington, DC: Author.

Ansbacher, H. L. (1964). An introduction to the Torchbook edition. In A. Adler, *Problems of neurosis: A book of case histories* (H. L. Ansbacher, Ed.). New York: Harper & Row.

Ansbacher, H. L. (1977). Individual Psychology. In R. J. Corsini (Ed.), *Current personality theories* (pp. 45–82). Itasca, IL: F. E. Peacock.

Ansbacher, H. L. (1978). Essay: Adler's sex theories. In A. Adler, *Cooperation between the sexes: Writings on women, love and marriage, sexuality and its disorders* (H. L. Ansbacher & R. R. Ansbacher, Eds.) (pp. 248–412). New York: Jason Aronson.

Ansbacher, H. L. (1992a). Alfred Adler, pioneer in prevention of mental disorders. *Individual Psychology: The Journal of Adlerian Theory, Research & Practice, 48,* 3–34.

Ansbacher, H. L. (1992b). Alfred Adler's concepts of community feeling and of social interest and the relevance of community feeling for old age. *Individual Psychology: The Journal of Adlerian Theory, Research & Practice, 48,* 402–412.

Aristotle. (1941). *Metaphysica* [*The Metaphysics*] (W. D. Ross, Trans.). In R. McKeon (Ed.), *The basic works of Aristotle* (pp. 689–926). New York: Random House. (Original work published circa 350 B. C. E.)

Baumeister, R. F., & Leary, M. R. (1995). The need to belong: Desire for interpersonal attachments as fundamental human motivation. *Psychological Bulletin, 117,* 497–529.

Beecher, W., & Beecher, M. (1986). *Beyond success and failure: Ways to self-reliance and maturity* (rev. ed.). Dallas: Beecher Foundation. (Original work published 1966)

Binder, J. L. (2004). *Key competencies in brief dynamic psychotherapy: Clinical practice beyond the manual.* New York: Guilford.

Bitter, J. R., & Main, F. O. (Eds.). (2011). Adlerian family therapy [Special issue]. *Journal of Individual Psychology, 67.*

Brown, B. (2007). *I thought it was just me (but it isn't): Telling the truth about perfectionism, inadequacy, power.* New York: Gotham Books.

Carlson, J., & Maniacci, M. P. (Eds.). (2012). *Alfred Adler revisited.* New York: Routledge.

Carlson, J., & Slavik, S. (Eds.). (1997). *Techniques in Adlerian psychology.* Washington, DC: Accelerated Development.

Carlson, J., & Sperry, L. (Eds.). (1998). *The disordered couple.* Bristol, PA: Brunner/Mazel.

Carlson, J., & Sperry, L. (Eds.). (1999). *The intimate couple.* Philadelphia: Brunner/Mazel.

Carlson, J., Sperry, L., & Lewis, J. (1997). *Family therapy: Ensuring treatment efficacy.* Pacific Grove, CA: Brooks/Cole.

Carlson, J., Sperry, L., & Lewis, J. (2005). *Family therapy techniques: Integration and tailoring.* New York: Brunner/Routledge.

Carlson, J. Watts, R. E., & Maniacci, M. (2006). *Adlerian therapy: Theory and practice.* Washington, DC: American Psychological Association.

Chandler, C. K. (Ed.). (1995). Counseling homosexuals and bisexuals [Special issue]. *Individual Psychology: The Journal of Adlerian Theory, Research & Practice, 51.*

Christensen, O. C., & Schramski, T. G. (Eds.). (1983). *Adlerian family counseling: A manual for counselor, educator, and psychotherapist.* Minneapolis: Educational Media Corporation.

Clark, A. J. (2002). *Early recollections: Theory and practice in counseling and psychotherapy.* New York: Brunner/Routledge.

Corsini, R. J. (1966). *Role playing in psychotherapy: A manual.* Chicago: Aldine.

Corsini, R. J. (1971). Group psychotherapy. In A. G. Nikelly (Ed.), *Techniques for behavior change: Applications of Adlerian theory* (pp. 111–115). Springfield, IL: Charles C. Thomas.

Dagley, J. C. (2000). Adlerian family therapy. In A. M. Horne (Ed.), *Family counseling and therapy* (3rd ed., pp. 366–419). Itasca, IL: F. E. Peacock.

de Shazer, S. (1988). *Clues: Investigating solutions in brief therapy.* New York: Norton.

Dewey, E. A. (1971). Family atmosphere. In A. G. Nikelly (Ed.), *Techniques for behavior change: Applications of Adlerian theory* (pp. 41–47). Springfield, IL: Charles C. Thomas.

Dinkmeyer, D., & Carlson, J. (1984). *Time for a better marriage.* Circle Pines, MN: American Guidance Service.

Dinkmeyer, D., & Carlson, J. (1989). *Taking time for love: How to stay happily married.* New York: Prentice Hall.

Dinkmeyer, D., Sr., McKay, G. D., & Dinkmeyer, D., Jr. (1997). *The parent's handbook: Systematic training for effective parenting (STEP).* Circle Pines, MN: American Guidance Service.

Dreikurs, R. (1946). *The challenge of marriage.* New York: Dell, Sloan, and Pearce.

Dreikurs, R. (1950). *Fundamentals of Adlerian psychology.* New York: Greenberg. (Original work published 1933)

Dreikurs, R. (1967). *Psychodynamics, psychotherapy, and counseling.* Chicago: Alfred Adler Institute.

Dreikurs, R. (1971). *Social equality: The challenge of today.* Chicago: Adler School of Professional Psychology.

Dreikurs, R. (1997). Family counseling: A demonstration. In J. Carlson & S. Slavik (Eds.), *Techniques in Adlerian psychology* (pp. 466–484). Washington, DC: Accelerated Development. (Original work published 1972)

Dreikurs, R., Shulman, B. H., & Mosak, H. H. (1984). *Multiple psychotherapy: The use of two therapists with one client.* Chicago: Alfred Adler Institute.

Dreikurs, R., & Soltz, V. (1964). *Children: The challenge.* New York: Dell, Sloan, and Pearce.

Dreikurs, S. E. (1986). *Cows can be purple: My life and art therapy* (N. Catlin & J. W. Croake, Eds.). Chicago: Alfred Adler Institute.

Eckstein, D., Aycock, K. J., Sperber, M. A., McDonald, J., Van Wiesner III, V., Watts, R. E., & Ginsburg, P. (2010). A review of 200 birth-order studies: Lifestyle characteristics. *Journal of Individual Psychology, 66,* 408–434.

Ellenberger, H. F. (1970). *The discovery of the unconscious: The history and evolution of dynamic psychiatry.* New York: Basic Books.

Evans, T. D., & Dinkmeyer, D., Jr. (Eds.). (1993). Marriage and couples counseling [Special issue]. *Individual Psychology: The Journal of Adlerian Theory, Research, & Practice, 3 & 4.*

Forer, L., & Still, H. (1976). *The birth order factor: How your personality is influenced by your place in the family.* New York: Pocket Books.

Freud, S. (1965). *New introductory lectures on Psychoanalysis* (J. Strachey, Ed. & Trans.). New York: Norton. (Original work published 1933)

Gold, L. (1981). Life style and dreams. In L. Baruth & D. Eckstein (Eds.), *Life style: Theory, practice and research* (2nd ed., pp. 24–30). Dubuque, IA: Kendall/Hunt.

Gottman, J. M. (1999). *The marriage clinic: A scientifically based marital therapy.* New York: Norton.

Grunwald, B. B., & McAbee, H. V. (1999). *Guiding the family: Practical counseling techniques* (2nd ed.). Philadelphia: Accelerated Development.

Hayes, S. C., & Follette, V. M., & Linehan, M. M. (Eds.). (2004). *Mindfulness and acceptance: Expanding the cognitive-behavioral tradition.* New York: Guilford.

Hoffman, E. (1994). *The drive for self: Alfred Adler and the founding of Individual Psychology.* Reading, MA: Addison-Wesley.

Huber, C. H., & Baruth, L. G. (1981). *Coping with marital conflict: An Adlerian approach to succeeding in marriage.* Champaign, IL: Stipes.

Kern, R. M., Gormley, L., & Curlette, W. L. (2008). BASIS-A inventory empirical studies: Research findings from 2000 to 2006. *Journal of Individual Psychology, 64,* 280–309.

Kern, R. M., Hawes, E. C., & Christensen, O. C. (Eds.). (1989). *Couples therapy: An Adlerian perspective.* Minneapolis: Educational Media Corporation.

Kern, R., Stoltz, K., Gottlieb-Low, H., & Frost, L. (2009). The therapeutic alliance and early recollections. *Journal of Individual Psychology, 65,* 110–122.

Kopp, R. R. (1995). *Metaphor therapy: Using client-generated metaphors in psychotherapy.* New York: Brunner/Mazel.

Kottman, T. (1995). *Partners in play: An Adlerian approach to play therapy.* Alexandria, VA: American Counseling Association.

Leman, K. (1985). *The birth order book: Why you are the way you are.* New York: Dell.

Leman, K. (1995). *Bringing up kids without tearing them down.* Nashville: Nelson.

Lombardi, D. L. (1973). Eight avenues of life style consistency. *Individual Psychologist, 10,* 5–9.

Mahoney, M. J. (1980). Psychotherapy and the structure of personal revolutions. In M. J. Mahoney (Ed.), *Psychotherapy process: Current issues and future directions* (pp. 157–180). New York: Plenum.

Manaster, G. J., & Corsini, R. J. (1982). *Individual Psychology: Theory and practice.* Itasca, IL: F. E. Peacock.

Main, F. (1986). *Perfect parenting and other myths.* Minneapolis: CompCare.

Maniacci, M. P. (1996a). An introduction to brief therapy of the personality disorders. *Individual Psychology: The Journal of Adlerian Theory, Research & Practice, 52,* 158–168.

Maniacci, M. P. (1996b). Mental disorders due to a general medical condition and other cognitive disorders. In L. Sperry & J. Carlson (Eds.), *Psychopathology and psychotherapy: From DSM-IV diagnosis to treatment* (2nd ed., pp. 51–75). Muncie, IN: Accelerated Development.

Maniacci, M. P. (1998). The psychotic couple. In J. Carlson & L. Sperry (Eds.), *The disordered couple* (pp. 57–81). Bristol, PA: Brunner/Mazel.

Maniacci, M. P. (1999). Clinical therapy. In R. E. Watts & J. Carlson (Eds.), *Interventions and strategies in counseling and psychotherapy* (pp. 59–85). Philadelphia: Accelerated Development.

Maniacci, M. P. (2002). The DSM and Individual Psychology: A general comparison. *Journal of Individual Psychology, 58,* 356–362.

Maniacci, M. P. (2012). An introduction to Alfred Adler. In J. Carlson & M. P. Maniacci (Eds.), *Alfred Adler revisited* (pp. 1–10). New York: Routledge.

Maniacci, M. P., & Carlson, J. (1991). A model for Adlerian family interventions with the chronically mentally ill. *American Journal of Family Therapy, 19,* 237–249.

Maniacci, M. P., & Sackett-Maniacci, L. (2002). The use of the *DSM-IV* in treatment planning: An Adlerian view. *Journal of Individual Psychology, 58,* 388–397.

McKay, G. D., & Dinkmeyer, D. (1994). *How you feel is up to you: The power of emotional choice.* San Luis Obispo, CA: Impact.

Mosak, H. H. (1977). *On purpose.* Chicago: Alfred Adler Institute.

Mosak, H. H. (1995). Adlerian psychotherapy. In R. J. Corsini & D. Wedding (Eds.), *Current psychotherapies* (5th ed., pp. 51–94). Itasca, IL: F. E. Peacock.

Mosak, H. H. (1997). Life style assessment: A demonstration focused on family constellation. In J. Carlson & S. Slavik (Eds.), *Techniques in Adlerian psychology* (pp. 39–55). Washington, DC: Accelerated Development.

Mosak, H. H., & DiPietro, R. (2006). *Early recollections: Interpretative methods and applications.* New York: Routledge.

Mosak, H. H., & Maniacci, M. P. (1993). Adlerian child psychotherapy. In T. R. Kratochwill & R. J. Morris (Eds.), *Handbook of psychotherapy with children and adolescents* (pp. 162–184). Boston: Allyn & Bacon.

Mosak, H. H., & Maniacci, M. P. (1998). *Tactics in counseling and psychotherapy.* Itasca, IL: F. E. Peacock.

Mosak, H. H., & Maniacci, M. P. (1999). *A primer of Adlerian psychology: The analytic- behavioral-cognitive psychology of Alfred Adler.* Philadelphia: Accelerated Development.

Mosak. H. H., & Maniacci, M. P. (2010). The case of Roger. In D. Wedding & R. J. Corsini (Eds.), *Case studies in psychotherapy* (7th ed., pp. 12–31). Belmont, CA: Brooks/Cole.

Mosak, H. H., & Maniacci, M. P. (2011). Adlerian psychotherapy. R. J. Corsini & D. Wedding (Eds.), *Current psychotherapies* (9th ed., 67–112). Belmont, CA: Brooks/Cole.

Mozdzierz, G. J., Peluso, P. R., & Lisiecki, J. (2009). *Principles of counseling and psychotherapy: Learning the essential domains and nonlinear thinking of master practitioners.* New York: Routledge.

Nelsen, J. (1996). *Positive discipline* (rev. ed.). New York: Ballantine.

Newman, M., & Berkowitz, B., with Owen, J. (1971). *How to be your own best friend.* New York: Ballantine.

Nietzsche, F. (1967). *The will to power* (W. Kaufman & R. J. Hollingdale, Trans. ; W. Kaufman, Ed.). New York: Vintage. (Original work published 1901)

Nikelly, A. G. (Ed.). (1971). *Techniques for behavior change: Applications of Adlerian theory.* Springfield, IL: Charles C. Thomas.

Oberst, U. E., & Stewart, A. E. (2003). *Adlerian psychotherapy: An advanced approach to Individual Psychology.* New York: Brunner/Routledge.

Orgler, H. (1963). *Alfred Adler: The man and his works: Triumph over the inferiority complex.* New York: Mentor Books. (Original work published 1939)

Peluso, P. R., Peluso, J. P., Buckner, J. P., Kern, R. M., & Curlette, W. (2009). Measuring lifestyle and attachment: An empirical investigation linking Individual Psychology and attachment theory. *Journal of Counseling and Development, 87,* 394–403.

Popkin, M. (1987). *Active parenting: Teaching cooperation, courage, and responsibility.* New York: Harper & Row.

Powers, R. L., & Griffith, J. (1987). *Understanding life-style: The psycho-clarity process.* Chicago: Americas Institute of Adlerian Studies.

Rasmussen, P. R. (2010). *The quest to feel good.* New York: Routledge.

Sackett-Maniacci, L. A. (1999). *Lifestyle factors of chronic migraine headache sufferers.* Unpublished doctoral dissertation, Adler School of Professional Psychology, Chicago.

Seligman, M. E. P. (2011). *Flourish: A visionary new understanding of happiness and well-being.* New York: Free Press.

Sherman, R. (1999). Family therapy: The art of integration. In R. Watts & J. Carlson (Eds.), *Interventions and strategies in counseling and psychotherapy* (pp. 101–134). Philadelphia: Accelerated Development.

Sherman, R., & Dinkmeyer, D. (1987). *Systems of family therapy: An Adlerian integration.* New York: Brunner/Mazel.

Sherman, R., & Fredman, N. (1986). *Handbook of structured techniques in marriage and family therapy.* New York: Brunner/Mazel.

Shulman, B. H. (1973). *Contributions to Individual Psychology.* Chicago: Alfred Adler Institute.

Shulman, B. H., & Mosak, H. H. (1977). Birth order and ordinal position: Two Adlerian views. *Journal of Individual Psychology, 33,* 114–121.

Shulman, B. H., & Mosak, H. H. (1988). *Manual for life style assessment.* Muncie, IN: Accelerated Development.

Sperry, L. (Ed.). (1989). Varieties of brief therapy [Special issue]. *Individual Psychology: The Journal of Adlerian Theory, Research & Practice, 1 & 2.*

Sperry, L. (1995). *Handbook of diagnosis and treatment of DSM-IV personality disorders.* New York: Brunner/Mazel.

Sperry, L. (Ed.). (2002). *DSM-IV in clinical practice* [Special issue]. *Journal of Individual Psychology, 58.*

Sperry, L., & Carlson, J. (1991). *Marital therapy: Integrating theory and technique.* Denver: Love Publishing.

Starr, A. (1977). *Rehearsal for living: Psychodrama: Illustrated therapeutic techniques.* Chicago: Nelson-Hall.

Sweeney, T. J. (2009). *Adlerian counseling and psychotherapy: A practitioner's approach* (5th ed.). New York: Routledge.

Vaihinger, H. (1965). *The philosophy of "as if."* (C. K. Ogden, Trans.). London: Routledge, Kegan, Paul. (Original work published 1911)

Wallin, D. J. (2007). *Attachment in psychotherapy.* New York: Guilford.

Watts, R. E. (Ed.). (2003). *Adlerian, cognitive, and constructivist therapies: An integrative dialogue.* New York: Springer.

Watts, R. E., & Carlson, J. (Eds.). (1999). *Interventions and strategies in counseling and psychotherapy.* Philadelphia: Accelerated Development.

West, G. K. (1986). *Parenting without guilt: The predictable and situational misbehaviors of childhood.* Springfield, IL: Charles C. Thomas.

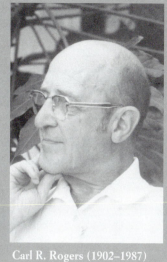

Carl R. Rogers (1902–1987)
© Bettmann/CORBIS

4 | CLIENT–CENTERED THERAPY

Nathaniel J. Raskin, Carl R. Rogers, and Marjorie C. Witty

OVERVIEW

On December 11, 1940, at a meeting of the Psi Chi chapter at the University of Minnesota, Carl Ransom Rogers presented his ideas about psychotherapy. Somewhat surprised by the impassioned debate following his presentation, Rogers realized his ideas were getting at something new. Thus, client-centered therapy was born.

By the 1950s, Rogers's evolving views, along with those of other humanistic psychologists, mounted a challenge to the prevailing psychoanalytic and behavioral paradigms. In this way, what came to be called the *third force* emerged on the scene in the field of psychology. Today, a half-century later, Rogers is considered to be among the most eminent psychologists of the 20th century and is the psychologist most named by other psychotherapists as having influenced their practice.

Ironically, in the field of clinical psychology, the approach is scarcely visible in many doctoral training programs. Still radical after all these years, client-centered therapy invites us to envision the human being as a *person*: self-determining and self-realizing, a sovereign subject.

In response to the pessimism of some who fear that the approach is being eclipsed by treatment manuals, empirically supported treatments, and the like, renowned Austrian person-centered therapist and scholar Peter Schmid responds:

> I do not share this view at all. . . . On the contrary, I am even convinced that the essence of the person-centered approach has not yet been sounded out by far, let alone has it been put into effect, in its radicalism, its profound humanism and in

its critical potential, a potential towards emancipation. Carl Rogers's positions and visions are not at all outdated, they have not even been caught up with. (Schmid, 2000, p. 12)

Basic Concepts

The Person

The animating vision of client-centered therapy consists in the claim that the human being is a *person*. Although this may seem obvious, actually there are many contexts where our social roles, gender, race, ethnicity, social class, or ability may diminish our personhood. This ethical claim differentiates client-centered therapy from approaches based on a medical model that reduces persons to instances of diagnoses—for example, the "alcoholic," the "schizophrenic," the "borderline," and so on (Schmid, 2003, p. 108). Personhood is an ethical claim that signifies that human beings should not be used as means to others' ends. All human beings are nonreducible "ends" in themselves, inherently deserving of dignity and respect.

Pointing out that almost all therapy theories focus on the therapist and may be considered "therapist-centric," Arthur Bohart cites an African proverb to illustrate this imbalance. "Until lions have their own historians, all tales of hunting will glorify the hunter." For Bohart, the client in therapy actively uses or "operates" on aspects of the therapeutic environment and the therapy process that are most personally useful. The client is not a passive receptacle for the therapist's attitudes but is an active agent interacting with and co-creating what is most productive for him or her as a unique person in the situation (Bohart, 2008; Bohart & Tallman, 1999).

Motivation

The actualizing tendency concept central to Rogers's motivational theory was originally advanced by Kurt Goldstein, a German neurologist who worked with brain-injured soldiers. His holistic theory of personality emphasized that individuals must be understood as totalities striving to actualize themselves (Goldstein, 1934/1959).

Based on Goldstein's theory and his own observations of clients, Rogers postulated that all living organisms are dynamic processes motivated by the inherent tendency to maintain and enhance themselves. This actualizing tendency, an axiom in client-centered theory, functions continually, directionally, and holistically throughout all subsystems of the organism (Bohart, 2007; Bozarth & Brodley, 1991; Brodley, 1999c/2011; Rogers, 1951, p. 487; Rogers, 1963).

Rogers (1980) speculated that the actualizing tendency is part of a more general formative tendency, observable in the syntropy of the universe manifesting increasing complexity, order, and interrelatedness observable in stars, crystals, and microorganisms as well as in human beings. In this view, persons and all living organisms are thought to be evolving toward greater complexity, fulfilling those potentials that preserve and enhance themselves.

It is important to note that Rogers's theory of the actualizing tendency is biological in nature, not moral. Even when people make self-destructive choices, the actualizing tendency is hypothesized to function in a constant and directional manner but may be distorted by environmental factors (Merry, 2004, pp. 23–24). Theoretically, if the goodness of fit between the person and her environment were perfect, the person would develop toward Rogers's view of the fully functioning person (Rogers, 1961, pp. 183–187), increasingly open to new experience, capable of living in the present moment, and trusting her own experiencing process as a guide for living.

Human Nature

The famous dictum attributed to Clyde Kluckhohn—that "each person is in some respect like every other person, like some other persons, and in some respects like no other person"—is helpful in getting at Rogers's understanding of human nature. At first glance, Rogers's theoretical view of human nature is universal: All human infants need positive regard (each person is like all persons). Within the therapeutic relationship, however, each person is entirely unique (each of us is like no other person).

Rogers can thus be described as both a scientist and a phenomenologist, depending on whether he is engaged in trying to organize the data of research and probe the findings for general statements or working as a therapist with a unique person in which general statements are basically irrelevant to that encounter. (Van Belle, 1980).

Certainly, Rogers's theory of personality is cast in terms of universally applicable constructs. For example, "As the awareness of self emerges, the individual develops a need for positive regard. This need is universal in human beings, and in the individual, is pervasive and persistent" (Rogers, 1959b, p. 223).

Rogers posits that every organism possesses an inherent *organismic valuing process*—and only to the extent that the emerging self of the person can assimilate his or her lived experiencing can congruence or wholeness be achieved. For Rogers, *congruence*, the state of wholeness and integration within the experience of the person, is the hallmark of psychological adjustment. Congruence is the antithesis of defensiveness and rigidity.

In spite of Rogers's belief in the individuality and uniqueness of each person, Rogers's theory is framed as universally descriptive—that is, "all persons are like no other persons." His position is grounded in objectivist, realist assumptions. Although each client's narrative from session to session is unique, and the client him- or herself is a fluid process changing over time, Rogers states that the process of becoming more congruent in client-centered therapy is a predictable outcome and can be observed in all therapy relationships that provide the therapeutic conditions.

Barbara Held, philosopher and practitioner, compares the realist assumptions undergirding client-centered theory as contrasted with antirealist, postmodern approaches such as narrative therapy:

> [E]ven the humanistic therapy movement advanced by Rogers, a movement which emphasizes the unique, subjective (or phenomenal) perspective of each individual therapy client, nonetheless propounds perfectly general laws of problem causation and problem resolution, laws that are, moreover, taken to be fully realist. For example, that movement makes reality claims about how the failure to symbolize and integrate experience in awareness damages the self-concept and thus leads to a host of problems. (Rogers, 1961). . . . These failures are posited by each theoretical system as nothing less than the real or true (general) cause of all problems defined within that system. (Held, 1995, p. 21)

Rogers's view of human nature has been characterized as both optimistic and naïve. Critics confuse his theory of the actualizing tendency with a belief in the goodness of persons. Rogers, however, did not view humans (or any living organisms) as inherently good or evil. Nor was he naïve about our human capacity for destructiveness (see Schmid, 2013, pp. 42–43). As he accompanied clients who suffered from a myriad of problems, he asserted that, in the course of his work, he was consistently heartened to find that clients moved in positive, prosocial directions when provided with a climate of respect, unconditional positive regard, and empathic understanding. He states

> In short, organisms are always seeking, always initiating, always "up to something." There is one central source of energy in the human organism. This source is a

trustworthy function of the whole system rather than of some portion of it; it is most simply conceptualized as a tendency toward fulfillment, toward actualization, involving the maintenance and enhancement of the organism. (Rogers, 1980, p. 123)

The Therapist

Client-centered therapists trust the person's inner resources for growth and self-realization, in spite of biologically based conditions or impairments, psychological limitations, trauma, or oppressive or environmental conditions and limitations. The therapist's trust in the client's inherent growth tendency and right to self-determination is expressed, in practice, in the therapist's "nondirective attitude" (Brodley, 1997/2011; Raskin, 1947/2005, 1948).

Client-centered psychotherapy has the metagoal of providing the conditions that will allow the person to pursue his or her own purposes, aims, and goals. While participating in this emancipatory process, the therapist cannot employ means that disempower the client without falling into contradiction (see O'Hara, 2006, p. 121).

This foundational attitude crucially informs the therapist's intentions. The therapist's nondirective attitude does not imply passivity or the lack of responsiveness; it does not inhibit the freedom of the client-centered therapist. As it represents our ethical commitment to the egalitarian nature of the therapy, it is not an expression of orthodoxy as some authors have claimed (see Cain, 2010, p. 45) but is rather a *moral compass* that guides our course without dictating the route. It is nonauthoritarian and attuned to protecting the autonomy of the client. As challenging today as it was in 1951, Rogers states,

[t]he primary point of importance here is the attitude held by the counselor toward the worth and the significance of the individual. How do we look upon others? Do we see each person as having worth and dignity in his[1] own right? If we do hold this point of view at the verbal level, to what extent is it operationally evident at the behavioral level? Do we tend to treat individuals as persons of worth, or do we subtly devalue them by our attitudes and behavior? Is our philosophy one in which respect for the individual is uppermost? Do we respect his capacity and his right to self-direction, or do we basically believe that his life would be best guided by us? To what extent do we have a need and a desire to dominate others? Are we willing for the individual to select and choose his own values, or are our actions guided by the conviction (usually unspoken) that he would be happiest if he permitted us to select for him his values and standards and goals? (Rogers, 1951, p. 20)

To undertake to develop as a client-centered therapist, one must be willing to take on the discipline of learning to be an open, authentic, empathic person in the relationship. Rogers described this empathic orientation as a *way of being* (Rogers, 1980).

In client-centered therapy, congruence, unconditional positive regard, and empathic understanding are neither techniques nor aspects of a professional role. An aspect of therapist development, these attitudes must first be consonant with the therapist's own values and beliefs. Rogers was not out to train client-centered therapists; he wanted them to find ways of working that were authentic to their own values and personalities. Rogers states,

. . . no student can or should be trained to become a client-centered therapist. If the attitudes he discovers within himself, if the hypotheses which in his experience are effective in dealing with people, happen to coincide in important ways with the

[1] A note on pronouns. Rogers typifies the largely male culture of psychology in the 1940s and 1950s in his reliance on the male pronoun. We have kept his use of male pronouns intact while noting that his consciousness of issues of race and gender was challenged in the 1960s by his daughter, Natalie Rogers, and other feminists and antiracist activists at the Center for the Study of the Person, including Maureen O'Hara, Gay Leah Swenson Barfield, Maria Villas Bowen, Suzanne Spector, and others.

client-centered orientation, then that is an interesting indication of the generality of those experiences, but no more. It is far more important that he be true to his own experiences than that he should coincide with any known therapeutic orientation. The basic reliance is upon the capacity of the student-counselor to develop himself into an effective therapist. (Rogers, 1951, p. 433)

The Relationship

Psychotherapy outcome research supports Rogers's hypothesis (1957) that the therapeutic relationship accounts for a significant percentage of the variance in positive outcome in all theoretical orientations of psychotherapy (Asay & Lambert, 1999, p. 31; Elliott, Bohart, Watson & Greenberg, 2011; Patterson, 1984).

Within the specific context of client-centered therapy, the therapist's embodiment of the therapeutic attitudes engenders a climate of freedom and safety. Within this climate, the client is free to participate in the situation in any way he or she wishes to. Active narration of whatever is most present is accepted—and silence is as well. The client propels the process. Bohart elucidates the client's active, self-healing activities; in concert with the therapist-provided conditions, these promote positive change. In this interactive model, *the client actively co-constructs the therapy* (Bohart, 2004, p. 108).

Because both the therapist and the client are unique persons, the relationship that develops between them cannot be prescribed or predicted in advance. It is a unique encounter premised on the response of the therapist to a person who seeks help. Client-centered therapists tend to be spontaneously responsive and accommodating to the requests of clients whenever possible. This willingness to accommodate requests—by answering questions, by changing a time, or making a phone call on behalf of a client—originates in the therapist's basic trust in and respect for the client and her aims and goals (Brodley, 2011a; Moon & Rice, in press).

On a practical level, practitioners of client-centered therapy trust that individuals and groups are fully capable of articulating and pursuing their own goals. This has special meaning in relation to children, students, and workers, who are often viewed as requiring constant guidance and supervision. The client-centered approach endorses the person's right to choose or reject therapy, to choose a therapist whom he or she thinks may be helpful (sometimes a person of the same age, race, gender, or sexual orientation), to choose the frequency of sessions and the length of the therapeutic relationship, to decide what needs to be explored, and to be the architect of the therapy process itself.

Similarly, when the therapeutic conditions are present in a group, and when the group is trusted to find its own way of being, group members tend to develop processes that are right for them and to resolve conflicts within the time constraints in the situation (Rogers, 1970).

The Core Conditions

Congruence, unconditional positive regard, and empathic understanding of the client's internal frame of reference are the three therapist-provided conditions in client-centered therapy (Rogers, 1959b). A large literature investigating the efficacy of what have grown to be called "the core conditions" has accumulated since Rogers postulated his theory (Cooper, Watson & Hölldampf, 2011; Elliott, 2001; Elliott & Freire, 2010; Patterson, 1984). Although they are theoretically distinguishable, these three attitudes function holistically as a gestalt in the experience of the therapist (Rogers, 1957). Arguments that "unconditional positive regard is impossible!" fail to recognize that Rogers's therapeutic attitudes exist on a dynamic continuum within each therapist with each client. The point for us as learners is to examine and reflect on the barriers within us that keep us from experiencing the attitudes.

Congruence.   Congruence represents the therapist's ongoing process of assimilating, integrating, and symbolizing the flow of experiences in awareness. Rogers states, "To me being congruent means that I am aware of and willing to represent the feelings I have at the moment. It is being real and authentic in the moment" (Rogers cited in Baldwin, 1987, p. 51).

A psychotherapist who is aware of the inner flow of experiencing and who is acceptant toward these inner experiences can be described as integrated and whole. Thus, even when the therapist experiences a lack of empathic understanding or a loss of unconditional positive regard, if these experiences are allowed into awareness without denial or distortion, the therapist is in a state of congruence (Brodley, 2001/2011b, p. 57). However, the diminished level of the conditions implies a lessening of the potency of the therapeutic environment.

The therapist's inner state of congruence usually manifests itself in a perceptible transparency or genuineness and in the behavioral quality of relaxed openness. As therapist congruence persists over time, the client learns that the therapist's apparent openness is genuine and that the therapist is not covertly "up to" anything such as making covert diagnostic judgments or having reactions that are off-limits to the client (Brodley, 2011b; Moon, 2005).

Unconditional Positive Regard.   The therapist enters into a relationship with the client hoping to experience unconditional positive regard for the client. This construct refers to a warm appreciation or nonjudgmental prizing of the other person. The therapist accepts the client's thoughts, feelings, wishes, intentions, theories, and attributions about causality as unique, human, and appropriate to his or her current experience. Ideally, the therapist's regard for the client will not be affected by particular choices, opinions, or behaviors—even when the behaviors are immoral or repugnant to the therapist. Complete, unswerving unconditionality is an ideal, but in seeking to realize this ideal attitude, therapists find that their acceptance, respect, and appreciation for clients deepen with the growth of understanding. *Tout comprendre, c'est tout pardonner:* "To understand all is to pardon all."

The therapist's ability to experience unconditional positive regard toward a particular client, which is reliably present over time, is a developmental process involving a commitment to be aware of and to explore judgmental reactions and to learn to inhibit critical responses that we often allow to emerge in common life situations. The novice therapist makes a commitment to expand his or her capacity for acceptance, to challenge his or her automatic judgments and biases, and to approach each client as a unique person doing the best he or she can *under the circumstances as they perceive them and that are affecting them even though they may not be aware of them* (Bozarth & Brodley, 1986, emphasis added).

Empathic Understanding of the Client's Frame of Reference.   Empathic understanding for the client-centered therapist is a complex process. It is an attitude of wishing to grasp the client's expressions, meanings, and narrative. This implies both openness to the client's communications, including any negative or critical reactions of the client, and a willingness to suspend one's own opinions, prejudices, and theories, including Rogers's theories. This practice of empathic understanding places the client's own expression and meanings at the center of the process as the therapist follows with understanding. The client is the author of her own life and the architect of the therapy.

The empathic attitude in Rogers's theory of therapy does not specify a particular response form. This is a widely misunderstood point. Rogers did not advocate repeating back what the client said. This kind of shallow, literal, and simplistic kind of parroting has no place in client-centered therapy. Occasionally, when a client's statement is very obscure, the therapist may literally reiterate the statement, but most of the time the therapist is trying to grasp the "point" the client is trying to make, and this leads to empathic understanding responses that capture the client's intention, agency, emotional associations, and so on. It is helpful to novice therapists to simply try to take in the client's "point" and to express this point spontaneously and in their own words. A simplistic focus on feeling words rarely results in accurate empathic responding.

The Client

Basic concepts on the client side of the process include self-concept, locus of evaluation, and experiencing. In focusing on what is important to the person seeking help, client-centered therapists soon discovered that the person's perceptions and feelings about self were of central concern (Raimy, 1948; Rogers, 1951, 1959b). A major component of one's self-concept is self-regard, which is often lacking in clients who seek therapeutic help. Some of the earliest psychotherapy research projects showed that when clients were rated as successful in therapy, their attitudes toward self became significantly more positive (Sheerer, 1949). More recent research underscores this important aspect of positive therapy outcome.

Rogers's group also found that clients tended to progress along a related dimension termed locus of evaluation. As they gained self-esteem, they tended to shift the basis for their standards and values from other people to themselves. People commonly began therapy overly concerned with what others thought of them—that is, their locus of evaluation was external. With success in therapy, their attitudes toward others, as toward themselves, became more positive, and they were less dependent on others for their values and standards (Raskin, 1952). These clients may be described as having moved from an external locus of evaluation to an internal locus of evaluation, and thus are more genuinely self-determining. Ryan and Deci have developed a theory of self-determination which has garnered substantial support:

> Comparisons between people whose motivation is authentic (literally, self-authored or endorsed) and those who are merely externally controlled for an action typically reveal that the former, relative to the latter, have more interest, excitement, and confidence which in turn is manifest both as enhanced performance, persistence, and creativity . . . and as heightened vitality . . . , self-esteem . . . , and general well-being. . . . This is so even when people have the same level of perceived competence or self-efficacy for the activity.

A third central concept in client-centered therapy is experiencing, a dimension along which many but not all clients improved (Rogers, Gendlin, Kiesler, & Truax, 1967), shifting from a rigid mode of experiencing self and world to one of greater openness and flexibility.

The therapeutic attitudes and the three client constructs described in this section have been carefully defined, measured, and studied in scores of research projects relating therapist practice to the outcome of psychotherapy. There is considerable evidence that when clients perceive unconditional positive regard and empathic understanding in a relationship with a congruent therapist, their self-concepts become more positive and realistic, they become more self-expressive and self-directed, they become more open and free in their experiencing, their behavior is rated as more mature, and they cope more effectively with stress (Rogers, 1986a).

Other Systems

Rogers's theory and research have, in turn, stimulated developments in theory and practice among his students and colleagues such as Barbara Temaner Brodley, Eugene Gendlin, Fred Zimring, Nat Raskin, Julius Seeman, and Maureen O'Hara.

Theories that claim a direct relation to Rogers's psychological theory and are sufficiently systematized to stand alone include Prouty's *pre-therapy* (Prouty, 1994), Gendlin's *experiential* or *focusing-oriented therapy* (Gendlin, 1996), Greenberg's *emotion-focused therapy* (EFT; also termed *process-experiential*) (Greenberg, 2002), and *integrative models* espoused by Bohart (2005) and Worsley (2004).

Although too numerous to review in this text, significant developments in person-centered theory and practice have come to the fore within the last 25 years. The emergence of critical theory, feminist critique, and social constructionism have inspired contemporary client-centered theorists in explicating connections between ethical-political analysis and the values in Rogers's theory. Currently, a fundamental point of contention concerns applying the approach to persons in diagnostic categories as opposed to rejecting the medical model in full (Proctor, Cooper, Sanders, & Malcolm, 2006). Although some person-centered practitioners argue for an acceptance of "illness" in the person-centered approach, Sanders has argued that construing clients' distress and affliction as "illness" leads to situating pathology inside the person, stigmatizing and marginalizing him or her and failing to perceive and attack the social roots of problems (Sanders, 2007; Van Blarikom, 2006, 2007).

Burstow (1987) has problematized the egalitarian nature of the person-centered approach as has Gillian Proctor (2002) in her analysis of power. Peggy Natiello (1994) grounds her client-centered work in feminist principles, framing the therapy relationship as a collaboration between therapist and client (Natiello, 1994). Maureen O'Hara has written on the emancipatory potential of the person-centered approach, comparing it to the work of Portuguese educator Paolo Freire (O'Hara, 2006), Carol Wolter-Gustafson (Wolter-Gustafson, 2004; 1999), and Gillian Proctor (2002), all of whom have produced critical analyses of power and relationality in psychotherapy practice and the client-centered approach.

Theory development includes Barbara Temaner Brodley's resurrection and exegesis of the nondirective attitude. Her theorizing has been enormously influential in preserving Rogers's theory and practice. Jerold Bozarth's reconceptualization of the "necessary and sufficient" conditions, Barry Grant's advocacy for an "ethics-only" approach to client-centered practice, Pete Sanders's politicization of the approach, Dave Mearn's work on relational depth, Mick Cooper's existential approach, and Peter Schmid's ethics-based dialogical encounter based on the philosophy of Emanual Levinas are all representative of new growth. Defending the approach from the charges of its having no empirical support, Elliott and Freire (2010) have taken a crucial role in reviewing the evidence for the efficacy and effectiveness of client centered and experiential- and process-directive therapies.

Focusing-Oriented Therapy

Eugene Gendlin's philosophy of experiencing led to his development of *experiential therapy*, later called *focusing-oriented therapy*, which locates the experiencing process in the body. Gendlin theorizes that bodily felt sensing is the source of a profound intricacy of experience. Only the "right" words can capture this edge of intricacy and when the person has expressed the "right" words, there is a release in the body, the feeling of "That's exactly it!"

Gendlin developed a series of steps to help the person learn to focus attention in the body. Through an acceptant listening to bodily sensing, particular images and words emerged that carried forward the experiencing process in what Gendlin termed a *felt-shift*. His approach has had enthusiastic support both here and internationally and has been applied in a variety of settings in addition to one-to-one therapy.

It is interesting to note that Rogers's references to the sensory and visceral flow within the body predate Gendlin's focusing theory. Ikemi (2005) observes that Rogers stressed the centrality of bodily experience in 1951, before his association with Gendlin. Rogers states, "This experience of discovering within oneself present attitudes and *emotions which have been viscerally and physiologically experienced,* but which have never been recognized in consciousness, constitutes one of the deepest and most significant phenomena of therapy" (Rogers, 1951, p. 76).

Gendlin's theory of experiencing and the nature of personality change shifted the site of change from the therapist's implementation of the therapeutic attitudes in Rogers's theory to the experiencing process in the client. If the level of experiencing is viewed as the crucial therapeutic variable, then attempting to deepen the level of experiencing is a logical procedure. This leads the therapist to attend to the bodily aspects of the client's experiencing and to the level of the experiencing process. Although experiential and focusing-oriented therapists believe that the correlation of experiencing level with outcome is uncontestable, a number of client-centered therapists report successful outcomes with clients who do not exhibit self-reflective awareness or focused experiencing (see Brodley, 1988, 1990).

Client-centered therapists acknowledge that the construct of focusing may capture phenomena observed in their therapy but do not advocate trying to stimulate more focused experiencing because it involves directiveness and a move away from encountering the person as a whole. In this way, the focusing approach diverges from client-centered therapy. At the same time, focusing-oriented therapy endorses the relationship conditions as crucial to creating an environment of safety that enables the client to make contact with the bodily felt sensing process, and they do not advocate teaching focusing within the therapy relationship (see Brodley, 1990; Gendlin, 1990).

Emotion-Focused Therapy

This approach to therapy was stimulated by the work of Laura North Rice, who studied with Rogers's colleagues at the University of Chicago just after Rogers had left for the University of Wisconsin. Rice's innovation of the "evocation function of the therapist" aimed at heightening the client's experience in the direction of more vivid feeling, resulting in more direct access to emotional experience (Greenberg, Rice, & Elliott, 1993). Collaborating with Rice at York University, Leslie Greenberg and Robert Elliott innovated emotion-focused therapy as a process-experiential approach. Client content was not the focus of the therapy but rather the deepening and intensifying of affect.

According to Cain (2010), EFT blends client-centered therapy with Gendlin's focus on experiencing, existentialism, and Gestalt methods. EFT is considered an "empirically supported humanistic treatment" that postulates that clients' difficulties stem from both dysregulation and avoidance of affect. Unable to contact and process emotions, the client is aided by the EFT therapist in bringing blocked experience to the foreground through identifying emotional triggers, two-chair work taken from Gestalt therapy, and the therapist's coaching. Maintaining a link to client-centered roots, Greenberg stresses that "the client and the quality of the relationship always take precedence over the therapeutic tasks proposed, methods, or goals" (Cain, 2010, p. 53).

Prouty's Pre-Therapy.   Garry Prouty studied with Gene Gendlin and was highly influenced by the theory of experiencing. His innovative work with both developmentally disabled persons and persons diagnosed as psychotic or schizophrenic led him to formulate the principles and practice of pre-therapy. Prouty claimed that normative therapeutic response modes were insufficient with these populations of persons who had much difficulty both in relating to others and communicating comprehensibly. As the first of Rogers's necessary and sufficient conditions states that two persons are in contact, Prouty's methods aim at stimulating and restoring contact with persons who are severely withdrawn and uncommunicative.

Persons who cannot self-represent in therapy may respond to Prouty's forms of response. These innovations include contact reflections in which the therapist mirrors the posture or gestures or facial expression of the client, saying, for instance, "You're standing by the window with your hand over your eyes." These simple, literal responses may help bring the client into interaction with the therapist so that eventually some trust may be established and more self-generated expression may occur (Prouty, 1994). Other client-centered theorists, including Margaret Warner in the United States and Lisbeth Sommerbeck in Denmark, have worked with hospitalized persons with psychotic symptoms (Sommerbeck, 2003; Warner, 2002).

Having reviewed several newer developments that have sprung up *within* the person-centered framework, we will briefly assess two approaches which overlap in some significant ways with the person-centered position: the positive psychology movement that emerged in 1999 and the feminist therapy movement growing out of the women's liberation movement in the early 1970s.

Positive Psychology.   The First Positive Psychology Summit was held in 1999, with an International Positive Psychology Summit occurring in 2002. This emergence of the positive psychology movement inaugurated by Martin Seligman (Seligman & Csikszentmihalyi, 2000) reprised some central tenets of client-centered theory and humanistic psychology more broadly. Both Seligman and Csikszentmihalyi argue that clinical psychology has long stressed illness, pathology, and "treatment"—that is, a medical model. They attribute this development in large part to postwar economic incentives for research and treatment of impairment and psychopathology in the form of National Institute of Mental Health grants. They have argued strongly for this being the "right time" for American psychologists to accentuate the positive. Topics such as "flow" experiences, happiness, subjective well-being, optimism, instrinsic motivation, and self-determination have attracted many eminent researchers and psychologists.

The overarching theme of positive psychology can be expressed as the desirability of focusing on clients' strengths as the engine of change. The client's strengths, when consciously attended to, are thought to catalyze positive emotional states. These emotions function not merely as outcomes but also as generators of change (Fitzpatrick & Stalikas, 2008). This focus on strength, potential, and resilience of persons constitutes an important point of convergence with the person-centered theory of the *actualizing tendency* inherent in the human organism's design. Bohart and Tallman's *How Clients Make Therapy Work,* published in 1999, focuses precisely on the client as an active agent of change with the potential for self-righting (restoring oneself to health and balance). Since the positive psychology movement was announced in 1999, it appears that Bohart and Tallman's ideas converged with—in fact, anticipated—the growth of positive psychology.

The second point of overlap in the two approaches is Rogers's commitment to applying scientific methods to the phenomena he observed in the process of psychotherapy. Seligman and Csikszentmihalyi have stressed the centrality of a "hard" science approach as positive psychology develops its research: "We are, unblushingly, scientists first. The work we seek to support and encourage must be nothing less than replicable, cumulative, and objective" (Seligman & Csikszentmihalyi, 2001, pp. 89–90). In a bid to position their movement as the standard bearer for legitimate "science," Seligman and Czikszentmihalyi (2000) initially claimed that "humanistic psychology did not attract much of a cumulative empirical base. . . . [I]t emphasized the self and encouraged a self-centeredness" (p. 7). The charge that the humanistic therapy movement in the 1960s did not attract a research base and encouraged narcissism and unscientific self-help outraged many humanistic psychologists. Bohart and Greening respond:

> We wish that Seligman and Czikszentmihalyi (2000) themselves had done a more scholarly job of investigating humanistic psychology. Neither the theory nor practice of humanistic psychology is narrowly focused on the narcissistic self or on individual fulfillment. (Bohart & Greening, 2001, p. 81)

While lauding the reemergence of a strength-based vision of the person capable of self-direction, well-being and intrinsic self-determination, Lambert and Erekson joined in the complaint that positive psychologists seem unaware of the historical research base in client-centered therapy, including the strong support for the efficacy of the approach.

> It is important in this context to note the substantial research base on the efficacy and effectiveness of client-centered therapy for diminishing symptoms of pathology and enhancing client well-being. The efficacy of client-centered psychotherapy for the client rests on 50 years of outcome and process research with a notable number of studies measuring changes in positive emotional states. (Lambert & Erekson, 2008, p. 224)

Lambert and Erekson continue their critique in response to the notion that clients should be steered away from negative emotions:

> What would appear to be at odds with the current emphasis on positive emotions, from the perspective of traditional client-centered psychotherapy, is the idea that something needs to be added to or sharpened in therapy in order to increase the likelihood of positive feelings emerging in the client. Certainly in this context most client-centered therapists would not imagine an advantage for the client in turning the client's attention away from feelings that are present in favor of directing the client toward subset of positive feelings. (Lambert & Erekson, 2008, p. 223)

While acknowledging the impressive growth of studies of positive psychology, Joseph and Linley (2006) also caution that if the positive psychology movement continues to ground itself in a medical model with positive interventions such as "happiness exercises for depression," the attempt to transcend the "illness" focus will fail. Rather than transcending the medical model approach of "applying appropriate treatments to disorders," positive psychology's interventions may be assimilated as just more "tools" in the therapy "toolkit." Readers are encouraged to check out the evidence for the claims of the positive psychology researchers and to review the critiques as well (Held, 2002; 2005; Joseph & Linley, 2006; Kristjánsson, 2010; Lambert & Erekson, 2008; Sugarman, 2007; Yen, 2010).

Feminist Psychotherapy.   The rise of the second wave of feminism in the late 1960s, consciousness-raising groups, which were unfacilitated, spontaneous gatherings of women, were revelatory for their women members (Brown, 1994). As women activists in the civil rights struggle and other progressive causes found that their own views, goals, and insights were subordinated to male leaders, their common experience of invisibility, inequality, and discrimination led to activism on many fronts. Issues that had never been discussed openly were made public: forced sterilization of poor women, rape, domestic violence, economic discrimination, child sexual abuse, heteronormative images of women, and exclusion from athletics. All of these and more provoked collective action. From radicals to reformists, feminism was a pluralistic, many-faceted phenomenon.

Women in the academy at that time mounted scathing critiques of blatant discrimination against women within the ranks and went further to unmask the sexist ideology of male dominance. Harvard-trained experimental psychologist Naomi Weisstein published her seminal critique of the field of clinical psychology in "*Kinder, Küche, Kirche as Scientific Fact: Psychology Constructs the Female*" (Weisstein, 1970). In this classic and still timely critique, Weisstein exposed psychology as a bastion of practices that, both explicitly and implicitly, enforced social control of women.

Deconstructing and challenging social role expectations, economic subordination, political disempowerment, and violence against women as a strategy of social control and intimidation, women moved from expressing what they had heretofore believed were unique, individual problems to respecting their experiences and recognizing that individual experiences were political through and through.

Drawn to the women's movement, women therapists turned their critical attention to the dominant therapeutic paradigms and theoretical schools, giving rise to challenges to the authority of the male founders. Feminist therapists stood the field of psychology on its head, exposing diagnostic categories oppressive to women, practices in therapy that reinscribed male authority, and the nonexistent evidentiary base for essentialist formulations of women's biological nature. The Freudian assertion that "Anatomy is destiny" became a target for critique. A real revolution was underway.

Mainstream psychology theories, however, continued to locate women's problems within the individual psyche. Whether "conflicts" arise from narcissictic injuries, anxious attachment style, or dysfunctional cognitive schemata to Rogers's "conditions of worth," traditional theorists confidently asserted that psychological problems could be traced to an intrapsychic source.

The economic incentives for professionals and academics were obvious. Under this model of causation, women *needed* individual, lengthy, and expensive treatment for their "complexes," lack of "adjustment" to their female roles, sexual "frigidity," and the like. Practitioners in what has been called the "misery business" held their particular techniques out as the answer to the pathologies women suffered.

Feminist critics argued that psychology's constructs mask the fact that one's perceived experiences are socially constructed. Kitzinger and Perkins (1993) argue that

> experience is always perceived through an (implicit or explicit) theoretical framework within which it gains meaning. Feelings and emotions are not simply immediate, unsocialized, self-authenticating responses. They are socially constructed and presuppose certain social norms. Experience is never "raw;" it is embedded in a social web of interpretation and reinterpretation. In encouraging and perpetuating the notion of pure, unsullied presocialized "experience" welling up from inside, therapists have disguised or obscured the social roots of our "inner selves." (Kitzinger & Perkins, 1993, pp. 191–192)

Psychologists for the most part represented a bastion of male authority in their espousal of essentialist narratives of internal pathogens, reductionist analyses of "what women want," and prescriptions of what they *should* want (see Gergen & Kaye, 1992, p. 169). As a response, feminist therapy addresses ethics and advocates more than one-to-one models of change. Many women's problems are rooted not in their psyches but in the social structures that oppress them. Rodis and Strehorn explain:

> Feminism clearly and uncompromisingly asserts that the psychology relationship and the therapeutic process must be centered in a dialogue about justice, both social and interpersonal; feminism claims that, even as most client problems are the

product of some injustice, the reaffirmation of justice as a moral ideal and the establishment of a more just society as a functional reality will bring about positive change. (Lerman & Porter, 1990; Prilleltensky & Walsh-Bowers, 1993; Rodis & Strehorn, 1997)

The ongoing problem that feminist theorists have faced is the move from reaction and critique to the development of innovative ways of working with other women. This movement progresses from traditional models that are largely "supportive" and nurturing to models that energize women's resistance. Today, feminist therapists integrate and adapt psychoanalytic, interpersonal, humanist, systems, and topical approaches such as trauma therapy as defining of feminist practice.

To circumvent, overcome, and contradict the prevailing models of therapy that are not explicitly critical or even aware of the power issues within the therapy context, feminist practitioners confront difficulty in leaping into a wholly new model. As Gergen has pointed out,

> [by] implication (and practice) the ultimate aim of most schools of therapy is hegemonic. All other schools of thought, and their associated narratives, should succumb. Psychoanalysts wish to eradicate behavior modification; cognitive-behavioral therapists see systems therapy as misguided and so on. Yet, the most immediate and potentially injurious consequences are reserved for the client. For in the end, the structure of the procedure furnishes the client a lesson in inferiority. (Gergen & Kaye, 1992, p. 171)

Client-centered feminist therapists counter Gergen's claim. We argue that the client-centered commitment to the client's reality as perceived, from a standpoint of acceptant neutrality avoids replacing the client's version of being-in-the-world with a hegemonic, theoretically based version. We avoid reassurance and confrontation of our clients precisely in order to empower them and not place them in a position to be "educated." In this respect, we would argue that client-centered practice is consonant with the feminist therapy's aims of empowerment of all of our clients. At the same time, we agree that although therapy can assist clients in numerous ways, it does not substitute for collective action for social change. The institution of therapy reinforces the deeply rooted idea that psychological problems are frequently superficial manifestations of underlying "disorders" that are individual in nature.

HISTORY

Precursors

One of the most powerful influences on Carl Rogers was learning that traditional child-guidance methods in which he had been trained did not work very well. At Columbia University's Teachers College, he had been taught testing, measurement, diagnostic interviewing, and interpretive treatment. This was followed by an internship at the psychoanalytically oriented Institute for Child Guidance, where he learned to take exhaustive case histories and do projective personality testing. It is important to note that Rogers originally went to a Rochester child-guidance agency believing in this diagnostic, prescriptive, professionally impersonal approach, and only after actual experience did he conclude that it was not effective. As an alternative, he tried listening and following the client's lead rather than assuming the role of the expert. This worked better, and he discovered some theoretical and applied support for this alternative approach in the work of Otto Rank and his followers at the University of Pennsylvania School of Social Work and the Philadelphia Child Guidance Clinic.

One particularly important event was a three-day seminar in Rochester with Rank (Rogers & Haigh, 1983). Another was his association with a Rankin-trained social worker, Elizabeth Davis, from whom "I first got the notion of responding almost entirely to the feelings being expressed. What later came to be called the reflection of feeling sprang from my contact with her" (Rogers & Haigh, 1983, p. 7).

Rogers's therapy practice and later his theory grew out of his own experience. At the same time, several links to Otto Rank are apparent in Rogers's early work. Aspects of Rankian theory bear a close relationship to principles of nondirective therapy. Rank explicitly, eloquently, and repeatedly rejected therapy by technique and interpretation:

> Every single case, yes every individual hour of the same case, is different, because it is derived momentarily from the play of forces given in the situation and immediately applied. My technique consists essentially in having no technique, but in utilizing as much as possible experience and understanding that are constantly converted into skill but never crystallized into technical rules which would be applicable ideologically. There is a technique only in an ideological therapy where technique is identical with theory and the chief task of the analyst is interpretation (ideological), not the bringing to pass and granting of experience. (1945, p. 105)

Rank is obscure about his actual practice of psychotherapy, particularly the amount and nature of his activity during the treatment hour. Unsystematic references in *Will Therapy, and Truth and Reality* (1945) reveal that, despite his criticism of educational and interpretive techniques and his expressed value of the patient being his or her own therapist, he assumed a position of undisputed power in the relationship.

Beginnings

Carl Ransom Rogers was born in Oak Park, Illinois, on January 8, 1902. His parents believed in hard work, responsibility, and religious fundamentalism and frowned on activities such as drinking, dancing, and card playing. The family was characterized by closeness and devotion but did not openly display affection. While in high school, Carl worked on the family farm, and he became interested in experimentation and the scientific aspect of agriculture. He entered the University of Wisconsin, following his parents and older siblings, as an agriculture major. Rogers also carried on his family's religious tradition. He was active in the campus YMCA and was chosen to be one of 10 American youth delegates to the World Student Christian Federation's conference in Peking, China, in 1922. At that time he switched his major from agriculture to history, which he thought would better prepare him for a career as a minister.

After graduating from Wisconsin in 1924 and marrying Helen Elliott, a childhood friend, he entered the Union Theological Seminary. Two years later, and in part as a result of taking several psychology courses, Rogers moved "across Broadway" to Teachers College, Columbia University, where he was exposed to what he later described as "a contradictory mixture of Freudian, scientific, and progressive education thinking" (Rogers & Sanford, 1985, p. 1374).

After Teachers College, Rogers worked for 12 years at a child-guidance center in Rochester, New York, where he soon became an administrator as well as a practicing psychologist. He began writing articles and became active at a national level. His book *The Clinical Treatment of the Problem Child* was published in 1939, and he was offered a professorship in psychology at Ohio State University. Once at Ohio State, Rogers began to teach newer ways of helping problem children and their parents.

In 1940, Rogers was teaching an enlightened distillation of the child-guidance practices described in *The Clinical Treatment of the Problem Child*. From his point of view, this approach represented a consensual direction in which the field was moving and was evolutionary rather than revolutionary. The clinical process began with an assessment, including testing children and interviewing parents; assessment results provided the basis for a treatment plan. In treatment, nondirective principles were followed.

Rogers's views gradually became more radical. His presentation at the University of Minnesota on December 11, 1940, entitled "Some Newer Concepts in Psychotherapy," is the single event most often identified with the birth of client-centered therapy. Rogers decided to expand this talk into a book titled *Counseling and Psychotherapy* (1942). The book, which included an electronically recorded eight-interview case, described the generalized process in which a client begins with a conflict situation and a predominance of negative attitudes and moves toward insight, independence, and positive attitudes. Rogers hypothesized that the counselor promoted such a process by avoiding advice and interpretation and by consistently recognizing and accepting the client's feelings. Research corroborating this new approach to counseling and psychotherapy was offered, including the first (Porter, 1943) of what soon became a series of pioneering doctoral dissertations on the process and outcomes of psychotherapy. In a very short time, both an entirely new approach to psychotherapy and the field of psychotherapy research were born. This approach and its accompanying research led to the eventual acceptance of psychotherapy as a primary professional function of clinical psychologists.

After serving as director of counseling services for the United Service Organizations during World War II, Rogers was appointed professor of psychology at the University of Chicago and became head of the university's counseling center. The 12 years during which Rogers remained at Chicago were a period of tremendous growth in client-centered theory, philosophy, practice, research, applications, and implications.

In 1957, Rogers published a classic paper entitled "The Necessary and Sufficient Conditions of Therapeutic Personality Change." *Congruence, unconditional positive regard*, and *empathic understanding* of the client's internal frame of reference were cited as three essential therapist-offered conditions of therapeutic personality change. This theoretical statement applied to all types of therapy, not just the client-centered approach, and its impact on the field cannot be overstated. It was followed by the most comprehensive and rigorous formulation of his theory of therapy, personality, and interpersonal relationships (Rogers, 1959b).

Rogers's philosophy of the "exquisitely rational" nature of the behavior and growth of human beings was further articulated and related to the thinking of Søren Kierkegaard, Abraham Maslow, Rollo May, Martin Buber, and others in the humanistic movement whose theories were catalyzing a "third force" in psychology, challenging the dominance of behaviorism and psychoanalysis.

At Ohio State, there was a sense that client-centered principles had implications beyond the counseling office. When Rogers moved to the University of Chicago, this was made most explicit by the empowerment of students and the counseling center staff. Shlien remarks that on the first day of the staff meeting, Rogers listed his and all members' salaries on the board and asked if people were satisfied with the numbers! This was unheard of in the staid atmosphere of the academic hierarchy and shows Rogers as the protofeminist that he was. About half of Rogers's *Client-Centered Therapy* (1951) was devoted to applications of client-centered therapy, with additional chapters on play therapy, group therapy, training of therapists, leadership, and administration.

In 1957, Rogers accepted a professorship in psychology and psychiatry at the University of Wisconsin. With the collaboration of associates and graduate students, a massive research project was mounted, based on the hypothesis that hospitalized schizophrenics would respond to a client-centered approach (Rogers et al., 1967). Two relatively clear conclusions emerged from a complex maze of results: (1) The most successful patients were those who had experienced the highest degree of accurate empathy, and (2) it was the client's, rather than the therapist's, judgment of the therapy relationship that correlated more highly with success or failure. This finding corresponds to recent investigations of the core conditions. Bohart and Tallman state:

> Findings abound that the client's perceptions of the relationship or alliance, more so than the therapist's correlate highly with therapeutic outcome. . . . Clients ratings of empathy also correlate as highly, or more highly, with outcome as do ratings of objective observers. . . . The client's ratings of the collaborative nature of the relationship also correlate with outcome more than the therapist's. (Bohart & Tallman cited in Cooper et al., 2010, p. 106)

Rogers left the University of Wisconsin and full-time academia and began living in La Jolla, California, in 1964. He was a resident fellow for four years at the Western Behavioral Sciences Institute and then, starting in 1968, at the Center for Studies of the Person. In more than two decades in California, Rogers wrote books on a person-centered approach to teaching (*Freedom to Learn for the 80s*, 1983) and educational administration, on encounter groups (*Carl Rogers on Encounter Groups*, 1970), on marriage and other forms of partnership, and on the "quiet revolution" that he believed would emerge with a new type of "self-empowered person" (*On Personal Power*, 1977). Rogers believed this revolution had the potential to change "the very nature of psychotherapy, marriage, education, administration, and politics" (Rogers, 1977). These books were based on observations and interpretations of hundreds of individual and group experiences.

A special interest of Rogers and his associates was the application of a person-centered approach to international conflict resolution. This resulted in trips to South Africa, Eastern Europe, and the Soviet Union, as well as meetings with Irish Catholics and Protestants and with representatives of nations involved in Central American conflicts (Rogers & Ryback, 1984). In addition to Rogers's books, a number of valuable films and videotapes have provided data for research on the basic person-centered hypothesis that individuals and groups who have experienced empathy, congruence, and unconditional positive regard will go through a constructive process of self-directed change.

Current Status

Since 1982, biennial international forums on the person-centered approach have met in Mexico, Austria, the United Kingdom, the United States, Brazil, the Netherlands, Greece, and South Africa. Alternating with these meetings have been international conferences on client-centered and experiential psychotherapy in Belgium, Scotland, Austria, Portugal, and the United States.

In September 1986, five months before his death, Rogers attended the inaugural meeting of the Association for the Development of the Person-Centered Approach (ADPCA) held at International House on the campus of the University of Chicago. David Cain, a person-centered therapist and a friend of Carl's, had encouraged him to allow the emergence of organizations. To that point, Rogers had been mostly opposed to anything smacking of centralization of power or bureaucracy. This meeting, which turned out to be the last Carl Rogers attended, was the beginning of the ADPCA and the journal *Person-Centered Review*, which David Cain edited.

The organization has maintained its robust health in spite of always challenging and sometimes fractious annual meetings. The ADPCA meets annually and can be accessed online at www.adpca.org. The association is composed of persons in a variety of occupations. Educators, nurses, psychologists, students, artists, and business consultants are all part of this growing community of persons interested in the potential of the approach.

Another idea for a workshop on the person-centered approach was developed during the first meeting of the ADPCA. The workshop, organized by Jerold Bozarth, professor emeritus at University of Georgia, and several graduate students, began a week after Carl Rogers's death on February 4, 1987. It was held in Warm Springs, Georgia, February 11–15, 1987, at the Rehabilitation Institute, where Franklin Roosevelt was treated after being stricken with polio.

Workshops have been held annually at Warm Springs since 1987, and the nonfacilitated, nondirective climate has been maintained over the years. The workshop consists of unplanned meetings of the whole community and is not organized around papers or workshop sessions. This may be the only entirely self-directed group experience available to interested persons.

These organizations have been largely attended by white, middle-class persons, with genders pretty evenly represented, along with those of fluid gender identities. Increasingly, our ranks include African Americans and Latinos and Latinas as well as a small representation of Japanese and Chinese members. The age range spans from the early 20s to persons in their 80s. We also have international attendees when meetings are in the United States, and many Americans attend the overseas forums.

In 1992, the *Person-Centered* Review was replaced by the *Person-Centered Journal*, coedited by Jerold Bozarth and Fred Zimring; this journal is still published today with editors selected at the annual meetings of the ADPCA.

In 2000, the World Association for Person-Centered and Experiential Psychotherapy and Counseling (WAPCEPC) was founded at the International Forum for the Person-Centered Approach in Lisbon, Portugal. This association consists of psychotherapists, researchers, and theorists from many countries, and it actively seeks to reassert the revolutionary nature of a person-centered approach. Association activities, conference schedules, and membership information may be found online at www.pce-world .org. This organization has launched the peer-reviewed journal *Person-Centered and Experiential Psychotherapy* (PCEP), which publishes empirical, qualitative, and theoretical articles of broad interest to humanistic practitioners and researchers. Full-text articles are available online for the PCEP back to 2001. For a more thorough review of the current status of the person-centered approach, see Howard Kirschenbaum's and April Jourdan's (2005) article "The Current Status of Carl Rogers and the Person-Centered Approach."

PERSONALITY

Theory of Personality

Rogers moved from a lack of interest in psychological theory to the development of a rigorous 19-proposition "theory of therapy, personality, and interpersonal relationships" (Rogers, 1951). On one level, this signified a change in Rogers's respect for theory. On another, this comprehensive formulation can be understood as a logical evolution. His belief in the importance of the child's conscious attitudes toward self and self-ideal was central to the test of personality adjustment he devised for children (Rogers, 1931). The portrayal of the client's growing through a process of reduced defensiveness and of self-directed expansion of self-awareness was described in a paper on the processes of therapy (Rogers, 1940).

Rogers expanded his observations into a theory of personality and behavior that he described in *Client-Centered Therapy* (1951). This theory is based on the following 19 basic propositions:

1. Every individual exists in a continually changing world of experience of which he or she is the center.

2. The organism reacts to the field as it is perceived. For the individual, this perceptual field is "reality."

3. The organism reacts as an organized whole to this phenomenal field.

4. The organism has one basic tendency and striving—to actualize, maintain, and enhance the experiencing organism.

5. Behavior is basically the goal-directed attempt of the organism to satisfy its needs as experienced in the field as perceived.

6. Emotion accompanies and in general facilitates such goal-directed behavior, the kind of emotion being related to the seeking versus the consummatory aspects of the behavior, and the intensity of the emotion being related to the perceived significance of the behavior for the maintenance and enhancement of the organism.

7. The best vantage point for understanding behavior is from the internal frame of reference of the individual.

8. A portion of the total perceptual field gradually becomes differentiated as the self.

9. As a result of interaction with the environment, and particularly as a result of evaluational interaction with others, the structure of self is formed—an organized, fluid, but consistent conceptual pattern of perceptions of characteristics and relationships of the "I" or the "me," together with values attached to these concepts.

10. The values attached to experiences and the values that are a part of the self-structure in some instances are values experienced directly by the organism, and in some instances they are values introjected or taken over from others but perceived in distorted fashion as though they had been experienced directly.

11. As experiences occur in the life of the individual, they are (a) symbolized, perceived, and organized into some relationship to the self; (b) ignored because there is no perceived relationship to the self-structure; or (c) denied symbolization or given a distorted symbolization because the experience is inconsistent with the structure of the self.

12. Most of the ways of behaving that are adopted by the organism are those that are consistent with the concept of self.

13. Behavior may, in some instances, be brought about by organismic experiences and needs that have not been symbolized. Such behavior may be inconsistent with the structure of the self, but in such instances the behavior is not "owned" by the individual.

14. Psychological maladjustment exists when the organism denies to awareness significant sensory and visceral experiences, which consequently are not symbolized and organized into the gestalt of the self-structure. When this situation exists, there is a basis for potential psychological tension.

15. Psychological adjustment exists when the concept of the self is such that all the sensory and visceral experiences of the organism are or may be assimilated on a symbolic level into a consistent relationship with the concept of self.

16. Any experience that is inconsistent with the organization or structure of self may be perceived as a threat. The more of these perceptions there are, the more rigidly the self-structure is organized to maintain itself.

17. Under certain conditions, involving primarily complete absence of any threat to the self-structure, experiences that are inconsistent with it may be perceived and examined and the structure of self revised to assimilate and include such experiences.

18. When the individual perceives all his sensory and visceral experiences and accepts them into one consistent and integrated system, then he is necessarily more understanding of others and more accepting of others as separate individuals.

19. As the individual perceives and accepts into his self-structure more of his organismic experiences, he finds that he is replacing his current value system—based so largely on introjections that have been distortedly symbolized—with a continuing organismic valuing process (Rogers, 1951, pp. 481–533).

Rogers comments that

This theory is basically phenomenological in character, and relies heavily upon the concept of the self as an explanatory construct. It pictures the end-point of personality development as being a basic congruence between the phenomenal field of experience and the conceptual structure of the self—a situation which, if achieved, would represent freedom from internal strain and anxiety, and freedom from potential strain; which would represent the maximum in realistically oriented adaptation; which would mean the establishment of an individualized value system having considerable identity with the value system of any other equally well-adjusted member of the human race. (1951, p. 532)

Further investigations of these propositions were conducted at the University of Chicago Counseling and Psychotherapy Research Center in the early 1950s in carefully designed and controlled studies. Stephenson's (1953) Q-sort technique was used to measure changes in self-concept and self-ideal during and following therapy and in a no-therapy control period. Many results confirmed Rogers's hypotheses. For example, a significant increase in congruence between self and ideal occurred during therapy, and changes in the perceived self resulted in better psychological adjustment (Rogers & Dymond, 1954).

Rogers's personality theory has been described as growth-oriented rather than developmental. Although this description is accurate, it does not acknowledge Rogers's sensitivity to the attitudes with which children are confronted, beginning in infancy:

While I have been fascinated by the horizontal spread of the person-centered approach into so many areas of our life, others have been more interested in the vertical direction and are discovering the profound value of treating the infant, during the whole birth process, as a person who should be understood, whose communications should be treated with respect, who should be dealt with empathically. This is the new and stimulating contribution of Frederick Leboyer, a French obstetrician who . . . has assisted in the delivery of at least a thousand infants in what can only be called a person-centered way. (Rogers, 1977, p. 31)

Rogers goes on to describe the infant's extreme sensitivity to light and sound, the rawness of the skin, the fragility of the head, the struggle to breathe, and the like, along with the specific ways in which Leboyer has taught parents and professionals to provide a beginning life experience that is caring, loving, and respectful.

This sensitivity to children was further expressed in Rogers's explanation of his fourth proposition: The organism has one basic tendency and striving—to actualize, maintain, and enhance the experiencing organism.

The whole process (of self-enhancement and growth) may be symbolized and illustrated by the child's learning to walk. The first steps involve struggle, and usually pain. Often it is true that the immediate reward involved in taking a few steps is in no way commensurate with the pain of falls and bumps. The child may, because of the pain, revert to crawling for a time. Yet the forward direction of growth is more powerful than the satisfactions of remaining infantile. Children will actualize themselves, in spite of the painful experiences of so doing. In the same way, they will become independent, responsible, self-governing, and socialized, in spite of the pain which is often involved in these steps. Even where they do not, because of a variety of circumstances, exhibit the growth, the tendency is still present. Given the opportunity for clear-cut choice between forward-moving and regressive behavior, the tendency will operate. (Rogers, 1951, pp. 490–491)

One of Rogers's hypotheses about personality (proposition 8) was that a part of the developing infant's private world becomes recognized as "me," "I," or "myself." Rogers described infants, in the course of interacting with the environment, as building up concepts about themselves, about the environment, and about themselves in relation to the environment.

Rogers's next suppositions are crucial to his theory of how development may proceed either soundly or in the direction of maladjustment. He assumes that very young infants are involved in "direct organismic valuing" with very little or no uncertainty. They have experiences such as "I am cold, and I don't like it," or "I like being cuddled," which may occur even though they lack descriptive words or symbols for these organismic experiences. The principle in this natural process is that the infant positively values those experiences that are perceived as self-enhancing and places a negative value on those that threaten or do not maintain or enhance the self.

This situation changes once children begin to be evaluated by others (Holdstock & Rogers, 1983). The love they are given and the symbolization of themselves as lovable children become dependent on behavior. To hit or to hate a baby sibling may result in a child being told that he or she is bad and unlovable. The child, to preserve a positive self-concept, may distort experience.

> It is in this way . . . that parental attitudes are not only introjected, but . . . are experienced . . . in distorted fashion, as if based on the evidence of one's own sensory and visceral equipment. Thus, through distorted symbolization, expression of anger comes to be "experienced" as bad, even though the more accurate symbolization would be that the expression of anger is often experienced as satisfying or enhancing. . . . The "self" which is formed on this basis of distorting the sensory and visceral evidence to fit the already present structure acquires an organization and integration which the individual endeavors to preserve. (Rogers, 1951, pp. 500–501)

This type of interaction may sow the seeds of confusion about self, self-doubt, and disapproval of self, as well as reliance on the evaluation of others. Rogers indicated that these consequences may be avoided if the parent can accept the child's negative feelings and the child as a whole while refusing to permit certain behaviors such as hitting the baby.

Variety of Concepts

Various terms and concepts appear in the presentation of Rogers's theory of personality and behavior that often have a unique and distinctive meaning in this orientation.

Experience

In Rogers's theory, the term *experience* refers to the private world of the individual. At any moment, some experience is conscious; for example, we feel the pressure of the keys against our fingers as we type. Some experiences may be difficult to bring into awareness, such as the idea "I am an aggressive person." People's actual awareness of their total experiential field may be limited, but each individual is the only one who can know it completely.

Reality

For psychological purposes, reality is basically the private world of individual perceptions, although for social purposes, reality consists of those perceptions that have a high degree of consensus among local communities of individuals. Two people will agree on the reality that a particular person is a politician. One sees her as a good woman who wants to help people and, on the basis of this reality, votes for her. The other person's reality is that the politician appropriates money to win favor, so this person votes against her. In therapy, changes in feelings and perceptions will result in changes in reality as perceived. This is particularly fundamental as the client is more and more able to accept "the self that I am now."

The Organism's Reacting as an Organized Whole

A person may be hungry but, because of a report to complete, skips lunch. In psychotherapy, clients often become clearer about what is important to them, resulting in behavioral changes directed toward the clarified goals. A politician may choose not to run for office because he decides that his family life is more important. A client with a disabling condition is more open to the changed circumstances of her life with the illness and is better able to care for herself in terms of rest and self-care.

The Organism's Actualizing Tendency

This is a central tenet in the writings of Kurt Goldstein, Hobart Mowrer, Harry Stack Sullivan, Karen Horney, and Andras Angyal, to name just a few. The child's painful struggle to learn to walk is an example. It is Rogers's belief and the belief of most other personality theorists that, in the absence of external force, individuals prefer to be healthy rather than sick, to be free to choose rather than having choices made for them, and in general to further the optimal development of the total organism. Deci and Ryan's (1985, 1991) formulation of self-determination theory (SDT) has stimulated many recent empirical studies investigating situations that support or constrain intrinsic motivation, which is a natural feature of human living. Ryan and Deci describe this human capacity:

> Perhaps no single phenomenon reflects the positive potential of human nature as much as intrinsic motivation, the inherent tendency to seek out novelty and challenges, to extend and exercise one's capacities, to explore, and to learn. . . . [T]he evidence is now clear that the maintenance and enhancement of this inherent propensity requires supportive conditions, as it can be fairly readily disrupted by various nonsupportive conditions. . . . [T]he study of conditions which facilitate versus undermine intrinsic motivation is an important first step in understanding sources of both alienation and liberation of the positive aspects of human nature. (Ryan & Deci, 2000, p. 70)

In Rogers's theory, the actualizing tendency functions as an axiom and is not subject to falsification. In the therapy situation, it is a functional construct for the therapist, who can conceive of the client as attempting to realize self and organism, especially when the client's behavior and ways of thinking appear self-destructive or irrational. In these situations, the client-centered therapist's trust in the client's "self-righting" capacities (Bohart, 2004) and self-regulatory capacities may be sorely tested, but holding to the hypothesis of the actualizing tendency supports the therapist's efforts to understand and maintain unconditionality toward the client (Brodley, 1999c/2011).

The Internal Frame of Reference

This is the perceptual field of the individual. It is the way the world appears to us from our own unique vantage point, given the whole continuum of learnings and experiences we have accumulated along with the meanings attached to experience and feelings. From the client-centered point of view, apprehending this internal frame provides the fullest understanding of why people behave as they do. It is to be distinguished from external judgments of behavior, attitudes, and personality.

The Self, Concept of Self, and Self–Structure

These terms refer to the

> organized, consistent, conceptual gestalt composed of perceptions of the character-istics of the "I" or "me" and the perceptions of the relationships of the "I" or "me" to others and to various aspects of life, together with the values attached to these perceptions. It is a gestalt available to awareness although not necessarily in aware-ness. It is a fluid and changing process, but at any given moment it . . . is at least partially definable in operational terms. (Meador & Rogers, 1984, p. 158)

Symbolization

This is the process by which the individual becomes aware or conscious of an experi-ence. There is a tendency to deny symbolization to experiences at variance with the concept of self; for example, people who think of themselves as truthful will tend to re-sist the symbolization of an act of lying. Ambiguous experiences tend to be symbolized in ways that are consistent with self-concept. A speaker lacking in self-confidence may symbolize a silent audience as unimpressed, whereas one who is confident may symbol-ize such a group as attentive and interested.

Psychological Adjustment or Maladjustment

Congruence, or its absence, between an individual's sensory and visceral experiences and his or her concept of self defines whether a person is psychologically adjusted or maladjusted. A self-concept that includes elements of weakness and imperfection facilitates the symbolization of failure experiences. The need to deny or distort such experiences does not exist and therefore fosters a condition of psychological adjustment. If a person who has always seen herself as honest tells a white lie to her daughter, she may experience discomfort and vulnerability. For that moment, there is incongruence between her self-concept and her behavior. Integration of the alien behavior—"I guess sometimes I take the easy way out and tell a lie"—may restore the person to congruence and free the person to consider whether she wants to change her behavior or her self-concept. A state of psychological adjustment means that the organism is open to his or her organismic experiencing as trustworthy and admissible to awareness.

Organismic Valuing Process

This is an ongoing process in which individuals freely rely on the evidence of their own senses for making value judgments. This is in contrast to a fixed system of introjected values characterized by "oughts" and "shoulds" and by what is supposed to be right or wrong. The organismic valuing process is consistent with the person-centered hypoth-esis of confidence in the individual and, even though established by each individual, it makes for a highly responsible socialized system of values and behavior. The responsibil-ity derives from people making choices on the basis of their direct, organismic process-ing of situations, in contrast to acting out of fear of what others may think of them or what others have taught them is "the way" to think and act.

The Fully Functioning Person

Rogers defined those who can readily assimilate organismic experiencing and who are capable of symbolizing these ongoing experiences in awareness as "fully functioning" persons, able to experience all of their feelings, afraid of none of them, allowing awareness to flow freely in and through their experiences. Seeman (1984) has been involved in a long-term research program to clarify and describe the qualities of such optimally functioning individuals. These empirical studies highlight the possession of a positive self-concept, greater physiological responsiveness, and an efficient use of the environment.

PSYCHOTHERAPY

Theory of Psychotherapy

Rogers's theory of therapeutic personality change posits that if a congruent therapist *experiences* unconditional positive regard and empathic understanding of the client's internal frame of reference, and if the client *perceives* the therapist's attitudes, then the client will respond with constructive changes in personality organization (Rogers, 1957, 1959b). *Congruence* is fundamental to the other two therapeutic conditions. Watson points out the following:

> If the client perceives the therapist as ungenuine, then the client will not perceive the therapist as communicating the other two conditions. It follows from this hypothesis that the client's perception of the therapist's congruence is one of the necessary and sufficient conditions for effective therapy. (Watson, 1984, p. 19)

When the core conditions are realized to some degree by the therapist (of any theoretical orientation), studies demonstrate that these qualities may be perceived by the client within the first several interviews. Changes in self-acceptance, immediacy of experiencing, directness of relating, and movement toward an internal locus of evaluation may occur in short-term intensive workshops or even in single interviews.

Empathic Understanding of the Client's Internal Frame of Reference

Empathic understanding in client-centered therapy is an active, immediate, continuous process involving the therapist's cognitive processes, affective responses, and expressive behavior. To correct a common misperception of the approach, Rogers is referring to an attitude, not a behavior. The theory does not specify or prescribe any particular way of responding to or being with the client! Raskin, in an oft-quoted paper written in 1947, describes this process:

> At this level, counselor participation becomes an active experiencing with the client of the feelings to which he gives expression, the counselor makes a maximum effort to get under the skin of the person with whom he is communicating, he tries to get *within* and to live the attitudes expressed instead of observing them, to catch every nuance of their changing nature; in a word, to absorb himself completely in the attitudes of the other. And in struggling to do this, there is simply no room for any other type of counselor activity or attitude; if he is attempting to live the attitudes of the other, he cannot be diagnosing them, he cannot be thinking of making the process go faster. Because he is another, and not the client, the understanding is not spontaneous but must be acquired, and this through the most intense, continuous and active attention to the feelings of the other, to the exclusion of any other type of attention. (Raskin, 1947/2005, pp. 6–7)

The accuracy of the therapist's overt empathic understanding responses has often been emphasized, but more important is the therapist's inner experience of empathic reception of the world of the client with the intent to check these emerging understandings with the client in the spirit of willingness to be corrected. This creates a process in which the therapist gets closer and closer to the client's meanings and feelings, developing an ever-deepening relationship based on respect for and understanding of the other person. Brodley (1994/2011) has documented the high proportion (often as high as 80% to 90%) of "empathic understanding responses" in Rogers's therapy transcripts. Brodley's research has shown that Rogers's therapy was highly consistent throughout his career and did not waver from his trust in the client and his commitment to the principle of nondirectivity. Rogers, however, did not ask that other therapists mimic his response repertoire. His responses were, he said, only ways that he had discovered to be helpful. Others might find unique and personal ways of being in relationship.

Unconditional Positive Regard

Other terms for this condition are *warm acceptance*, *nonpossessive caring*, and a *nonjudgmental openness* to the client as a person, his or her behaviors, beliefs, and values. Biases and prejudices go with us into the therapy room, but within that relationship, the therapist makes every effort to be aware of evaluative or judgmental responses and to set them aside. If the reactions are troublesome and threaten unconditional positive regard, then the responsible therapist takes up the basis of the judgments within the consultative relation with a trusted supervisor.

> When the therapist is experiencing a positive, nonjudgmental, acceptant attitude toward whatever the client is at that moment, therapeutic movement or change is more likely. It involves the therapist's willingness for the client to be whatever immediate feeling is going on—confusion, resentment, fear, anger, courage, love, or pride. . . . When the therapist prizes the client in a total rather than a conditional way, forward movement is likely. (Rogers, 1986a, p. 198)

Congruence

Rogers regarded congruence as

> the most basic of the attitudinal conditions that foster therapeutic growth. [It] does not mean that the therapist burdens the client with all of his or her problems or feelings. It does not mean that the therapist blurts out impulsively any attitudes that come to mind. It does mean, however, that the therapist does not deny to himself or herself the feelings being experienced and that the therapist is willing to express and to be open about any persistent feelings that exist in the relationship. It means avoiding the temptation to hide behind a mask of professionalism. (Rogers & Sanford, 1985, p. 1379)

Relationship Therapeutic Conditions

Three other conditions that pertain to the client—in addition to the "therapist-offered" conditions of empathy, congruence, and unconditional positive regard—are included in this list of all six of the necessary and sufficient conditions. It is very important to understand that Rogers's *if-then* statements listed here pertain to all therapies, not just client-centered therapy. Bozarth identifies this paper as Rogers's "integrative" statement as opposed to his later explicitly client-centered theory in the 1959 theoretical statement (Bozarth, 1996).

1. Two persons are in psychological contact.
2. The first, whom we shall term the *client*, is in a state of incongruence, being vulnerable or anxious (although see Ehrbar, 2004, p. 158).
3. The second person, whom we shall term the *therapist*, is congruent or integrated in the relationship.
4. The therapist experiences unconditional positive regard for the client.
5. The therapist experiences an empathic understanding of the client's internal frame of reference and endeavors to communicate this experience to the client.
6. The communication to the client of the therapist's empathic understanding and unconditional positive regard is to a minimal degree achieved (Rogers, 1957, p. 96).

Rogers described the first two as preconditions for therapy. The sixth condition, the perception by the client of the conditions offered by the therapist, is sometimes overlooked but is essential. Research relating therapeutic outcome to empathy, congruence, and unconditional positive regard based on external judgments of these variables supports the person-centered hypothesis. If the ratings are done by clients themselves, then the relationship to outcome is stronger. Orlinsky and Howard (1978) reviewed 15 studies relating client perception of empathy to outcome and found that 12 supported the critical importance of client-perceived empathy.

Orlinsky, Grawe, and Parks (1994), updating the original study by Orlinsky and Howard (1986), summarized findings from 76 studies investigating the relationship between positive regard and therapist affirmation and outcome. Out of 154 findings from these studies, 56% showed the predicted positive relationship, and when patients' ratings were used, the figure rose to 65%. As Watson (1984) points out, the theory requires the client's perception of the attitudes, so in any outcome research, the client is the most legitimate judge of the therapist's attitudes (Watson, 1984, p. 21).

Significantly, in an updated meta-analysis, Elliott et al. (2011) found that "client-perceived empathy predicted outcome better than observer- or therapist-rated empathy" (Elliott et al., 2011, p. 44). These findings represent the tip of the iceberg, however. Literally hundreds of studies have been generated since Rogers published his foundational paper in 1957.

Process of Psychotherapy

The practice of client-centered therapy is a distinctive practice by virtue of a thoroughgoing respect for the client as the architect of the therapy (Raskin, 1947/2005; Rogers, 1951; Witty, 2004). This commitment to the nondirective attitude differentiates client-centered therapy from all models of therapy that formulate a priori goals for the client. This foundational attitude distinguishes the approach from other person-centered process-directive therapies such as emotion-focused, focusing-oriented, existential, and experiential orientations within the humanistic framework.

In the client-centered approach, therapy begins immediately, with the therapist trying to understand the client's world in whatever way the client wishes to share it. The first interview is not used to take a history, arrive at a diagnosis, determine whether the client is treatable, or establish the length of treatment.

The therapist respects clients, allowing them to proceed in whatever way is comfortable for them, listening without prejudice and without a private agenda. The therapist is open to either positive or negative feelings, to either speech or silence. The first hour may be the first of hundreds or it may be the only one; this is for the client to determine.

If the client has questions, the therapist tries to recognize and respond to whatever feelings are implicit in the questions. "How am I going to get out of this mess?" may be the expression of the feeling "My situation seems hopeless." The therapist will convey recognition and acceptance of this statement. If this question is actually a plea for suggestions, then the therapist first clarifies the question. If the therapist has an answer, then he or she will give it. Often, we may not really have an answer, in which case the therapist explains why. Either one simply doesn't know or doesn't yet have sufficient understanding to formulate an answer.

There is a willingness to stay with the client in moments of confusion and despair. Reassurance and advice giving are most often not helpful and may communicate a subtle lack of confidence in the client's own approach to his or her life difficulties. Brodley and other client-centered practitioners (1999a/2011) agree that the attitude that leads the therapist to reassure and support the client is often a reflection of the therapist's own anxiety. There are no rules, however; in some cases, spontaneous reassurances may be given. It depends on the relationship and on the freedom and confidence of the therapist.

Principled nondirectiveness in practice requires that the therapist respond to the client's direct questions simply out of respect (Brodley, 2011d; Grant, 1990). In the case example later in this chapter, there are examples of the therapist responding directly to the client's questions. Learning to answer questions in ways that are consistent with nondirectiveness is an aspect of client-centered therapy as a discipline because in everyday life we are often eager to assert our own frame of reference and readily jump in with answers. Brodley explains:

> The nondirective attitude in client-centered work implies that questions and requests should be respected as part of the client's rights in the relationship. These rights are the client's right to self-determination of his or her therapeutic content and process, and the client's right to direct the manner of the therapist's participation within the limits of the therapist's philosophy, ethics, and capabilities. The result of the therapist's respect towards these client rights is a collaborative relationship (see Natiello, 1994).

This conception of the client's rights in the relationship is radically different from that of other clinical approaches. In other approaches, to a greater or lesser extent depending on the theory, the therapist paternalistically decides whether or not it will be good for the client to have his or her questions answered or requests honored. The client-centered approach eschews decision making for the client (Brodley, 1997/2011, p. 24).

Regard is also demonstrated through discussion of options such as group therapy and family therapy, in contrast to therapists of other orientations who "put" the client in a group or make therapy conditional on involvement of the whole family. In this approach, the client is a vital partner in determining the nature of the therapy, the frequency, and the length of time he or she wishes to invest in the work. On all issues pertaining to the client, the client is regarded as the best expert.

In a paper given at the first meeting of the American Academy of Psychotherapists in 1956, Rogers (1959a) presented "a client centered view" of "the essence of psychotherapy." He conceptualized a "molecule" of personality change, hypothesizing that "therapy is made up of a series of such molecules, sometimes strung rather closely together, sometimes occurring at long intervals, always with periods of preparatory experiences in between" (p. 52). Rogers attributed four qualities to such a "moment of movement":

1. It is something that occurs in this existential moment. It is not a thinking about something—it is an experience of something at this instant in the relationship.

2. It is an experiencing that is without barriers, inhibitions, or holding back.

3. The past "experience" has never been completely experienced.

4. This experience has the quality of being acceptable and capable of being integrated with the self-concept.

Mechanisms of Psychotherapy

Broadly speaking, two theoretical perspectives try to account for change in the person's concept of self that ultimately results in more effective functioning. The traditional paradigm, which is common to most psychotherapies, including client-centered therapy, asserts that change is the product of "unearthing" hidden or denied feelings or experiences that distort the concept of self, resulting in symptoms of vulnerability and anxiety.

In the course of development, most children learn that their worth is conditional on good behavior, moral or religious standards, academic or athletic performance, or undecipherable factors they can only guess at. In the most severe cases, the child's subjective reality is so consistently denied as having any importance to others that the child doubts the validity of his or her own perceptions and experiences. Rogers describes this process as "acquiring conditions of worth" and the resulting self as "incongruent." For persons whose own attempts at self-definition and self-regulation have met with harsh conditions of worth, the act of voicing a preference or a feeling or an opinion is the first step in establishing selfhood and personal identity. From the perspective of the traditional theory, such a person has suppressed his or her own feelings and reactions habitually for long periods of time. The popularized image is one of a "murky swamp" of unexplored "forgotten" experiences.

There arises, however, the issue of how "feelings" that heretofore have been "hidden" or "not in awareness" exist as "entities." The traditional model has pictured these problematic feelings paradoxically as both existent (coming from the past) and yet nonexistent until symbolized in awareness (felt for the first time when expressed). This paradox requires resolution because logic demands it and because of the issue of where to direct our empathic understanding when we are listening to clients' narratives.

Fred Zimring, a colleague of Rogers, clarifies the problem: "If the therapist attends to material not in the client's awareness, the therapist is not in the client's internal frame of reference and so would not be fulfilling an important 'necessary' condition" (Zimring, 1995, p. 36). In addition, how can we know what is not in the client's awareness until the client tells us? Zimring presents a new paradigm that unifies Rogers's theory of the necessary and sufficient conditions with the therapeutic practice of empathic understanding, which avoids the problematic notion of hidden or unknown feelings. A much abbreviated version of his work is summarized here.

Zimring asserts that human beings become persons only through interaction with other persons and that this process takes place within a particular culture. If you were born into a Western culture, the notion of the "buried conflict" is part of your cultural legacy. There is some pathological entity "inside" that needs to be brought into the light of awareness. Whether it is the wounded "inner child" or "repressed memories" or one's "abandonment issues," the underlying assumption holds that until one is able to make the unconscious conscious, psychological maladjustment will persist.

By contrast, Zimring posits that each of us does, in fact, live within a phenomenological context akin to Rogers's notion of the inner frame of reference but that that context is always "under construction." The self in this sense is a perspective that crystallizes and dissolves constantly in each moment of each new situation. It is a dynamic property arising from interactions between the person and the situation rather than a static, private entity. Zimring explains:

> [The] old paradigm assumes that our experience is determined by inner meanings and reactions. Thus, if we feel bad, it is assumed that we are not aware of some

internal meaning which is affecting our experience. In the new paradigm our experience is seen as having a different source: experience is seen as coming from the context in which we are at the moment. We feel differently when in one context rather than in the other. (Zimring, 1995, p. 41)

Zimring explains that in the Western context, we tend to think in terms of an "inside" and an "outside." But actually we construct both the subjective, reflexive internal world and the objective, everyday world; that is, we interact with our own unique internal representations of both of these contexts. Persons differ in their awareness and access to the inner subjective context. This is understandable given Rogers's explication of the ways in which the person's absorption of harsh conditions of worth tend to degrade or erase the significance of subjective experience. Zimring (1995) gives an example of a client he was working with who had little access to the subjective context at all:

> Most of the time these people see themselves as part of the objective world. When forced to describe something that may have subjective dimensions, they will emphasize the objective aspect of the thing described. A man described how he cried on the anniversary of his daughter's death. When asked how he felt when he was crying, he responded, "I hoped I could stop." In the client-centered situation, this person may be seen as the "difficult" client (the difficulty is not in the client but rather in the therapist's unrealistic expectation that the client "should" be talking about a subjective world). In other therapy contexts, this client is seen as defensive. The present analysis gives rise to a different description. Here, this client is seen as not having developed a reflexive, subjective world. (p. 42)

Because, within the subjective context, "it is the quality of the reaction to which we are attending, its fresh presentness, personal relevance, and aliveness" (Zimring, 1995, p. 41), we are, in that moment, free from the defining criteria of the objective context that is governed by logic, causation, success, or failure. Experience of the subjective context gives access to the inner locus of evaluation and the freedom from moralistic or pathologizing judgments (in the specific way Zimring is defining it). We can enter the objective context in our own inner representations, for instance, by picturing being blamed for losing a championship game by missing the last free throw and how we might deal with such a humiliating disappointment. But it is only when "I" attend to my feeling of disappointment with myself instead of reacting to the "me" that I can be said to have access to the subjective context and to allow the feeling to change.

Thus, Zimring is describing two different types of internal contexts: (1) the objective context that is stressed in our culture as significant and meaningful and (2) the subjective context having little real-world value. Thinking of oneself as an object, as "me," is to inhabit an objective transactional state, whereas while thinking as a subject, as "I," is to inhabit a subjective transactional state. Client-centered therapists, by attending to and carefully attempting to understand the person's narrative (even though the narrative may be a story of what happened to the "me" at the basketball game), tacitly validate the subjective context, eventually strengthening the person's subjective context itself and access to it.

> The theory presented here assumes the self to be existing in the discourse that occurs in reaction to the phenomenological and social context, assumes a self that exists in perspective and in action, rather than a self that exists as an entity that determines action. This view of self implies a new view of the processes of change of self. This view is that the self changes from a change in perspective and discourse not from a discovery of the hidden, true self. . . . [T]he self changes, as feelings do, when we develop a new context. (Zimring, 1995, p. 47)

For some clients, establishing contact with their own subjective inner context within the facilitative interpersonal context of client-centered therapy may prove a difficult transition that may take time. Eventually, their access to that context and their ability to express it may increase. The self (the "I") that was available to the person only within therapy begins to appear in other contexts. An Asian American woman client of the third author recently said, "I was actually facing up to my father's anger. He was yelling at me that I was 'unfriendly,' meaning I wasn't doing what he wanted me to do. I could hardly recognize myself!"

It now is clearer why the client's perception of the therapist-provided conditions is so critical in achieving progress in therapy. Validation of the client's internal frame of reference (or, in Zimring's terms, the *subjective context*) is a serendipitous by-product of the process of interaction between the client who is communicating and the therapist's empathic responses. As the client perceives him- or herself as being received as unique and particular, as not being "made into an instance of anything else, be it a social category, a psychological theory, a moral principle, or whatever" (Kitwood, 1990, p. 6), the person's experience of being a self is strengthened and changed. Zimring explains that empathic understanding allows the client to "change from being in the Me to being in the I state which also grows the I":

> [W]e are responding to the unique aspects of the person, to those aspects in which we are most individual. In responding to these, in checking with the person to see if our responses are valid, in our assumption that these unique aspects of the person are important truths, we are demonstrating our belief in the validity of the person's intentions and inner world. Once this happens, once people begin to believe in the validity of their intentions and inner world, of their internal frame of reference, they begin to respond from an internal rather than from an external frame of reference. When we see ourselves as I or agent rather than Me or object, our experience changes. (Zimring, 2000, p. 112)

Client-centered therapy, in common with other therapeutic approaches, aims to enhance the life functioning and self-experience of clients. Unlike other therapies, however, client-centered therapy does not use techniques, treatment planning, or goal setting to achieve these ends. Brodley states:

> It may seem strange, but the therapeutic benefits of client-centered work are serendipitous in the sense that they are not the result of the therapist's concrete intentions when he or she is present with or expressively communicating with the client. The absence of intentional goals pursued for clients seems to me to be essential for some of the therapeutic benefits of the approach. Specifically, the nondirectivity inherent in the therapist's expressive attitude helps protect the client's autonomy and self-determination. It has the effect of promoting the client's experience as the architect of the therapy. . . . Client-centeredness, in its nondirectivity and expressiveness—being profoundly nondiagnostic and concretely not a means to any ends—has an exceptional power to help without harming. (Brodley, 2000/2011, pp. 137–138; emphasis added)

APPLICATIONS

Who Can We Help?

Because client-centered therapy is not problem-centered but person-centered, clients are not viewed as instances of diagnostic categories who come into therapy with "presenting problems" (Mearns, 2003). When the therapist meets the other person as a human being worthy of respect, it is the emergent collaborative relationship that heals, not the application of the correct "intervention" to the "disorder" (Natiello, 2001). Of course, clients come to therapy for a reason, and often the reason involves "problems" of some kind. But the point is that problems are not assumed and are not viewed as instances of a priori categories. Mearns clarifies this stance:

> Each person has a unique "problem" and must be treated as unique. The definition of the problem is something the client does, gradually symbolizing different facets under the gentle facilitation of the therapist; the client's work in "defining the problem" is the therapy. This is the same reasoning behind Carl Rogers's statement that the therapy is the diagnosis. "In a very meaningful and accurate sense, therapy is diagnosis, and this diagnosis a process which goes on in the experience of the client, rather than in the intellect of the clinician." (Mearns, 2003, p. 90; Rogers, 1951, p. 223)

This philosophy of the person leads us in the direction of appreciating each person as a dynamic whole. Human lives are processes evolving toward complexity, differentiation, and more effective self–world creation. In contrast, the medical model sees persons in terms of "parts"—as problematic "conflicts," "self-defeating" behaviors, or "irrational cognitions." Proponents of client-centered therapy see problems, disorders, and diagnoses as constructs that are generated by processes of social and political influence in the domains of psychiatry, pharmaceuticals, and third-party payers as much as by bona fide science.

Another common misconception of client-centered therapy concerns the applicability of the approach. Critics from outside the humanistic therapies dismiss this approach as (1) biased toward white, Western, middle-class, verbal clients and thus ineffective for clients of less privileged social class, clients of color, or those who live in collectivist cultures; (2) superficial, limited, and ineffective, particularly with "severe disorders" such as axis II personality disorders; and (3) using only the technique of "reflection" and thus failing to offer clients "treatments" of proven effectiveness. Students of this approach who wish to investigate both the critiques and the refutations are referred to several recent works: Bozarth's *Person-Centered Therapy: A Revolutionary Paradigm* (1998); Brian Levitt's *Embracing Non-Directivity* (2005); and Moodley, Lago, and Talahite's *Carl Rogers Counsels a Black Client* (2004). In their analysis of Rogers's work with a black client, Mier and Witty defend the adequacy of the theory insofar as constructs such as experiencing and the client's internal frame of reference are held to apply universally. Tension or limitations in cross-cultural therapy dyads arise from the personal limitations and biases of the therapist (Mier & Witty, 2004, p. 104).

In therapy, some clients may define self fundamentally by their group identity—for example, family or kinship relations, religion, or tribal customs. At some points in their lives, many persons may define themselves in terms of other types of group affiliation (e.g., "I am a transsexual," "I am a trauma survivor," "I'm a stay-at-home Mom"). These definitions of self tend to emerge in the therapy relationship and are accepted and understood as central to the client's personal identity. However, it is an error to suppose that client-centered therapists aim to promote autonomy, independence, or other Western social values such as individualism and self-reliance. Respect for and appreciation of clients precludes therapists' formulating goals. Consultation offers the opportunity for therapists to examine biases of all types and to progress toward greater openness and acceptance of clients' culture, religious values, and traditions.

Feminist scholars of therapy both within the humanistic tradition and from the psychodynamic traditions have criticized client-centered therapy as focusing only on the individual without educating the client to the political context of her problems. Although it is true that client-centered therapists do not have psychoeducational goals for clients, these writers fail to recognize the ways in which social and political perspectives emerge in client-centered relationships. The recent work of Wolter-Gustafson (2004) and Proctor and Napier (2004) shows the convergence between the client-centered approach and the more recent "relational" and feminist therapies.

In an interview with Baldwin shortly before his death in 1987, Rogers made the following statement that illustrates the consistency with which he endorsed the nondirective attitude: "[T]he goal has to be within myself, with the way I am. . . . [Therapy is effective] when the therapist's goals are limited to the process of therapy and not the outcome" (quoted in Baldwin, 1987, p. 47).

Occasionally, clients who are veterans of the mental health system may have incorporated clinical diagnoses into their self-concepts and may refer to themselves in those terms. For example, "I guess I suffer from major depression. My psychiatrist says I'm like a plane flying with only one engine." Even though client-centered therapists do not view clients through a diagnostic lens, this self-description is to be understood and accepted like any other aspect of the client's self-definition. Note that this kind of self-categorization can be an instance of an external locus of evaluation in which a naïve and uncritical client has taken a stock label and applied it to him- or herself. Or, conversely, it may represent a long, thoughtful assessment of one's experience and history, thus being a more truly independent self-assessment. If the client describes herself as "crazy" or "psychotic," the client-centered therapist would not say, "Oh, don't be so hard on yourself. You're not crazy." We put our confidence in the process of the therapy over time to yield more self-accepting and accurate self-appraisals on the part of the client rather than telling the client how to think because his or her thinking is clearly wrong.

Although client-centered therapy is nondiagnostic in stance, client-centered therapists work with individuals diagnosed by others as psychotic, developmentally disabled, panic disordered, bulimic, and the like, as well as with people simply seeking a personal growth experience. This assumption that the therapy is generally applicable to anyone, regardless of diagnostic label, rests on the belief that the person is always more—that it is the person's expression of self and his or her relation between self and disorder, self and environment, that we seek to understand. Rogers states unequivocally that the diagnostic process is unnecessary and "for the most part, a colossal waste of time" (Kirschenbaum & Henderson, 1989, pp. 231–232). Rogers elaborates on the issue:

> Probably no idea is so prevalent in clinical work today as that one works with neurotics in one way, with psychotics in another; that certain therapeutic conditions must be provided for compulsives, others for homosexuals, etc. . . . I advance the concept that the essential conditions of psychotherapy exist in a single configuration, even though the client or patient may use them very differently . . . [and that] it is [not] necessary for psychotherapy that the therapist have an accurate psychological diagnosis of the client. . . . [T]he more I have observed therapists . . . the more I am forced to the conclusion that such diagnostic knowledge is not essential to psychotherapy. (Kirschenbaum & Henderson, 1989, pp. 230–232)

When therapists do not try to dissuade clients from asking direct questions by suggesting that clients should work on finding their own answers, clients may occasionally request help from the therapist. Although there is some disagreement within the person-centered therapeutic community about answering questions, many client-centered therapists believe that following the client's self-direction logically requires responding to the client's direct questions. Depending on the question, such therapists might offer their thinking, which could include diagnostic observations, in the interest of providing the client with access to alternatives, including pharmacotherapy, behavioral interventions, and the like. But, crucially, these offerings emerge from the client's initiative, and therapists have no stake in gaining "compliance" from the client with their offerings.

Client-centered therapists have worked successfully with a myriad of clients with problems in living, including those of psychogenic, biogenic, and sociogenic origins.

The common thread is the need to understand the client's relationship to the problem, illness, or self-destructive behavior; to collaborate with the client in self-healing and growth; and to trust that the client has the resources to meet the challenges he or she faces. No school of psychotherapy can claim to cure schizophrenia or alcoholism or to extract someone from an abusive relationship. But within a partnership of respect and acceptance, the client's inner relation to the behavior or negative experience changes in the direction of greater self-acceptance and greater self-understanding, which often leads to more self-preserving behavior.

In spite of the stereotype of client-centered therapy as applicable only to "not-too-severe" clients, several client-centered scholars and practitioners have written about the success of this approach with clients whose lives have been severely afflicted with "mental illness." For example, Garry Prouty's work with clients who are described as "psychotic" is described in his book *Theoretical Evolutions in Person-Centered/Experiential Therapy* (1994). In her book *The Client-Centered Therapist in Psychiatric Contexts: A Therapist's Guide to the Psychiatric Landscape and its Inhabitants*, Danish clinician Lisbeth Sommerbeck (2003) presents the issues she deals with as a client-centered therapist in a psychiatric setting in which her colleagues treat "patients" from the traditional medical model.

In contrast to long-term therapy, the current trend with persons diagnosed with schizophrenia has focused on social skills training, occupational therapy, and medication. It is rare for such a person to experience the potency of a client-centered relationship in which she or he is not being prodded to "comply" with a medication regimen, to exhibit "appropriate" behavior and social skills, and to follow directives that are supposedly in the person's interest as defined by an expert. In the client-centered relationship, the person can express her or his own perceptions that the medication isn't helping without the immediate response "But you know that if you stop the medication, you will end up back in the hospital." This respect of the person's inner experience and perceptions empowers the person as someone with authority about self and experience. This is not to deny the positive aspects of skills training, psychotropic medications, and psychiatry. If medications and programs really do help, then clients can be trusted to elect to use them; if they are forced to do so by their families and therapists and by institutions of the state, then they are being treated paternalistically, as less than fully capable of deciding their own course in life.

A case that stuck in Rogers's memory over the years was that of Jim Brown, also known as "Mr. Vac," who was part of the Wisconsin study of chronically mentally ill patients (Bozarth, 1996; Rogers et al., 1967). In the course of a detailed description of two interviews with this patient, a "moment of change" is described in which the patient's hard shell is broken by his perception of the therapist's warmth and caring, and he pours out his hurt and sorrow in anguished sobs. This breakthrough followed an intense effort by Rogers, in two interviews a week for the better part of a year, to reach this 28-year-old man, whose sessions were filled with prolonged silences of as long as 20 minutes. Rogers stated, "We were relating as two . . . genuine persons. In the moments of real encounter the differences in education, in status, in degree of psychological disturbance, had no importance—we were two persons in a relationship" (Rogers et al., 1967, p. 411). Eight years later, this client telephoned Rogers and reported continued success on his job and general stability in his living situation, and he expressed appreciation for the therapeutic relationship with Rogers (Meador & Rogers, 1984).

This account emphasizes the person-centered rather than problem-centered nature of this approach. Rogers often stated his belief that what was most personal was the most universal. The client-centered approach respects the various ways in which people deal with fear of being unlovable, fear of taking risks, fear of change and loss, and the myriad nature of problems in living. Understanding the range of differences among us, Rogers saw that people are deeply similar in our wish to be respected and loved; our hope for belonging, for being understood; and our search for coherence, value, and meaning in our lives.

Client-centered therapists are open to a whole range of adjunctive sources of help and provide information to clients about those resources if asked. These would include self-help groups, other types of therapy, exercise programs, medication, and the like limited only by what the therapist knows about and believes to be effective and ethical. The attitude toward these psychoeducational procedures and treatments is not one of urging the client to seek out resources of any kind but rather to suggest them in a spirit of "You can try it and see what you think." The client is always the ultimate arbiter of what is and is not helpful and of which professionals and institutions are life enhancing and which are disempowering.

Because the therapist is open to client initiatives, clients may at times wish to bring in a partner, spouse, child, or other person with whom they are having a conflict. Client-centered therapists are flexible and are often open to these alternative ways of working collaboratively with clients. The ethical commitment, however, is to the client, and it may be appropriate to refer others for couple or family therapy within the client-centered framework. Several authors (including Nathaniel Raskin, Ferdinand van der Veen, Kathryn Moon and Susan Pildes, John McPherrin, Ned Gaylin, and Noriko Motomasa) have written about working with couples and families in the person-centered and client-centered approach.

This lack of concern with a person's "category" can be seen in person-centered cross-cultural and international conflict resolution. Empathy is provided in equal measure for Catholics and Protestants in Northern Ireland (Rogers & Ryback, 1984) and for blacks and whites in South Africa (Rogers, 1986b). Conflict resolution is fostered when the facilitator appreciates the attitudes and feelings of opposing parties, and then the stereotyping of one side by the other is broken down by the protagonists' achievement of empathy. Marshall Rosenberg, a student of Rogers at the University of Wisconsin, has developed an important approach to conflict that he calls "nonviolent communication" (Rosenberg, 2003). This approach to communication implements the client-centered conditions in ways that do not dehumanize the other person or group.

Treatment

First off, client-centered therapists eschew the term *treatment* because of the implication that "therapy" is a medical treatment instead of a metaphor. Psychotherapy is conversation (Szasz, 1978/1988)! That said, the person-centered approach has been described particularly in the context of individual psychotherapy with adults, its original domain. The broadening of the *client-centered* designation to *the person-centered approach* stemmed from the applicability of client-centered principles to any situation in which the welfare and psychological growth of persons is a central aim. People who have institutional responsibility learn—often by trial and error—to implement the core conditions guided by the principle of nondirectiveness.

For example, a recent graduate student in clinical psychology described going to the cell of an inmate he was seeing in therapy on his therapy practicum. He addressed the man as "Mr." and invited him to join him for the hour, giving him the power to refuse to talk if he didn't want to or feel up to it. This courteous treatment was such a contrast to the ways the man was treated by the prison guards that he wrote the student a long letter after the conclusion of the therapy, expressing his gratitude for being treated like a human being. Thus, even when clients are involuntarily mandated to "treatment," it is possible to function consistently from the core conditions.

Play Therapy

Rogers deeply admired Jessie Taft's play therapy with children at the Philadelphia Child Guidance Clinic, and he was specifically impressed by her ability to accept the negative feelings verbalized or acted out by the child, which eventually led to positive attitudes in the child. One of Rogers's graduate student associates, Virginia Axline, formulated play therapy as a comprehensive system of treatment for children. Axline shared Rogers's deep conviction about self-direction and self-actualization and was also passionate about helping fearful, inhibited, sometimes abused children develop the courage to express long-buried emotions and to experience the exhilaration of being themselves. She used play when children could not overcome the obstacles to self-realization by words alone.

Axline made major contributions to research on play therapy, group therapy with children, schoolroom applications, and parent–teacher as well as teacher–administrator relationships. She also demonstrated the value of play therapy for poor readers, for clarifying the diagnosis of mental retardation in children, and for dealing with race conflicts in young children (Axline, 1947; Rogers, 1951).

Ellinwood and Raskin (1993) offer a comprehensive chapter on client-centered play therapy that starts with the principles formulated by Axline and shows how they have evolved into practice with parents and children. Empathy with children and adults, respect for their capacity for self-directed change, and the congruence of the therapist are emphasized and illustrated. More recently, Kathryn Moon has clarified the nondirective attitude in client-centered work with children (Moon, 2002).

Client-Centered Group Process

Beginning as a one-to-one method of counseling in the 1940s, client-centered principles were being employed in group therapy, classroom teaching, workshops, organizational development, and concepts of leadership less than 10 years later. Teaching, intensive groups, and peace and conflict resolution exemplify the spread of the principles that originated in counseling and psychotherapy.

Classroom Teaching

In Columbus, while Rogers was beginning to espouse the nondirective approach, he accepted the role of the expert who structured classes and graded students. At Chicago, he began to practice a new philosophy, which he later articulated in *Freedom to Learn*:

> I ceased to be a teacher. It wasn't easy. It happened rather gradually, but as I began to trust students, I found they did incredible things in their communication with each other, in their learning of content material in the course, in blossoming out as growing human beings. Most of all they gave me courage to be myself more freely, and this led to profound interaction. They told me their feelings, they raised questions I had never thought about. I began to sparkle with emerging ideas that were new and exciting to me, but also, I found, to them. I believe I passed some sort of crucial divide when I was able to begin a course with a statement something like this: "This course has the title 'Personality Theory' (or whatever). But what we do with this course is up to us. We can build it around the goals we want to achieve, within that very general area. We can conduct it the way we want to. We can decide mutually how we wish to handle these bugaboos of exams and grades. I have many resources on tap, and I can help you find others. I believe I am one of the resources, and I am available to you to the extent that you wish. But this is our class. So what do we want to make of it?" This kind of statement said in effect, "We are free to

learn what we wish, as we wish." It made the whole climate of the classroom completely different. Though at the time I had never thought of phrasing it this way, I changed at that point from being a teacher and evaluator, to being a facilitator of learning—a very different occupation. (Rogers, 1983, p. 26)

The change was not easy for Rogers. Nor was it easy for students who were used to being led and who thus experienced the self-evaluation method of grading as strange and unwelcome.

The Intensive Group

The early 1960s witnessed another important development: the intensive group. Rogers's move to California in 1964 spurred his interest in intensive groups, and in 1970 he published a 15-step formulation of the development of the basic encounter group. Rogers visualized the core of the process, the *basic encounter*, as occurring when an individual in the group responds with undivided empathy to another in the group who is sharing and also not holding back. Rogers conceptualized the leader's or facilitator's role in the group as exemplifying the same basic qualities as the individual therapist; in addition, he thought it important to accept and respect not only the group as a whole but also the individual members. An outstanding example of the basic encounter group can be seen in the film *Journey into Self*, which shows very clearly the genuineness, spontaneity, caring, and empathic behavior of co-facilitators Rogers and Richard Farson (McGaw, Farson, & Rogers, 1968).

Peace and Conflict Resolution

Searching for peaceful ways to resolve conflict between larger groups became the cutting edge of the person-centered movement in the 1980s. The scope of the person-centered movement's interest in this arena extends from interpersonal conflicts to conflicts between nations. In some instances, opposing groups have met in an intensive format with person-centered leadership. This has occurred with parties from Northern Ireland, South Africa, and Central America. A meeting in Austria on the "Central American Challenge" included a significant number of diplomats and other government officials (Rogers, 1986c). A major goal accomplished at this meeting was to provide a model of person-centered experiences for diplomats in the hope that they would be strengthened in future international meetings by an increased capacity to be empathic. Rogers (1987) and his associates also conducted workshops on the person-centered approach in Eastern Europe and the Soviet Union.

Rogers offered a person-centered interpretation of the Camp David Accords and a proposal for avoiding nuclear disaster (Rogers & Ryback, 1984). One notion is central to all these attempts at peaceful conflict resolution: When a group in conflict can receive and operate under conditions of empathy, genuineness, and caring, then negative stereotypes of the opposition weaken and are replaced by personal, human feelings of relatedness (Raskin & Zucconi, 1984).

Evidence

Although clients almost never ask us to produce empirical evidence to support our claim that client-centered therapy will succeed in helping them, the question is entirely legitimate and one we should be capable of answering. To be a therapist is to represent oneself as a professional who is successful at helping. If one fails to help, then there is an ethical responsibility to give the client an accounting for the failure (Brodley, 2011c).

Although the medical model of "treatment" is antithetical to client-centered philosophy and practice, objective, empirical research is not. Humanistic scholars see the links between theoretical models of therapy, research methods, and the practice of therapy as complex, plural, and not inevitable because they necessarily issue from differing philosophies of science and epistemologies. The fundamental question is posed: What is the relationship between scientific research findings and practice? What should the relationship be?

Evidence for the Approach

Carl Rogers was a committed researcher and student of the therapy process, and he received the Distinguished Scientific Contribution Award from the American Psychological Association in 1957. He said that it was the award he valued over all others.

Client-centered scholars and researchers continue to be interested in finding answers to the questions of the efficacy and effectiveness of the client-centered approach. However, there have been almost no large-scale quantitatively focused studies in recent decades, even though theoretical, philosophical, ethical, and naturalistic qualitative studies have burgeoned in the *Person-Centered Review* and *The Person-Centered Journal*, the *Person-Centered and Experiential Psychotherapy Journal*, and the *Journal of Humanistic Psychology*, and other journals. Research in process-experiential therapy is an exception, as is the research being conducted in Germany (Eckert, Hoger, & Schwab, 2003). Client-centered therapy also has strong support, albeit indirect support, from "common-factors" research efforts (Wampold, 2007).

Common Factors

Saul Rosenzweig (1936) first hypothesized that outcome in psychotherapy might be the result of factors that all therapies have in common (such as the personal characteristics of the therapist, the resources of the client, and the potency of the therapeutic relationship), rather than to techniques specific to theoretical orientations. This hypothesis was termed the *Dodo Bird conjecture*.

The character of the Dodo Bird appears in *Alice in Wonderland*. The animals decided to have a race to dry off after they were soaked by Alice's tears. Because they ran in all directions, the race had to be suspended. The animals appealed to the Dodo Bird for a decision. The Dodo Bird ruled as follows: "Everybody has won and all must have prizes!" The conclusion that all major psychotherapies, in fact, yield comparable effect sizes (measures of effectiveness) is often referred to as the *Dodo Bird effect*.

Decades of meta-analyses strongly support the Dodo Bird effect, refuting the idea that specific schools of therapy and their specific techniques are more important than the common factors (Elliott, 1996, 2002; Lambert, 2004; Luborsky, Singer, & Luborsky, 1975; Smith & Glass, 1977; Wampold, 2006). It is interesting to note that even therapies based on radically different philosophies and values show similar effect sizes in terms of successful outcome in studies using widely varying outcome measures.

The elements that constitute outcome can be categorized as either *therapeutic* or *extratherapeutic*. In the first category, we find effects that issue from the therapist, the therapeutic relationship, and the specific techniques associated with the particular therapeutic orientation. In the case of client-centered therapy, not only the therapist's experienced attitudes and communication of the attitudes but also the client's perception of these attitudes are hypothesized to be the necessary and sufficient conditions that are causal factors leading to positive outcome.

Therapeutic effects also include the effects of specific techniques that are sometimes used by nondirective client-centered therapists if clients suggest their use and if the therapist is competent in the particular technique. Asay and Lambert's 1999 study estimated that the variance in outcome attributed to therapeutic factors is approximately 30%; that attributed to techniques was about 15%. Placebo or expectancy effects represent 15% of the variance in outcome (client variables account for the remaining 40%). This describes a situation in which the client has reason to expect that the therapy is going to make a positive difference in his or her life situation and experience simply by virtue of undertaking the therapy process with some degree of commitment.

Extratherapeutic factors include the environment of the client, the various vulnerabilities and problems he or she is dealing with, the presence or absence of adequate social support, and any particular events (such as losses or other changes) that influence the course of therapy. This category also includes client factors described by Bohart, such as the person's own creative resources and ability to direct his or her decisions, resilience or hardiness, life experience in solving problems in living, and the client's own active use of the therapy experience (Bohart, 2006, pp. 223–234). This factor is estimated at 40% of the overall variance. Clearly, the client and the numerous variables that make up the internal and external realities of the client's situation contribute greatly to the therapy outcome equation (Bohart, 2004).

If a client is not in therapy voluntarily, is hostile toward the process and the therapist, and is noncommittal about attending sessions, then the likelihood of positive outcome diminishes. By contrast, a client who enters the relationship feeling a strong need to obtain help, who is open and willing to give therapy a try, who is consistent in following through in attending sessions, and who is capable of relating to the therapist is much more likely to benefit from the experience. This tradition of what is called *common-factors research* has yielded strong, highly consistent findings supportive of the therapy relationship as a principal source of therapeutic change. Such research has also found that techniques, though not negligible, contribute much less to the actual outcome. Many clinicians, however, have resisted the common-factors position, insisting that their techniques are the difference that makes the difference.

Along with many others who support a contextual or common-factors position, Bozarth (2002) opposes the idea that specific techniques (most often cognitive behavioral or other behavioral approaches) are crucial to therapeutic success. Further, he argues that this idea, which he calls the *specificity myth*—that is, the belief that specific disorders require specific "treatments"—is a fiction. Bruce Wampold's (2001) book *The Great Psychotherapy Debate*, in which he reviews and reanalyzes many meta-analytic studies, supports Bozarth's assessment. Wampold concludes that the famous Dodo Bird verdict has been robustly and repeatedly confirmed. Wampold reiterates his findings in a more recent review (2006).

Despite the work of Wampold and others, resistance to the Dodo Bird verdict continues. New schools of thought and accompanying techniques produce income and status in the field of psychology, leading to a proliferation of "treatments" for an ongoing proliferation of "disorders" on which various practitioners announce themselves as experts. But in the big picture of psychotherapy outcome, the evidence strongly supports a contextual model of therapy in which, as Wampold points out, the specific ingredients are important only as aspects of the entire healing context (2001, p. 217).

Evidence for the Core Conditions

The client-centered approach can confidently claim evidentiary support for the core conditions and for the impact on outcome when the client's perception of the conditions is used as an outcome measure (this was part of Rogers's original hypothesis that the client must perceive the therapist-experienced conditions in order to derive benefit).

Truax and Mitchell's (1971) analysis of 14 studies with 992 total participants studied the association between the core conditions and outcome. Sixty-six significant findings correlated positively with outcome, and there was one significant negative correlation (Kirschenbaum & Jourdan, 2005, p. 41).

C. H. Patterson's "Empathy, Warmth, and Genuineness: A Review of Reviews" (1984) critiques conclusions from many studies of the core conditions conducted in the 1970s and 1980s. Patterson concludes that in many studies in which client-centered therapy was either the experimental or the control condition, the therapists were not experienced client-centered therapists. Researchers either knowingly or unknowingly equated client-centered therapy with active listening or simple repeating back what the client says, and consequently the therapy did not meet the requirements of the theory of the conditions necessary for change in psychotherapy. In spite of this, many studies produced positive results supporting the approach. Patterson speculates that the measures of outcome would probably have been substantially more significant had the therapists involved been committed to working from Rogers's premise and had developed their ability to realize the attitudinal conditions (Patterson, 1984). His review also notes the bias against client-centered therapy in many reviews in spite of the actual positive evidence under review.

Orlinsky and Howard (1986) reviewed numerous studies focusing on relationship variables and clients' perception of the relationship. They found that generally between 50% and 80% of the substantial number of findings in this area were significantly positive, indicating that these dimensions were very consistently related to patient outcome. This was especially true when process measures were based on patients' observations of the therapeutic relationship (Orlinsky & Howard, 1986, p. 365).

Orlinsky, Grawe, and Parks (1994), updating the original study by Orlinsky and Howard, summarized findings from 76 studies investigating the relationship between positive regard and therapist affirmation and outcome. Out of 154 findings from these studies, 56% showed the predicted positive relationship; when patients' ratings were used, the figure rose to 65%.

Bohart, Elliott, Greenberg, and Watson (2002) conducted a large meta-analytic study of empathy and outcome, surveying studies from 1961 through 2000. These studies involved 3,026 clients and yielded 190 associations between empathy and outcome. A medium effect size of 0.32 was found, which indicates a meaningful correlation. With regard to these last two studies, we must remember that studies of only one of the core conditions do not test Rogers's client-centered model of therapy; rather, all six of the necessary and sufficient conditions must be accounted for in the research design (Watson, 1984). Even so, positive correlations between outcome and empathy and between outcome and positive regard are partially supportive of the model.

A recent study by process-experiential researchers illustrates some of the difficulties in assessing client-centered therapy. Greenberg and Watson's (1998) study of experiential therapy for depression compares process-experiential interventions (in the context of the core conditions) to the client-centered relationship conditions. Basically, the study showed the equivalence of the relationship conditions with process-experiential interventions for depression. Although process directivity received some support in long-term follow-up, the treatments did not differ at termination or at 6-month follow-up (Greenberg & Watson, 1998). Once again, however, because the "client-centered" experimental condition in this study was operationalized with a manual, the comparison condition does not represent client-centered therapy. Bohart comments about this particular study:

It is true, in a sense, that client-centered therapy has been manualized (Greenberg & Watson, 1998). I have personally seen these manuals. They are very well done, but what they create is an excellent analogue of client-centered therapy mapped into a different intellectual universe. They do not fully represent client-centered therapy as I understand it. Again, the very concept of following a manual is antithetical to the basic nature of client-centered therapy. To manualize an approach like client-centered therapy reminds me a little bit of Cinderella's sister who tries to fit into the glass slipper by cutting off part of her foot. One can do it, and one can even make it fit, but would it not be better to find a scientific glass slipper that truly fits the phenomenon being studied instead of mangling it to fit it into one that doesn't? (Bohart, 2002, p. 266)

In pointing out the problems with studying client-centered therapy not as a treatment package but as a unique relationship, we are not denying the importance of finding adequate ways to conduct research on this approach (see Mearns & McLeod, 1984). Newer models are emerging from the humanistic research community that hold promise for more adequate assessments of this model, such as Elliott's single-case hermeneutic design, Bohart's adjudicational model, Rennie's studies of client experience while in the therapy hour, and many qualitative studies that have emerged in the past two decades.

Most recently, Elliott and Freire (2010; 2008; Elliott, 2002) conducted an expanded meta-analysis of humanistic therapies (including client-centered, process-experiential, focusing-oriented, and emotion-focused therapies) that assessed nearly 180 outcome studies. Their analyses examined 203 client samples from 191 studies, 14,000 people overall. Their findings follow.

1. Person-centered and experiential therapies are associated with large pre–post change. Average effect size was 1.01 standard deviations (considered a very large effect).

2. Posttherapy gains in person-centered therapies are stable; they are maintained over early (less than 12 months) and late (12 months) follow-ups.

3. In randomized clinical trials with untreated control clients, clients who participate in person-centered and experiential therapies generally show substantially more change than comparable untreated clients (controlled effect size of 0.78 standard deviations).

4. In randomized clinical trials with comparative treatment control clients, clients in humanistic therapies generally show amounts of change equivalent to clients in non-humanistic therapies, including cognitive-behavior therapy (CBT) (Elliott, 2002, pp. 71–72; Elliott & Freire, 2008).

Elliott and Freire conclude that their meta-analytic studies show strong support for person-centered and experiential therapy, even when compared to cognitive behavioral approaches. In some studies in which CBT appears to have an edge over person-centered therapy, this advantage disappeared when researcher allegiance (experimenter bias) was controlled for.

Evidence for the Self–Determining Client

The work of Ryan and Deci and colleagues supports the view of the person as intrinsically motivated toward autonomy, competence, and relatedness—that is, the active client as described by Bohart and Tallman (1999). The literature focusing on subjective well-being, hardiness and resilience, and self-determination and psychological well-being supports the image of the active, generative, meaning-making person whom Rogers observed in his own therapy, which led him to postulate the actualizing tendency as the sole motive in human life.

Empirically Supported Treatments

In 1995, a Society of Clinical Psychology (Division 12) Task Force on Promotion and Dissemination of Psychological Procedures of the American Psychological Association (now known as the APA Division 12 Science and Practice Committee) was charged with identifying those "treatments" that warranted the description "empirically validated." This initiative followed similar efforts in medicine to identify "best practices." The reasoning behind the effort to identify best practices for particular disorders such as bulimia, obsessive–compulsive disorder, depression, and generalized anxiety disorder, among others, seems straightforward. Are certain types of therapy more effective than others in helping people suffering with these problems? When this question and its implications are explored in depth, however, many difficulties arise, and addressing them has led to greater clarity about the epistemological assumptions informing research studies.

The *empirically supported treatment* (EST) movement urges use of the "gold standard" research design used by pharmaceutical companies when testing the efficacy of new medications. This design calls for random sampling of subjects and random assignment to experimental and control groups using double-blind procedures so that neither the clinician nor the patient knows which group receives the active medication. Because double-blind procedures are not possible in testing therapeutic efficacy (the therapist is aware of which treatment is "active"), there is the immediate confound of researcher allegiance unless therapists committed to one orientation are compared to therapists equally committed to another.

Additional difficulties arise in deciding what the control will consist of and how it will be administered. Wampold (2001) argues that any control group must be a bona fide psychological treatment, not just a wait-list or group case-management condition. Attrition from randomization is a common problem in randomized clinical trials (RCTs). Elliott (1998) has raised the issue of underpowered studies in which the numbers of subjects are too low to outweigh allegiance effects and other threats to validity.

As Wampold (2006) cautions, the fact that a "treatment" has not met the criteria to be labeled an empirically supported treatment does not mean that many therapeutic approaches are not just as effective as those treatments that have been studied using the task force's criteria. Wampold (2001) argues as follows:

> Simply stated, the conceptual basis of the EST movement is embedded in the medical model of psychotherapy and thus favors treatments more closely aligned with the medical model, such as behavioral and cognitive treatments. . . . As a result of this medical model bias, humanistic and dynamic treatments are at a distinct disadvantage, regardless of their effectiveness. . . . In the larger context . . . giving primacy to an EST ignores the scientific finding that all treatments studied appear to be uniformly beneficial as long as they are intended to be therapeutic. . . . Although apparently harmless, the EST movement has immense detrimental effects on the science and practice of psychotherapy, as it legitimates the medical model of psychotherapy when in fact treatments are equally effective. (pp. 215–216)

From the point of view of client-centered therapy research, the problem with many studies that focus on only one of the core conditions is that the client-centered model Rogers proposed is not being tested. Rogers proposed that the therapist-provided conditions and attitudes function holistically as a single gestalt, with the client perceiving the levels of the presence of the conditions in a succession of percepts and related inferences about the therapist's relation to her or him. Many studies of empathy, particularly those from other orientations, are, we believe, studying a somewhat different condition. A congruent, nondirective client-centered therapist who has no goals for the client, who is experiencing some level of positive regard, and who aims to empathically understand the communications of the client from within the frame of reference of the client is a different phenomenon from the therapist who deliberately sets out to establish a "therapeutic alliance" in order to establish bonds, tasks, and goals. Indeed, Rogerian therapy is a wholly different phenomenon from studies in which "nondirective therapy" is used as a control and the therapist uses empathic responses. These studies show nothing valid (pro or con) about true client-centered therapy. In spite of these methodological flaws and definitional differences, studies from a psychodynamic perspective also support the association between positive regard and outcome (Farber & Lane, 2002, p. 191).

Strong support exists for empathic understanding and positive regard, whereas the results of studies of congruence are more ambiguous. Part of the problem in studying congruence results from confusion about definitions. Many researchers, including person-centered investigators, seem to define congruence behaviorally as achieving transparency through self-disclosure. In fact, although Rogers advocated for client-centered therapists' freedom to be real and personal in the relationship, he didn't advocate saying whatever comes into one's mind. Only when the therapist has a "persistent feeling" should he or she consider raising the issue with the client. The necessity of maintaining the other core conditions influences how and when the therapist brings in his or her own frame of reference.

In research, congruence should be defined as an inner state of integration that naturally fluctuates throughout a session, in concert with the experienced attitudes of unconditional positive regard and empathy. The therapeutic attitudes combine into a gestalt as the therapist attends to the narrative of the client. Therapist congruence must be assessed primarily by the therapist; the client may evaluate whether he or she perceived the therapist as sincere, genuine, and transparent, but those evaluations are inferences based on the therapist's verbal and nonverbal behavior, not on congruence itself. Watson (1984) has argued that Rogers's 1957 hypothesis (which he intended to apply to all therapies) has not really been tested adequately. With some few exceptions, this is still the case nearly three decades after Watson's meticulous examination of the data available on client-centered therapy in 1984.

Alternatives to the strategies of studying persons as objects, as the final repository of the action of independent variables, are humanistic research paradigms in which clients are co-investigators of the therapy process. Guidelines detailing these approaches can be found in a document produced by a Task Force for the Development of Practice Recommendations for the Provision of Humanistic Psychosocial Services from the American Psychological Association's Division of Humanistic Psychology (2005).

For a more comprehensive survey (from the humanistic side) of the issues involved in the EST controversy, see Bohart (2002); Elliott, Greenberg, and Lietaer (2004); Kirschenbaum and Jourdan (2005); Norcross, Beutler, and Levant (2006); Wampold (2001, 2006); and Westen, Novotny, and Thompson-Brenner (2004), among others. A recent book edited by Norcross, Beutler, and Levant, *Evidence-based Practices in Mental Health: Debate and Dialogue on the Fundamental Questions* (2006), is a wide-ranging collection of articles debating the EST movement and challenging the RCT research model, as well as arguing for its continuing significance.

Psychotherapy in a Multicultural World

If the reader has followed Rogers's arguments against the "specificity hypothesis," it will come as no surprise to find that client-centered therapists have reacted with skepticism to arguments supporting the necessity of culture-specific approaches to each racial, cultural or ethnic group, gender identity, sexual orientation, or social class identity. Attempts to sensitize student therapists to cultural differences have often led to simplistic stereotypes about differing groups. We argue that within-group differences may exceed between-group differences, that groups' self-definitions are constantly under construction, and that, similarly, group members are usually members of multiple groups leading to ever-increasing permutations of identity (Patterson, 1996).

A client-centered approach does not assume "difference" except as the client asserts how he or she experiences self as different. At the same time, those of us working from this approach understand that each person is completely unique in terms of what his or her history, ethnicity, religion or lack of it, and racial identity mean. The task, as always, is empathic understanding of the client's communicated meanings about self and about the world he or she perceives and constructs.

Does this mean that client-centered therapy has a "one size fits all" approach? The answer is complex. We answer "Yes" to the extent that uniqueness of the person is universal. We answer "no" to counteract the prevalent color-blind assertion that "We're all human beings!" This seemingly benign assertion has masked many covert biases that therapists whose master statuses are dominant and "unmarked" have carried into therapy. The multicultural therapy movement has served to sensitize and challenge this kind of status-quo thinking and practice. Client-centered therapists are just as prone to bias as therapists of differing theoretical orientations. We suspect that there is a qualitative difference in the empathic understanding process of the therapist who has been challenged on his or her biases and the therapist who is still denying them. Research has yet to be done regarding this contention, but it seems to us very likely that the quality and depth of empathy are affected by the therapist's own growth of understanding about his or her location in the various social hierarchies of dominance.

Our basic practice remains true to the core conditions no matter who our client may be. We also assert that our ability to form an initial therapeutic relationship depends on our own openness to and appreciation of and respect for all kinds of difference.

CASE EXAMPLE

It has always been characteristic of the person-centered approach to illustrate its principles with verbatim accounts. This has the advantage of depicting the interaction between therapist and client exactly and gives readers the opportunity to agree or differ with the interpretation of the data. The following interview took place in Szeged, Hungary, at a Cross-Cultural Workshop, in July 1986. John Shlien, former colleague and student of Rogers, had convened a group to learn about client-centered therapy, and Dr. Barbara Temaner Brodley, who had practiced client-centered therapy for more than 30 years at that time, volunteered to do a demonstration interview. A young European woman who had recently earned a master's degree in the United States volunteered to be the client. There were several English-speaking participants in the observing group and 8 or 10 Hungarians. The Hungarian participants clustered together in a corner so as not to disturb the interview while they were receiving a simultaneous translation. The interview was scheduled for 20 minutes, more or less, depending on the client's wishes.

The Demonstration Interview[2]

Barbara: Before we start I'd like to relax a little bit. Is that all right with you? (Spoken to the Client) I would like to say to the group that I'm going to attempt to empathically understand my client, to do pure empathic following. As I have the need, I will express my empathic understanding of what she says, and expresses, to me about her concerns and herself. (Turns to Client) I want you to know that I am also willing to answer any questions that you might ask. (C: O.K.) If it happens that you have a question.

C1:   You are my first woman therapist. Do you know that?
T1:   I didn't know.

[2] Reproduced with permission from Fairhurst (1999).

C2: And that's important for me because . . . uh . . . it sort of relates to what I'm going to talk about. Which has been going on in my mind since I decided to spend the summer in Europe. (T: Uhm-hm) Um . . . I spent the last two years in the United States studying, and (pause) when I left ******* in 1984, I was not the same person I am right now.

T2: Something has happened to you.

C3: A lot of things have happened to me! (laughs). And, I'm coming back to Europe this summer primarily to see my parents again. When I had left ******* two years ago, I had left in a state of panic. Promising almost never to go back. Promising never to see them again. And . . .

T3: Escaping and going to something.

C4: Yeah, yeah, yeah. Getting away from . . . and I had never expected that I would reach this point, that I would be able to go back and see them again.

T4: Uhm-hm. You were so sure, then.

C5: I was angry. (T: Uhm-hmm) I was so angry. And it's good for me that I'm taking all this time before I go back to *******. I mean this workshop now, and then I'm going to travel. And then I'm going to go to ******* at a certain point in August. (T: Uhm-hmm) But sometimes, I just, I'm struck by the fact that, gosh, I'm going to see them again, and how would that be? How will that be?

T5: You're making it gradual and yet at a certain point you will be there, (C: Uh-huh) and what will that be? (C: Uh-huh) Is? . . . you have, uh, an . . . anticipation or fear (C: Yeah) or (C: Yeah) something like that.

C6: Yeah, and I guess . . . I was thinking about my mother the other day, and . . . I realized, in the States, I realized that she and I had a very competitive relationship. And . . . it was interesting, but three days ago in Budapest I saw a lady in the street who reminded me of my mother. But my mother—not at the age which she has right now—but my mother 20 years from now. And, I don't know why. I was so struck by that because I saw my mother being old and, and, weak. So she was not this powerful, domineering person that she used to be in ******* who I was so much afraid of.

T6: Uhm-hm. But old and weakened and diminished . . .

C7: Diminished. That's the word. (T: Uhm-hm.) That's the word. (Begins to cry).

T7: It moved you to think of that, that she would (C: Yeah.) be so weak and diminished.

C8: And I think there was something in that lady's eyes that reminded me of my mother which (voice breaks; crying) I was not aware of when I was in *******. And it was fear. (T: Uh-huh) I saw fear in the woman's eyes. (T: Fear) Yeah. And, I was not aware of that.

T8: You mean, when you saw this woman who resembled your mother but 20 years from now, you saw in this woman's eyes something you had not realized was, in fact, in the eyes of your mother. (C: Yeah) And that was the quality of fear. And that had some great impact on you.

C9: Yeah. Because I felt that this woman needed me. (Crying) (Pause) It feels good that I am crying now. (T: Uhm-hm) I'm feeling very well that I am crying . . .(T: Uhm-hm)

T9: (Pause) It was a sense of your mother in the future, and that your mother will need you.

C10: You got it! The future stuff. It's not the present stuff. (Pause) It feels right here. (She places her hand over her abdomen.)

T10: The feeling is that your mother will have—has—fear and will have great need for you, (C: Yeah.) later on.

C11: Yeah. (Pause) And as I am going back to *******, I don't know if I'm ready to, if I'm ready to take care of her. I don't know if I'm ready to see that need expressed by her. (Continuing to cry)

T11: Uhm-hm, uhm-hm, uhm-hm. (Pause) You're afraid that when you get there, that will be more present in her. Or you will see it more than you did before, now that you've seen this woman. And that that will be a kind of demand on you, and you're afraid you're not ready to meet that.

C12: That's it, yeah, and it's gotten too much for me. Or, right now in Hungary, I perceive it as being too much. (Crying continues)

T12: Uhm-hm. At least, you're saying you're not sure how you will feel there, but it feels now like if that comes forth, if you see that, you, you, won't be able to . . . (C: Take it.) respond—be able to take it.

C13: Yeah, yeah. It was interesting. I kept looking at her, you know. And it's like I was staring at her and she was staring at me. She was Hungarian. She didn't know why I was looking at her and I didn't know why I was looking at her either. But it's like I wanted to take all of her in, and make her mine, and prepare myself. And suddenly I realized that all this anger I had was gone. There was nothing left. It was gone. (Crying)

T13: Uhm-hm. You mean, as you and this older woman looked at each other, and you had the meaning that it had for you about your mother, you wanted to—at that moment—you wanted to take her in and to give to her. To somehow have her feel that you were receiving her.

C14: Yeah. (Expressed with a note of reservation)

T14: The important thing is that . . . out of that you realized that you weren't afraid of your mother anymore, you weren't afraid of her dominance or . . .

C15: Yeah. Yeah.

T15: And that's a kind of incredible—(C: Discovery)—discovery and an incredible phenomenon that that (C: Yeah) fear and oppression could drop away so suddenly.

C16: And I guess, another feeling that I had also was, I felt sorry for her.

T16: Your mother.

C17: Yeah. (Pause) And I don't like feeling sorry for her at all. (Crying) I used to a lot. For a long time when I loved somebody I used to feel sorry for them at the same time. I couldn't split those two things. (Pause) I don't know what I'm trying to say right now . . . I don't know if I'm trying to say that I felt that I was loving her or that I was feeling sorry for her or both.

T17: There's a quality—pity . . . or feeling sorry for her that was strong but which you did not like. And then you don't know whether there was a quality of love that was part of that pity?

C18: Yeah.

T18: So both the feelings are mixed and confusing (C: Yeah) and then the reactions of—of having the sympathy and then having the (C: Uh-huh) pulling back (C: Uh-huh) from it.

C19: And I don't know if the woman did really resemble my mother or if it was my wish to make her resemble my mother. Maybe I'm ready (pause) ready to get there. I'm ready to see my mother as a person, and not—I can't put a word because I don't know how I was perceiving my life so far. But I had never perceived her as a woman in the street, just a woman, just another woman in the street, (her voice quakes with feeling) vulnerable and anxious and needy, and scared (softly).

T19: And you don't know whether you had changed and therefore saw—experienced this woman from the change, of being open to seeing all of that in your mother. (C: That's right) Or whether she really—when you looked at her—looked very much like your mother and how she would look. Is that right? (C: Yeah) You don't know which?

C20: Yeah.

T20: I guess then, that the really important thing is that you saw her, your mother, in your mind through this woman in a completely new way, as a person, as vulnerable, as afraid, as in need.

C21: Uhm-hm, uhm-hm. And that made me feel more human . . .

T21: Made you feel more human. (C: Uh-huh) To see her as more human (C: Also) made you feel more human in yourself.

C22: Yeah.

T22: Uhm-hm, because the force of how she had been to you—the tyrant or something . . .

C23: She had a lot of qualities. Some of them I don't remember anymore.

T23: But not a whole person to you, not a vulnerable person.

C24: Uhm-hm. (Pause) I said at the beginning that you were my first woman therapist. (T: Uhm-hm) I was avoiding women therapists like hell. (T: Uhm-hm) All the therapists I had were men so far and now I know why. I can't put why to words but I know why.

T24: That some of your feelings about her made you avoid a woman therapist and choose men?

C25: Yeah. (Pause) And lots of other things. But at this point, um, I, I'm perceiving everybody as another person, and that makes me feel more of a person as well.

T25: Uhm-hm. You're perceiving everybody (C: Everybody) as more rounded . . . um . . . (C: Yeah) including the therapist.

C26: Therapists were big—were a big thing for me for a long time. Very big authority figures and stuff like that. (T: Uhm-hm) So I guess I was afraid that a woman therapist—a woman therapist was very threatening to me. (T: Uhm-hm) Four years ago, three years ago. But at this point I feel everybody's a person.

T26: Everybody's a person. So that among the many transformations that have occurred since you left home (C: Yeah) for the United States. That's a big one. (C: That was . . .) That people have become persons to you instead of figures of various sorts.

C27: Absolutely true. I mean that's absolutely right. And it happened after I left *****.

T27: Uhm-hm.

C28: And I feel . . . (Looking toward group).

T28: And you feel it's about time?

C29: (Client nods.) Thank you.

T29: You're welcome. Thank you. (Client leans towards therapist and they embrace with affection and smiles.)

C30: Thank you very much. (They continue to embrace.)

Brodley comments about the interview:

When I evaluate client-centered therapy interviews, I make a basic distinction between errors of understanding and errors of attitude. Errors of attitude occur when the therapist's intentions are other than maintaining congruence, unconditional positive regard and empathic understanding or other than a nondirective attitude. For example, when the therapist is distracted and failing to try to empathically understand the client. Or when the therapist is emotionally disturbed and unsettled. Or when the therapist has lost unconditional acceptance and reveals this in the tone or content of his communications. Errors of understanding occur when the therapist is attempting to acceptantly and empathically understand, but misses or misinterprets what the client is getting at and trying to express. In this brief interview my volunteer client was in her mid-[20s] and I was in my late [50s] when the interview took place. It is impossible to know how much influence on the content of the interview resulted from my age being close to the client's mother's age. I do know that we had a good chemistry, were attracted to each other. The client and I had briefly encountered each other the evening before the interview and after the interview, she told me she had experienced a positive reaction to me (as I had toward her) and that she volunteered because I was to be the therapist. In the session I was emotionally open to her and felt strong feelings as she unfolded her narrative. One of our Hungarian observers told me after the interview, "now I understand client-centered therapy" because he saw tears in my eyes as I worked with her. (Brodley, 1999b; cited in Fairhurst, 1999, pp. 85–92)

Commentary

This interview illustrates, in concrete form, several principles of the process of client-centered therapy. The client's first statement, "You are my first woman therapist" precedes her direct question "Did you know that?" Barbara responds immediately, "I didn't know." Clearly, the client is implying that interacting with her first woman therapist is significant to her. Whereas some therapists might have immediately answered the question with another question, such as "Why is that significant?" client-centered therapists, in keeping with the nondirective attitude, do not prompt or lead their clients. The client here is free to pursue why it is significant or not to do so. She does say that Barbara's being a woman is important "because it sort of relates to what I'm going to talk about" but does not explain it more fully until later in the interview. And even then, she has a new awareness that she cannot really put into words. In C25, she states, "I said at the beginning that you were my first woman therapist. I was avoiding women therapists like hell. All the therapists I had were men so far and now I know why. I can't put why to words but I know why."

Commitment to nondirectiveness should not be understood as a tense, conscious inhibiting of what one might wish to say to a client. As therapists mature in the approach, the nondirective attitude is often described as involving an experience of relief. The therapist who has formerly felt responsible for the interaction trusts the client to decide how much to disclose and when to disclose it. In this interview, the client clearly directs the conversation toward a concern of great moment to her—the trip she will be making in a matter of weeks to see her parents, whom she had promised herself never to see again. She explains that she has been in the United States for the preceding two years as she studied for a master's degree and had not returned to her home country or her family. She explains that she had left home in a state of intense anger toward her parents—and now she is wondering how it will be to see them after this absence that was more a voluntary exile than simply a peaceful time away.

During this part of the interview, the therapist makes several empathic remarks following responses to check her understanding of the content of the story and also the client's immediate meaning. It is not until the therapist tentatively grasps the point of the client's narrative that it becomes possible to experience empathic understanding. In T5, the therapist says, "You're making it [the return trip] gradual and yet at a certain point you will be there and what will that be . . . you have an anticipation or fear or something like that." This response is accepted, and the client moves on to tell of the encounter she had three days earlier in which her attention was captured by an older woman in the streets of Budapest. Although it is unclear to the client why she associated this older woman with her own mother, she reports being strongly affected by the spontaneous perception of her mother in the future as old and weak. "So she was not this powerful, domineering person that she used to be in [her country] who I was so much afraid of." The therapist's response in which she says "old and weakened and diminished" is an example of an accurate empathic response that exactly captures the client's immediate experiencing. This is an important difference between recounting an emotion (as the client had earlier when she recalled how angry she had been on leaving her home and her parents) and the direct experiencing of the emotion. After the therapist's response, she replies, "Diminished. That's the word. That's the word." At this moment, she has access to deeply sensed though unidentified emotions.

Client-centered therapy, in this way, spontaneously stimulates the unfolding of the inner experiencing of the client. In experiential terms, the "felt sense" has been symbolized and is carried forward, allowing a new gestalt of experiencing to arise (Gendlin, 1961). But unlike process-directive and emotion-focused therapists' aims, the therapist was not aiming to produce focusing, nor was she trying to "deepen the felt sense" or do anything except understand what the client was communicating. In this way, the powerful focusing effects that frequently occur in client-centered therapy are serendipitous and unintended. The stance of the nondirective therapist is expressive, not instrumental (Brodley, 2000/2011). Barbara's use of the term *diminished* captures the client's perception of her mother in the future, and the client begins to weep.

As she moves further into the experience of her perception of the older woman, the client tells Barbara that what she saw in the woman's eyes was fear—a fear that she now realizes had been present in her own mother's eyes, although at the time she had seen it without being aware of having seen it, an instance of what Rogers has termed *subception*. Barbara checks her understanding of this event, which occurred only days earlier and involved a stranger in the present but someone who, for the client, represented her mother in the future, noting that the client's perception of fear in the woman's eyes "had some great impact on you." The client responds with immediacy and deep feeling: "Yeah, because I felt that this woman needed me," and she continues to cry. With her immediate experiencing openly available to her, she notes, "It feels good that I am crying now. I'm feeling very well that I am crying." A moment later she places her hand over her abdomen saying "It feels right here," letting the therapist know that she is having a direct, bodily awareness of her experiencing and that it feels good to her to allow herself to cry.

We infer that the therapist's embodiment of the therapeutic conditions has facilitated the deeply felt expression of this experience. It is also possible to infer, although we can't be sure, that the fact that the client has been to several male therapists indicates that Rogers's second condition (that the person be vulnerable and anxious) may apply to the client because of the risk she is taking to work with a woman for the first time, even though this is a single therapy session. She may be vulnerable regarding this experience, but she is actively seeking an opportunity for personal growth in the possibly intimidating setting of a public workshop.

Another way to look at this experience is in terms of its complexity. The client is feeling and expressing both sorrow and pity for her mother in the future and, at the same moment, is aware of a sense of well-being or fullness in the expression of the pain. Clients can be trusted to relate what is meaningful to them, moving toward the points they wish to bring out that embody meaning. At the same time as they are giving "content," they are experiencing themselves expressing meaning, and so there is a self-reflexive aspect of the communication that may remain implicit. In this instance, the client makes her relation to her own experiencing and expression explicit. The aim of empathic understanding is not so much to catch the underlying implicit feeling as much as to fully grasp both the narrative and the client's inner relation to what is being expressed. The agency or intentions of the person are to be understood simultaneously with the explicit content (Brodley, 2000/2011; Zimring, 2000).

In the next part of the interview, the client reveals that as she stood looking at the Hungarian woman, and as she felt like taking the woman in and preparing herself, she recognized that her anger toward her parents had dissipated entirely. She says, "Suddenly I realized that all this anger I had was gone. There was nothing left. It was gone." In this instance, she is recounting a powerful experience she had had a few days before the interview. And shortly she relates that she felt sorry for her mother in the midst of this perception—a feeling she did not welcome had previously been unable to discriminate from love. In C20, there is what Rogers calls a *moment of movement* in which the client says, "I don't know if the woman did really resemble my mother or if it was my wish to make her resemble my mother. Maybe I'm ready . . . (pause) . . . ready to get there. I'm ready to see my mother as a person . . . I had never perceived her as a woman in the street, just a woman, just another woman in the street vulnerable and anxious and needy and scared."

The chance encounter with the Hungarian woman stimulated the client's recognition that her perception of her mother has shifted from someone she had resisted, feared, and seen as a figure of authority to someone whom she is perhaps ready to encounter as a human being who is "just a woman, just another woman in the street." The result of this shift is enhancing to her sense of herself as a person. In C26 she says, "But at this point, I'm perceiving everybody as another person, and that makes me feel more of a person as well." One way to look at this interview is that there is movement from not being sure she is ready to see her mother's need to "maybe I'm ready . . . (pause) . . . ready to get there." It is possible that as she interacts with the therapist in this climate of acceptance and empathic understanding, she begins to feel more of her own strength and coping capacity.

Another aspect of this situation is the client's fear of women therapists, which is clearly related to her fear of and anger toward her mother. Again, it is possible that in her immediate interaction with a woman therapist onto whom she has projected negative feelings in the past she experiences quite different emotions and reactions: the warm acceptance and presence of a real woman therapist. This allows a restoration of personal congruence in that we infer she is not reacting with anxiety and fear in the interview. This integrative experience may directly interact with the reorganization she experiences toward the feared mother from the past to the vulnerable, human mother in the future who will need her. Thus, she may be experiencing a greater sense of autonomy; she is no longer in the grip of anger, and she is now ready or almost ready to encounter her mother as a vulnerable person. As Ryan and Deci point out, autonomy may be thought of in terms of volition as well as in terms of independence (Ryan & Deci, 2000, p. 74). The client's increasing sense of her freedom and her emerging sense of readiness to return leads to an increase in personal authority or power, as well as to an increased sense of her own humanity as someone who is at last perceiving other persons not as "figures" but simply as individual human beings. The client appears to have greater access to her own inner subjective context and, within the psychologically facilitative environment of the client-centered core conditions, to have become more of an authentic person in her own right.

When the client-centered therapy process persists over time, clients are likely to experience a deepening sense of self-authority and personal power. They become more capable of resistance to external authority, particularly when it is unjust, and more capable of deep connections with others. These changes in self-concept lead to more effective learning and problem solving and to enhanced openness to life.

SUMMARY

The central hypothesis of the person-centered approach postulates that individuals have within themselves vast resources for self-understanding and for altering their self-concepts, behavior, and attitudes toward others. These resources are mobilized and released in a definable and facilitative psychological climate. Such a climate is created by a psychotherapist who is empathic, caring, and genuine.

Empathy, as practiced in the person-centered approach, consists of a consistent, unflagging appreciation for the experience of the client. It involves a continuous process of checking with the client to see whether understanding is complete and accurate. It is carried out in a manner that is personal, natural, and free-flowing; it is not a mechanical kind of reflection or mirroring. Caring is characterized by a profound respect for the individuality of the client and by nonpossessive, warm, acceptant caring or unconditional positive regard. Genuineness is marked by congruence between what the therapist feels and says and by the therapist's willingness to relate on a person-to-person basis rather than through a professionally distant role.

The impetus given to psychotherapy research by the person-centered approach has resulted in substantial evidence that demonstrates that changes in personality and behavior occur when a therapeutic climate is provided and used by an active, generative client. Two frequent results of successful client-centered therapy are increased self-esteem and greater openness to experience. Trust in the perceptions and the self-directive capacities of clients expanded client-centered therapy into a person-centered approach to education, group process, organizational development, and conflict resolution.

When Carl Rogers began his journey in 1940, psychotherapy was dominated by individuals who practiced in a manner that encouraged a view of themselves as experts. Rogers created a way of helping in which the therapist was a facilitator of a process that was directed by the client. More than half a century later, the person-centered approach remains unique in the magnitude of its trust in the client and in its unwavering commitment to the sovereignty of the human person.

Counseling CourseMate Website:

See this text's Counseling CourseMate website at www.cengagebrain.com for learning tools such as chapter quizzing, videos, glossary flashcards, and more.

ANNOTATED BIBLIOGRAPHY AND WEB RESOURCES

Barrett-Lennard, G. T. (1998). *Carl Rogers's helping system: Journey and substance.* London: Sage Publications.

This is a comprehensive and scholarly presentation of the person-centered approach to psychotherapy and human relations. It starts with the beginnings of client-centered therapy and the social, political, and economic milieu of the 1920s and 1930s, and it continues with a description of early practice and theory; detailed examinations of the helping interview and the course of therapy; applications to work with children and families and use with groups; education; conflict resolution and the building of community; and research and training. It concludes with a retrospective and prospective look at this system of helping.

Bozarth, J. (1998). *Person-centered therapy: A revolutionary paradigm.* Ross-on-Wye, UK: PCCS Books.

A collection of 20 revised and new papers by one of the movement's outstanding teachers and theoreticians. This book is divided into the following sections: Theory and Philosophy, The Basics of Practice, Applications of Practice, Research, and Implications. It reflects on Carl Rogers's theoretical foundations, emphasizes the revolutionary nature of these foundations, and offers extended frames for understanding this radical approach to therapy.

Raskin, N. J. (2004). *Contributions to client-centered therapy and the person-centered approach.* Ross-on-Wye, UK: PCCS Books.

This collection of Raskin's articles includes empirical studies, historical accounts of theoretical developments in the person-centered approach, and a personal description of Raskin's own growth as a person and therapist. It is a broad, incisively written compendium of articles by one of the founders of the approach.

Rogers, C. R. (1951). *Client-centered therapy.* Boston: Houghton Mifflin.

This book describes the orientation of the therapist, the therapeutic relationship as experienced by the client, and the process of therapy. It expands and develops the ideas expressed in the earlier book *Counseling and Psychotherapy* (1942).

Rogers, C. R. (1961). *On becoming a person.* Boston: Houghton Mifflin.

Perhaps Rogers's best-known work, this book helped make his personal style and positive philosophy known globally. The book includes an autobiographical chapter and sections on the helping relationship; the ways in which people grow in therapy; the fully functioning person; the place of research; the implications of client-centered principles for education, family life, communication, and creativity; and the impact on the individual of the growing power of the behavioral sciences.

Rogers, C. R. (1980). *A way of being.* Boston: Houghton Mifflin.

As the book jacket states, this volume "encompasses the changes that have occurred in Dr. Rogers's life and thought during the decade of the seventies in much the same way *On Becoming a Person* covered an earlier period of his life. The style is direct, personal, clear—the style that attracted so many readers to the earlier book." In addition to important chapters on theory, there is a large personal section, including chapters on what it means to Rogers to listen and to be heard and one on his experience of growing as he becomes older (he was 78 when the book was published). An appendix contains a chronological bibliography of Rogers's publications from 1930 to 1980.

Web Sites

Association for the Person-Centered Approach (ADPCA): www.adpca.org

British Association for the Person-Centered Approach: www.bapca.co.uk

Center for the Studies of the Person: www.centerfortheperson.org/

World Association for Person-Centered and Experiential Psychotherapy and Counseling (WAPCEPC): www.pce-world.org

CASE READINGS

Ellis, J., & Zimring, F. (1994). Two therapists and a client. *Person-Centered Journal, 1*(2), 77–92.

This article contains the transcripts of short interviews by two therapists with the same client. Because 8 years intervened between the interviews, these typescripts permit a glimpse of the changes in the client over the period, as well as allow for comparison of the style and effect of two client-centered therapists.

Knight, T. A. (2007). Showing clients the doors: Active problem-solving in person-centered psychotherapy. *Journal of Psychotherapy Integration, 17*(1), 111–124. [Reprinted in D. Wedding & R. J. Corsini (Eds.) (2011). *Case studies in psychotherapy* (6th ed.). Belmont, CA: Cengage.]

This case illustrates the ways in which a therapist can maintain a nondirective and person-centered approach while still responding to the expressed needs of clients who present with circumscribed problems they expect to solve.

Raskin, N. J. (1996). The case of Loretta: A psychiatric inpatient. In B. A. Farber, D. C. Brink, & P. M. Raskin, *The psychotherapy of Carl Rogers: Cases and commentary* (pp. 33–56). New York: Guilford.

This is one of the few verbatim recordings of a therapy interview with a psychotic patient, and it provides a concrete example of the application of client-centered therapy to a psychiatric inpatient diagnosed as paranoid schizophrenic. The interview shows a deeply disturbed individual responding positively to the therapist-offered conditions of empathy, congruence, and unconditional positive regard. It is especially dramatic because another patient can be heard screaming in the background while the interview is taking place.

Rogers, C. R. (1942). The case of Herbert Bryan. In C. R. Rogers, *Counseling and psychotherapy* (pp. 261–437). Boston: Houghton Mifflin.

This may be the first publication of a completely recorded and transcribed case of individual psychotherapy that illustrates the new nondirective approach. After each interview, Rogers provides a summary of the client's feelings and additional commentary.

Rogers, C. R. (1961). The case of Mrs. Oak. In C. Rogers, *On becoming a person.* Boston: Houghton Mifflin.

This classic case study documents a client's personal growth during a series of therapy sessions with Carl Rogers.

Rogers, C. R. (1967). A silent young man. In C. R. Rogers, G. T. Gendlin, D. V. Kiesler, & C. Truax (Eds.), *The therapeutic*

relationship and its impact: A study of psychotherapy with schizophrenics (pp. 401–406). Madison: University of Wisconsin Press.

This case study consists of two transcribed interviews that were conducted by Rogers as part of a year-long treatment of a very withdrawn hospitalized schizophrenic patient who was part of a client-centered research project on client-centered therapy with a schizophrenic population.

Witty, M. C. (2013). Client-centered therapy with David: A sojourn in loneliness. In D. Wedding & R. J. Corsini (Eds.), *Case studies in psychotherapy* (7th ed.). Belmont, CA: Cengage.

This case study includes a brief history of a man diagnosed with schizophrenia in his early 20s. In addition to a theoretical conceptualization from a phenomenological view of the client, the study includes a verbatim transcription of a therapy session, including the therapist's own critique of her work.

REFERENCES

American Psychological Association Division of Humanistic Psychology. (2005). *Recommended principles and practices for the provision of humanistic psychosocial services: Alternative to mandated practice and treatment guidelines.* Retrieved from www.apa.org/divisions/div32/draft.html.

Asay, T. P., & Lambert, M. J. (1999). The empirical case for the common factors in therapy: Quantitative findings. In M. A. Hubble, B. L. Duncan, & S. D. Miller (Eds.), *The heart and soul of change: What works in therapy* (pp. 23–55). Washington, DC: American Psychological Association.

Axline, V. M. (1947). *Play therapy.* Boston: Houghton Mifflin.

Baldwin, M. (1987). Interview with Carl Rogers on the use of the self in therapy. In M. Baldwin & V. Satir (Eds.), *The use of self* (pp. 45–52). New York: The Haworth Press.

Bohart, A. C. (2002). A passionate critique of empirically supported treatments and the provision of an alternative paradigm. In J. C. Watson, R. N. Goldman, & M. S. Warner (Eds.), *Client-centered and experiential psychotherapy in the 21st century: Advances in theory, research, and practice* (pp. 258–277). Ross-on-Wye, UK: PCCS Books.

Bohart, A. C. (2004). How do clients make empathy work? *Person-Centered and Experiential Psychotherapies, 3*(2), 102–116.

Bohart, A. C. (2005). Can you be integrative and a person-centered therapist at the same time? *Person-Centered and Experiential Psychotherapies, 11*(1), 1–13.

Bohart, A. C. (2006). The active client. In J. C. Norcross, L. E. Beutler, & R. F. Levant (Eds.). *Evidence-based practices in mental health: Debate and dialogue on the fundamental questions* (pp. 218–226). Washington, DC: American Psychological Association.

Bohart, A. C. (2007). The actualizing person. In M. Cooper, M. O'Hara, P. F. Schmid & G. Wyatt (Eds.), *The handbook of person-centered psychotherapy and counselling* (pp. 47–63). Houndmills, UK: Palgrave Macmillan.

Bohart, A. C. (2008). How clients self-heal in psychotherapy. In B. E. Levitt (Ed.), *Reflections on human potential:*

Bridging the person-centered approach and positive psychology (pp. 175–186). Ross-on-Wye, Wales: PCCS Books.

Bohart, A. C. & Greening, T. (2001). Humanistic psychology and positive psychology. *American Psychologist, 56*(1), p. 81.

Bohart, A. C., & Tallman, K. (1999). *How clients make therapy work: The process of active self-healing.* Washington, DC: American Psychological Association.

Bohart, A. C., Elliott, R., Greenberg, L. S., & Watson, J. C. (2002). Empathy. In J. C. Norcross (Ed.), *Psychotherapy relationships that work: Therapist contributions and responsiveness to patients* (pp. 89–108). New York: Oxford University Press.

Bozarth, J. D. (1996). The integrative statement of Carl Rogers. In R. Hutterer, G. Pawlowsky, P. F. Schmid, & R. Stipsits (Eds.), *Client-centered and experiential psychotherapy: A paradigm in motion* (pp. 25–34). Berlin: Peter Lang.

Bozarth, J. D. (1998). *Client-centered therapy: A revolutionary paradigm.* Ross-on-Wye, UK: PCCS Books.

Bozarth, J. D. (2002). Empirically supported treatment: Epitome of the "specificity myth." In J. C. Watson, R. N. Goldman, & M. S. Warner (Eds.), *Client-centered and experiential psychotherapy in the 21st century: Advances in theory, research, and practice* (pp. 168–181). Ross-on-Wye, UK: PCCS Books.

Bozarth, J. D. & Brodley, B. T. (1986/1993). The core values and theory of the person-centered approach. Paper presented at first annual meeting of the Association for the Person-Centered Approach, Chicago, September 3–7. Published (1993) as Les valeurs essentieles de l'approche centrée sur la personne. The core values of the person-centered approach (in French and English) in *Le Journal du PCAII* (pp. 1– 25). (Person-centered Approach Institute International—France.)

Bozarth, J. D. & Brodley, B. T. (1991). Actualization: A functional concept in client-centered therapy. In A. Jones & R. Crandall (Eds.), *Handbook of Self-Actualization.* [Special Issue]. *Journal of Social Behavior and Personality, 6*(5), 45–59.

Brodley, B. T. (1988). Does early-in-therapy experiencing level predict outcome? A review of research. Unpublished manuscript. Revision of a discussion paper prepared for presentation at second annual meeting of the Association for the Development of the Person-Centered Approach, May 26–30.

Brodley, B. T. (1990). Client-centered and experiential: Two different therapies. In G. Lietaer, J. Rombauts, & R. Van Balen (Eds.), *Client-centered and experiential psychotherapy in the nineties* (pp. 87–107). Leuven, Belgium: Leuven University Press. Also published in K. A. Moon, M. C. Witty, B. Grant, & B. Rice (Eds.). (2011). *Practicing client-centered therapy: Selected writings of Barbara Temaner Brodley* (pp. 289–308). Ross-on-Wye, UK: PCCS Books.

Brodley, B. T. (1994). Some observations of Carl Rogers's behavior in therapy interviews. *Person-Centered Journal, 1*(2), 37–47. Also published in K. A. Moon, M. C. Witty, B. Grant, & B. Rice (Eds.). (2011). *Practicing client-centered therapy: Selected writings of Barbara Temaner Brodley* (pp. 313–327). Ross-on-Wye, UK: PCCS Books.

Brodley, B. T. (1997). The nondirective attitude in client-centered therapy. *Person-Centered Journal, 4*(1), 18–30. Also published in K. A. Moon, M. C. Witty, B. Grant, & B. Rice (Eds.). (2011). *Practicing client-centered therapy: Selected writings of Barbara Temaner Brodley* (pp. 47–62). Ross-on-Wye, UK: PCCS Books.

Brodley, B. T. (1999a). Reasons for responses expressing the therapist's frame of reference in client-centered therapy. *Person-Centered Journal, 6*(1), 4–27. Also published in K. A. Moon, M. C. Witty, B. Grant, & B. Rice (Eds.). (2011). *Practicing client-centered therapy: Selected writings of Barbara Temaner Brodley* (pp. 207–238). Ross-on-Wye, UK: PCCS Books.

Brodley, B. T. (1999b). A client-centered demonstration in Hungary. In I. Fairhurst (Ed.), *Women writing in the person-centered approach* (pp. 85–92). Ross-on-Wye, UK: PCCS Books.

Brodley, B. T. (1999c). The actualizing concept in client-centered theory. *Person-Centered Journal, 6*, 108–120. Also published in K. A. Moon, M. C. Witty, B. Grant, & B. Rice (Eds.). (2011). *Practicing client-centered therapy: Selected writings of Barbara Temaner Brodley* (pp. 153–170). Ross-on-Wye, UK: PCCS Books.

Brodley, B. T. (2000). Client-centered: An expressive therapy. In J. Marques-Teixeira & S.Antunes (Eds.), *Client centered and experiential psychotherapy* (pp. 133–147). Linda a Velha, Portugal: Vale & Vale. Also published in K. A. Moon, M. C. Witty, B. Grant, & B. Rice (Eds.). (2011). *Practicing client-centered therapy: Selected writings of Barbara Temaner Brodley* (pp. 180–193). Ross-on-Wye, UK: PCCS Books.

Brodley, B. T. (2011a). Considerations when responding to questions and requests in client-centered therapy. In K.A. Moon, M.C. Witty, B. Grant, & B. Rice (Eds.), *Practicing client-centered therapy: Selected writings of Barbara Temaner Brodley* (pp. 239–240). Ross-on-Wye, UK: PCCS Books.

Brodley, B. T. (20011b). Congruence and its relation to communication in client-centered therapy. In K. A. Moon, M. C. Witty, B. Grant, & B. Rice (Eds.). (2011). *Practicing client-centered therapy: Selected writings of Barbara Temaner Brodley* (pp. 73–102). Ross-on-Wye, UK: PCCS Books.

Brodley, B. T. (2011c). *Ethics in psychotherapy.* In K. A. Moon, M. C. Witty, B. Grant, & B. Rice (Eds.), *Practicing client-centered therapy: Selected writings of Barbara Temaner Brodley* (pp. 33–46). Ross-on- Wye, UK: PCCS Books.

Brodley, B. T. (2011d). The nondirective attitude in client-centered therapy. In K. Moon, M.C. Witty, B. Grant, & B. Rice (Eds.). (2011). Practicing client-centered therapy: Selected writings of Barbara Temaner Brodley (pp. 47–70). Ross-on-Wye, UK: PCCS Books.

Brown, L. S. (1994). *Subversive dialogues: Theory in feminist therapy.* New York: Basic Books.

Burstow, B. (1987). Humanistic psychotherapy and the issue of equality. *Journal of Humanistic Psychology, 27*(1), 9–25.

Cain, D. J. (2010). *Person-centered psychotherapies.* Washington, DC: American Psychological Association.

Cooper, M., Watson, J. C., & Hölldampf, D. (Eds.). (2010). *Person-centered and experiential therapies work: A review of the research on counseling, psychotherapy, and related practices.* Ross-on-Wye, UK: PCCS Books.

Deci, E. L., & Ryan, R. M. (1985). *Intrinsic motivation and self-determination in human behavior.* New York: Plenum.

Deci, E. L., & Ryan, R. M. (1991). A motivational approach to self: Integration in personality. In R. Dienstbier (Ed.), *Nebraska Symposium on Motivation: Perspectives on motivation, 38,* 237–288. Lincoln: University of Nebraska Press.

Eckert, J., Hoger, D., & Schwab, R. (2003). Development and current state of the research on client-centered therapy in the German-language region. *Person-Centered and Experiential Psychotherapies, 2*(2), 3–18.

Ellinwood, C. G., & Raskin, N. J. (1993). Client centered/humanistic psychotherapy. In T. R. Kratochwill & R. J. Morris (Eds.), *Handbook of psychotherapy with children and adolescents* (pp. 258–287). Boston: Allyn & Bacon.

Elliott, R. (1996). Are client-centered/experiential therapies effective? A meta-analysis of outcome research. In U. Esser, H. Pabst, & G. W. Speierer (Eds.), *The power of the person-centered approach* (pp. 125–138). Koln, Germany: GwG Verlag.

Elliott, R. (1998). Editor's introduction: A guide to the empirically supported treatments controversy. *Psychotherapy Research, 8*(2), 115–125.

Elliott, R. (2001). Research on the effectiveness of humanistic therapies: A meta-analysis. In D. J. Cain & J. Seeman (Eds.), *Humanistic psychotherapies: Handbook of research and practice* (pp. 57–81). Washington, DC: American Psychological Association.

Elliott, R. (2002). The effectiveness of humanistic therapies: A meta-analysis. In D. J. Cain & J. Seeman (Eds.), *Humanistic psychotherapies: Handbook of research and practice* (pp. 57–81). Washington, DC: American Psychological Association.

Elliott, R., Bohart, A. C., Watson, J. C., & Greenberg, L. S. (2011). Empathy. *Psychotherapy, 48*(1) 43–49.

Elliott, R. & Freire, E. (2008, November). Person-centered and experiential therapies are highly effective: Summary of the 2008 meta-analysis. *Person-Centered Quarterly,* 1–3.

Elliott, R. & Freire, E. (2010). The effectiveness of person-centered and experiential therapies: A review of the meta-analyses. In M. Cooper, J. C. Watson, & D. Hölldampf (Eds.), *Person-centered and experiential therapies work: A review of the research on counseling, psychotherapy, and related practices* (pp. 1–15). Ross-on-Wye, UK: PCCS Books.

Elliot, R., Greenberg, L. S., & Lietaer, G. (2004). Research on experiential psychotherapies. In M. J. Lambert (Ed.), *Bergin and Garfield's handbook of psychotherapy and behavior change* (5th ed., pp. 493–539). New York: Wiley.

Ehrbar, R. D. (2004). Taking context and culture into account in the core conditions: A feminist person-centered approach. In G. Proctor & M. B. Napier (Eds.), *Encountering Feminism* (pp. 154–165). Ross-on-Wye, UK: PCCS Books.

Fairhurst, I. (Ed.). (1999). *Women writing in the person-centered approach*. Ross-on-Wye, UK: PCCS Books.

Farber, B. A., Brink, D. C., & Raskin, P. M. (1996). *The psychotherapy of Carl Rogers: Cases and commentary* (pp. 33–56). New York: Guilford.

Farber, B. A., & Lane, J. S. (2002). Positive regard. In J. C. Norcross (Ed.), *Psychotherapy relationships that work: Therapist contributions and responsiveness to patients* (pp. 175–194). New York: Oxford University Press.

Fitzpatrick, M. R., & Stalikas, A. (2008). Positive emotions as generators of therapeutic change. *Journal of Psychotherapy Integration, 18*(2), 137-154.

Gendlin, E. T. (1990). The small steps of the therapy process: How they come and how to help them come. In G. Lietaer, J. Rombauts & R. Van Balen (Eds.), *Client-centered and experiential psychotherapy in the nineties* (pp. 205–224). Leuven, Belgium: Leuven University Press.

Gendlin, E. T. (1961). Experiencing: A variable in the process of therapeutic change. *American Journal of Psychotherapy 15*, 233–245.

Gendlin, E. T. (1996). *Focusing-oriented psychotherapy*. New York: Guilford Press.

Gergen, K. J., & Kaye, J. (1992). Beyond narrative in the negotiation of therapeutic meaning. In S. McNamee & K. J. Gergen (Eds.), *Therapy as social construction* (pp. 166–185). Thousand Oaks, CA: Sage Publications.

Goldstein, K. (1959). *The organism: A holistic approach to biology derived from psychological data in man*. New York: American Book. (Original work published 1934)

Grant, B. (1990). Principled and instrumental non-directiveness in person-centered and client-centered therapy. *Person-Centered Review, 5*: 77–88. Reprinted in D. J. Cain (Ed) (2002). *Classics in the person-centered approach* (pp. 371–377). Ross-on-Wye, UK: PCCS Books.

Greenberg, L. S. (2002). *Emotion-focused therapy: Coaching clients to work through their feelings*. Washington, DC: American Psychological Association.

Greenberg, L. S., Rice, L. N., & Elliott, R. (1993). *Facilitating emotional change*. New York: Guilford.

Greenberg, L. S., & Watson, J. (1998). Experiential therapy of depression: Differential effects of client-centered relationship conditions and process experiential interventions. *Psychotherapy Research, 8*(2), 210–224.

Held, B. S. (1995). *Back to reality: A critique of postmodern theory in psychotherapy*. New York: W.W. Norton.

Held, B. S. (2002). The tyranny of the positive attitude in America: Observation and speculation. *Journal of Clinical Psychology, 58*(9), 965–992.

Held, B. S. (2005). The "virtues of positive psychology." *Journal of Theoretical and Philosophical Psychology, 25*(1), 1–34.

Ikemi, A. (2005). Carl Rogers and Eugene Gendlin on the bodily felt sense: What they share and where they differ. *Person-Centered and Experiential Psychotherapies, 4*(1), 31–32.

Holdstock, T. L., & Rogers, C. R. (1983). Person-centered theory. In R. J. Corsini & A. J. Marsella (Eds.), *Personality theories, research, and assessment*. Itasca, IL: F.E. Peacock.

Joseph, S., & Linley, P.A. (2006). Positive psychology versus the medical model?: Comment. *American Psychologist, 61*(4), 332–333. doi: 10.1037/0003-066x.60.4.332

Kirschenbaum, H., & Henderson, V. L. (Eds.). (1989). *The Carl Rogers reader*. Boston: Houghton Mifflin.

Kirschenbaum, H., & Jourdan, A. (2005). The current status of Carl Rogers and the person-centered approach. *Psychotherapy: Theory, Research, Practice, Training, 42*(1), 37–51.

Kristjánsson, K. (2010). Positive psychology, happiness, and virtue: The troublesome conceptual issues. *Review of General Psychology, 14*(4), 296–310.

Kitwood, T. (1990). Psychotherapy, postmodernism, and morality. *Journal of Moral Education, 19*(1), 3–13.

Kitzinger, C., & Perkins, R. (1993). *Changing our minds: Lesbian feminism and psychology*. New York: New York University Press.

Lambert, M. J. (Ed.). (2004). *Bergin and Garfield's handbook of psychotherapy and behavior change* (5th ed.). New York: Wiley.

Lambert, M. J., & Erekson, D. M. (2008). Positive psychology and the humanistic tradition. *Journal of Psychotherapy Integration, 18*(2), 222–232. Doi: 10.1037/1053-0479.18.2.222

Lerman, H., & Porter, N. (Eds.). (1990). Feminist Therapy Institute code of ethics. *Feminist Ethics in Psychotherapy*, 37–40.

Levitt, B. E. (Ed.). (2005). *Embracing non-directivity: Reassessing person-centered theory and practice in the 21st century*. Ross-on-Wye, UK: PCCS Books.

Lietaer, G., Rombauts, J., & Van Balen, R. (1990). *Client-centered and experiential in the nineties*. Leuven, Belgium: Leuven University Press.

Luborsky, L., Singer, B., & Luborsky, L. (1975). Comparative studies of psychotherapies: Is it true that "everyone has won and all must have prizes"? *Archives of General Psychiatry, 32*, 995–1008.

McGaw, W. H., Farson, R. E., & Rogers, C. R. (Producers). (1968). *Journey into self* [Film]. Berkeley: University of California Extension Media Center.

McNamee, S. & Gergen, K. J. (Eds.) (1992). *Therapy as social construction*. Thousand Oaks, CA: Sage Publications.

Meador, B. D., & Rogers, C. R. (1984). Client-centered therapy. In R. J. Corsini (Ed.), *Current psychotherapies* (3rd ed., pp. 142–195). Itasca, IL: F.E. Peacock.

Mearns, D. (2003). Problem-centered is not person-centered. *Person-Centered and Experiential Psychotherapies, 3*(2), 88–101.

Mearns, D., & McLeod, J. (1984). A person-centered approach to research. In R. F. Levant & J. M. Shlien (Eds.), *Client-centered therapy and the person-centered approach: New directions in theory, research, and practice* (pp. 370–389). New York: Praeger.

Merry, T. (2004). Classical client-centered therapy. In P. Sanders (Ed.), *The tribes of the person-centered nation: A introduction to the schools of therapy related to the person-centered approach* (pp. 21–44). Ross-on-Wye, UK: PCCS Books.

Mier, S., & Witty, M. (2004). Considerations of race and culture in the practice of non-directive client-centered therapy. In R. Moodley, C. Lago, & A. Talahite (Eds.), *Carl Rogers counsels a black client* (pp. 85–104). Ross-on-Wye, UK: PCCS Books.

Moodley, R., Lago, C., & Talahite, A. (Eds.) (2004). *Carl Rogers counsels a black client*. Ross-on-Wye, UK: PCCS Books.

Moon, K. (2002). Nondirective client-centered work with children. In J. C. Watson, R. N. Goldman, & M. S. Warner (Eds.), *Client-centered and experiential psychotherapy in the 21st century: Advances in theory, research, and practice* (pp. 485–492), Ross-on-Wye, UK: PCCS Books.

Moon, K. A. (2005). Non-directive therapist congruence in theory and practice. In B. E. Levitt (Ed.), *Embracing nondirectivity: Reassessing person-centered theory and practice for the 21st century* (pp. 261–280). Ross-on-Wye, UK: PCCS Books.

Moon, K. A. & Rice, B. (in press). The nondirective attitude in client-centered practice: A few questions. *Person-Centered and Experiential Psychotherapies.*

Moon, K. A., Witty, M. C., Grant, B., & Rice, B. (Eds.) (2011). *Practicing client-centered therapy: Selected writings of Barbara Temaner Brodley*. Ross-on-Wye, UK: PCCS Books.

Natiello, P. (1994). The collaborative relationship in psychotherapy. *The Person-Centered Journal, 1*(2), 11–17.

Natiello, P. (2001). *The person-centered approach: A passionate presence*. Ross-on-Wye, UK: PCCS Books.

Norcross, J. C., Beutler, L. E., & Levant, R. F. (Eds.). (2006). *Evidence-based practices in mental health: Debate and dialogue on the fundamental questions*. Washington, DC: American Psychological Association.

O'Hara, M. (2006). The radical humanism of Carl Rogers and Paulo Freire: Considering the person-centered approach as a form of conscientização. In G. Proctor, M. Cooper, P. Sanders, & B. Malcolm (Eds.), *Politicizing the person-centered approach: An agenda for social change* (pp. 115–126). Ross-on-Wye:UK: PCCS Books Ltd.

Orlinsky, D. E., & Howard, K. L. (1978). The relation of process to outcome in psychotherapy. In S. L. Garfield & A. E. Bergin (Eds.), *Handbook of psychotherapy and*

behavior change: An empirical analysis (2nd ed., pp. 283–329). New York: Wiley.

Orlinsky, D. E., & Howard, K. L. (1986). A generic model of psychotherapy. *Journal of Integrative and Eclectic Psychotherapy, 6,* 6–28.

Orlinsky, D. E., Grawe, K., & Parks, B. K. (1994). Process and outcome in psychotherapy: *Noch einmal*. In S. L. Garfield & A. E. Bergin (Eds.), *Handbook of psychotherapy and behavior change* (4th ed., pp. 270–376). New York: Wiley.

Patterson, C. H. (1984). Empathy, warmth, and genuineness in psychotherapy: A review of reviews. *Psychotherapy, 21,* 431–438.

Patterson, C. H. (1996, January–February). Multicultural counseling: From diversity to universality. *Journal of Counseling and Development, 74.*

Porter, E. H., Jr. (1943). The development and evaluation of a measure of counseling interview procedures. *Educational and Psychological Measurement, 3,* 105–126.

Prilleltensky, I., & Walsh-Bowers, R. (1993). Psychology and the moral imperative. *Journal of Theoretical and Philosophical Psychology, 13,* 2, 90–102.

Proctor, G. (2002). *The dynamics of power in counselling and psychotherapy: Ethics, politics, and practice.* Ross-on-Wye, UK: PCCS Books.

Proctor, G., & Napier, M. (2004). *Encountering feminism: Intersections between feminism and the person-centered approach.* Ross-on-Wye, UK: PCCS Books.

Proctor, G., Cooper, M., Sanders, P., & Malcolm, B. (Eds.). (2006). *Politicizing the person-centered approach: An agenda for social change.* Ross-on-Wye, UK: PCCS Books.

Prouty, G. (1994). *Theoretical evolutions in person-centered/experiential therapy: Applications to schizophrenic and retarded psychoses.* Westport, CT: Praeger.

Raimy, V. C. (1948). Self-reference in counseling interviews. *Journal of Consulting Psychology, 12,* 153–163.

Rank, O. (1945). *Will therapy, and truth and reality.* New York: Knopf.

Raskin, N. J. (1948). The development of nondirective therapy. *Journal of Consulting Psychology, 12,* 92–110.

Raskin, N. J. (1952). An objective study of the locus-of-evaluation factor in psychotherapy. In W. Wolff & J. Precker (Eds.), *Personality monographs: Vol. 3. Success in psychotherapy* (pp. viii, 215–238). New York: Grune & Stratton.

Raskin, N. J. (2004). *Contributions to client-centered therapy and the person-centered approach.* Ross-on-Wye, UK: PCCS Books.

Raskin, N. J. (2005). The nondirective attitude. *Person-Centered Journal, 12*(1–2), 5–22. (Original work published 1947)

Raskin, N. J., & Zucconi, A. (1984). *Peace, conflict resolution, and the person-centered approach.* Program presented at annual convention of the American Psychological Association, Toronto.

Rodis, P. T., & Strehorn, K. C. (1997). Ethical issues for psychology in the postmodernist era: Feminist psychology and multicultural therapy (MCT). *Journal of Theoretical and Philosophical Psychology 17*(1), 13–31.

Rogers, C. R. (1931). *Measuring personality adjustment in children nine to thirteen.* New York: Teachers College, Columbia University, Bureau of Publications.

Rogers, C. R. (1939). *The clinical treatment of the problem child.* Boston: Houghton Mifflin.

Rogers, C. R. (1940). The process of therapy. *Journal of Consulting Psychology, 4,* 161–164.

Rogers, C. R. (1942). *Counseling and psychotherapy.* Boston: Houghton Mifflin.

Rogers, C. R. (1951). *Client-centered therapy.* Boston: Houghton Mifflin.

Rogers, C. R. (1957). The necessary and sufficient conditions of therapeutic personality change. *Journal of Consulting Psychology, 21,* 95–103.

Rogers, C. R. (1959a). The essence of psychotherapy: A client-centered view. *Annals of Psychotherapy, 1,* 51–57.

Rogers, C. R. (1959b). A theory of therapy, personality and interpersonal relationships as developed in the client-centered framework. In S. Koch (Ed.), *Psychology: A study of science: Vol. 3. Formulations of the person and the social context* (pp. 184–256). New York: McGraw-Hill.

Rogers, C. R. (1961). *On becoming a person.* Boston: Houghton Mifflin.

Rogers, C. R. (1963). The actualizing tendency in relation to "motive" and to consciousness. In M. Jones (Ed.), *Nebraska Symposium on Motivation* (pp. 1–24). Lincoln, NE: University of Nebraska Press.

Rogers, C. R. (1970). *On encounter groups.* New York: Harper & Row.

Rogers, C. R. (1977). *Carl Rogers on personal power.* New York: Delacorte Press.

Rogers, C. R. (1980). *A way of being.* Boston: Houghton Mifflin.

Rogers, C. R. (1983). *Freedom to learn for the 80s.* Columbus, OH: Charles E. Merrill.

Rogers, C. R. (1986a). Client-centered therapy. In I. L. Kutash & A. Wolf (Eds.), *Psychotherapist's casebook: Therapy and technique in practice* (pp. 197–208). San Francisco: Jossey-Bass.

Rogers, C. R. (1986b). The dilemmas of a South African white. *Person-Centered Review, 1,* 15–35.

Rogers, C. R. (1986c). The Rust workshop: A personal overview. *Journal of Humanistic Psychology, 26,* 23–45.

Rogers, C. R. (1987). Inside the world of the Soviet professional. *Journal of Humanistic Psychology, 27,* 277–304.

Rogers, C. R., & Dymond, R. F. (Eds.). (1954). *Psychotherapy and personality change.* Chicago: University of Chicago Press.

Rogers, C. R., Gendlin, G. T., Kiesler, D. V., & Truax, C. (Eds.). (1967). *The therapeutic relationship and its impact: A study of psychotherapy with schizophrenics.* Madison: University of Wisconsin Press.

Rogers, C. R., & Haigh, G. (1983). I walk softly through life. *Voices: The art and science of psychotherapy, 18,* 6–14.

Rogers, C. R., & Ryback, D. (1984). One alternative to nuclear planetary suicide. In R. F. Levant & J. M. Shlien (Eds.), *Client-centered therapy and the person-centered approach: New directions in theory, research, and practice* (pp. 400–422). New York: Praeger.

Rogers, C. R., & Sanford, R. C. (1985). Client-centered psychotherapy. In H. I. Kaplan, B. J. Sadock, & A. M. Friedman (Eds.), *Comprehensive textbook of psychiatry* (4th ed., pp. 1374–1388). Baltimore: William & Wilkins.

Rosenberg, M. B. (2003). *Nonviolent communication: A language of life.* Encinitas, CA: Puddle Dancer Press.

Rosenzweig, S. (1936). Some implicit common factors in diverse methods of psychotherapy. *American Journal of Orthopsychiatry, 6,* 412–415.

Ryan, R. M., & Deci, E. L. (2000). Self-determination theory and the facilitation of intrinsic motivation, social development, and well-being. *American Psychologist, 55*(1), 68–78.

Sanders, P. (2007). Schizophrenia is not an illness: A response to van Blarikom. *Person-Centered and Experiential Psychotherapies. 6*(2), 112–128.

Schmid, P. F. (2000). Prospects on further developments in the person-centered approach. In J. Marques-Teixeira & S. Antunes (Eds.), *Client-centered and experiential psychotherapy,* (pp. 11–31). Linda a Velha, Portugal: Vale &Vale Editores, LDA.

Schmid, P. F. (2003). The characteristics of a person-centered approach to therapy and counseling: Criteria for identity and coherence. *Person-Centered and Experiential Psychotherapies, 2*(2), 104–120.

Schmid, P. F. (2013). Whence the evil? A personalistic and dialogic perspective. In A. C. Bohart, B. S. Held, E. Mendelowitz, and K. J. Schneider (Eds.), *Humanity's dark side: Evil, destructive experience, and psychotherapy.* (pp. 35–55). Washington, DC: American Psychological Association.

Seeman, J. (1984). The fully functioning person: Theory and research. In R. F. Levant & J. M. Shlien (Eds.), *Client-centered therapy and the person-centered approach: New directions in theory, research, and practice* (pp. 131–152). New York: Praeger.

Seligman, M. E. P. & Csikszentmihalyi, M. (2000, January). Positive psychology: An introduction. *American Psychologist,* 5–14.

Seligman, M. E. P., & Csikzentmihalyi, M. (2001, January). "Positive psychology: An introduction." Reply. *American Psychologist,* 89–90.

Sheerer, E. T. (1949). An analysis of the relationship between acceptance of and respect for others in ten counseling cases. *Journal of Consulting Psychology, 13,* 169–175.

Smith, M. L., & Glass, G. V. (1977). Meta-analysis of psychotherapy outcome studies. *American Psychologist, 32,* 752–760.

Sommerbeck, L. (2003). *The client-centered therapist in psychiatric contexts: A therapist's guide to the psychiatric landscape and its inhabitants.* Ross-on-Wye, UK: PCCS Books.

Stephenson, W. V. (1953). *The study of behavior.* Chicago: University of Chicago Press.

Sugarman, J. (2007). Practical rationality and the questionable promise of positive psychology. *Journal of Humanistic Psychology, 47*(2), 175–197.

Szasz, T. S. (1988). *The myth of psychotherapy: Mental healing as religion, rhetoric, and repression.* Garden City, NY: Anchor Press/Doubleday. (Original work published in 1988 by Syracuse University Press)

Truax, C. B., & Mitchell, K. M. (1971). Research on certain therapist interpersonal skills in relation to process and outcome. In A. E. Bergin & S. L. Garfield (Eds.), *Handbook of psychotherapy and behavior change: An empirical analysis* (pp. 299–344). New York: Wiley.

Van Belle, H. A. (1980). *Basic intent and therapeutic approach of Carl R. Rogers: A study of his view of man in relation to his view of therapy, personality, and interpersonal relations.* Toronto: Wedge Publishing Foundation.

Van Blarikom, J. (2006). A person-centered approach to schizophrenia. *Person-Centered and Experiential Psychotherapies, 5*(3), 155–173.

Van Blarikom, J. (2007). Is there a place for illness in the person-centered approach? A response to Sanders. *Person-Centered and Experiential Psychotherapies, 6*(3), 205–209.

Wampold, B. E. (2001). *The great psychotherapy debate: Models, methods, and findings.* Mahwah, NJ: Lawrence Erlbaum Associates.

Wampold, B. E. (2006). Not a scintilla of evidence to support empirically supported treatments as more effective than other treatments. In J. C. Norcross, L. E. Beutler, & R. F. Levant (Eds.), *Evidence-based practices in mental health: Debate and dialogue on the fundamental questions* (pp. 299–307). Washington, DC: American Psychological Association.

Wampold, B. E. (2007, November). Psychotherapy: The Humanistic (and effective) treatment. *American Psychologist,* 857–873.

Warner, M. S. (2002). Luke's dilemmas: A client-centered/experiential model of processing with a schizophrenic thought disorder. In J. C. Watson, R. N. Goldman, & M. S. Warner (Eds.), *Client-centered and experiential psychotherapy in the 21st century: Advances in theory, research, and practice* (pp. 459–472). Ross-on-Wye, UK: PCCS Books.

Watson, N. (1984). The empirical status of Rogers's hypotheses of the necessary and sufficient conditions for effective psychotherapy. In R. F. Levant & J. M. Shlien (Eds.), *Client-centered therapy and the person-centered approach: New directions in theory, research, and practice* (pp. 17–40). New York: Praeger.

Westen, D., Novotny, C. M., & Thompson-Brenner, H. (2004). The empirical status of empirically supported psychotherapies: Assumptions, findings, and reporting in controlled clinical trials. *Psychological Bulletin, 130*(4), 631–663.

Weisstein, N. (1970). Kinder, küche, und kirche as scientific law: Psychology constructs the female. In R. Morgan (Ed.), *Sisterhood is powerful: An anthology of writings from the women's liberation movement* (pp. 228–245). New York: Random House.

Witty, M. C. (2004). The difference directiveness makes: The ethics and consequences of guidance in psychotherapy. *The Person-Centered Journal, 11,* 22–32.

Witty, M. C. (2013). Client-centered therapy with David: A sojourn in loneliness. In D. Wedding & R. J. Corsini (Eds.), *Case studies in psychotherapy* (7th ed.). Belmont, CA: Cengage.

Wolter-Gustafson, C. (1999). The power of the premise: Reconstructing gender and human development with Rogers' theory. In I. Fairhurst (Ed.), *Women writing in the person-centered approach* (pp. 199–214), Ross-on-Wye, UK: PCCS Books.

Wolter-Gustafson, C. (2004). Towards convergence: Client-centered and feminist assumptions about epistemology and power. In G. Proctor & M. B. Napier (Eds.), *Encountering feminism: Intersections between feminism and the person-centered approach* (pp. 97–115), Ross-on-Wye, UK: PCCS Books.

Worsley, R. (2004). Integrating with integrity. In P. Sanders (Ed.), *The tribes of the person-centered nation* (pp. 125–147). Ross-on-Wye, UK: PCCS Books.

Yen, J. (2010). Authorizing happiness: Rhetorical demarcation of science and society in historical narratives of positive psychology. *Journal of Theoretical and Philosophical Psychology, 30*(2), 67–78.

Zimring, F. M. (1995). A new explanation for the beneficial results of client-centered therapy: The possibility of a new paradigm. *Person-Centered Journal, 2*(2), 36–48.

Zimring, F. M. (2000). Empathic understanding grows the person. *Person-Centered Journal, 7*(2), 101–113.

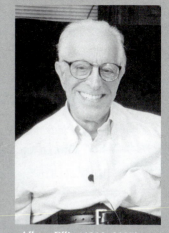

Albert Ellis (1913–2007)
Photo courtesy of Dr. Debbie Joffe Ellis

5 | RATIONAL EMOTIVE BEHAVIOR THERAPY

Albert Ellis and Debbie Joffe Ellis

OVERVIEW

Rational emotive behavior therapy (REBT), a theory of personality and a method of psychotherapy developed in the 1950s by clinical psychologist Albert Ellis, holds that when a highly charged emotional consequence (C) follows a significant activating event (A), event A may seem to, but actually does not, cause C. Instead, emotional consequences are largely created by B—the individual's *belief system*. When an undesirable emotional consequence occurs, such as severe anxiety, this usually involves the person's irrational beliefs, and when these beliefs are effectively disputed (at point D), by challenging them rationally and behaviorally, the disturbed consequences are reduced. From its inception, REBT has viewed cognition and emotion integratively, with thought, feeling, desires, and action interacting with each other. It is therefore a comprehensive cognitive-affective-behavioral theory and practice of psychotherapy (Ellis, 1962, 1994; Ellis & Harper, 1997; Ellis & Ellis, 2011).

Formerly known as *rational emotive therapy* (RET), this approach is more accurately referred to as *rational emotive behavior therapy* (REBT). From the beginning, REBT considered the importance of both mind and body or of thinking, feeling, wanting (contents of the mind according to psychology) and of behavior (the operations of the body). It is a holistic approach. It has stressed that personality change can occur in both directions: Therapists can talk with people and attempt to change their minds so that they will behave differently, or they can help clients change their behaviors and thus modify their thinking. As stated in several early writings on REBT that are reprinted in *The Albert Ellis Reader* (Ellis & Blau, 1998) and in more recent writings such as *Rational Emotive Behavior Therapy* (Ellis & Ellis, 2011), REBT theory states that humans rarely change a profound self-defeating belief unless they act against it. Thus, it is most accurately called *rational emotive behavior therapy*.

Basic Concepts

The main propositions of REBT can be described as follows:

1. *People are born with a potential to be rational (self-constructive) as well as irrational (self-defeating).* They have predispositions to be self-preserving, to think about their thinking, to be creative, to be sensuous, to be interested in other people, to learn from their mistakes, and to actualize their potential for life and growth. They also tend to be self-destructive, to be short-range hedonists, to avoid thinking things through, to procrastinate, to repeat the same mistakes, to be superstitious, to be intolerant, to be perfectionistic and grandiose, and to avoid actualizing their potential for growth.

2. *People's tendency to irrational thinking, self-damaging habituations, wishful thinking, and intolerance is frequently exacerbated by their culture and their family group.* Their suggestibility (or conditionability) is greatest during their early years because they are dependent on and highly influenced by family and social pressures.

3. *Humans perceive, think, emote, and behave simultaneously.* They are, therefore, at one and the same time cognitive, conative (purposive), and motoric. They rarely act without implicit thinking. Their sensations and actions are viewed in a framework of prior experiences, memories, and conclusions. People seldom emote without thinking because their feelings include and are usually triggered by an appraisal of a given situation and its importance. People rarely act without simultaneously perceiving, thinking, and emoting because these processes provide reasons for acting. For this reason, it is usually desirable to use a variety of perceptual-cognitive, emotive-evocative, and behavioralistic-reeducative methods (Bernard & Wolfe, 1993; Ellis, 1962, 1994, 2001a, 2001b, 2002, 2003a; Ellis & Ellis, 2011; Walen, DiGiuseppe, & Dryden, 1992).

4. *Even though all the major psychotherapies employ a variety of cognitive, emotive, and behavioral techniques, and even though all (including unscientific methods such as witch doctoring) may help individuals who have faith in them, they are probably not all equally effective or efficient.* Highly cognitive, active-directive, homework-assigning, and discipline-oriented therapies such as REBT are likely to be more effective, usually in briefer periods and with fewer sessions.

5. *REBT emphasizes the philosophy of unconditional acceptance: specifically, unconditional self-acceptance (USA), unconditional other acceptance (UOA), and unconditional life acceptance (ULA).* This is explained in *The Myth of Self-Esteem* (Ellis, 2005a). The humanistic principle of unconditional acceptance holds this assumption regarding human worth: I exist, I deserve to exist, I am a fallible human, and I can choose to accept myself unconditionally with my flaws and mistakes with or without great achievements—simply because I am alive, simply because I exist. It says that conditional self-esteem is one of the greatest of all human disturbances because it leads to people praising themselves when they do well and are approved by others and damning themselves if they don't do well and others disapprove of them. Rating traits and behaviors can be beneficial because it allows one to learn from mistakes and to improve and grow, but to overgeneralize and rate one's whole

worth, being, and totality as "good" or "bad" is inaccurate and harmful. A person's totality is too complex and ephemeral to define and measure. Hence, USA, not self-esteem, is recommended in REBT.

UOA holds that people condemn others' iniquitous thoughts, feelings, and actions but accept the others as fallible humans—just as they are. ULA encourages acceptance of adversities that we neither create nor can change—such as deaths of loved ones, physical disabilities, hurricanes, and floods.

REBT recognizes that life contains inevitable suffering as well as pleasure and that accepting the unpleasant circumstances that can't be changed can lead to emotional stability, self-actualization, and great fulfillment.

6. *Rational emotive behavior therapists do not believe a warm relationship between client and counselor is a necessary or a sufficient condition for effective personality change, although it is quite desirable.* They stress unconditional acceptance of and close collaboration with clients, but they also actively encourage clients to unconditionally accept themselves with their inevitable fallibility. In addition, therapists may use a variety of practical methods, including didactic discussion, behavior modification, bibliotherapy, audiovisual aids, and activity-oriented homework assignments. To discourage clients from becoming unduly dependent, therapists often use hard-headed methods of convincing them that they had better resort to self-discipline and self-direction.

7. *Rational emotive behavior therapy uses role playing, assertion training, desensitization, humor, operant conditioning, suggestion, support, and a whole bag of other "tricks."* As Arnold Lazarus points out in his "multimodal" therapy (Lazarus, 1989), such wide-ranging methods are effective in helping clients achieve deep-seated cognitive change. REBT is not just oriented toward symptom removal, except when it seems that this is the only kind of change likely to be accomplished. It is designed to help people examine and change some of their basic values—particularly those that keep them disturbed. If clients seriously fear failing on the job, REBT not only helps them give up this particular symptom but also tries to show them how to minimize their basic "awfulizing" tendencies.

The usual goal of REBT is to help people reduce their underlying symptom-creating propensities. There are two basic forms of rational emotive behavior therapy: general REBT, which is almost synonymous with cognitive-behavior therapy, and preferential REBT, which not only includes general REBT but also emphasizes a profound philosophical change. General REBT tends to teach clients rational or healthful behaviors. Preferential REBT teaches them how to dispute irrational ideas and unhealthful behaviors and to become more creative, scientific, and skeptical thinkers.

8. *REBT holds that most neurotic problems involve unrealistic, illogical, self-defeating thinking and that if disturbance-creating ideas are vigorously disputed by logico-empirical and pragmatic thinking, they can be minimized.* No matter how defective people's heredity may be, and no matter what trauma they may have experienced, the main reason why they usually now overreact or underreact to adversities (at point A) is that they *now* have some dogmatic, irrational, unexamined beliefs (at point B). Because these beliefs are unrealistic, they will not withstand rational scrutiny. They are often deifications and devilifications of themselves and others, and they tend to wane when empirically checked, logically disputed, and shown to be impractical. Thus, a woman with severe emotional difficulties does not merely believe it is undesirable if her lover rejects her. She tends to believe, also, that (a) it is awful; (b) she cannot stand it; (c) she should not, *must* not be rejected; (d) she will never be accepted by a desirable partner; (e) she is a worthless person because one lover has rejected her; and (f) she deserves to be rejected for being so worthless.

Such common covert hypotheses are illogical, unrealistic, and destructive. They can be revealed and disputed by a rational emotive behavior therapist who shows clients how to think more flexibly and scientifically, and the rational emotive therapist is partly that: an exposing and skeptical scientist.

9. *REBT shows how activating events or adversities (A) in people's lives contribute to but do not directly cause emotional consequences (C); these consequences stem from people's interpretations of the activating events or adversities—that is, from their unrealistic and overgeneralized beliefs (B) about those events.* The "real" cause of upsets, therefore, lies mainly in people, not in what happens to them (even though gruesome experiences obviously have considerable influence over what people think and feel). REBT provides clients with several powerful insights. Insight number one is that a person's self-defeating behavior usually follows from the interaction of A (adversity) and B (belief about A). Disturbed consequences (C) therefore usually follow the formula A–B–C.

Insight number two is the understanding that although people have become emotionally disturbed (or have *made* themselves disturbed) in the past, they are *now* upset because they keep indoctrinating themselves with similar constructed beliefs. These beliefs do not continue because people were once "conditioned" and so now hold them "automatically." No! People still, here and now, actively reinforce them, and their current active self-propagandizations and constructions keep those constructed beliefs alive. Unless people fully admit and face their own responsibilities for the continuation of their dysfunctional beliefs, it is unlikely that they will be able to uproot them.

Insight number three acknowledges that *only hard work and practice* will correct irrational beliefs—and keep them corrected. Insights 1 and 2 are not enough! Commitment to repeated rethinking of irrational beliefs and repeated actions designed to undo them will likely extinguish or minimize them.

10. *Historically, psychology was considered a stimulus–response (S–R) science.* Later, it became evident that similar stimuli produce different responses in different people. This was presumed to mean that something between the S and the R is responsible for such variations.

An analogy may be helpful. If you hit the same billiard ball from the same spot with exactly the same force and let it bounce off the side of the billiard table, that ball will always come back to exactly the same spot. Otherwise, no one would play billiards. Therefore, hitting the billiard ball is the stimulus (S) and the movement of the ball is the response (R). However, suppose there were a tiny person inside a billiard ball who could have some control over the direction and velocity of the ball after it was hit. Then the ball could move to different locations because the tiny person inside could guide it to a certain extent.

An analogous concept was introduced into psychology in the late 1800s by James McKeen Cattell, an American psychologist studying with Wilhelm Wundt in Leipzig, Germany. In so doing, he launched an entirely different kind of psychology known as *idiographic psychology,* in contrast to the *nomothetic psychology* that Wundt and his students were working on. Wundt and his followers were looking for average behavior, or S–R behavior, and were discounting individual variations. The truth was, according to them, the average. Cattell disagreed, and he introduced a psychology that acknowledged the importance of recognizing *individual differences.* As a result, the S–R concept changed to S–O–R. The O stood for "organism," but what it really meant was that the ball (or the person) had a mind of its own and that it did not go precisely where a ball with no mind of its own would go, because O had some degree of independence.

REBT includes precisely the same concept. RE represents the contents of the mind: rationality and emotions. REBT therapists attempt to change people's thinking and feelings (let's call the combination the *philosophy* of a person), with the goal of enabling them to change their behavior via a new understanding (rationality) and a new set of feelings (emotions) about self and others. By showing their clients how to combine thinking and feeling, REBT therapists have given the little man in the billiard ball the ability to change directions. When the ball is hit (confronted with particular stimuli) again, it no longer goes where it used to go.

In REBT, we want to empower individuals by changing their thinking and feelings to act differently—in a manner desired by the client, the therapist, and society. At the same time, REBT encourages people to act differently—this is where the B (for "behavior") comes in—and thereby to think and feel differently. The interaction goes both ways! Thinking, feeling, and behaving seem to be separate human processes, but as Ellis said in his first paper on REBT in 1956, which he presented at the annual American Psychological Association convention held in Chicago that year, they actually go together holistically and inevitably influence each other (Ellis, 1958). When you think, you feel and act; when you feel, you think and act; and when you act, you think and feel. That is why REBT uses many cognitive, emotive, and behavioral methods to help clients change their disturbances.

Other Systems

REBT differs from psychoanalytic schools of psychotherapy by eschewing free association, compulsive gathering of material about the client's history, and most dream analysis. It is not concerned with the presumed sexual origins of disturbance or with the oedipal complex. When transference does occur in therapy, the rational therapist is likely to attack it, showing clients that transference phenomena tend to arise from the irrational belief that they must be loved by the therapist (and others). Although REBT practitioners are much closer to modern neoanalytic schools such as those of Karen Horney, Erich Fromm, Harry Stack Sullivan, and Franz Alexander than to the Freudian school, they employ considerably more persuasion, philosophical analysis, homework-activity assignments, and other directive techniques than practitioners of these schools.

REBT overlaps significantly with Adlerian theory, but it departs from the Adlerian practices of stressing early childhood memories and insisting that social interest is the heart of therapeutic effectiveness. REBT is more specific than Adler's Individual Psychology in disclosing, analyzing, and disputing clients' concrete internalized beliefs and is closer in this respect to general semantic theory and philosophical analysis than to Individual Psychology. It is also much more behavioral than Adlerian therapy.

Adler (1931, 1964) contended that people have basic fictional premises and goals and that they generally proceed quite logically on the basis of these false hypotheses. REBT, on the other hand, holds that people, when disturbed, may have both irrational premises and illogical deductions from these premises. Thus, in Individual Psychology, a male who has the unrealistic premise that he *should* be the king of the universe but actually has only mediocre abilities is shown that he is "logically" concluding that he is an utterly inferior person. But in REBT this same individual, with the same irrational premise, is shown that in addition to his "logical" deduction, he may be making several other illogical conclusions. For example, he may be concluding that (1) he should be king of the universe because he was once king of his own family; (2) his parents will be impressed by him only if he is outstandingly achieving and *therefore* he must achieve outstandingly; (3) if he cannot be king of the universe, then he might as well do nothing and get nowhere in life; and (4) he deserves to suffer for not being the noble king that he should be.

REBT has much in common with parts of the Jungian therapeutic outlook, especially in that it views clients holistically, holds that the goals of therapy include growth and achievement of potential as well as relief of disturbed symptoms, and emphasizes enlightened individuality. However, REBT deviates radically from Jungian treatment because Jungians are preoccupied with dreams, fantasies, symbol productions, and the mythological or archetypal contents of their clients' thinking—most of which the REBT practitioner deems a waste of time.

REBT is in close agreement with person-centered or relationship therapy in some ways: They both emphasize what Carl Rogers (1961) calls *unconditional positive regard* and what in rational emotive psychology is called *full acceptance, unconditional acceptance,* or *tolerance*. Rational therapists differ from Rogerian therapists in that they actively *teach* (1) that blaming is the core of much emotional disturbance; (2) that it leads to dreadful results; (3) that it is possible, though difficult, for humans to learn to avoid rating themselves even while continuing to rate their performances; and (4) that they can give up self-rating by challenging their grandiose (*must*urbatory), self-evaluating assumptions and by deliberately risking (through homework activity assignments) possible failures and rejections. The REBT practitioner is more active-directive and more emotive-evocative than the person-centered practitioner (Ellis, 1962, 2001a, 2001b; Ellis & Ellis, 2011; Hauck, 1992).

REBT is in many respects an existential, phenomenologically oriented therapy because its goals overlap with the usual existentialist goals of helping clients to define their own freedom, cultivate individuality, live in dialogue with others, accept their experiencing as highly important, be fully present in the immediacy of the moment, and learn to accept limits in life (Ellis, 2001b, 2002, 2005a, 2010). Many who call themselves existential therapists, however, are rather anti-intellectual, prejudiced against the technology of therapy, and confusingly nondirective, whereas REBT makes much use of incisive logical analysis, clear-cut techniques (including behavior modification procedures), and directiveness and teaching by the therapist.

REBT has much in common with behavior modification. Many behavior therapists, however, are mainly concerned with symptom removal and ignore the cognitive aspects of conditioning and deconditioning. REBT is therefore closer to cognitive and multimodal therapists such as Aaron Beck, Arnold Lazarus, and Donald Meichenbaum. Martin A. Seligman, one of the founders of the Positive Psychology movement, has said of Ellis (Bernard, Froh, DiGiuseppe, Joyce, & Dryden, 2010), "He is an unsung hero of Positive Psychology."

REBT, CT, and CBT

REBT, cognitive therapy (CT), as developed by Aaron T. Beck, and cognitive behavior therapy (CBT) have much in common. Over time, CBT has become more eclectic and integrative, and CT has changed in the past two to three decades (Ellis, 2003c), making CT and REBT more similar than they were earlier. However, significant differences remain, and the unique aspects of REBT merit its continued standing as a major therapy and theory. Ellis disagreed with the hybridization and blending of REBT into more general CBT (Ellis, 2010), as some writers and practitioners have done in recent years, particularly since his death in 2007.

The main differences between REBT and CT today are:

- REBT strongly holds, in its theory and practice, the primacy of demandingness, specifically emphasizing *shoulds* and tacit *musts*. REBT practitioners assume their clients practically always have explicit and implicit "musts" that contribute to their emotional disturbances, and practitioners sometimes will quickly get to clients' core beliefs in the first session so that the clients clearly identify and start modifying these beliefs.

- REBT emphasizes philosophizing more than CT does (Ellis, 2003c, 2005b; Padesky & Beck, 2003, 2005). It works to help people with disturbances make profound life-enhancing ideational and philosophic change. Somewhat like Buddhism, it encourages healthy use of the mind to facilitate greater happiness. REBT uses cognitive methods with strong emotional and behavioral overtones; it uses emotional-evocative techniques with powerful thinking and behaving; and it uses its behavioral techniques with forceful thinking and emotions. It integrates its cognitive and emotive and behavioral methods—and applies them with great vigor.

- REBT emphasizes the benefits of incorporating the practice of unconditional acceptance—specifically, (1) unconditional self-acceptance (USA), (2) unconditional other acceptance (UOA), and (3) unconditional life acceptance (ULA). It also encourages the adopting of the philosophy of constructivism, of the approach of "feeling better *and* getting better," of the philosophy of commitment and effort, the emphasis on humor, and of having distinct meaning and purpose in life.

- REBT practitioners tend to use their techniques more directly, forcefully, strongly and quickly than cognitive therapists. To test whether forceful, determined, and vigorous REBT is more effective than nondirective REBT and CT, it would be most beneficial to create experiments and study which method is more effective with different kinds of clients.

HISTORY

Precursors

The philosophical origins of rational emotive behavior therapy go back to such Asian philosophers as Confucius, Lao-Tsu, and Buddha and especially to ancient Greek philosophers such as Epicurus and the Greek and Roman stoic philosophers Epictetus and Marcus Aurelius. Although most early stoic writings have been lost, their essence has come down to us through Epictetus, who in the first century a.d. wrote in *The Enchiridion*, "People are disturbed not by things, but by the view which they take of them."

The modern psychotherapist who was the main precursor of REBT was Alfred Adler. "I am convinced," he stated, "that *a person's behavior springs from his ideas*" (1964, italics in original). According to Adler,

> The individual . . . does not relate himself to the outside world in a predetermined manner, as is often assumed. He relates himself always according to his own interpretation of himself and of his present problem. . . . It is his attitude toward life which determines his relationship to the outside world. (1964)

Adler (1931) put the A–B–C or *stimulus–organism–response* (S–O–R) theory of human disturbance neatly: No experience is a cause of success or failure. We do not suffer from the shock of our experiences—the so-called trauma—but we make out of them just what suits our purposes. We are self-determined by the meaning we give to our experiences, and it is almost a mistake to view particular experiences as the basis of our future life. Meanings are not determined by situations, but we determine ourselves by the meanings we give to situations. In his first book on Individual Psychology, Adler's motto was *Omnia ex opinione suspense sunt* ("Everything depends on opinion").

Paul DuBois, using persuasive forms of psychotherapy, was another important precursor of REBT. Alexander Herzberg was one of the inventors of homework assignments. Hippolyte Bernheim, Andrew Salter, and a host of other therapists have employed hypnosis and suggestion in a highly active-directive manner. Frederick Thorne created what he called *directive therapy*. Franz Alexander, Thomas French, John Dollard, Neal Miller, Wilhelm Stekel, and Lewis Wolberg all practiced forms of psychoanalytic psychotherapy that diverged so far from the Freudian therapy that they resemble active-directive therapy more closely and are in many ways precursors of REBT.

In addition, a large number of individuals during the 1950s, when REBT was first being formulated, independently began to arrive at some theories and methodologies that significantly overlap with the methods outlined by Ellis (1962). These theorists include Eric Berne, Jerome Frank, George Kelly, Abraham Low, E. Lakin Phillips, Julian Rotter, and Joseph Wolpe.

Beginnings

After practicing psychoanalysis for several years during the late 1940s and early 1950s, Ellis discovered that no matter how much insight his clients gained or how well they seemed to understand events from their early childhood, they rarely lost their symptoms and still retained tendencies to create new ones. He realized that this was because they were not merely indoctrinated with irrational, mistaken ideas of their own worthlessness when they were young but also *constructed* dysfunctional demands on themselves and others and kept *reindoctrinating* themselves with these commands (Ellis, 1962, 2001b, 2002, 2003a, 2004a, 2010; Ellis, D. J. 2010a).

Ellis also discovered that as he pressed his clients to surrender their basic irrational premises, they often tended to resist giving up these ideas. This was not, as the Freudians hypothesized, because they hated the therapist or wanted to destroy themselves or were still resisting parent images but because they *naturally*, one might say *normally*, tended to *must*urbate. They insisted (1) that they *must* do well and win others' approval, (2) that other people *must* act considerately and fairly, and (3) that environmental conditions *must* be gratifying and free of frustration. Ellis concluded that humans are *self-talking, self-evaluating,* and *self-construing.* They frequently take strong preferences, such as desires for love, approval, success, and pleasure, and misleadingly *define* them as needs. They thereby create many of their "emotional" difficulties.

People are not exclusively the products of social learning. Their so-called pathological symptoms are the result of *bio*social processes. *Because they are human,* they tend to have strong, irrational, and empirically misleading ideas; as long as they hold on to these ideas, they tend to be what is commonly called "neurotic." These irrational ideologies are not infinitely varied or hard to discover. They can be listed under a few major headings and, once understood, quickly uncovered by REBT analysis.

Ellis also discovered that people's irrational assumptions were so biosocially deep rooted that weak methods were unlikely to budge them. Passive, nondirective methodologies (such as reflection of feeling and free association) rarely changed them. Warmth and support often helped clients live more "happily" with unrealistic notions. Suggestion or "positive thinking" sometimes enabled them to cover up and live more "successfully" with underlying negative self-evaluations. Abreaction and catharsis frequently helped them to feel better but tended to reinforce rather than eliminate their demands. Classic desensitizing sometimes relieved clients of anxieties and phobias but did not undermine their anxiety-arousing, phobia-creating fundamental meanings and philosophies.

What *did* work effectively, Ellis found, was an active-directive, cognitive-emotive behavioral attack on major self-defeating "musts" and commands. The essence of effective psychotherapy, according to REBT, is full tolerance (i.e., unconditional acceptance) of oneself and of others as *persons,* combined with a campaign against one's self-defeating *ideas, traits,* and *performances.*

As Ellis abandoned his previous psychoanalytic approaches, he obtained better results (Ellis, 1962, 2010). Other therapists who began to employ REBT also found that when they switched to its procedures, more progress was made in a few weeks than had been made in months or years of prior treatment (Ellis, 2002; Lyons & Woods, 1991; Walen et al., 1992).

Current Status

When members of the Society of Clinical Psychology were asked to name the most influential person in the history of psychotherapy, the individuals most often listed were Carl Rogers, Albert Ellis, and Sigmund Freud in that order (Corsini, 2005). This survey gives some indication of the stature of Albert Ellis in the eyes of his colleagues. In the 1980s, a similar survey done in Canada rated Albert Ellis as the number one influential figure.

At the opening session of the American Psychological Association's 2013 convention in Honolulu, Hawaii, Albert Ellis was posthumously presented the APA Award for Outstanding Lifetime Contributions to Psychology. This was a fitting tribute to Albert Ellis, and the award was presented during the 100th anniversary of the year of his birth. Other distinguished psychologists who have received this award include Albert Bandura, B. F. Skinner, Kenneth B. Clark, Herbert Simon, and Daniel Kahneman.

The Albert Ellis Institute, a nonprofit scientific and educational organization, was founded by Albert Ellis in 1959 to teach the principles of healthy living. With headquarters in New York City and affiliates in several cities in the United States and other countries, it disseminated the rational emotive behavioral approach through (1) adult education courses and workshops in the principles of rational living, (2) postgraduate training programs, (3) moderately priced clinics for individual and group therapy, and (4) special books, monographs, pamphlets, audiovisual materials, and the *Journal of Rational-Emotive and Cognitive-Behavior Therapy*.

Ironically, Albert Ellis had a strained relationship with the Albert Ellis Institute from 2004. In 2005, the Board of Trustees of the Albert Ellis Institute removed Ellis from the board and dismissed him from all duties at the institute. The mission statement was changed, without the approval of Ellis: The former mission tied the Institute to the promotion and teaching of rational emotive behavior therapy; the new mission promoted the benefits of both rational emotive and cognitive behavioral therapies. Ellis opposed the hybridization of REBT and cognitive behavior therapy (Ellis, 2010), and he wanted the Institute bearing his name be dedicated to spreading REBT and conducting research on REBT.

From that time until May 2006, Ellis continued to give workshops in a rented space next door to the institute. Nothing but severe illness and ultimately death could stop him from working and helping others. In January 2006, the New York State Supreme Court in Manhattan ruled that the board was wrong in ousting Ellis at a meeting from which Ellis had been excluded. The judge's decision reinstated him to the board. The judge called the institute's position regarding Dr. Ellis "disingenuous," citing case law saying that such a "dismissal, accomplished without notice of any kind or the right of confrontation, is offensive and contrary to our fundamental process of democratic and legal procedure, fair play and the spirit of the law."

Only hours after giving an inspiring Friday Night Workshop (he had been presenting these famous workshops for over four decades) in May 2006, Ellis was hospitalized with aspiration pneumonia. For the next 14 months, he made every effort to recover with remarkable determination and courage. He conducted workshops with students from his hospital bed and within his rehabilitation facility and also gave interviews (Ramirez, 2006), worked on his writings, updated his chapter in *Current Psychotherapies*, and helped others. He was often experiencing great pain and increasing health complications, and despite his incredible and heroic battle to continue, he died peacefully, in the arms of his wife, on July 24, 2007.

The REBT Network was established in 2006, and EllisREBT was established in 2012 to promote rational emotive behavior therapy and the works of Dr. Albert Ellis. These organizations are in no way associated with the Albert Ellis Institute. In 2006, Ellis stated that the Albert Ellis Institute was following a program that was in many ways inconsistent with the theory and practice of REBT. The REBT network has a register of psychotherapists who have received training in REBT. In addition, thousands of other therapists primarily follow REBT principles, and a still greater number use some major aspects of REBT in their work. Cognitive restructuring, employed by almost all cognitive-behavior therapists today, stems mainly from REBT. REBT practitioners also include many other emotive and behavioral methods, with particular emphasis on unconditional acceptance, on disputing irrational beliefs with vigor, and on developing greater *high frustration tolerance* (HFT).

In 2004, Albert Ellis married Australian psychologist Debbie Joffe, whom he called "the greatest love of my life" and whom he trusted to carry on his work (Ellis, 2010). She worked closely with Dr. Ellis in every aspect of his work until his death and continues to write and give presentations and workshops on REBT throughout North and South America and across the globe. She also works with clients in private practice, and she is dedicated to continuing the work of her husband. She is currently completing a manuscript on REBT and Buddhism that she and her husband were working on before his death and writing about the application of REBT to help people address issues of aging and coping with grief.

In April 2012, the first Albert Ellis Professional Learning Center was opened in South Australia (Bruce, 2012). The Learning Center teaches the principles of REBT and *rational emotive behavior education* (REBE) to students, parents, teachers, health-care professionals, and others.

Anyone interested in learning more about the life of Albert Ellis and the history of REBT will benefit from reading *Rational Emotive Behavior Therapy—It Works for Me—It Can Work for You* (Ellis, 2004a) and his autobiography, *All Out!* (Ellis, 2010).

PERSONALITY

Theories of Personality

Physiological Basis of Personality

REBT emphasizes the biological aspects of human personality. Obliquely, some other systems do this, too, saying something like this: "Humans are easily influenced by their parents during early childhood and thereafter remain similarly influenced for the rest of their lives unless some intervention, such as years of psychotherapy, occurs to enable them to give up this early suggestibility and to start thinking much more independently." These psychotherapeutic systems implicitly posit an "environmentalist's" position, which is actually physiologically and genetically based, because only a *special, innately predisposed* kind of person would be so prone to be "environmentally determined."

Although REBT holds (1) that people are born constructivists and have considerable resources for human growth and (2) that they are in many important ways able to change their social and personal destinies, it also holds (3) that they have powerful innate tendencies to think irrationally and to defeat themselves (Ellis, 1976, 2001b, 2003a, 2004b).

Most such human tendencies may be summarized by stating that humans are born with a tendency to want, to "need," and to condemn (1) themselves, (2) others, and (3) the world when they do not immediately get what they supposedly "need." They consequently tend to think "childishly" (or "humanly") all their lives and are able only with real effort to achieve and maintain "mature" or realistic behavior. This is not to deny, as Abraham Maslow and Carl Rogers have pointed out, that humans have impressive self-actualizing capacities. They do, and these also are strong inborn propensities. But, alas, people frequently defeat themselves by their inborn and acquired self-sabotaging ways.

A great deal of evidence shows that people's basic personality or temperament has strong biological, as well as environmental, influences. People are born, as well as reared, with greater or lesser degrees of demandingness, and therefore they can change from demanding to *desiring* only with great difficulty. If their demandingness is largely acquired rather than innate, they still seem to have difficulty in ameliorating this tendency toward disturbance. REBT emphasizes that people nonetheless have the *choice* of changing their dysfunctional behaviors and specifically shows them many ways of doing so. It particularly stresses flexible thinking and behaving that helps them remove the rigidities to which they often easily fall victim.

Social Aspects of Personality

Humans are reared in social groups and spend much of their lives trying to impress other people, live up to others' expectations, and outdo the performances of other people. On the surface, they are "ego-oriented," "identity-seeking," or "self-centered." Even more important, however, they usually define their "selves" as "good" or "worthwhile" when they believe that others accept and approve of them. It is realistic and sensible for people to find or fulfill themselves in their interpersonal relations and to have a good amount of what Adler calls "social interest." For, as John Donne beautifully expressed it, no one is an island unto himself or herself. The healthy individual finds it enjoyable to love and be loved by significant others and to relate to almost everyone he or she encounters. In fact, the better one's interpersonal relations are, the happier one is likely to be.

However, what is called *emotional disturbance* is frequently associated with caring *too much* about what others think. This stems from people's belief that they can accept themselves *only* if others think well of them. When disturbed, they escalate their desire for others' approval, and the practical advantages that normally go with such approval, into an absolutistic *dire need* to be liked, and in so doing they become anxious and prone to depression. Given that we have our being in the world, as the existentialists point out, it is quite *important* that others to some degree value us. But it is our tendency to exaggerate the importance of others' acceptance in a way that often leads to self-denigration (Ellis, 1962, 2001a, 2002, 2005a; Ellis & Harper, 1997; Hauck, 1992).

Psychological Aspects of Personality

How, specifically, do people become psychologically disordered? According to REBT, they usually needlessly upset themselves as follows: When individuals feel upset at point C after experiencing an obnoxious adversity at point A, they almost always convince themselves of irrational beliefs (B), such as "I *can't stand* adversity! It is *awful* that it exists! It *shouldn't exist!* I am a *worthless person* for not being able to get rid of it!" This set of beliefs is irrational for several reasons:

1. People *can* stand obnoxious adversities, even though they may never like them.
2. Adversities are hardly awful, because *awful* is an essentially indefinable term, with surplus meaning and little empirical referent. By calling the noxious events awful, the disturbed individual means they are (a) highly inconvenient and (b) totally inconvenient, disadvantageous, and unbeneficial. But what noxious stimuli can, in point of fact, be totally inconvenient, disadvantageous, and unbeneficial? Or as bad as it could be?
3. By holding that the unfortunate happenings in their lives *absolutely should not* exist, people really imply that they have godly power and that whatever they *want* not to exist *must* not. This hypothesis is, to say the least, highly dubious!

4. By contending that they are *worthless persons* because they have not been able to ward off unfortunate events, people hold that they should be able to control the universe and that because they are not succeeding in doing what they cannot do, they are obviously worthless. (What drivel!)

The basic tenet of REBT is that emotional *upsets,* as distinguished from feelings of sorrow, regret, annoyance, and frustration, largely stem from irrational beliefs. These beliefs are irrational because they magically insist that something in the universe *should, ought,* or *must* be different from the way it is. Although these irrational beliefs are ostensibly connected with reality (the adversity at point A), they are dogmatic ideas beyond the realm of empiricism. They generally take the form of the statement "Because I want something, it is not only desirable and preferable that it exist, but it absolutely should, and it is awful when it doesn't!" No such proposition, obviously, can be substantiated. Yet such propositions are devoutly held, every day, by literally billions of humans. That is how incredibly disturbance prone most people are!

Once people become emotionally upset—or, rather, upset themselves!—a peculiar thing frequently occurs. Most of the time, they know they feel anxious, depressed, or otherwise agitated, and they also know their symptoms are undesirable and (in our culture) socially disapproved. For who approves or respects highly agitated or "crazy" people? They therefore make their emotional consequence (C) or symptom into another activating event or adversity (A) and create a secondary symptom (C2) about this new A!

Thus, if you originally start with something like A ("I did poorly on my job today") and B ("Isn't that horrible!"), you may wind up with C (feelings of anxiety, worthlessness, and depression). You may now start all over with A2 ("I feel anxious and depressed, and worthless!"). Then you proceed to B2 ("Isn't *that* horrible!"). Now you end up with C2: even greater feelings of anxiety, worthlessness, and depression. In other words, once you become anxious, you frequently make yourself anxious about *being* anxious; once you become depressed, you make yourself depressed about *being* depressed; and so on. You now have two consequences or symptoms for the price of one, and you often go around and around, in a vicious cycle of (1) condemning yourself for doing poorly at some task, (2) feeling guilty or depressed because of this self-condemnation, (3) condemning yourself for your feelings of guilt and depression, (4) condemning yourself for condemning yourself, (5) condemning yourself for seeing your disturbances and still not eliminating them, (6) condemning yourself for going for psychotherapeutic help and still not getting better, (7) condemning yourself for being more disturbed than other individuals,(8) concluding that you are without question hopelessly disturbed and that nothing can be done about it; and so on, in an endless spiral.

No matter what your original self-condemnation is about—and it hardly matters what it was, because your adversity (A) is often not that important—you eventually tend to end up with a chain of disturbed reactions only obliquely related to the original "traumatic events" of your life. That is why dramatic psychotherapies are often misleading—they overemphasize "traumatic events" rather than self-condemnatory attitudes *about* these events—and that is why these therapies fail to help with any secondary disturbance, such as being anxious about being anxious. Most major psychotherapies also concentrate either on A (the adversities) or on C (the emotional consequences) and rarely consider B (the belief system), which is a vital factor in creating self-disturbance.

Even assuming, moreover, that adversities and emotional consequences are important, as in posttraumatic stress disorder (PTSD), for instance, there is not too much we can do by concentrating our therapeutic attention on them (Ellis & Ellis, 2011). The adversities belong to the past. There is nothing anyone can do to *change* the past.

As for clients' present feelings, the more we focus on them, the worse they are likely to feel. If we keep talking about their anxiety and getting clients to reexperience this feeling, they can become still more anxious. The best way to interrupt their disturbed process is usually to help them to focus on their anxiety-creating belief system—point B—because that is the main (though not the only) cause of their disturbance.

If, for example, a male client feels anxious during a therapy session and the therapist reassures him that there is nothing for him to be anxious about, he may achieve a palliative "solution" to his problem by thinking, "I am afraid that I will act foolishly right here and now, and wouldn't that be awful! No, it really wouldn't be awful, because *this* therapist will accept me, anyway." He may thereby temporarily decrease his anxiety.

Or the therapist can concentrate on the past adversities in the client's life that are presumably making him anxious—by, for instance, showing him that his mother used to point out his deficiencies, that he was always afraid of speaking to authority figures who might disapprove of him, and that, *therefore,* because of all his prior and current fears, in situations A1, A2, A3, . . . , A11, he is *now* anxious with the therapist. Whereupon the client might convince himself, "Ah! Now I see that I am generally anxious when I am faced with authority figures. No wonder I am anxious even with my own therapist!" In which case, he might feel better and temporarily lose his anxiety.

It would be better, however, for the therapist to show this client that he was anxious as a child and is still anxious with authority figures because he has always believed, and still believes, that he *must* be approved, that it is *awful* when an authority figure disapproves of him. Then the anxious client would tend to become diverted from concentrating on A (criticism by an authority figure) and from C (his feelings of anxiety) to a consideration of B (his irrational belief system). This diversion would help him become immediately nonanxious because when he is focusing on "What am I telling myself (at B) to *make myself* anxious?" he cannot focus on the self-defeating, useless thought "Wouldn't it be terrible if I said something stupid to my therapist and if even he disapproved of me!" He would begin actively to dispute (at point D) his irrational beliefs, and he could not only temporarily change them (by convincing himself, "It would be *unfortunate* if I said something stupid to my therapist and he disapproved of me, but it would hardly be *terrible* or *catastrophic!*") but also tend to have a much weaker allegiance to these self-defeating beliefs the next time. Thus, he would obtain, by the therapist's helping him to focus primarily on B rather than on A and C, curative and preventive, rather than merely palliative, results in connection with his anxiety.

This is the basic personality theory of REBT: Humans largely create their own emotional consequences. They appear to be born with a distinct proneness to do so, and they learn, through social conditioning, to exaggerate (rather than to minimize) that proneness. They nonetheless have considerable ability to understand what they foolishly believe to cause their distress (because they have a unique talent for thinking about their thinking) and to train themselves to change their self-sabotaging beliefs (because they also have a unique capacity for self-discipline or self-reconditioning). If they *think* and *work* hard at understanding and contradicting their *must*urbatory belief systems, they can make amazing curative and preventive changes. And if they are helped to zero in on their crooked thinking and unhealthy emoting and behaving by a highly active-directive homework-assigning therapist, they are more likely to change their beliefs than if they work with a dynamically oriented, client-centered, conventional existential therapist or with a classical therapist who emphasizes behavior modification.

Although REBT is mainly a theory of personality change, it is also a personality theory in its own right (Ellis, 1994, 2001b, 2002).

Variety of Concepts

Ellis largely agrees with (1) Sigmund Freud that the pleasure principle (or short-range hedonism) tends to run most people's lives; (2) Karen Horney and Erich Fromm that cultural influences as well as early family influences tend to play a significant part in bolstering people's irrational thinking; (3) Alfred Adler that fictitious goals tend to order and run human lives; (4) Gordon Allport that when individuals begin to think and act in a certain manner, they find it very difficult to think or act differently, even when they want very much to do so; (5) Ivan Pavlov that our species' large cerebral cortex provides humans with a secondary signaling system through which they often become cognitively conditioned; (6) Jerome Frank that people are exceptionally prone to the influence of suggestion; (7) Jean Piaget that active learning is much more effective than passive learning; (8) Anna Freud that people frequently refuse to acknowledge their mistakes and resort to defenses and rationalizations to cover up underlying feelings of shame and self-deprecation; and (9) Abraham Maslow and Carl Rogers that humans, however disturbed they may be, have great untapped capacity for growth.

On the other hand, REBT has serious differences with certain aspects of many popular personality theories.

1. It opposes the Freudian concept that people have clear-cut libidinous instincts that, if thwarted, must lead to emotional disturbances. It also objects to the view of William Glasser and many other therapists that all humans *need* to be approved and to succeed—and that if these needs are blocked, they cannot possibly accept themselves or be happy. REBT instead posits strong human desires that become needs or necessities only when people foolishly define them as such.

2. REBT places the oedipal complex as a relatively minor subheading under people's major irrational belief that they absolutely have to receive the approval of their parents (and others), that they *must not* fail (at lusting or almost anything else), and that when they are disapproved of and when they fail, they are worthless. Many so-called sexual problems—sexual inadequacy, severe inhibition, and obsessive–compulsive behavior—partly result from people's irrational beliefs that they *need* approval, success, and immediate gratification.

3. REBT holds that people's environment, particularly their childhood parental environment, *reaffirms* but does not always *create* strong tendencies to think irrationally and to be disturbed. Parents and culture teach children standards and values, but they do not always teach them "musts" about these values. People naturally and easily add rigid commands to socially inhibited standards.

4. REBT looks skeptically at anything mystical, devout, transpersonal, or magical when these terms are used in the strict sense. It maintains that reason itself is limited, ungodlike, and absolute (Ellis, 1962, 1994). It holds that humans may in some ways transcend themselves or experience altered states of consciousness—for example, hypnosis—that may enhance their ability to know themselves and the world and to solve some of their problems (Ellis, D. J. 2010a). REBT does not, however, believe that people can transcend their humanness and become superhuman. They can become more adept and competent, but they still remain fallible and in no way godly. REBT holds that minimal disturbance goes with people's surrendering all pretensions to superhumanness and accepting, while still disliking, their own and the world's limitations.

5. For REBT, no part of a human is to be reified into an entity called the unconscious, although it holds that people have many thoughts, feelings, and even acts of which they are unaware. These "unconscious" or tacit thoughts and feelings are, for the most part, slightly below the level of consciousness, are not often

deeply repressed, and can usually be brought to consciousness by brief, incisive probing. Thus, suppose a wife is angrier with her husband than she is aware of and that her anger is motivated by the unconscious grandiose thought, "After all I've done for him he *absolutely should* be having sex with me more frequently!" A rational emotive behavior therapist (who suspects that she has these unconscious feelings and thoughts) can usually induce her to (a) hypothesize that she is angry with her husband and look for some evidence with which to test that hypothesis and (b) check herself for grandiose thinking whenever she feels angry. In the majority of instances, without resorting to free association, dream analysis, analyzing the transference relationship, hypnosis, or other presumably "depth-centered" techniques for revealing unconscious thoughts and feelings, REBT practitioners can reveal these in short order—sometimes in a matter of minutes. They show the client her unconsciously held attitudes, beliefs, and values and, in addition, teach the client how to bring her self-defeating, hidden ideas to consciousness and actively dispute them.

People often see how REBT differs significantly from psychoanalysis, Rogerianism, Gestalt therapy, and orthodox behavior therapy but have difficulty seeing how it differs from more closely related schools such as Adler's Individual Psychology. REBT agrees with nearly all of Adlerian theory but has a more hardheaded and behavior-oriented practice (Ellis, 1994; Ellis & Dryden, 1997; Ellis & MacLaren, 1998). It also ignores most of the Adlerian emphasis on early childhood memories and the importance of birth order. But the basic mistakes that Adlerians emphasize are similar to the irrational beliefs of REBT.

REBT overlaps with Beck's cognitive therapy in several ways, but it also differs in significant ways.

1. It usually disputes clients' irrational beliefs more actively, directly, quickly, and forcefully than does CT.

2. It emphasizes absolutist *musts* more than CT and holds that most major irrationalities implicitly stem from dogmatic *shoulds* and *musts*.

3. It uses psychoeducational approaches—such as books, pamphlets, audiovisual materials, talks, and workshops—as intrinsic elements and stresses their use more than CT does.

4. It clearly distinguishes between healthy negative feelings (e.g., sadness and frustration) and unhealthy negative feelings (e.g., depression and hostility).

5. REBT emphasizes several emotive-evocative methods—such as shame-attacking exercises, rational emotive imagery, and *strong* self-statements and self-dialogues—that CT often neglects.

6. REBT favors in vivo desensitization, preferably done implosively, more than CT does.

7. REBT often uses penalties as well as reinforcements to help people do their homework (Ellis, 2001b, 2002, 2003a).

8. It emphasizes profound philosophical and *unconditional* acceptance of oneself, other people, and the world more than CT does (Ellis, 2005a).

REBT is humanistic and to some degree existentialist. It first tries to help people minimize their emotional and behavioral disturbances, but it also encourages them to make themselves happier than they normally are and to strive for more self-actualization and human growth (Ellis, 1994). It is closer in some respects to Rogers's (1961) person-centered approach than to other therapies in that it mainly emphasizes unconditional self-acceptance as well as unconditional other acceptance no matter how well or how badly people may perform (Ellis, 2001a, 2002, 2003a, 2005a; Ellis & Blau, 1998; Ellis & Ellis, 2011; Ellis & Harper, 1997; Hauck, 1992).

PSYCHOTHERAPY

Theory of Psychotherapy

According to the theory of REBT, neurotic disturbance occurs when individuals demand that their wishes be satisfied, that they succeed and be approved, that others treat them fairly, and that the universe be more pleasant. When people's demandingness (and not their desirousness) gets them into emotional trouble, they tend to alleviate their pain in both inelegant and elegant ways.

Distraction

Just as a whining child can be temporarily diverted by receiving a piece of candy, so can adult demanders be transitorily sidetracked by distraction. Thus, a therapist who sees someone who is afraid of being rejected (that is, one who demands that significant others accept him) can try to divert him into activities such as sports, aesthetic creation, a political cause, yoga exercises, meditation, or preoccupation with the events of his childhood. While the individual is so diverted, he will not be so inclined to demand acceptance by others and to make himself anxious. Distraction techniques are mainly palliative, given that distracted people are still demanders and that they will probably return to their destructive commanding once they are not diverted.

Satisfaction of Demands

If a client's insistences are always catered to, she or he will tend to feel better (but will not necessarily get better). To arrange this kind of "solution," a therapist can give her or his love and approval, provide pleasurable sensations (for example, put the client in an encounter group to be hugged or massaged), teach methods of having demands met, or give reassurance that the client eventually will be gratified. Many clients will feel immensely better when accorded this kind of treatment, but they may well have their demandingness reinforced rather than minimized.

Magic and Mysticism

A boy who demands may be assuaged by magic—for example, by his parents saying that a fairy godmother will soon satisfy his demands. Similarly, adolescent and adult demanders can be led to believe (by a therapist or someone else) that their therapist is a kind of magician who will take away their troubles merely by listening to what bothers them. These magical solutions sometimes work beautifully by getting true believers to feel better and give up disturbed symptoms, but they rarely work for any length of time and frequently lead to eventual disillusionment.

Minimization of Demandingness

The most elegant solution to the problems resulting from irrational demandingness is to help individuals become less demanding. As children mature, they normally become less childish and less insistent that their desires be immediately gratified. REBT encourages clients to achieve minimal demandingness and maximum tolerance.

REBT practitioners may at times use temporary "solutions" such as distraction, satisfying the client's "needs," and even (on rare occasions) "magic." But they realize that these are low-level, inelegant, palliative solutions that are mainly to be used with clients who refuse to accept a more elegant and permanent resolution. The therapist prefers to strive for the highest-order solution: minimizing *must*urbation, perfectionism, grandiosity, and low frustration tolerance.

In REBT, therapists help clients to minimize their absolutistic core philosophies by using cognitive, emotive, and behavioristic procedures.

1. REBT cognitively attempts to show clients that giving up perfectionism can help them lead happier, less anxiety-ridden lives. It teaches them how to recognize their *shoulds, oughts,* and *musts;* how to separate rational (preferential) from irrational (absolutistic) beliefs; how to be logical and pragmatic about their own problems; and how to accept reality, even when it is pretty grim. REBT is oriented toward helping disturbed people philosophize more effectively and thereby uncreate the needless problems they have constructed. Not only does it employ a one-to-one Socratic-type dialogue between the client and the therapist, but also it encourages members in group therapy to discuss, explain, and reason with other ineffectually thinking clients. It teaches logical and semantic precision—that a man's being rejected does not mean that he will always be rejected and that a woman's failure does not mean she cannot succeed. It helps clients to keep asking themselves whether the worst things that could happen would really be as bad as they melodramatically fantasize they would be.

2. REBT emotively employs various means of dramatizing preferences and *musts* so that clients can clearly distinguish between the two. Thus, the therapist may employ *role playing* to show clients how to adopt different ideas; *humor* to reduce disturbance-creating ideas to absurdity; *unconditional acceptance* to demonstrate that clients are acceptable, even with their unfortunate traits; and *strong disputing* to persuade people to give up some of their "crazy thinking" and replace it with more efficient notions. The therapist may also encourage clients, either in individual or group counseling, to take risks (for example, telling another group member what they really think of him or her) that will prove to be not that risky; to reveal themselves (for example, by sharing the details of their sexual problems); to convince themselves that others can accept them with their failings; and to get in touch with their "shameful" feelings (such as hostility) so that they can zero in on exactly what they are telling themselves to create these feelings. Experiential exercises are used to help clients overcome denial of their feelings and then work at REBT's ABCDs (the D refers to disputation) to change their self-defeating emotions. The therapist may also use pleasure-giving techniques, not merely to satisfy clients' unreasonable demands for immediate gratification but also to show them they are capable of doing many pleasant acts that they wrongly think they cannot do, and that they can seek pleasure for its own sake, even though others may frown on them for doing so.

3. *Behavior therapy* is employed in REBT not only to help clients become habituated to more effective ways of performing but also to help change their cognitions. Thus, their demandingness that they perform beautifully may be whittled away by their agreeing to do risk-taking assignments such as asking a desired person for a date, deliberately failing at some task (for example, making a real attempt to speak badly in public), imagining themselves in failing situations, and throwing themselves into unusual activities that they consider especially dangerous. Clients' demandingness that others treat them fairly and that the world be kind may be challenged by the therapist's encouraging them to stay in poor circumstances and teach themselves, at least temporarily, to accept them; to take on hard tasks (such as enrolling in college);

to imagine themselves having a rough time at something and making themselves not feel terribly upset or having to "cop out" of it; to allow themselves to do a pleasant thing, such as go to a movie or see their friends, only after they have done unpleasant but desirable tasks, such as studying French or finishing a report for their boss; and so on. REBT often employs operant conditioning to reinforce people's efforts to change undesirable behavior (e.g., smoking or overeating) or to change irrational thinking (e.g., condemning themselves when they smoke or overeat).

REBT accepts that there are many kinds of psychological treatment and that most of them work to some degree. An elegant system of therapy includes (a) economy of time and effort, (b) rapid symptom reduction, (c) effectiveness with a large percentage of different kinds of clients, (d) depth of solution of the presenting problems, and (e) lastingness of the therapeutic results. Philosophically, REBT combats absoluteness and ruthlessly persists at undermining childish demandingness—the main element of much neurotic disturbance (Ellis, 1962, 1994, 2002). It theorizes that if people learn to only strongly prefer that their desires be fulfilled instead of grandiosely insisting on it, they can make themselves remarkably less disturbed and less disturbable (Ellis, 1999, 2001a, 2001b, 2002).

Process of Psychotherapy

REBT helps clients acquire a more realistic, tolerant philosophy of life. Because some of its methods are similar to methods used by other therapists, they are not detailed in this section. Most of the space here is devoted to the cognitive-persuasive aspects of REBT, one of its most distinguishing characteristics.

REBT practitioners generally do not spend a great deal of time listening to the client's history, encouraging long tales of woe, sympathetically getting in tune with emotionalizing, or carefully and incisively reflecting feelings. They may use all these methods, but they generally keep them short because they consider most long-winded dialogues a form of indulgence therapy in which the client may be helped to *feel* better but rarely to *get* better. Even when these methods work, they are often inefficient and sidetracking (Ellis, 2001a).

Similarly, the rational emotive behavior therapist makes little use of free association, dream analysis, interpretations of the transference relationship, explanations of the client's current symptoms in terms of past experiences, disclosure, analysis of the so-called oedipal complex, and other dynamically directed interpretations or explanations. When they are employed at all, they are used to help clients see some of their basic irrational ideas.

Thus, if a male therapist notes that a female client rebels against him just as she previously rebelled against her father during childhood, he will not interpret the current rebelliousness as stemming from the prior pattern but instead will probably say something like this:

> It looks like you frequently hated your father because he kept forcing you to follow certain rules you considered arbitrary and because you kept convincing yourself, "My father isn't being considerate of me and he *ought* to be! I'll get even with him!" I think you are now telling yourself approximately the same thing about me. But your angry rebelliousness against your father was senseless because (a) he was not a *total bastard* for perpetrating a bastardly act; (b) there was no reason why he *ought* to have been considerate of you (although there were several reasons why it *would have been preferable* if he had been); and (c) your getting angry at him and trying to "get even with him" would not, probably, encourage him to act more kindly but would actually induce him to be more cruel.

You consequently confused—as most children will—being displeased with your father's behavior with being "righteously" angry at him, and you needlessly made yourself upset about his real or imagined unfair treatment of you. In my case, too, you may be doing much the same thing. You may be taking the risks that I encourage you to take and insisting that they arc too onerous (when in fact, they are only onerous), and after assuming that I am wrong in suggesting them (which I indeed may be), you are condemning me for my supposedly wrong deeds. Moreover, you are quite possibly assuming that I am "wrong" and a "louse" for being wrong because I resemble, in some ways, your "wrong" and "lousy" father.

But this is another illogical conclusion (that I resemble him in all ways) and an irrational premise (that I, like your father, am a *bad person* if I do a wrong act). So you are not only *inventing* a false connection between me and your father, but you are creating today, as you have done for many years now, a renewed *demand* that the world be an easy place for you and that everyone *ought* to treat you fairly. Now, how can you challenge these irrational premises and illogical deductions?

REBT practitioners often employ a rapid-fire active-directive-persuasive-philosophical methodology. In most instances, they quickly pin clients down to a few basic dysfunctional beliefs. They challenge them to try to defend these ideas; show that they contain illogical premises that cannot be substantiated logically; analyze these ideas and actively dispute them; vigorously show why they cannot work and why they will almost inevitably lead to more disturbance; reduce these ideas to absurdity, sometimes in a humorous manner; explain how they can be replaced with more rational philosophies; and teach clients how to think scientifically so that they can observe, logically parse, and minimize any subsequent irrational ideas and illogical deductions that lead to self-defeating feelings and behaviors.

When working with certain clients who have suffered extreme traumas (such as incest, rape, child abuse, or other violent situations), REBT practitioners may well be quite empathic and go more slowly before doing any vigorous disputing of clients' dysfunctional beliefs about these traumatic events or about anything else in their lives.

To show how REBT is sometimes, but hardly always, actively and directively done, the following is a verbatim transcript of a session with a 25-year-old single woman, Sara, who worked as the head of a computer-programming section of a firm and who, without any traumatic or violent history, was very insecure and self-denigrating.

T-1:   What would you want to start on first?

C-1:   I don't know. I'm petrified at the moment!

T-2:   You're petrified—of what?

C-2:   Of you!

T-3:   No, surely not of me—perhaps of yourself!

C-3:   [Laughs nervously.]

T-4:   Because of what I am going to do to you?

C-4:   Right! You are threatening me, I guess.

T-5:   But how? What am I doing? Obviously, I'm not going to take a knife and stab you. Now, in what way am I threatening you?

C-5:   I guess I'm afraid, perhaps, of what I'm going to find out—about me.

T-6:   Well, so let's suppose you find out something dreadful about you—that you're thinking foolishly or something. Now why would that be awful?

C-6:   Because I, I guess I'm the most important thing to me at the moment.

T-7:   No, I don't think that's the answer. It's, I believe, the opposite! You're really the least important thing to you. You are prepared to beat yourself over the head if I tell you that you're acting foolishly. If you were not a self-blamer, then you wouldn't care what I said. It would be important to you—but you'd just go around correcting it. But if I tell you something really negative about you, you're going to beat yourself mercilessly. Aren't you?

C-7:   Yes, I generally do.

T-8:   All right. So perhaps that's what you're really afraid of. You're not afraid of me. You're afraid of your own self-criticism.

C-8:   [Sighs.] All right.

T-9:   So why do you have to criticize yourself? Suppose I find you're the worst person I ever met? Let's just suppose that. All right, now *why* would you have to criticize yourself?

C-9:   [Pause.] I'd have to. I don't know any other behavior pattern, I guess, in this point of time. I always do. I guess I think I'm just a shit.

T-10: Yeah. But that, that isn't so. If you don't know how to ski or swim, you could learn. You can also learn not to condemn yourself, no matter what you do.

C-10: I don't know.

T-11: Well, the answer is: You don't know how.

C-11: Perhaps.

T-12: I get the impression you're saying, "I have to berate myself if I do something wrong." Because isn't that where your depression comes from?

C-12: Yes, I guess so. [Silence.]

T-13: Now, what are you *mainly* putting yourself down for right now?

C-13: I don't seem quite able, in this point of time, to break it down very neatly. The form [that our clinic gets clients to fill out before their sessions] gave me a great deal of trouble. Because my tendency is to say *everything,* I want to change everything; I'm depressed about everything, etc.

T-14: Give me a couple of things, for example.

C-14: What I'm depressed about? I, uh, don't know that I have any purpose in life. I don't know what I—what I am. And I don't know in what direction I'm going.

T-15: Yeah, but that's—so you're saying, "I'm ignorant!" [Client nods.] Well, what's so awful about being ignorant? It's too bad you're ignorant. It would be nicer if you weren't—if you *had* a purpose and *knew* where you were going. But just let's suppose the worst: for the rest of your life you didn't have a purpose and you stayed this way. Let's suppose that. Now, why would *you* be so bad?

C-15: Because everyone *should* have a purpose!

T-16: Where did you get the *should?*

C-16: 'Cause it's what I believe in. [Silence.]

T-17: I know. But think about it for a minute. You're obviously a bright woman. Now, where did that *should* come from?

C-17: I, I don't know! I'm not thinking clearly at the moment. I'm too nervous! I'm sorry.

T-18: Well, but you *can* think clearly. Are you now saying, "Oh, it's hopeless! I can't think clearly. What a shit I am for not thinking clearly!" You see: you're blaming yourself for *that.*

[From C-18 to C-26 the client upsets herself about not reacting well to the session, but the therapist shows her that this is not overly important and calms her down.]

C-27: I can't imagine existing, uh, or that there would be any reason for existing without a purpose!

T-28: No, but the vast majority of human beings don't have much purpose.

C-28: [Angrily.] All right, then, I should not feel bad about it.

T-29: No, no, no! Wait a minute, now. You just *jumped.* [Laughs.] You jumped from one extreme to another! You see, you said a sane sentence and an *insane* sentence. Now, if we could get you to separate the two—which you're perfectly able to do—you would solve the problem. What you really mean is "It *would be better* if I had a purpose. Because I'd be happier." Right?

C-29: Yes.

T-30: But then you magically jump to "Therefore I *should!*" Now do you see the difference between "It *would be better* if I had a purpose" and "I *should,* I *must,* I've *got to*"?

C-30: Yes, I do.

T-31: Well, what's the difference?

C-31: [Laughs.] I just said that to agree with you!

T-32: Yes! See, that won't be any good. We could go on that way forever, and you'll agree with me, and I'll say, "Oh, what a great woman! She agrees with me." And then you'll go out of here as nutty as you were before!

C-32: [Laughs, this time with genuine appreciation and good humor.]

T-33: You're perfectly able, as I said, to think—to stop giving up. That's what you've done most of your life. That's why you're disturbed. Because you refuse to think. And let's go over it again: "It would be better if I had a purpose in life; if I weren't depressed, etc., etc. If I had a good, nice, enjoyable purpose." We could give reasons why it would be better. "It's fairly obvious why it would be better!" Now, why is that a magical statement, that "I *should* do what would be better"?

C-33: You mean, why do I feel that way?

T-34: No, no. It's a belief. You feel that way because you believe that way.

C-34: Yes.

T-35: If you believed you were a kangaroo, you'd be hopping around and you'd *feel* like a kangaroo. Whatever you *believe,* you feel. Feelings largely come from your beliefs. Now, I'm temporarily forgetting about your feelings, because we really can't change feelings without changing beliefs. So I'm showing you; you have two beliefs—or two feelings, if you want to call them that. One, "It would be better if I had a purpose in life." Do you agree? [Client nods.] Now that's perfectly reasonable. That's quite true. We could prove it. Two, "Therefore I *should* do what would be better." Now those are two different statements. They may seem the same, but they're vastly different. Now, the first one, as I said, is sane. Because we could prove it. It's related to reality. We can list the advantages of having a purpose—for almost anybody, not just for you.

C-35: [Calm now, and listening intently to T's explanation.] Uh-huh.

T-36: But the second one, "Therefore I *should* do what would be better," is crazy. Now, why is it crazy?

C-36: I can't accept it as a crazy statement.

T-37: Because who said you *should?*

C-37: I don't know where it all began! Somebody said it.

T-38: I know, but I say whoever said it was screwy!

C-38: [Laughs.] All right.

T-39: How could the world possibly have a *should?*

C-39: Well, it does.

T-40: But it *doesn't!* You see, that's what emotional disturbance is: believing in *shoulds, oughts,* and *musts* instead of *it would be betters.* That's exactly what makes people neurotic! Suppose you said to yourself, "I wish I had a dollar in my pocket right now," and you had only 90 cents. How would you feel?

C-40:   Not particularly upset.

T-41:   Yes, you'd be a little disappointed. It would be better to have a dollar. But now suppose you said, "I should, I must have a dollar in my pocket at all times," and you found you had only 90 cents. Now, how would you feel?

C-41:   Then I would be terribly upset, following your line of reasoning.

T-42:   But not because you had only 90 cents.

C-42:   Because I thought I should have a dollar.

T-43:   THAT'S RIGHT! The should. And what's more, let's just go one step further. Suppose you said, "I must have a dollar in my pocket at all times." And you found you had a dollar and 10 cents. Now how would you feel?

C-43:   Superb, I guess!

T-44:   No—anxious!

C-44:   [Laughs.] You mean I'd be guilty: "What was I doing with the extra money?"

T-45:   No.

C-45:   I'm sorry, I'm not following you. I—

T-46:   Because you're not thinking. Think for a minute. Why, if you said, "I must have a dollar, I should have a dollar," and you had a dollar and 10 cents, would you still be anxious? Anybody would be. Now why would anybody be anxious if they were saying, "I've got to have a dollar!" and they found they had a dollar and 10 cents?

C-46:   Because it violated their should. It violated their rule of what they thought was right, I guess.

T-47:   Well, not at the moment. But they could easily lose 20 cents.

C-47:   Oh! Well.

T-48:   Yeah! They'd still be anxious. You see, because must means, "At all times I must—"

C-48:   Oh, I see what you mean! All right. I see what you mean. They could easily lose some of the money and would therefore feel insecure.

T-49:   Yeah. Most anxiety comes from musts.

C-49:   [Long silence.] Why do you create such an anxiety-ridden situation initially for someone?

T-50:   I don't think I do. I see hundreds of people and you're one of the few who makes this so anxiety-provoking for yourself. The others may do it mildly, but you're making it very anxiety-provoking. Which just shows that you may carry must into everything, including this situation. Most people come in here very relieved. They finally get to talk to somebody who knows how to help them, and they're very happy that I stop the horseshit, and stop asking about their childhood, and don't talk about the weather, etc. And I get *right away* to what bothers them. I tell them in 5 minutes. I've just explained to you the secret of most emotional disturbance. If you really followed what I said, and used it, you'd never be disturbed about practically anything for the rest of your life!

C-50:   Uh-huh.

T-51:   Because practically every time you're disturbed, you're changing it would be better to a must! That's all neurosis is! Very, very simple. Now, why should I waste your time and not explain this—and talk about irrelevant things?

C-51:   Because perhaps I would have followed your explanation a little better if I hadn't been so threatened initially.

T-52:   But then, if I pat you on the head and hold back, etc., then you'll think for the rest of your life you have to be patted on the head! You're a bright woman!

C-52:   All right—

T-53: That's another should. "He should pat me on the head and take it slowly—then a shit like me can understand! But if he goes fast and makes me think, oh my God I'll make an error—and that is awful!" More horseshit! You don't have to believe that horseshit! You're perfectly able to follow what I say—if you stop worrying, "I should do perfectly well!" For that's what you're basically thinking, sitting there. Well, why should you do perfectly well? Suppose we had to go over it 20 times before you got it?

C-53: I don't *like* to appear stupid!

T-54: No. See. Now you're lying to yourself! Because again you said a sane thing—and then you added an insane thing. The sane thing was, "I don't like to appear stupid, because it's *better* to appear bright." But then you immediately jumped over to the insane thing: "And it's *awful* if I appear stupid—"

C-54: [Laughs appreciatively, almost joyously.]

T-55: "—I *should* appear bright!" You see?

C-55: [With conviction.] Yes.

T-56: The same crap! It's always the same crap. Now if you would look at the crap—instead of "Oh, how stupid I am! He hates me! I think I'll kill myself!"—then you'd be on the road to getting better fairly quickly.

C-56: You've been listening! [Laughs.]

T-57: Listening to what?

C-57: [Laughs.] Those wild statements in my mind, like that, that I make.

T-58: That's right! Because I know that you have to make those statements—because I have a good *theory.* And according to my theory, people wouldn't usually get upset *unless* they made those nutty statements to themselves.

C-58: I haven't the faintest idea why I've been so upset—

T-59: But you *do* have the faintest idea. I just told you.

C-59: All right, I know!

T-60: Why are you upset? Report it to me.

C-60: I'm upset because I know, I—the role that I envisioned myself being in when I walked in here and what I [Laughs, almost joyously] and what I would do and should do—

T-61: Yeah?

C-61: And therefore you forced me to violate that. And I don't like it.

T-62: "And isn't it *awful* that I didn't come out greatly! If I had violated that needed role *beautifully,* and I gave him the *right* answers immediately, and he beamed, and said, 'Boy, what a bright woman, this!' then it would have been all right."

C-62: [Laughing good-humoredly.] Certainly!

T-63: Horseshit! You would have been exactly as disturbed as you are now! It wouldn't have helped you a bit! In fact, you would have gotten nuttier! Because then you would have gone out of here with the same philosophy you came in here with: "That when I act well and people pat me on the head and say, 'What a great woman I am!' then everything is rosy!" It's a nutty philosophy! Because even if I loved you madly, the next person you talk to is likely to hate you. So I like brown eyes and he likes blue eyes or something else. So you're then dead! Because you really think: "I've got to be *accepted!* I've got to act intelligently!" Well, why?

C-63: [Very soberly and reflectively.] True.

T-64: You see?

C-64: Yes.

T-65: Now, if you will learn that lesson, then you've had a very valuable session. Because you *don't* have to upset yourself. As I said before, if I thought you

were the worst shit who ever existed, well, that's my *opinion*. And I'm entitled to it. But does it make you a turd?

C-65:   [Reflective silence.]

T-66:   *Does* it?

C-66   No.

T-67:   *What* makes you a turd?

C-67:   *Thinking* that you are.

T-68:   That's right! Your *belief* that you are. That's the only thing that could ever
do it. And you never have to believe that. See? You control your thinking.
I control *my* thinking—*my* belief about you. But you don't have to be affected by that. You *always* control what you think. And you believe you
don't. So let's get back to that depression. The depression, as I said before,
stems from self-castigation. That's where it comes from. Now what are you
castigating yourself for?

C-68:   Because I can't live up to it—there's a basic conflict in what people appear
to think I am and what I think I am.

T-69:   Right.

C-69:   And perhaps it's not fair to blame other people. Perhaps I thrust myself into
a leader's role. But, anyway, my feeling right now is that all my life I've been
forced to be something that I'm not, and the older I get, the more difficult
this *façade,* huh, this *appearance,* uh— that the veneer is becoming thinner
and thinner and thinner, until I just can't do it anymore.

T-70:   Well, but really, yeah, I'm afraid you're a little wrong. Because oddly enough,
almost the opposite is happening. You are thrust into this role. That's right:
the role of something of a leader. Is that correct?

C-70:   Yes.

T-71:   And *they* think you're filling it.

C-71:   Everyone usually does.

T-72:   And it just so happens they're *right.*

C-72:   But it's taking more and more out of me.

T-73:   Because you're not doing something else. You see, you are fulfilling *their* expectations of you. Because, obviously, they wouldn't think you are a leader,
they'd think you were nothing if you *were* acting like a nonleader. So you are
fulfilling their expectations. But you're not fulfilling your own idealistic and
impractical expectations of leadership.

C-73:   [Verging on tears.] No, I guess I'm not.

T-74:   You see, that's the issue. So therefore you *are* doing O. K. by them—by your
job. But you're not being an angel, you're not being *perfect!* And you *should*
be, to be a real *leader.* And therefore you're a *sham!* You see? Now, if you
give up those nutty expectations of yourself and go back to their expectations, you're in no trouble at all. Because obviously you're doing all right by
them and *their* expectations.

C-74:   Well, I haven't been. I had to, to give up one very successful situation. And,
uh, when I left, they thought it was still successful. But I just couldn't go on—

T-75:   "Because I must, I must *really* be a leader in *my* eyes, be pretty *perfect."* You
see, "If I satisfy the world, but I know I did badly, or less than I *should,* then
I'm a slob! And they haven't found me out, so that makes me a *double* slob.
Because I'm pretending to them to be a nonslob when I really am one!"

C-75:   [Laughs in agreement, then grows sober.] True.

T-76:   But it's all your silly *expectations.* It's not *them.* And oddly enough,
you are—even with your *handicap,* which is depression, self-deprecation,
etc. —you're doing remarkably well. Imagine what you might do *without*

this nutty handicap! You see, you're satisfying them while you're spending most of your time and energy flagellating yourself. Imagine what you might do *without* the self-flagellation! Can you see that?

C-76:   [Stopped in her self-blaming tracks, at least temporarily convinced, speaks very meaningfully.] Yes.

Mechanisms of Psychotherapy

From the foregoing partial protocol (which consumed about 15 minutes of the first session with the client), it can be seen that the therapist tries to do several things:

1.   No matter what *feelings* the client brings out, the therapist tries to get back to her main irrational *ideas* that probably lie behind these feelings—especially her ideas that it would be *awful* if someone, including him, disliked her.

2.   The therapist does not hesitate to contradict the client, using evidence from the client's own life and from his knowledge of people in general.

3.   He usually is one step *ahead* of her—tells her, for example, that she is a self-blamer before she has said that she is. Knowing, on the basis of REBT theory, that she has *shoulds, oughts,* and *musts* in her thinking if she becomes anxious, depressed, and guilty, he helps her to admit these *shoulds* and then dispute them (T-16, T-17).

4.   He uses the strongest philosophical approach he can think of: "Suppose," he keeps saying to her, "the *worst* thing happened and you really did do badly and others hated you, would you *still* be so bad?" (T-15). He assumes that if he can convince her that *none* of her behavior, no matter how execrable, denigrates *her,* he has helped her to make a *deep* attitudinal change.

5.   He is not thrown by her distress (C-17) and is not too sympathetic about these feelings, but he *uses* them to try to prove to her that, right now, she still believes in foolish ideas and thereby upsets herself. He does not dwell on her "transference" feelings. He interprets the *ideas* behind these feelings, shows her why they are self-defeating, and indicates why his acting sympathetically would probably reinforce her demanding philosophy instead of helping her change it.

6.   He not only is fairly stern with her but also shows full acceptance and demonstrates confidence in her abilities, especially her constructive ability to change herself.

7.   Instead of merely *telling* her that her ideas are irrational, he keeps trying to get her to see this for herself (T-36). He wants her not merely to accept or parrot *his* rational philosophies but also to think them through. He does, however, explain some relevant psychological processes, such as the way the client's feelings largely derive from her thinking (T-35, T-68).

8.   He deliberately, on several occasions, uses strong language (T-18, T-50). This is done (a) to help loosen up the client; (b) to show that he, the therapist, is a down-to-earth human being; and (c) to give her an emotive jolt or shock so his words may have a more dramatic effect. Note that in this case, the client first calls herself a "shit" (C-9).

9.   Although hardly sympathetic to her ideas, he is really quite empathic. Rational emotive behavior therapists are usually attuned to the client's unexpressed thoughts (her negative ideas about herself and the world) rather than to her superficial feelings (her perceptions that she is doing poorly or that others are abusing her). They empathize with the client's *feelings* and with the *beliefs* that underlie these feelings. This is a two-pronged form of empathy that many therapies miss out on.

10. The therapist keeps checking the client's ostensible understanding of what he is teaching her (T-65, T-66, T-67).

11. The therapist—as is common in early sessions of REBT—does most of the talking and explaining. He gives the client plenty of opportunity to express herself but uses her responses as points of departure for further teaching. He tries to make each "lecture" brief and trenchant and to relate it specifically to her problems and feelings. Also, at times he stops to let ideas sink in.

As can be seen from the first part of this initial REBT session, the client does not receive feelings of love and warmth from the therapist. Transference and countertransference spontaneously occur, but they are quickly analyzed, the philosophies behind them are revealed, and they tend to evaporate in the process. The client's deep feelings (shame, self-pity, weeping, anger) clearly exist, but the client is not given too much chance to revel in these feelings or to abreact strongly about them. As the therapist points out and attacks the ideologies that underlie these feelings, they swiftly change and are sometimes almost miraculously transformed into other, contradictory feelings (such as humor, joy, and reflective contemplation). The therapist's "coolness," philosophizing, and encouraging insistence that the client can feel something besides anxiety and depression help change her destructiveness into constructive feelings. That is why REBT is a constructivist rather than a purely rationalist kind of therapy (Ellis, 1994, 1999, 2001a, 2001b, 2002).

What the client does seem to experience, as the session proceeds, is (1) full acceptance of herself, in spite of her poor behavior; (2) renewed confidence that she can do certain things, such as think for herself; (3) the belief that it is her own perfectionistic *shoulds* that are upsetting her and not the attitudes of others (including the therapist); (4) reality testing, in her starting to see that even though she performs inefficiently (with the therapist and with some of the people she works with), she can still recover, try again, and probably do better in the future; and (5) reduction of some of her defenses in that she can stop blaming others (such as her therapist) for her anxiety and start to admit that she is doing something herself to cause it.

In these 15 minutes, the client is getting only *glimmerings* of these constructive thoughts and feelings. The REBT intent, however, is that she will *keep* getting insights—that is, *philosophical* rather than merely *psychodynamic* insights—into the self-causation of her disturbed symptoms; that she will use these insights to change some of her most enduring and deep-seated ways of thinking about herself, about others, and about the world; and that she will thereby eventually become ideationally, emotionally, and behaviorally less self-defeating. Unless she finally makes an *attitudinal* (as well as symptom-reducing) change, although she may be helped to some degree, she will still be far from the ideal REBT goal of making a basic and lasting personality change.

APPLICATIONS

Who Can We Help?

It is easier to state what kinds of problems are *not* handled than what kinds *are* handled in REBT. Individuals who are out of contact with reality, in a highly manic state, seriously autistic or brain injured, or in the lower ranges of mental deficiency are not normally treated by REBT therapists (or by most other practitioners). They are referred for medical treatment, for custodial or institutional care, or for behavior therapy along operant conditioning lines.

Most other individuals with difficulties are treated with REBT. These include (1) clients with maladjustment, moderate anxiety, or marital problems; (2) those with sexual difficulties;

(3) run-of-the-mill "neurotics"; (4) individuals with character disorders; (5) truants, juvenile delinquents, and adult criminals; (6) borderline personalities and others with personality disorders; (7) overt psychotics, including those with delusions and hallucinations, when they are under medication and somewhat in contact with reality; (8) individuals with higher-grade mental deficiency; and (9) clients with psychosomatic problems.

Although varying types of problems are treated with REBT, no claim is made that they are treated with equal effectiveness. As is the case with virtually all psychotherapies, the REBT approach is more effective with clients who have a single major symptom (such as sexual inadequacy) than with seriously disordered clients (Ellis, 2001b, 2002). This is consistent with several hypotheses of REBT theory: that the tendency toward emotional distress is partly inborn and not merely acquired, that individuals with serious aberrations are more innately predisposed to have rigid and crooked thinking than are those with lesser aberrations, and that these clients consequently are less likely to make major advances. Moreover, REBT emphasizes commitment to changing one's thinking and to doing homework activity assignments, and it is clinically observable that many of the most dramatically symptom-ridden individuals (such as those who are severely depressed) tend to do considerably less work and more shirking (including shirking at therapy) than those with milder symptoms. Nevertheless, seasoned REBT practitioners claim they get better results with a wide variety of clients than do therapists from other schools of psychological thought (Ellis, 1994; Lyons & Woods, 1991; McGovern & Silverman, 1984; Silverman, McCarthy, & McGovern, 1992).

REBT is applicable for preventive purposes. Rational emotive procedures are closely connected to the field of education and have enormous implications for emotional prophylaxis (Ellis, 2003b). A number of clinicians have shown how they have helped prevent normal children from eventually becoming seriously disturbed. Evidence shows that when nondisturbed grade school pupils are given, along with regular elements of an academic education, a steady process of REBT education, they can learn to understand themselves and others and learn to live more rationally and happily in this difficult world (Ellis & Bernard, 2006; Ellis & Ellis, 2011; Vernon, 2001).

Treatment

REBT employs virtually all forms of individual and group psychotherapy. Some of the main methods are described in this section.

Individual Therapy

Most clients with whom REBT is practiced are seen for individual sessions, usually on a weekly basis, for from 5 to 50 sessions. They generally begin their sessions by telling the most upsetting feelings or consequences (C) that they have experienced during the week. REBT therapists then discover what adversities (A) occurred before clients felt so badly and help them to see what rational beliefs and what irrational beliefs (B) they hold in connection with these adversities. They teach clients to dispute (D) their irrational beliefs and often agree on concrete homework activity assignments to help with this disputing. They then check up in the following session, sometimes with the help of an REBT Self-Help Report Form, to see how the clients have tried to use the REBT approach during the week. If clients work at REBT, they arrive at an effective new philosophy (E)—which they reach through *effort* and *exercise.*

In particular, REBT therapists try to show clients how to (1) minimize anxiety, guilt, and depression by unconditionally accepting themselves; (2) alleviate their anger, hostility, and violence by unconditionally accepting other people; and (3) reduce their low frustration tolerance and inertia by learning to accept life unconditionally even when it is grim (Ellis, 2001a; Ellis, 2005a; Ellis & Blau, 1998; Ellis & Ellis, 2011; Fuller et al., 2010; McCracken et al., 2008).

When working with individuals on issues of addiction, it is important to recognize that not all addicts are alike, that many factors contribute to people's addictiveness, that people with personality disorders may be more prone to addiction, and that many such clients may have multiple addictions and dual diagnoses (Ellis & Ellis, 2011; Ellis, D. J. 2010b; Velten & Penn, 2010).

Group Therapy

REBT is particularly applicable to group therapy. Because group members are taught to apply REBT procedures to one another, they can help others learn the procedures and get practice (under the direct supervision of the group leader) in applying them. In group work, moreover, there is usually more opportunity for the members to agree on homework assignments (some of which are to be carried out in the group itself), to get assertiveness training, to engage in role playing, to interact with other people, to take verbal and nonverbal risks, to learn from the experiences of others, to interact thera-peutically and socially with each other in after-group sessions, and to have their behavior directly observed by the therapist and other group members (Ellis, 2001b; Ellis & Dryden, 1997).

REBT Workshops, Rational Encounter Marathons, and Intensives

REBT has successfully used marathon encounter groups and large-scale, one-day intensive workshops that include many verbal and nonverbal exercises, dramatic risk-taking procedures, evocative lectures, personal encounters, homework assignments, and other emotive and behavioral methods. Research studies have shown that these workshops, marathons, and intensive workshops have beneficial, immediate, and lasting effects (Ellis & Dryden, 1997; Ellis & Joffe, 2002).

Brief Therapy

REBT is naturally designed for brief therapy. It is preferable that individuals with severe disturbances come to individual or group sessions or both for at least 6 months. But for individuals who are going to stay in therapy for only a short while, REBT can teach them, in 1 to 10 sessions, the A–B–C method of understanding emotional problems, seeing their main philosophical source, and beginning to change fundamental disturbance-creating attitudes (Ellis, 2001b).

This is particularly true for the person who has a specific problem—such as hostility toward a boss or sexual inadequacy—and who is not too *generally* disturbed. Such an individual can, with the help of REBT, be almost completely "cured" in a few sessions. But even clients with long-standing difficulties may be significantly helped as a result of brief therapy.

Two special devices often employed in REBT can help speed the therapeutic process. The first is to tape the entire session. These recordings are then listened to, usually several times, by the clients in their own home, car, or office so that they can more clearly see their problems and the rational emotive behavioral way of handling them. Many clients who have difficulty "hearing" what goes on during the face-to-face sessions (because they are too intent on talking themselves, are easily distracted, or are too anxious) are able to get more from listening to a recording of these sessions than from the original encounter.

Second, an REBT Self-Help Form is frequently used with clients to help teach them how to use the method when they encounter emotional problems between therapy sessions or after therapy has ended. This form is reproduced on pages 182–183.

Marriage and Family Therapy

From its beginning, REBT has been used extensively in marriage and family counseling (Ellis, 1962, 2001b; Ellis & Dryden, 1997; Ellis & Harper, 1997, 2003). Usually, marital or love partners are seen together. REBT therapists listen to their complaints about each other and then try to show that even if the complaints are justified, making themselves unduly upset is not. Work is done with either or both participants to minimize anxiety, depression, guilt, and (especially) hostility. As they begin to learn and apply the REBT principles, they usually become much less disturbed, often within a few sessions, and then are much better able to minimize their incompatibilities and maximize their compatibilities.

Sometimes, of course, they decide that they would be better off separated or divorced, but usually they decide to work at their problems to achieve a happier marital arrangement. They are frequently taught contracting, compromising, communication, and other relating skills. The therapist is concerned with both of them as individuals who can be helped emotionally, whether or not they decide to stay together. But the more they work at helping themselves, the better their relationship tends to become (Ellis, 2001b; Ellis & Crawford, 2000; Ellis & Harper, 2003). Albert Ellis and Debbie Joffe Ellis joyfully and successfully applied REBT in their lives and within their relationship (Eckstein, 2012; Eckstein & Ellis, 2011; Ellis, 2010).

In family therapy, REBT practitioners sometimes see all members of the same family together, see the children in one session and the parents in another, or see them all individually. Several joint sessions are usually held to observe the interactions among family members. Whether together or separately, parents are frequently shown how to accept their children and to stop condemning them, and children are similarly shown that they can accept their parents and their siblings. The general REBT principles of unconditionally accepting oneself and others are repeatedly taught. As is common with other REBT procedures, bibliotherapy supplements counseling with REBT materials such as *A Guide to Rational Living* (Ellis & Harper, 1997), *A Rational Counseling Primer* (Young, 1974), *How to Make Yourself Happy and Remarkably Less Disturbable* (Ellis, 1999), *Feeling Better, Getting Better, Staying Better* (Ellis, 2001a), *The Myth of Self-Esteem* (Ellis, 2005a), and *Rational Emotive Behavior Therapy* (Ellis & Ellis, 2011).

The *setting* of REBT sessions is much like that for other types of therapy. Most individual sessions take place in an office, but there may well be no desk between the therapist and the client, and REBT therapists tend to be informally dressed and to use simple language. They tend to be more open, authentic, and less "professional" than the average therapist. The main special equipment used is an audio recorder. The client is likely to be encouraged to make a recording of the session to take home for replaying.

REBT therapists are highly active, give their own views without hesitation, usually answer direct questions about their personal lives, are quite energetic and often directive in group therapy, and do a good deal of speaking, particularly during early sessions. At the same time, they unconditionally accept clients. They may engage in considerable explaining, interpreting, and "lecturing" and may easily work with clients they personally do not like. Because they tend to have complete tolerance for all individuals, REBT therapists are often seen as warm and caring by their clients.

Resistance is usually handled by showing clients that they resist changing because they would like to find a magical, easy solution rather than work at changing themselves. Resistance is not usually interpreted as their particular feelings about the therapist. If a client tries to seduce a therapist, this is usually explained not in terms of "transference" but in terms of (1) the client's need for love, (2) normal attraction to a helpful person, and (3) the natural sex urges of two people who have intimate mental-emotional contact. If the therapist is attracted to the client, he or she usually admits the attraction but explains why it is unethical to have sexual or personal relations with a client (Ellis, 2002).

Evidence

REBT has directly or indirectly inspired scores of experiments to test its theories, and there are now hundreds of research studies that tend to validate its major theoretical hypotheses. More than 200 outcome studies have been published showing that REBT is effective in changing the thoughts, feelings, and behaviors of groups of individuals with various kinds of disturbances (DiGiuseppe, Terjesen, Rose, Doyle, & Vadalakis, 1998). These studies tend to show that REBT disputing and other methods usually work better than no therapy and are often more effective than other forms of psychotherapy (DiGiuseppe, Miller, & Trexler, 1979; Engels, Garnefski, & Diekstra, 1993; Haaga & Davison, 1993; Hajzler & Bernard, 1991; Jorn, 1989; Lyons & Woods, 1991; McGovern & Silverman, 1984; Silverman et al., 1992).

Applications of REBT to special kinds of clients have also been shown to be effective. It has yielded particularly good results with individuals who have anger disorders (Ellis, 2003a), with religious clients (Nielsen, Johnson, & Ellis, 2001), and with schoolchildren (Seligman, Revich, Jaycox, & Gillham, 1995).

In addition, hundreds of other outcome studies done by cognitive therapists—particularly by Aaron Beck (Alford & Beck, 1997) and his associates—also support the clinical hypothesis of REBT. Finally, more than 1,000 other investigations have shown that the irrationality scales derived from Ellis's original list of irrational beliefs significantly correlate with the diagnostic disorders with which these scales have been tested (Hollon & Beck, 1994; Woods, 1992). Although much has yet to be learned about the effectiveness of REBT and other cognitive-behavior therapies, the research results that exist are impressive.

Specific Studies

Many researchers have tested the main hypotheses of REBT, and the majority of their findings support central REBT contentions (Hajzler & Bernard, 1991; Lyons & Woods, 1991; McGovern & Silverman, 1984; Silverman et al., 1992). These research studies show that (1) clients tend to receive more effective help from a highly active-directive approach than from a more passive one; (2) efficient therapy includes activity-oriented homework assignments; (3) people largely choose to disturb themselves and can choose to surrender these disturbances; (4) helping clients modify their beliefs helps them to make significant behavioral changes; and (5) many effective methods of cognitive therapy exist, including modeling, role playing, skill training, and problem solving.

REBT in conjunction with medication is more effective than medication alone in certain conditions. This has been shown for conditions such as major depression (Macaskill & Macaskill, 1996) and dysthymic disorder (Wang, Jia, Fang, Zhu & Huang, 1999). REBT has been shown to be an effective adjunct with inpatients with schizophrenia (Shelley, Battaglia, Lucely, Ellis, & Opler, 2001), and it has also been shown superior to control conditions in the treatment of obsessive–compulsive disorder, social phobia, and social anxiety (Dryden & David, 2008).

Because REBT was the first of the cognitive-behavioral psychotherapies (CBTs), all of which incorporate aspects of REBT, the research programs of CBT—especially those of Aaron T. Beck's CT—serve to also support the efficacy of REBT's clinical applications. A comprehensive survey of meta-analyses that offer empirical validation for CBT in different clinical applications is found in Butler, Chapman, Forman, and Beck (2005).

Although it was the forerunner of all current cognitive-behavioral psychotherapies, REBT still offers a unique theory of emotional disturbance, one that is not completely shared by the other CBT psychotherapies. The uniqueness of REBT's model stems first of all from its claim that emotional disturbance arises from the human propensity to turn "preferences" into "demands." REBT hypothesizes that human "musts" precede Beck's (1976) "automatic thoughts" (Ellis & Whiteley, 1979).

In addition, hundreds of clinical and research papers present empirical evidence supporting REBT's main theories of personality. Many of these studies are reviewed in Ellis and Whiteley (1979). These studies tend to substantiate the following hypotheses:

1. Human thinking and emotion do not constitute two disparate or different processes but instead significantly overlap.

2. Although activating events or adversities (A) significantly contribute to emotional and behavioral consequences (C), people's beliefs (B) about A more importantly and more directly cause C.

3. The kinds of things people say to themselves, as well as the form in which they say these things, affect their emotions and behavior and often disturb them.

4. Humans not only think and think about their thinking but also think about thinking about their thinking. Whenever they have disturbances at C (consequence) after something unfortunate has happened in their lives at A (adversity), they tend to make C into a new A—to perceive and think about their emotional disturbances and thereby often create new ones.

5. People think about what happens to them not only in words, phrases, and sentences but also via images, fantasies, and dreams. Nonverbal cognitions contribute to their emotions and behaviors and can be used to change such behaviors.

6. Just as cognitions contribute to emotions and actions, emotions also contribute to or cause cognitions and actions, and actions contribute to or cause cognitions and emotions. When people change one of these three modalities of behaving, they concomitantly tend to change the other two (Ellis, 1994, 1998).

7. Uniquely among the schools of CBT, REBT uses a philosophical approach that attempts to promote an overall change in the client's belief system and philosophy of life, especially in regard to demandingness and nonacceptance (Ellis, 2005a; Ellis & Ellis, 2011), and to improve his or her functioning outside of psychotherapy (Ellis, 2004a). Furthermore, research has shown that REBT can be effectively done outside the therapeutic setting—for example, in public presentations—to the benefit of participating volunteers and their audience members (Ellis & Joffe, 2002). Various nonpsychotherapeutic applications of REBT have been summarized by Ellis and Blau (1998). Froh et al. (2007) documented that irrationality predicted lower levels of life satisfaction, but this relationship was at least partially mediated by interpersonal relations.

It is unfortunate that few substantial REBT studies have been conducted since the death of Ellis in 2007. Some articles document the efficacy of REBT, some describe REBT combined with CBT, a few blend it with the field of coaching, and Cohen (2007) incorporates concepts of positive psychology.

Several writers conclude that further exploration and future research is necessary. Advancing REBT as a theory and a practice will require new studies on (1) the basic REBT tenet that people largely disturb themselves by thinking in terms of absolutistic shoulds and musts; (2) specific studies addressing REBT used to treat anger, anxiety, depression, addiction and relationship issues; and (3) the relative effectiveness of core REBT procedures versus those of general CBT and other therapeutic systems.

Psychotherapy in a Multicultural World

It is important for all therapists to appreciate the multicultural aspects of psychotherapy because this is a vital issue (Sue & Sue, 2003). REBT has always taken a multicultural position and promotes flexibility and open-mindedness so that practitioners who use it can deal with clients who follow different family, religious, and cultural customs. This is because it practically never gets people to dispute or discard their cultural goals, values, and ideals but only their grandiose insistences that these goals *absolutely must* be achieved.

Suppose a client lives in an American city populated largely by middle-class white Protestant citizens, and she is a relatively poor, dark-skinned, Pakistani-born Muslim. She will naturally have some real differences with her neighbors and co-workers and may upset herself about these differences. Her REBT therapist would give her unconditional acceptance, even though the therapist was a member of the majority group in the client's region and viewed some of her views and leanings as "peculiar." Her cultural and religious values would be respected as being legitimate and good for her, in spite of her differences with her community's values.

This client would be supported in following her goals and purposes—as long as she was willing to accept the consequences of displeasing some of the townspeople by sticking to them. She could be shown, with REBT, how to refuse to put herself down if she suffered from community criticism, and her "peculiar" cultural and religious ways would be questioned only if they were so rigidly held that they interfered with her basic aims.

REBT Self-Help Form

A (ACTIVATING EVENTS OR ADVERSITIES)

- Briefly summarize the situation you are disturbed about (what would a camera see?)
- An A can be *internal* or *external*, *real* or *imagined*.
- An A can be an event in the *past*, *present*, or *future*.

IBs (IRRATIONAL BELIEFS)   D (DISPUTING IBs)

REBT Self-Help Form (*continued*)

To identify IBs, look for

- Dogmatic Demands
  (musts, absolutes, shoulds)
- Awfulizing
  (It's awful, terrible, horrible)
- Low Frustration Tolerance
  (I can't stand it)
- Self/Other Rating
  (I'm/he is/she is bad, worthless)

To dispute, ask yourself:

- Where is holding this belief getting me? Is it *helpful* or *self-defeating?*
- Where is the evidence to support the existence of my irrational belief? Is it *consistent with social reality?*
- Is my belief *logical?* Does it follow from my preferences?
- Is it really *awful* (as bad as it could be)?
- Can I really not *stand* it?

C (CONSEQUENCES)

Major unhealthy negative **emotions:**

Major self-defeating **behaviors:**

Unhealthy negative emotions include

- Anxiety
- Depression
- Rage
- Low Frustration Tolerance
- Shame/Embarrassment
- Hurt
- Jealousy
- Guilt

E (EFFECTIVE NEW PHILOSOPHIES)

E (EFFECTIVE EMOTIONS & BEHAVIORS)

New healthy
negative emotions:

New constructive
behaviors:

To think more rationally, strive for:

- Nondogmatic Preferences
  (wishes, wants, desires)
- Evaluating Badness
  (it's bad, unfortunate)
- High Frustration Tolerance
  (I don't like it, but I can stand it)
- Not Globally Rating Self or Others
  (I—and others—are fallible human beings)

Healthy negative emotions include:

- Disappointment
- Concern
- Annoyance
- Sadness
- Regret
- Frustration

Thus, if she flouted the social-sexual mores of her own religion and culture and concluded that she was worthless for not following them perfectly, she would be shown that it was her rigid demand that she *absolutely must* inflexibly adhere to them that was leading to her feelings of worthlessness and depression. If she changed her *must* to a *preference,* she could choose to follow or not to follow these cultural rules and not feel worthless and depressed.

REBT, then, has three main principles relevant to cross-cultural psychotherapy:

1. Clients can unconditionally accept themselves and other individuals and can achieve high frustration tolerance when faced with life adversities.

2. If the therapist follows these rules and encourages her or his clients to follow them and to lead a flexible life, multicultural problems may sometimes exist but can be resolved with minimum intercultural and intracultural prejudice.

3. Most multicultural issues involve bias and intolerance, which REBT particularly works against (see *The Road to Tolerance*, Ellis, 2004b).

Client Problems

No matter what the presenting problem may be, REBT therapists first help clients to express their disturbed emotional and behavioral reactions to their practical difficulties and to see and tackle the basic ideas or philosophies that underlie these reactions. This is apparent in the course of workshops for executives. In these workshops, the executives constantly bring up business, management, organizational, personal, and other problems. But they are shown that these practical problems often are tied to their self-defeating belief systems, and it is *this* problem that REBT mainly helps them resolve (Ellis, Gordon, Neenan, & Palmer, 1998).

Some individuals, however, may be so inhibited or defensive that they do not permit themselves to feel and therefore may not even be aware of some of their underlying emotional problems. Thus, the successful executive who comes for psychological help only because his wife insists they have a poor relationship and who claims that nothing really bothers him other than his wife's complaints may have to be jolted out of his complacency by direct confrontation. REBT group therapy may be particularly helpful for such an individual so that he finally expresses underlying anxieties and resentments and begins to acknowledge that he has emotional problems.

Extreme emotionalism in the course of REBT sessions—such as crying, psychotic behavior, and violent expressions of suicidal or homicidal intent—are naturally difficult to handle. But therapists handle these problems by their own, presumably rational philosophy of life and therapy, which includes these ideas: (1) Client outbursts make things difficult, but they are hardly *awful, terrible,* or *catastrophic.* (2) Behind each outburst is some irrational idea. Now, what is this idea? How can it be brought to the client's attention, and what can be done to help change it? (3) No therapist can possibly help every client all the time. If this particular client cannot be helped and has to be referred elsewhere or lost to therapy, this is unfortunate. But it does not mean that the therapist is a failure.

REBT therapists usually handle clients' profound depressions by showing them, as quickly, directly, and vigorously as possible, that they are probably creating or exacerbating their depression by (1) blaming themselves for what they have done or not done, (2) castigating themselves for being depressed and inert, and (3) bemoaning their fate because of the hassles and harshness of environmental conditions. Their self-condemnation is not only revealed but also firmly disputed, and in the meantime, the therapist may give clients reassurance and support, refer them for supplementary medication, speak to their relatives or friends to enlist their aid, and recommend temporary withdrawal from some activities. Through an immediate and direct disputing of clients' extreme self-deprecation and self-pity, the therapist often helps deeply depressed and suicidal people in a short period.

The most difficult clients are usually the chronic avoiders or shirkers who keep looking for magical solutions. These individuals are shown that no such magic exists; that if they do not want to work hard to get better, it is their privilege to keep suffering; and that they are not *terrible persons* for goofing off but could live much more enjoyably if they worked at helping themselves. To help them get going, a form of people-involved therapy, such as group therapy, is frequently a method of choice. Results with unresponsive clients are still relatively poor in REBT (and in virtually all other therapies), but persistence and vigor on the part of the therapist often eventually overcome this kind of resistance (Ellis, 1994, 2002; Ellis & Tafrate, 1998).

CASE EXAMPLE

This section is relatively brief because it concerns the 25-year-old computer programmer whose initial session was presented in this chapter (pp. 169–175). Other case material on this client follows.

Background

Sara came from an Orthodox Jewish family. Her mother died in childbirth when Sara was 2 years of age, so Sara was raised by a loving but strict and somewhat remote father and a dominating paternal grandmother. She did well in school but had few friends up to and through college. Although fairly attractive, she was always ashamed of her body, did little dating, and occupied herself mainly with her work. At age 25, she was head of a section in a data-processing firm. She was highly sexual and masturbated several times a week, but she had had intercourse with a man only once, when she was too drunk to know what she was doing. She had been overeating and overdrinking steadily since her college days. She had had 3 years of classical psychoanalysis. She thought her analyst was "a very kind and helpful man," but she had not really been helped by the process. She was quite disillusioned about therapy as a result of this experience and returned to it only because the president of her company, who liked her a great deal, told her that he would no longer put up with her constant drinking and insisted that she come to see Albert Ellis, the co-author of this chapter.

Treatment

Treatment continued for six sessions along the same lines indicated in the transcript previously in this chapter. This was followed by 24 weeks of REBT group therapy and a weekend-long rational encounter marathon.

Cognitively, the client was shown repeatedly that her central problem was that she devoutly believed she *had* to be almost perfect and that she *must not* be criticized in any major way by significant others. She was persistently shown, instead, how to refrain from rating her *self* but only to measure her *performances;* to see that she could never be, except by arbitrary definition, a "worm" even if she never succeeded in overcoming her overeating, compulsive drinking, and foolish symptoms; to see that it was highly desirable but not necessary that she relate intimately to a man and win the approval of her peers and her bosses at work; and first to accept herself *with* her hostility and then to give up her childish *demands* on others that led her to be so hostile to them. Although she devoutly believed in the "fact" that she and others *should* be extremely efficient and follow strict disciplinary rules, and although time and again she resisted the therapist's and the group members' assaults against her moralistic *shoulds,* she was finally induced to replace them, in her vocabulary as well as in her internalized beliefs, with *it would be betters.* She claimed to have completely overthrown her original religious orthodoxy, but she was shown that she had merely replaced it with an inordinate demand for certainty in her personal life and in world affairs, and she was finally induced to give this up, too (Ellis, 2003b).

Emotively, Sara was fully accepted by the therapist *as a person,* even though he strongly assailed many of her *ideas* and sometimes humorously reduced them to absurdity. She was assertively confronted by some of the group members, who helped her see how she was angrily condemning other group members for their stupidities and their shirking, and she was encouraged to accept these "bad" group members (as well as people outside the group) in spite of their inadequacies. The therapist and some of the others in her group and in the marathon weekend of rational encounter in which she participated used vigorous, down-to-earth language with her. This initially horrified Sara, but she later began to loosen up and use similar language. When she went on a drinking bout for a few weeks and felt utterly depressed and hopeless, two group members brought out their own previous difficulties with alcohol and drugs and showed how they had managed to get through that almost impossible period in their lives. Another member gave her steady support through many phone calls and visits. At times when she clammed up and sulked, the therapist and other group members pushed her to open up and voice her real feelings. Then they went after her defenses, revealed her foolish ideas (especially the idea that she had to be terribly hurt if others rejected her), and showed how these could be uprooted. During the marathon, she was able, for the first time in her life, to let herself be really touched emotionally by a man who, up to that time, was a perfect stranger to her, and this showed her that she could afford to let down her long-held barriers to intimacy and allow herself to love.

Behaviorally, Sara was given homework assignments that included talking to attractive men in public places and thereby overcoming her fears of being rejected. She was shown how to stay on a long-term diet (which she had never done before) by allowing herself rewarding experiences (such as listening to classical music) only when she had first maintained her diet for a certain number of hours. Through role playing with the therapist and other group members, she was given training in being assertive with people at work and in her social life without being aggressive (Ellis, 2003a).

Resolution

Sara progressed in several ways: (1) She stopped drinking completely, lost 25 pounds, and appeared to be maintaining both her sobriety and her weight loss; (2) she became considerably less condemnatory of both herself and others and began to make some close friends; (3) she had satisfactory sexual relations with three different men and began to date one of them steadily; and (4) she only rarely made herself guilty or depressed, accepted herself with her failings, and began to focus much more on enjoying herself than on rating herself.

Follow-Up

Sara had REBT individual and group sessions for 6 months and occasional follow-up sessions the next year. She married her steady boyfriend about a year after she had originally begun treatment, after having two premarital counseling sessions with him following their engagement. Two and a half years after the close of therapy, she and her husband reported that everything was going well in their marriage, at her job, and in their social life. Her husband seemed particularly appreciative of the use she was making of REBT principles and noted, "she still works hard at what she learned with you and the group and, frankly, I think that she keeps improving, because of this work, all the time." She smilingly and enthusiastically agreed.

SUMMARY

Rational emotive behavior therapy (REBT) is a comprehensive system of personality change that incorporates cognitive, emotive, and behavior therapy methods. It is based on a clear-cut theory of emotional health and disturbance, and the many techniques it employs are usually related to that theory. Its major hypotheses also apply to child rearing, education, social and political affairs, the extension of people's intellectual and emotional frontiers, and support of their unique potential for growth. REBT psychology is vigorous, empirically oriented, rational, and nonmagical. It fosters the use of reason, science, and technology. It is humanistic, existentialist, and hedonistic. It aims for reduced emotional disturbance as well as increased growth and self-actualization in people's intrapersonal and interpersonal lives.

REBT theory holds that people are biologically and culturally predisposed to choose, create, and enjoy but are also strongly predisposed to overconform, be suggestible, hate, and foolishly block their enjoying. Although they have remarkable capacities to observe, reason, imaginatively enhance their experiencing, and transcend some of their own essential limitations, they also have strong tendencies to ignore social reality, misuse reason, and invent absolutist *musts* that frequently sabotage their health and happiness. Because of their refusals to accept social reality, their continual *must*urbation, and their absorption in deifying and devilifying themselves and others, people frequently wind up with emotional disturbances.

When noxious stimuli occur in people's lives at point A (their adversities), they usually observe these events objectively and conclude, at point rB (their rational belief), that this event is unfortunate, inconvenient, and disadvantageous and that they wish it would change. Then they healthily feel at point C (the consequence) sad, regretful, frustrated, or annoyed. These healthy negative feelings usually help them to try to do something about their adversities to improve or change them. Their inborn and acquired hedonism and constructivism encourage them to have, in regard to adversities, rational thoughts ("I don't like this; let's see what I can do to change it") and healthy negative feelings (sorrow and annoyance) that enable them to reorder their environment and to live more enjoyably.

Very often, however, when similar adversities occur in people's lives, they observe these events intolerantly and grandiosely and conclude at point iB (their irrational beliefs), that these events are awful, horrible, and catastrophic; that they *must* not exist; and that they absolutely cannot stand them. They then self-defeatingly feel the consequence at point C of worthlessness, guilt, anxiety, depression, rage, and inertia. Their disturbed feelings usually interfere with their doing something constructive about the adversities, and they tend to condemn themselves for their unconstructiveness and to experience more feelings of shame, inferiority, and hopelessness. Their inborn and acquired self-critical, antihumanistic, and deifying and devilifying philosophies encourage them to have, in regard to unfortunate activating events, foolish thoughts ("How awful this is and I am! There's nothing I can do about it!") and dysfunctional feelings (hatred of themselves, of others, and of the world) that encourage them to whine and rant and live less enjoyably.

REBT is a cognitive-emotive-behavioristic method of psychotherapy uniquely designed to enable people to observe, understand, and persistently dispute their irrational, grandiose, perfectionistic *shoulds, oughts,* and *musts* and their *awfulizing.* It employs the logico-empirical method of science to encourage people to surrender magic, absolutes, and damnation; to acknowledge that nothing is sacred or all-important (although many things are exceptionally unpleasant and inconvenient); and to gradually teach themselves and to practice the philosophy of desiring rather than demanding and of working at changing what they can change and gracefully accepting what they cannot change about themselves, about others, and about the world (Ellis, 1994, 2002; 2005a; Ellis & Blau, 1998; Ellis & Ellis, 2011).

In conclusion, REBT is a holistic method of personality change that quickly and efficiently helps people resist their tendencies to be too conforming, suggestible, and anhedonic. It actively and didactically, as well as emotively and behaviorally, shows people how to abet and enhance one side of their humanness while simultaneously changing and living more happily with (and not repressing or squelching) another side. It is thus realistic and practical as well as idealistic and future oriented. It helps individuals more fully actualize, experience, and enjoy the here and now, but it also espouses long-range hedonism, which includes planning for their own (and others') future. It is what its name implies: rational *and* emotive *and* behavioral, realistic *and* visionary, empirical *and* humanistic—as, in all their complexity, are humans.

 Counseling CourseMate Website:

See this text's Counseling CourseMate website at www.cengagebrain.com for learning tools such as chapter quizzing, videos, glossary flashcards, and more.

ANNOTATED BIBLIOGRAPHY

Web Sites

Dr. Debbie Joffe Ellis: www.debbiejoffeellis.com

EllisREBT: www.ellisrebt.com

REBT Network, www.rebtnetwork.org

Books

Ellis, A. (1962). *Reason and emotion in psychotherapy.* Secaucus, NJ: Citadel.

The original seminal and groundbreaking book on rational emotive behavior therapy.

Ellis, A. (2004a). *Rational emotive behavior therapy—it works for me—it can work for you.* Amherst, NY: Prometheus Books.

This autobiographical book presents an excellent overview of the life and work of Albert Ellis.

Ellis, A. (2004b). *The road to tolerance: The philosophy of rational emotive behavior therapy.* Amherst, NY: Prometheus Books.

This book reviews the theoretical underpinnings of REBT and advocates tolerance for and patience with the all-too-common shortcomings of human beings.

Ellis, A. (2005a). *The myth of self-esteem.* New York: Prometheus Books.

The book provides an overview of Ellis's approach to life and psychotherapy and REBT's emphasis on unconditional acceptance, and it gives insight into the breadth of his intellect. Separate chapters deal with Jean-Paul Sartre, Martin Heidegger, Martin Buber, D. T. Suzuki, and Zen Buddhism.

Ellis, A. (2010). *All out! An autobiography.* Amherst, NY: Prometheus Books.

Albert Ellis's last work, this fascinating, candid, and substantial autobiography includes memorable episodes, descriptions of the important people in his life, the way he coped with difficulties, his developing of REBT, his love life, and personal reflections.

Ellis, A., & Dryden, W. (1997). *The practice of rational emotive behavior therapy.* New York: Springer.

This book presents the general theory and basic practice of rational emotive behavior therapy, with special chapters on how it is used in individual, couples, family, group, and sex therapy, and it gives many details about REBT therapy procedures.

Ellis, A., & Ellis, D. J. (2011). *Rational emotive behavior therapy.* Washington, DC: American Psychological Association.

This concise yet substantial book presents the main aspects of REBT in a clear and straightforward style; it is ideal for students, practitioners, and all others who are interested in knowing the essentials of the approach.

Ellis, A., & Harper, R. A. (1997). *A guide to rational living.* North Hollywood, CA: Wilshire Books.

This completely revised and rewritten version of the REBT self-help classic is one of the most widely read self-help books ever published, and it is often recommended by cognitive-behavior therapists to their clients. It is a succinct, straightforward approach to REBT based on self-questioning and homework and shows how readers can help themselves with various emotional problems.

CASE READINGS

Ellis, A. (1971). A twenty-three-year-old woman, guilty about not following her parents' rules. In A. Ellis, *Growth through reason: Verbatim cases in rational-emotive therapy* (pp. 223–286). Hollywood: Wilshire Books. [Reprinted in D. Wedding & R. J. Corsini (Eds.). (2013). *Case studies in psychotherapy.* Belmont, CA: Brooks/Cole.]

> Ellis presents a verbatim protocol of the first, second, and fourth sessions with a woman who comes for help because she is self-punishing, impulsive and compulsive, and afraid of males, has no goals in life, and is guilty about her relations with her parents. The therapist quickly zeroes in on her main problems and shows her that she need not feel guilty about doing what she wants to do in life, even if her parents keep upsetting themselves about her beliefs and actions.

Ellis, A. (1977). Verbatim psychotherapy session with a procrastinator. In A. Ellis & W. J. Knaus, *Overcoming procrastination* (pp. 152–167). New York: New American Library.

> Ellis presents a single verbatim session with a procrastinator who was failing to finish her doctoral thesis in sociology. He deals with her problems in a direct, no-nonsense manner typical of rational emotive behavior therapy, and she later reports that as a result of a single session, she finished her thesis, although she had previously been procrastinating on it for several years.

Ellis, A., & Dryden, W. (1996). Transcript of a demonstration session, with comments on the session by Windy Dryden and Albert Ellis. In W. Dryden, *Practical skills in rational emotive behavior therapy* (pp. 91–117). London: Whurr.

> Ellis presents a verbatim protocol with a therapist who volunteers to bring up problems of feeling inadequate as a therapist and as a person. Albert Ellis shows her some core beliefs leading to her self-downing and how to actively dispute and surrender these beliefs. Ellis and Windy Dryden then review the protocol to analyze its REBT aspects.

REFERENCES

Adler, A. (1931). *What life should mean to you.* New York: Blue Ribbon Books.

Adler, A. (1964). *Social interest: A challenge to mankind.* New York: Capricorn.

Alford, B. A., & Beck, A. T. (1997). *The integrative power of cognitive therapy.* New York: Guilford Press.

Beck, A. T. (1976). *Cognitive therapy and the emotional disorders.* New York: International Universities Press.

Bernard, M. E., Froh, J., DiGiuseppe, R., Joyce, M., & Dryden, W. (2010). Albert Ellis: Unsung hero of positive psychology. *Journal of Positive Psychology, 5* (4), 302–310.

Bernard, M. E., & Wolfe, J. W. (Eds.). (1993). *The RET resource book for practitioners.* New York: Institute for Rational-Emotive Therapy.

Bruce, K. (2012, April 17). World first centre to open in Whyalla. *Whyalla News*, . S. A., Australia.

Butler, A. C., Chapman, J. E., Forman, E. M., & Beck, A. T. (2005). The empirical status of cognitive-behavioral therapy: A review of meta-analyses. *Clinical Psychology Review, 26*(1), 17–31.

Cohen, E. (2007). *The new rational therapy: Thinking your way to serenity, success and profound happiness.* Lanham, MD: Rowman & Littlefield.

Corsini, R. J. (2005, January 5). The incredible Albert Ellis. [Review of the book *Rational emotive behavior therapy—It works for me—It can work for you.*] *PsycCRITIQUES: Contemporary Psychology—APA Review of Books, 50,* Article 2. Retrieved September 9, 2006, from the PsycCRITIQUES database.

DiGiuseppe, R. A., Miller, N. K., & Trexler, L. D. (1979). A review of rational-emotive psychotherapy outcome studies. In A. Ellis & J. M. Whiteley (Eds.), *Theoretical and empirical foundations of rational-emotive therapy* (pp. 218–235). Monterey, CA: Brooks/Cole.

DiGiuseppe, R. A., Terjesen, M., Rose, R., Doyle, K., & Vadalakis, N. (1998, August). *Selective abstractions errors in reviewing REBT outcome studies: A review of reviews.* Poster presented at the 106th Annual Convention of the American Psychological Association, San Francisco, CA.

Dryden, W., & David, D. (2008). Rational emotive behavior therapy: Current status. *Journal of Cognitive Psychotherapy: An International Quarterly, 22*(3), 195–209.

Eckstein, D. (2012). *The couple's match book: Techniques for lighting, rekindling, or extinguishing the flame.* Bloomington, IN: Trafford Publishing.

Eckstein, D., & Ellis, D. J. (2011). Up close and personal. *The Family Journal, 19*(4), 407–411.

Ellis, A. (1958). Rational Psychotherapy. *The Journal of General Psychology, 59*, 35–49.

Ellis, A. (1962). *Reason and emotion in psychotherapy.* Secaucus, NJ: Citadel.

Ellis, A. (1971). A twenty-three-year-old woman, guilty about not following her parents' rules. In A. Ellis, *Growth through reason: Verbatim cases in rational-emotive therapy* (pp. 223–286). Hollywood: Wilshire Books.

Ellis, A. (1976). The biological basis of human irrationality. *Journal of Individual Psychology, 32,* 145–168.

Ellis, A. (1977). Verbatim psychotherapy session with a procrastinator. In A. Ellis & W. J. Knaus, *Overcoming procrastination* (pp. 152–167). New York: New American Library.

Ellis, A. (1994). *Reason and emotion in psychotherapy* (rev. ed.). New York: Citadel.

Ellis, A. (1998). *How to control your anxiety before it controls you.* New York: Citadel.

Ellis, A. (1999). *How to make yourself happy and remarkably less disturbable.* San Luis Obispo, CA: Impact Publishers.

Ellis, A. (2001a). *Feeling better, getting better, staying better.* Atascadero, CA: Impact Publishers.

Ellis, A. (2001b). *Overcoming destructive beliefs, feelings, and behaviors.* Amherst, NY: Prometheus Books.

Ellis, A. (2002). *Overcoming resistance: A rational emotive behavior therapy integrative approach.* New York: Springer.

Ellis, A. (2003a). *Anger: How to live with it and without it* (rev. ed.). New York: Citadel Press.

Ellis, A. (2003b). *Sex without guilt in the twenty-first century.* Teaneck, NJ: Battleside Books.

Ellis, A. (2003c). Similarities and differences between rational emotive behavior therapy and cognitive therapy. *Journal of Cognitive Psychotherapy: An International Quarterly, 17* (3), 225–240.

Ellis, A. (2004a). *Rational emotive behavior therapy: It works for me, it can work for you.* Amherst, NY: Prometheus Books.

Ellis, A. (2004b). *The road to tolerance: The philosophy of rational emotive behavior therapy.* Amherst, NY: Prometheus Books.

Ellis, A. (2005a). *The myth of self-esteem.* Amherst, NY: Prometheus Books.

Ellis, A. (2005b). Discussion of Christine A. Padesky and Aaron T. Beck, "Science and philosophy: Comparison of cognitive Therapy and rational emotive behavior therapy." *Journal of Cognitive Psychotherapy: An International Quarterly, 19*(2), 181–189.

Ellis, A. (2010). *All out! An autobiography.* Amherst, NY: Prometheus Books.

Ellis, A., & Bernard, M. E. (Eds.). (2006). *Rational emotive behavioral approaches to childhood disorders: Theory, practice and research.* New York: Springer.

Ellis, A., & Blau, S. (Eds.). (1998). *The Albert Ellis reader.* Secaucus, NJ: Carol Publishing Group.

Ellis, A., & Crawford, T. (2000). *Making intimate connections.* Atascadero, CA: Impact Publishers.

Ellis, A., & Dryden, W. (1996). Transcript of demonstration session. Commentary on Albert Ellis' demonstration session by Windy Dryden and Albert Ellis. In W. Dryden, *Practical skills in rational emotive behavior therapy* (pp. 91–117). London: Whurr.

Ellis, A., & Dryden, W. (1997). *The practice of rational emotive behavior therapy.* New York: Springer.

Ellis, A., & Ellis, D. J. (2011). *Rational emotive behavior therapy.* Washington D.C.: American Psychological Association.

Ellis, A., Gordon, J., Neenan, M., & Palmer, S. (1998). *Stress counseling.* New York: Springer.

Ellis, A., & Harper, R. A. (1997). *A guide to rational living.* North Hollywood, CA: Melvin Powers.

Ellis, A., & Harper, R. A. (2003). *Dating, mating, and relating.* New York: Citadel.

Ellis, A., & Joffe, D. (2002). A study of volunteer clients who experience live sessions of rational emotive behavior therapy in front of a public audience. *Journal of Rational-Emotive and Cognitive-Behavior Therapy, 20,* 151–158.

Ellis, A., & MacLaren, C. (1998). *Rational emotive behavior therapy: A therapist's guide.* Atascadero, CA: Impact Publishers.

Ellis, A., & Tafrate, R. C. (1998). *How to control your anger before it controls you.* Secaucus, NJ: Birch Lane Press.

Ellis, A., & Whiteley, J. (1979). *Theoretical and empirical foundations of rational-emotive therapy.* Pacific Grove, CA: Brooks/Cole.

Ellis, D. J. (2010a). Albert Ellis, PhD: Master therapist, pioneer, humanist. *Psychological Hypnosis: American Psychological Association Bulletin of Division 30 (Society of Psychological Hypnosis), 19*(1), 7–12.

Ellis, D. J. (2010b). Theory, method, practice and Humor: Recipe for effective teaching of REBT as applied to people with co-occurring problems. *[Review of the book: REBT for people with co-occurring problems: Albert Ellis in the wilds of Arizona.]PsycCRITIQUES, 55(32).*

Engels, G. I., Garnefski, N., & Diekstra, R. F. W. (1993). Efficacy of rational-emotive therapy: A quantitative analysis. *Journal of Consulting & Clinical Psychology, 61,* 1083–1090.

Froh, J. J., Fives, C. K., Fuller, J. R., Jacofsky, M. D., Terjesen, M. D., & Yurkewicz, C. (2007). Interpersonal relationships and irrationality as predictors of life satisfaction. *Journal of Positive Psychology, 2*(1), 29–39.

Fuller, R. J., DiGiuseppe, R., O'Leary, S., Fountain, T., & Lang, C. (2010). An open trial of a comprehensive anger treatment program on an outpatient sample. *Behavioral and Cognitive Psychotherapy, 38*(4), 485–490.

Haaga, D. A. F., & Davison, G. C. (1993). An appraisal of rational-emotive therapy. *Journal of Consulting & Clinical Psychology, 61,* 215–220.

Hajzler, D., & Bernard, M. E. (1991). A review of rational emotive outcome studies. *School Psychology Studies, 6*(1), 27–49.

Hauck, P. A. (1992). *Overcoming the rating game: Beyond self-love—Beyond self-esteem.* Louisville, KY: Westminster/John Knox.

Hollon, S. D., & Beck, A. T. (1994). Cognitive and cognitive-behavioral therapies. In A. E. Bergin & S. L. Garfield (Eds.), *Handbook of psychotherapy and behavior change* (4th ed., pp. 428–466). New York: Wiley.

Jorn, A. F. (1989). Modifiability and neuroticism: A meta-analysis of the literature. *Australian and New Zealand Journal of Psychiatry, 23,* 21–29.

Lazarus, A. A. (1989). *The practice of multimodal therapy* . Baltimore, MD: The John Hopkins University Press.

Lyons, L. C., & Woods, P. J. (1991). The efficacy of rational-emotive therapy: A quantitative review of the outcome research. *Clinical Psychology Review, 11,* 357–369.

Macaskill, N. D., & Macaskill, A. (1996). Rational-emotive therapy plus pharmacotherapy versus pharmacotherapy alone in the treatment of high cognitive dysfunction depression. *Cognitive Therapy and Research, 20,* 575–592.

McCracken, J., Lindner, H., & Schiacchitano, L. (2008). The mediating role of secondary beliefs: Enhancing the understanding of emotional responses and illness perceptions in arthritis. *Journal of Allied Health, 37*(1), 30–37.

McGovern, T. E., & Silverman, M. S. (1984). A review of outcome studies of rational-emotive therapy from 1977 to 1982. *Journal of Rational-Emotive Therapy, 2*(1), 7–18.

Nielsen, S., Johnson, W. B., & Ellis, A. (2001). *Counseling and psychotherapy with religious persons.* Mahwah, NJ: Erlbaum.

Padesky, C. A., & Beck, A. T. (2003). Science and philosophy: Comparison of cognitive therapy and rational emotive behavior therapy. *Journal of Cognitive Psychotherapy: An International Quarterly, 17* (3), 211–224.

Padesky, C. A., & Beck, A. T. (2005). Response to Ellis' discussion of "Science and philosophy: Comparison of cognitive therapy and rational emotive behavior therapy." *Journal of Cognitive Psychotherapy: An International Quarterly*, 19(2), 187–189.

Ramirez, A. (2006. December 10). Despite illness and lawsuits, a famed psychotherapist is temporarily back in session. *The New York Times*, p. 52.

Rogers, C. R. (1961). *On becoming a person.* Boston: Houghton Mifflin.

Seligman, M. E. P., Revich, K., Jaycox, L., & Gillham, J. (1995). *The optimistic child.* Boston: Houghton Mifflin.

Shelley, A. M., Battaglia, J., Lucely, J., Ellis, A., & Opler, A. (2001). Symptom-specific group therapy for inpatients with schizophrenia. *Einstein Quarterly Journal of Biology and Medicine, 18,* 21–28.

Silverman, M. S., McCarthy, M., & McGovern, T. (1992). A review of outcome studies of rational-emotive therapy from 1982–1989. *Journal of Rational-Emotive and Cognitive-Behavior Therapy, 10*(3), 111–186.

Sue, D. W., & Sue, D. (2003). *Counseling with the culturally diverse.* New York: Wiley.

Velten, E., & Penn, P. E. (2010). *REBT for people with co-occurring problems: Albert Ellis in the wilds of Arizona.* Sarasota, FL: Professional Resource Press.

Vernon, A. (2001). *The passport program* (Vols. 1–3). Champaign, IL: Research Press.

Walen, S. R., DiGiuseppe, R., & Dryden, W. (1992). *A practitioner's guide to rational-emotive therapy* (2nd ed.). New York: Oxford.

Wang, C., Jia, F., Fang, R., Zhu, Y., & Huang, Y. (1999). Comparative study of rational-emotive therapy for 95 patients with dysthymic disorder. *Chinese Mental Health Journal, 13,* 172–183.

Woods, P. J. (1992). A study of belief and non-belief items from the Jones Irrational Beliefs Test with implications for the theory of RET. *Journal of Rational-Emotive and Cognitive-Behavior Therapy, 10,* 41–52.

Young, H. S. (1974). *A rational counseling primer.* New York: Albert Ellis Institute.

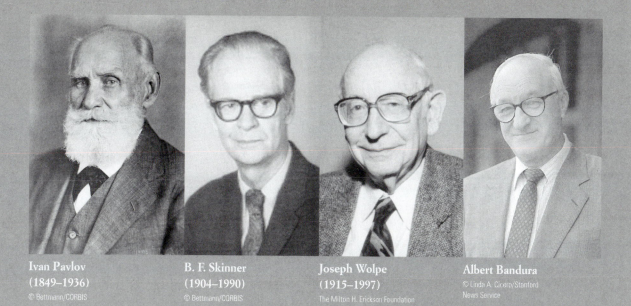

Ivan Pavlov
(1849–1936)
© Bettmann/CORBIS

B. F. Skinner
(1904–1990)
© Bettmann/CORBIS

Joseph Wolpe
(1915–1997)
The Milton H. Erickson Foundation

Albert Bandura
© Linda A. Cicero/Stanford
News Service

6 | BEHAVIOR THERAPY

Martin M. Antony

OVERVIEW

Basic Concepts

Since its beginnings in the mid-20th century, the scope of behavior therapy has evolved and expanded. Today, behavior therapy encompasses a wide range of strategies from progressive muscle relaxation to exposure therapy to mindfulness meditation. Behavior therapy aims to change factors in the environment that influence an individual's behavior as well as the ways in which individuals respond to their environment. Behavior therapists define the term *behavior* broadly to include motor behaviors, physiological responses, emotions, and cognitions. In fact, most practicing behavior therapists today refer to their work as *cognitive-behavior therapy* (CBT), and they use a blend of both traditional behavioral methods as well as cognitive methods, such as those described elsewhere in this book (see Chapter 5, Rational Emotive Behavior Therapy, and Chapter 7, Cognitive Therapy). Not only are behavior therapy strategies diverse, but also so are the therapists who use them. There is debate among behavioral practitioners regarding which strategies are most useful for which problems, and therapists often favor some strategies over others.

Despite the diversity among behavioral approaches, several features characterize behavior therapy in all of its forms (Antony & Roemer, 2011):

- *Behavior therapy focuses on changing behavior.* Behavior therapy aims to decrease the frequency of maladaptive behaviors, and increase the frequency of adaptive or helpful behaviors. Ultimately, the goal is to increase flexibility in the client's behavioral reper-toire so that the individual has a wider range of response options in any given situation.

- *Behavior therapy is rooted in empiricism.* Behavior therapists adopt a scientific, hypothesis-driven approach in their work. They speculate about the variables that contribute to a problem behavior, and they test out their assumptions through a range of behavioral-assessment methods. They collect data throughout treatment and revise their hypotheses as appropriate. They use evidence-based methods to evaluate the effects of their interventions throughout treatment.

- *Behaviors are assumed to have a function.* In behavior therapy, all behaviors "make sense" in the contexts in which they occur. Behaviors are believed to result, in part, from patterns of reinforcement and punishment from the environment. For exam-ple, a child who receives attention for problem behaviors (e.g., crying when having to go to school) but not for positive behaviors (leaving for school without making a scene) may increase the frequency of the problem behavior as a way of getting more attention. For the most part, behavioral problems are not seen as rooted in the indi-vidual; rather, they are seen as rooted in the environment or in the ways in which the individual and the environment interact. Because behavior therapists view problem behaviors as understandable given their context, clients are not blamed for their behaviors or their problems.

- *Behavior therapy emphasizes maintaining factors rather than factors that may have ini-tially triggered a problem.* Behavior therapy is not concerned with helping a client to identify and understand the early developmental events that may have set the stage for a problem. Instead, treatment focuses on changing the current determinants of behavior, which may include contingencies in the environment, as well as maladaptive learned behaviors (e.g., avoidance of feared situations, biased thinking, tantrums).

- *Behavior therapy is supported by research.* Behavior therapy (including CBT) is the most extensively researched form of psychotherapy, with hundreds of studies sup-porting its effectiveness for a wide range of problems, including anxiety disorders, depression, eating disorders, schizophrenia, addiction, behavioral disorders in chil-dren, and many others (Sturmey & Hersen, 2012).

- *Behavior therapy is active.* In behavior therapy, the therapist provides frequent ad-vice and suggestions (in other words, behavior therapy is a *directive* approach). The client is also actively engaged during the course of treatment, practicing behavioral strategies both within the session and between sessions for homework. For exam-ple, a client may practice relaxation exercises on a daily basis to reduce generalized anxiety and worry, or she or he may practice encountering enclosed places repeat-edly until fear decreases in order to overcome claustrophobia.

- *Behavior therapy is transparent.* A goal in behavior therapy is for clients to learn the skills necessary to eventually become their own therapists. Therefore, they are provided with a behavioral model by which to understand their problems, a de-tailed rationale for each strategy, and step-by-step instructions on how to use the behavioral techniques. Data collected during the course of behavioral assessment are readily shared with the client. The client is an active partner in the therapy pro-cess, including setting treatment goals and setting the agenda for each session.

Other Systems

Behavior therapy closely aligned with several other psychotherapies, particularly those that are directive and brief, such as cognitive therapy and rational emotive behavior therapy. In fact, practitioners in all three of these modalities often refer to themselves as *cognitive-behavioral therapists* and use strategies borrowed from all of these approaches, including traditional behavioral strategies (e.g., exposure to feared situations) and techniques initially developed by cognitively oriented therapists (examining and changing negative thinking patterns). Although the earliest forms of behavior therapy paid less attention to unobservable responses such as thoughts and emotions, many contemporary behavior therapists believe that one's thoughts play an important role in how the individual responds to the environment. Like behavior therapy, cognitive therapy and rational emotive behavior therapy are time limited, directive, transparent, evidence based, and active, and they focus on changing the factors thought to maintain psychological problems instead of working to understand factors that may have initially triggered a problem in the past.

At the other extreme, behavior therapy is perhaps most different from psychoanalysis (and other related *psychodynamic* approaches such as analytical psychotherapy). Psychoanalysis assumes that observable behavioral symptoms are a manifestation of unconscious conflicts and motivations, whereas behavior therapy takes behaviors at face value, for the most part. That's not to say that individuals are always conscious of why they behave the way they do. There is considerable evidence that humans process much information outside of their awareness, and behavior therapists accept that we are not always conscious of our motivations and assumptions. Nevertheless, behavior therapists do not accept many of the views about the unconscious that are held by those who practice psychoanalysis (e.g., the role of psychosexual conflicts, defense mechanisms, transference, and the idea that symbolism in dreams matters or can be validly interpreted by a therapist).

Compared to behavior therapy, psychoanalysis tends to be nondirective, less transparent, less evidence based, more reliant on interpretation by the therapist, and more focused on developing insight into early developmental contributors to a problem rather than its current maintaining factors. Unlike behavior therapists, psychoanalysts also assume that to deliver good psychotherapy, therapists must also have undergone their own psychoanalysis. In contrast, behavior therapists do not assume that undergoing one's own behavior therapy necessarily leads to better outcomes. Compared to behavior therapy, traditional psychoanalysis can be a much more expensive treatment, often occurring over many years (sometimes with several sessions per week), although short-term psychoanalytically oriented psychotherapies are also in wide use, especially in recent years.

Finally, psychoanalytic theory cannot explain the results of behavior therapy, which often contradict the principles of psychoanalysis. For example, psychoanalytic theory predicts that treatments focusing on changing symptoms (for example, exposure therapy for a phobia) will ultimately be ineffective because they target the surface manifestations and not the root cause of the problem. Psychoanalysts talk about *symptom substitution*, which refers to the underlying problem showing up in some other form when a surface symptom is treated. However, there is no evidence supporting the notion of symptom substitution. If anything, behavioral treatments lead to improvements in areas of functioning that were not directly targeted through the process of *generalization*, which is discussed later in this chapter.

Client-centered psychotherapy also differs from behavior therapy in that it is nondirective and does not include homework practices between sessions. Although behavior therapists traditionally paid little attention to the therapeutic relationship relative to therapists from other modalities, several of the concepts seen as critical in client-centered therapy (e.g., including having a therapist who is supportive, warm, trustworthy, and congruent) are now known to be important in all psychotherapies, including behavior therapy.

Behavior therapy shares features with several other psychotherapies. Like CBT, Adlerian psychotherapy emphasizes the importance of changing one's beliefs, particularly those that minimize one's self-worth, and it also uses several action-oriented techniques (e.g., task setting) that may overlap with some behavioral strategies. Adlerian therapy and behavior therapy also share the view that abnormal behavior is best construed in terms of "problems in living" rather than as evidence of illness. From a behavioral perspective, abnormal or maladaptive behaviors develop through the same methods as normative or adaptive behaviors.

Gestalt therapy uses some behavioral strategies as well, including role plays and strategies in which clients experience their emotions and feelings rather than try to control them. Like behavior therapy, interpersonal psychotherapy is a brief psychotherapy, is highly structured, and includes some behavioral strategies (e.g., social-skills training). Family therapies may also overlap with behavioral treatments; in fact, behavior therapy can be administered in a family context (typically referred to as *behavioral family therapy*).

HISTORY

Precursors

One of the earliest documented descriptions of the use of behavioral treatment involved a Roman scholar named Pliny the Elder, who lived more than 2,000 years ago. Pliny reportedly used spiders, strategically placed at the bottom of a drinker's glass, to treat alcoholism—a strategy that might now be referred to as *aversion therapy* (Franks, 1963). Another early account of a behavioral intervention involved the treatment of Victor of Aveyron (also known as the Wild Boy of Aveyron), who grew up in the 18th century without human contact until the age of 12. Victor was treated by Jean-Marc-Gaspard Itard (1962) using strategies that resemble what might now be referred to as *modeling*, *shaping*, and *reinforcement*.

Although these early writings show that behavioral strategies had been used in the distant past, there is no evidence that these early documented cases had any influence on the more recent development of behavior therapy in the 1950s. Rather, the roots of behavior therapy can be traced back to several events in the early to mid-1900s. The first of these is the launch of experimental research on the processes underlying learning, starting with Russian physiologist Ivan Pavlov's *classical conditioning* experiments in the early 1900s (Pavlov, 1927). Classical conditioning involves pairing two stimuli so that a neutral stimulus (e.g., a light or bell) comes to signal the occurrence of a second stimulus that is not neutral (e.g., food or shock). Pavlov was the first to demonstrate the process of classical conditioning when he showed that dogs could be taught to salivate in response to a previously neutral light or tone through the repeated pairing of the stimulus with food (Pavlov, 1927).

A second factor that set the stage for the development of behavior therapy was the rise of behaviorism in the United States, beginning with the work of John B. Watson, who first studied the process of classical conditioning in humans. In 1920, Watson and Rayner conducted their now classic experiment in which an infant named Albert learned to fear a white rat after the presence of the rat was paired with a loud noise (Watson & Rayner, 1920). Watson, who is often credited as the founder of *behaviorism*, believed that only observable behaviors should be the focus of psychology, and he rejected the notion that unobservable experiences such as emotions and thoughts be studied (Watson, 1913).

Several contemporary behavioral strategies were first described in the 1920s and 1930s as a direct result of early research on classical conditioning. For example, Mary Cover Jones (a student of John Watson) used a combination of *modeling* and *exposure* to treat a young boy who feared rabbits (Jones, 1924). Specifically, she had the child observe other children playing with rabbits and encouraged the boy to gradually approach and touch rabbits until he was no longer afraid. Similarly, Mowrer and Mowrer (1938) used classical conditioning principles to treat childhood bed-wetting. Their treatment involved placing a moisture-sensitive pad under the child's sheets and connecting the pad to a bell that rang every time the child urinated in bed. This treatment, known as the *bell and pad*, remains the most effective method for treating bed-wetting in children.

In addition to research on classical conditioning, another important contributor to the growth of behavior therapy involved research on *operant conditioning* (also known as *instrumental conditioning*), which is most frequently attributed to Edward Thorndike (1911) and later B. F. Skinner (1938). The principle of operant conditioning assumes that behavior is ultimately controlled by contingencies in the environment. Specifically, positive consequences (or *reinforcement*) increase the frequency of a given behavior, whereas negative consequences (or *punishment*) decrease the frequency of the behavior. These principles had direct implications for treating problem behavior. By changing patterns of reinforcement and punishment in an individual's environment, it became possible to change the individual's behavior. In fact, it was Skinner and colleagues who first used the term *behavior therapy* in an unpublished hospital report to refer to their use of operant-conditioning principles in the treatment of inpatients suffering from psychosis (Lindsley, Skinner, & Solomon, 1953).

A third factor that provided a context for the expansion of behavior therapy was the 1949 Boulder Conference on Graduate Education in Clinical Psychology, after which the field of psychology began to embrace a new *scientist-practitioner* model of training, emphasizing the importance of training psychologists to be both scientists and practitioners (Benjamin & Baker, 2000). As a result, many psychologists began to abandon psychoanalysis (the most influential psychotherapy at the time) in favor of approaches that could be more easily subjected to rigorous scientific study such as behavior therapy.

Beginnings

Behavior therapy emerged in the 1950s as research groups in South Africa, the United Kingdom, the United States, and Canada began to apply learning principles to behavioral problems (for accounts of the early days of behavior therapy, see Franks, 2001; Lazarus, 2001). In South Africa and the United Kingdom, the development of behavior therapy was mostly influenced by experimental research in the area of classical conditioning, whereas the roots of behavior therapy in North America grew out of operant-conditioning theory and research.

Joseph Wolpe, a physician in South Africa, first studied classical conditioning and learning theory as a medical student under the supervision of psychologists Leo Reyna, James Taylor, and Cynthia Adelstein. Inspired by his work in the area, Wolpe developed a form of treatment known as *systematic desensitization*, one of the earliest forms of exposure therapy to be formally researched. Systematic desensitization involves gradually confronting feared situations in imagination while simultaneously practicing progressive relaxation to relax the muscles of the body. Wolpe believed that by pairing feelings of relaxation with mental images of a feared situation that a client's fear would decrease because it is impossible to be both relaxed and frightened. Wolpe called the process underlying his treatment *reciprocal inhibition* (Wolpe, 1958). Although there is evidence supporting systematic desensitization, it is rarely recommended today. Instead, contemporary exposure-based treatments use exposure in real life (rather than exposure in imagination), and exposure is rarely paired with relaxation exercises because relaxation does not seem to add to the effectiveness of exposure (see Moscovitch, Antony, & Swinson, 2009).

Wolpe worked at the University of Witwatersrand in Johannesburg from the late 1940s until 1960. He then moved to the University of Virginia School of Medicine and then to Temple University in 1965. Throughout the 1950s, Wolpe trained his team (including psychologists Arnold Lazarus and Stanley Rachman, who themselves went on to make important contributions to the field of behavior therapy) to administer what they then referred to as *conditioning therapy* (Lazarus, 2001). It was Lazarus who first suggested in a 1957 team meeting to change the name of their approach from *conditioning therapy* to *behavior therapy*. Lazarus (1958) was also the first person to use the terms *behavior therapy* and *behavior therapist* in a published journal article (not realizing that Skinner has used the term in an unpublished report five years earlier). While at Temple University (in 1970), Wolpe launched the *Journal of Behavior Therapy and Experimental Psychiatry* with his mentor, Leo Reyna.

Meanwhile in the United Kingdom, German-born psychologist Hans Eysenck and his students studied behavioral treatments at the Institute of Psychiatry (Maudsley Hospital) in London. Behavior therapy was one of several domains in which Eysenck had an impact; he is also well known for his contributions to the field of personality theory. Eysenck founded the first behavior therapy journal in 1963, *Behaviour Research and Therapy*, and helped to popularize the term behavior therapy through his writings in the 1960s. Eysenck's students also made important contributions to the field of behavior therapy for years to come. For example, Stanley Rachman (who Eysenck recruited from Wolpe's group in South Africa) developed effective behavioral treatments for agoraphobia, obsessive–compulsive disorder (OCD), and several other anxiety-based problems, both in the United Kingdom and at the University of British Columbia in Canada. Cyril Franks, another one of Eysenck's students, moved to the United States in 1957, where he founded the Association for the Advancement of the Behavioral Therapies (AABT) in 1966, serving both as founding president and as the first editor of AABT's journal, *Behavior Therapy*. In 1967, AABT changed its name to the Association for Advancement of Behavior Therapy, and in 2005 the name was changed to the Association for Behavioral and Cognitive Therapies (ABCT) to reflect the evolution of behavior therapy to encompass cognitive approaches.

In North America, behavior therapy's roots were most closely associated with Skinner's work in the area of operant conditioning. Nathan Azrin (a student of Skinner) was one of the first people to develop treatments based on operant-conditioning principles. He helped establish the field of *applied behavior analysis*, developed reinforcement-based programs for treating substance-use disorders, and developed behavioral treatments for reversing unwanted habits. In collaboration with Teodoro Ayllon, a psychologist at the Saskatchewan Hospital in Canada, Azrin also developed a method known as *token economy* in which behavioral problems were managed through reinforcement of desirable behaviors by providing tokens that could later be exchanged for rewards (Ayllon & Azrin, 1968). Token economy became a popular method for managing disruptive behavior among psychiatric inpatients, especially before the widespread availability of effective psychotropic medications.

Current Status

The boundaries of behavior therapy began to expand with the introduction of cognitive techniques when Albert Ellis first started practicing what he called *rational psychotherapy* in 1955 (renamed *rational emotive therapy* in 1962 and then *rational emotive behavior therapy* in 1993; Ellis, 2001). Aaron Beck (the founder of *cognitive therapy*) and others (e.g., Donald Meichenbaum, Marvin Goldfried, Gerald Davison, Michael Mahoney) further developed effective strategies for changing negative thinking, contributing to the popularity of emerging cognitive approaches (Lazarus, 2001). Many behavior therapists (including Rachman and Lazarus) began to use integrative cognitive strategies into their work, and before long CBT was being practiced around the world. According to Lazarus (2001), the term cognitive-behavioral therapy was first introduced by Cyril Franks in his overview to the 1977 *Annual Review of Behavior Therapy* (Franks & Wilson, 1978), in which the transition of behavior therapy to CBT was discussed.

The work of Albert Bandura also had an important impact on the field of behavior therapy. Bandura noted that, in addition to learning through classical and operant conditioning, people also learn by observing others and that this process (often referred to as *social learning* or *modeling*) can contribute to both desirable and undesirable behaviors (Bandura, 1969). Today, modeling of desired behaviors (e.g., by parents, the therapist, or others) is often included in behavioral treatments. Bandura's model of social learning (currently referred to as *social-cognitive theory*) also incorporated the role of cognition (Bandura, 1986).

In the past decade, there has been a further shift, sometimes referred to as a "third wave" of behavior therapy (e.g., Hayes, Follette, & Linehan, 2004). This refers to the development of the *acceptance-based behavioral therapies*, which emphasize the importance of accepting unwanted thoughts, feelings, and emotions rather than trying to control or directly change them. These treatments include *acceptance and commitment therapy* (ACT; Hayes, Strosahl, & Wilson, 2012), *mindfulness-based cognitive therapy* (Segal, Williams & Teasdale, 2013), *dialectical behavior therapy* (Linehan, 1993), and other related approaches. Acceptance-based treatments (especially ACT) also involve teaching clients to become more aware of what is most important to them and to begin to shift their behaviors to live in a way that is more consistent with their values. It is too early to know whether acceptance-based approaches will catch on in the way that traditional behavior therapy and CBT did, although they are rapidly gaining both popularity and empirical support.

Today, behavioral treatments (including CBT) are among the most widely used approaches for managing psychological and behavioral problems. Treatment guidelines published by various professional associations (e.g., American Psychiatric Association), as well as independent government-funded agencies (such as the National Institute for Health and Clinical Excellence in the United Kingdom) consistently list behavioral therapies as the psychological treatments of choice for most forms of psychopathology. More than 20 scientific journals are now devoted to behavior therapy, and many countries around the world have their own professional associations for those who practice behavioral or cognitive-behavioral treatments. Behavior therapy is well entrenched, and there is every indication that it will continue to grow and evolve for years to come.

PERSONALITY

Theory of Personality

Trait theories of personality assume that each individual has unique, enduring patterns of behavior that can be observed across a wide range of situations and that these patterns can be understood in terms of specific personality characteristics—*traits*—that vary in intensity from low to high. Since psychologists first started studying personality, researchers have disagreed about the actual number of traits and about which traits are most important. For example, Gordon Allport, one of the first psychologists to systematically study personality traits, initially identified 18,000 words in the English dictionary that referred to personality traits (Allport & Odbert, 1936). This list was subsequently reduced by Allport to about 4,500 words, and later reduced further by Raymond Cattell, initially to 171 traits (Cattell, 1943) and later to 16 personality factors (Cattell, 1946, 1989).

Today, Costa and McCrae's (1992) *five-factor model* (or the "big five") is perhaps the most influential approach to describing core domains of personality, including *openness* (i.e., curious vs. cautious), *conscientiousness* (e.g., organized vs. careless or easygoing), *extraversion* (outgoing vs. solitary or reserved), *agreeableness* (compassionate vs. cold or unkind), and *neuroticism* (sensitive or anxious vs. secure or confident). Within each broad factor is assumed to be a cluster of associated, more narrowly focused traits.

Traditionally, behavioral approaches are restricted to the study of behavior (especially observable behavior) and the environmental conditions that influence behavior. For the most part, behaviorists reject traditional trait approaches to personality and are skeptical about their ability to predict behavior. Rather than explaining behavior in terms of stable characteristics or traits, behaviorists believe that behavior is influenced primarily by variables in the environment (reinforcement, punishment, classical conditioning, etc.) and that individuals behave differently across situations. For example, an individual might be outgoing in one situation and more reserved in another.

From a behavioral perspective, one's teacher, for example, might be expected to behave differently in front of a classroom than at home or the doctor's office or while driving in traffic. What does research tell us about the relationship between traits and behavior? In 1968, psychologist Walter Mischel reviewed the relevant research and found that studies consistently showed that behavior is primarily dependent on situational cues and that very little research supported the notion that people behave consistently across situations, challenging the classic notion of personality traits (Mischel, 1968).

However, a strict behavioral view is not completely supported by research either. Strong evidence supports the notion of individual temperaments that influence behavior. For example, Jerome Kagan and others have demonstrated that two types of temperament in infancy (inhibited, shy, or timid vs. uninhibited, sociable, or outgoing) are highly influenced by biology (e.g., genetics) and can predict the development of later behavior, depending on how they interact with events in the environment (e.g., Kagan, 1997).

Today, most behavior therapists acknowledge the importance of stable temperamental characteristics affecting behavior, and they assume that these patterns are influenced both by an individual's learning history and by biological makeup. At the same time, behaviorists recognize that much of our behavior varies across situations and is determined by immediate situational cues.

Variety of Concepts

Behavior therapy emphasizes the importance of learning, both in the development of behaviors, as well as the strategies for changing them. This section discusses concepts that underlie behavior therapy, including classical conditioning, operant conditioning, vicarious learning, and rule-governed behavior.

Classical Conditioning

Classical conditioning (also known as *Pavlovian conditioning* or *respondent conditioning*) is a form of learning in which one stimulus, a *conditioned stimulus* (CS), comes to signal the occurrence of a second stimulus, an *unconditioned stimulus* (US). A US is typically a stimulus that naturally causes a characteristic response, known as an *unconditioned response* (UR). For example, a shock (US) causes pain (UR), starvation (US) causes hunger (UR), and so on. By pairing a US and a CS, a person (or animal) comes to expect the occurrence of the US whenever exposed to the CS and eventually develops a *conditioned response* (CR) to encountering the CS alone. For example, a child who is bullied at school (US) will experience distress and emotional pain (UR). Later, even if the bullying has stopped, the same child may still experience fear and anxiety (CR) at school (CS).

Classical conditioning can sometimes explain why we experience negative emotions (e.g., fear, anger) in some situations and positive emotions (e.g., joy, love) in other situations. It can also help to explain why we approach some situations and avoid others. In fact, classical conditioning theory has been used to explain patterns of sexual arousal (e.g., cases where individuals become sexually aroused in the presence of inanimate objects such as shoes), hunger in response to particular environmental cues, cravings for drugs that are often triggered by particular situations, and a range of other experiences.

Extinction refers to presentation of the CS in the absence of the US so that the CR eventually stops occurring. Simply put, through the process of extinction, the CS no longer signals the occurrence of the US and therefore stops triggering a response. The principle of extinction has been used to explain the process of fear reduction through exposure to feared situations. By confronting a feared situation repeatedly in the absence of any negative consequence, a person stops responding to the situation with fear. However, through *reinstatement* (e.g., a subsequent repairing of the US and CS) a fear typically returns quickly. For example, someone who experiences a car accident after overcoming a fear of driving may experience a sudden and intense return of fear, suggesting the extinction doesn't erase previous learning.

Operant Conditioning

Operant conditioning is a form of learning in which the frequency, form, or strength of a behavior is influenced by its consequences. For example, a child who receives praise or rewards for having high standards and attending to details might become more perfectionistic than a child who is not rewarded for these behaviors. Reinforcement and punishment are the two primary methods through which operant conditioning operates.

Reinforcement. Reinforcement is a consequence that causes a behavior to increase in frequency or intensity. There are two types of reinforcement. *Positive reinforcement* occurs when a behavior is followed by a stimulus that is rewarding (e.g., food, money, attention). *Negative reinforcement* (or *escape*) occurs when a behavior is followed by the removal of an aversive stimulus. For example, an individual who pulls over on the highway during a panic attack is negatively reinforced for escaping because of the relief experienced after leaving the highway. Similarly, individuals who are dependent on alcohol or other drugs are negatively reinforced for their drug use whenever they use their preferred drug to reduce uncomfortable withdrawal symptoms.

Punishment. Punishment refers to any consequence that causes a behavior to decrease in frequency or intensity. Like reinforcement, punishment comes in two forms. *Positive punishment* occurs when a behavior is followed by an aversive consequence such as being hit, yelled at, or fired from a job. *Negative punishment* occurs when a behavior is followed by the removal of a desired stimulus such as a decrease in weekly allowance after misbehaving in school or not being allowed to eat dessert after refusing to eat one's vegetables.

Extinction. In the context of operant conditioning, extinction refers to a behavior that stops occurring because it is no longer followed by a positive consequence. For example, children learn to stop throwing tantrums when the tantrums are no longer reinforced (e.g., the child no longer gets what he or she wants as a result of the tantrum).

Discrimination Learning. Discrimination learning occurs when a response is reinforced or punished in one situation but not in another. Discrimination learning can explain why people behave differently in some situations than others. For example, an individual with OCD might feel compelled to engage in excessive hand washing at home but may be able to resist the urges to wash in public locations such as work or school.

Generalization.   Generalization refers to the occurrence of a learned behavior in situations other than those where the behavior was acquired. For example, an individual who is robbed while walking in the park late at night may develop a fear of being alone in other public situations and at other times of the day.

Vicarious Learning

Vicarious learning (also known as *observational learning*) refers to learning about environmental contingencies by watching the behavior of others. For example, witnessing a car accident may be enough to trigger a fear of driving even if an individual has not personally experienced an accident firsthand. Similarly, seeing others enjoy themselves while using cocaine may lead an adolescent to try cocaine for the first time.

Rule-Governed Behavior

People can also learn about contingencies indirectly through information that they hear or read without ever experiencing the contingencies firsthand, a process sometimes referred to as *rule-governed behavior* and *instructional learning*. For example, a person may learn to look to the left and the right before crossing the road as a result of parents explaining the dangers of crossing the street without first checking for oncoming traffic. Similarly, a person might develop a strong dislike of another individual whom he or she has never met simply because of gossip about the individual heard from others.

PSYCHOTHERAPY

Theory of Psychotherapy

Behavior therapy assumes that all behavior is learned through association, consequences, observation, or rules learned through communication and language. Therapy aims to help clients by providing corrective learning experiences that lead to changes in behavior, broadly defined (including cognitive, emotional, and physiological responses).

The learning that happens in behavior therapy is highly structured and active. Clients are expected to "do" things both within the therapy session and for homework. Examples include completing diaries to monitor eating, conducting exposure to feared situations, and practicing relaxation exercises. In fact, unlike many other forms of psychotherapy, much of the change that happens in behavior therapy is thought to occur as a result of homework practices completed between sessions. Clients are expected to apply what they learn during sessions in real-life situations—for example, at home, at work, and in day-to-day interactions with others.

The Therapeutic Relationship

Behavior therapists are sometimes faulted for ignoring the importance of the therapeutic relationship, and to some extent these charges are understandable. Behavior therapists have not emphasized the relationship between therapist and client, and some have argued that the therapeutic relationship is unimportant in behavior therapy. For example, Lang, Melamed, and Hart (1970) published a study on an automated procedure for administering systematic desensitization for the reduction of fear. In the abstract, they concluded that "an apparatus designed to administer systematic desensitization automatically was as effective as a live therapist in reducing phobic behavior, suggesting that desensitization is not dependent on a concurrent interpersonal interaction" (p. 220). Furthermore, there has been a growing literature supporting the use of computer-administered treatments and self-help treatments, which raises the question of whether the therapeutic relationship is important.

Despite these findings, there is a large body of research that is quite clear: A strong therapeutic relationship is indeed important across all forms of psychotherapy, including behavior therapy (Norcross, 2011). For example, therapist factors such as empathy, positive regard, congruence and genuineness, and self-disclosure have all been found to contribute to positive outcomes in psychotherapy. This is not surprising from a behavioral perspective. As reviewed by Antony and Roemer (2011), these characteristics might be expected to facilitate change because they provide immediate social reinforcement for desired behaviors, model desired interpersonal skills, and promote engagement in therapy, compliance with homework, and collaboration toward treatment goals.

Even in self-help treatments, there is evidence that the therapeutic relationship matters. For example, a study on the effectiveness of a self-help book on CBT for panic disorder found that self-help treatment was as effective as therapist-administered treatment, but only when the self-help book was combined with occasional meetings with a therapist to check on progress and compliance with treatment (Febbraro, Clum, Roodman, & Wright, 1999).

Behavioral strategies are generally effective when they are used as prescribed. The challenge in behavior therapy is to keep clients motivated so that they are fully engaged in treatment and so that they invest the time and energy needed to benefit from therapy. For those who are ambivalent about treatment, clients can be helped using techniques such as *motivational interviewing* (a client-centered approach designed to help clients explore and resolve sources of ambivalence about therapy) before starting behavioral treatment. Motivational interviewing has been used to improve outcomes during CBT for substance-use problems, eating disorders, anxiety disorders, and a range of other issues (Miller & Rollnick, 2013).

Process of Psychotherapy

Format and Structure of Behavior Therapy

Compared to most other forms of psychotherapy, the structure and format of behavior therapy is quite diverse. Therapy often consists of individual meetings with a therapist, but it may also be administered in groups or with families or couples. For example, in cases where family members subtly reinforce maladaptive behaviors, they may be invited to join one or more therapy sessions to learn strategies that will keep them from continuing to reinforce the client's problem behaviors. Behavioral interventions are usually administered by a therapist, but they may also be directed by others (e.g., parents, teachers, health-care professionals, prison guards). Treatment strategies can also be learned through self-help books, Internet-based programs, and other methods with minimal therapist contact.

Like other forms of psychotherapy, behavior therapy sessions often last about an hour, but it is not unusual for sessions to vary in length. For example, therapist-assisted exposure-therapy sessions may last longer than an hour, and group therapy sessions often last 90 minutes to 2 hours. Therapy sessions may occur in the therapist's office, but it is also not unusual for behavior therapists to meet with clients in other settings. For example, a behavior therapist based in the schools might visit a child's classroom for the purpose of behavioral observation and intervention. A therapist working with an individual who fears being in public places, such as restaurants or shopping malls, might visit these situations with the client during exposure-therapy sessions.

Behavior therapy is usually time limited. In the majority of studies, behavioral treatments are conducted over a period of 10 to 20 sessions, although the duration of treatment may vary. For example, phobias of animals can often be successfully treated in as little as one session (Hood & Antony, 2012). For other problems, such as borderline personality disorder, treatment may last a year or longer (Lynch, Trost, Salsman, & Linehan, 2007). Outside of the context of research studies (which typically have a predetermined number of sessions), treatment may last longer in routine clinical practice, depending on the patient's progress and the affordability of the treatment. Regardless of the duration, a goal of therapy is for the client to no longer be in therapy. Clients are taught strategies not only to change problem behaviors but also to maintain their improvements once treatment has ended.

Ethical Issues

A common misconception about behavior therapy is that it is coercive (e.g., that clients are forced to do things that they don't want to do). In practice, concerns about coercion that might be associated with behavior therapy are unfounded. As previously noted, behavior therapy is only likely to be effective when it is conducted in the context of a supportive therapeutic relationship. Many of the strategies used in behavior therapy depend on the client practicing the techniques, often on a daily basis, and treatment is unlikely to work unless the client is fully engaged and with a positive expectation that treatment will be helpful. Consider exposure therapy as an example. In exposure therapy, clients confront feared situations until they are no longer frightened. Although exposure to feared situations is an effective treatment for anxiety-based problems, positive outcomes depend on the client practicing regularly. A sense of perceived control in the situations is also important. In other words, clients who are forced to complete exposure practices or to take steps more quickly than they are willing are unlikely to benefit from treatment.

Of course, as is the case with any form of psychotherapy (and many other types of professional relationships), there is a power differential between the therapist and client and a potential for the therapist to influence the client in ways that are not in the client's best interest. Therapists need to be aware of their potential influence on the client and be careful to only make recommendations that are for the client's benefit.

Another ethical issue that arises in behavior therapy is the question of who determines the goals for treatment. There may be cases in which clients and therapists disagree about the most appropriate treatment goals. For example, a client presenting for treatment of insomnia may have sleep problems that are secondary to posttraumatic stress disorder (PTSD) but may refuse to discuss the issues surrounding the trauma, insisting that therapy focus on the sleep problems only. In such a case, the therapist would likely discuss with the client why addressing the trauma is important for improving the insomnia, but ultimately the client determines the treatment goals. There may be some cases in which the client has less input into the focus of treatment (e.g., a young child with behavior problems, an older adult with dementia who behaves violently, a client whose treatment is mandated by the courts). However, even in these cases, treatment is unlikely to be helpful unless the client and therapist have shared goals.

Behavior therapy differs from other forms of therapy in that sessions may include activities other than just talking in the therapist's office. For example, a client with an eating disorder might eat with the therapist. Or a client with a fear of riding the bus might practice riding buses with the therapist. It is important for the therapist to maintain clear professional boundaries at all times and for the client to fully understand the purpose of the activities being practiced in therapy (e.g., eating together for the purpose of overcoming an eating disorder is different than sharing a meal for the purpose of socializing). Therapists also must be careful to maintain confidentiality. For example, if therapy involves spending time in public places, it is possible that the therapist or client will encounter people they know from other settings. The therapist and client will often plan in advance how to handle such situations if they arise.

Mechanisms of Psychotherapy

Traditionally, behavior therapists relied on learning principles (e.g., reinforcement, punishment, extinction) to explain the effects of treatment. Increasingly, however, models based on information processing, emotional processing, and cognitive reappraisal have been advanced to explain the process by which clients change during behavior therapy. For example, Foa and colleagues' emotional-processing theory has changed the way in which many behavior therapists understand the mechanisms underlying exposure therapy (Foa & Kozak, 1986; Foa, Huppert, & Cahill, 2006). According to the model, fearful associations are stored in memory in a fear network comprised of a *stimulus* component (e.g., dog), a *response* component (e.g., fear), and a *meaning* component (e.g., I will get attacked). Conditioning experiences cause these components to become associated with one another so that experiencing any one of these elements (e.g., seeing a dog) makes it more likely that the other components (e.g., fear, thoughts about being attacked) will also be activated. According to the theory, exposure to feared situations works by (1) fully activating the fear network and (2) incorporating new, corrective information.

Predictors of Improvement

In recent years, research on behavior therapy has begun to focus on identifying factors that predict who will respond best to treatment. Although conclusions differ somewhat across studies, across problems, and across interventions, a few findings have emerged across several treatments and diagnostic groups. For example, some of the variables associated with worse outcomes following CBT for anxiety disorders include the presence of personality disorders, severe depression, more severe anxiety-disorder symptoms, more stressful life events, poorer insight into the excessiveness of the anxiety symptoms, poor motivation, negative patterns of communication among family members, and poor compliance with treatment (e.g., missing sessions; not completing homework). Similar factors have been found to affect outcomes for a range of other conditions as well (see Antony, Ledley, & Heimberg, 2005).

APPLICATIONS

Who Can We Help?

The effects of behavioral and cognitive-behavioral therapies have been demonstrated in hundreds of studies with just about every type of psychological problem, including anxiety disorders (Antony & Stein, 2009), depression (Cuijpers et al., 2012), substance-use disorders (Hallgren, Greenfield, Ladd, Glynn, & McCrady, 2012; Vedel & Emmelkamp, 2012), schizophrenia (Jones & Meaden, 2012), eating disorders (Touyz, Polivy, & Hay, 2008), sexual dysfunction (Wincze & Carey, 2001), sleep disorders (Smith, et al., 2002), borderline personality disorder (Kliem, Kröger, & Kosfelder, 2010), and problem gambling (Gooding & Terrier, 2009), among many others. Behavioral treatments are well supported in both adults and children and across a wide range of other specific groups.

A comprehensive review of the evidence regarding behavioral treatments is beyond the scope of this chapter. However, as an illustration, this section provides a brief discussion of which behavioral strategies have been found to be useful for anxiety disorders (with an emphasis on panic disorder and OCD), depression, substance-use disorders, and schizophrenia. Several excellent resources provide detailed reviews of the evidence concerning behavioral treatments (and other evidence-based approaches) for a wide range of disorders (e.g., Nathan & Gorman, 2007; Sturmey & Hersen, 2012).

Anxiety Disorders

Extensive research supports the use of behavioral therapies across all of the anxiety disorders (Antony & Stein, 2009; Olatunji, Cisler, & Deacon, 2010). For example, in panic disorder (a condition associated with unexpected panic attacks, worry about the consequences of panic, and avoidance of situations that trigger panic), evidence-based treatment often includes a combination of psychoeducation, exposure (both to feared situations and feared sensations), and cognitive reevaluation (for a review, see Koerner, Vorstenbosch, & Antony, 2012). In OCD, a problem associated with obsessions (intrusive, unwanted thoughts, images, and urges) and compulsions (behaviors that occur in response to obsessions that are designed to reduce anxiety or prevent harm), the most studied behavioral treatment is exposure (both in vivo and in imagination) combined with response prevention, although there are also recent studies supporting cognitive strategies (see Williams, Powers, & Foa, 2012).

Behavioral strategies (e.g., exposure, cognitive techniques, relaxation training, mindfulness- and acceptance-based strategies) have also been found to be effective to varying degrees across other anxiety-based disorders (e.g., generalized anxiety disorder, PTSD, social anxiety disorder, specific phobias), although there are some differences in which strategies are used in each disorder (for a review, see Antony & Stein, 2009). For example, although relaxation training is useful as a stand-alone treatment for generalized anxiety disorder, it is more likely to be used in combination with other strategies (or not at all) for the other anxiety disorders. For specific phobias, the primary evidence based approach is exposure to the phobic situation.

Depression

Behavioral and cognitive-behavioral approaches (e.g., behavioral activation, cognitive reappraisal, problem-solving training, social-skills training, mindfulness-based treatments) have been found to be effective for both the treatment of unipolar depression and the prevention of future depressive episodes (e.g., Cuijpers, van Straten, Andersson, & van Oppen, 2008; Piet & Houggard, 2011). Several non-CBT approaches are also quite effective for treating depression, including interpersonal psychotherapy, short-term psychodynamic psychotherapy, nondirective supportive psychotherapy, and couples therapy (Cuijpers et al., 2012). The effects of CBT on depression in bipolar disorder (sometimes referred to as *manic depressive disorder*) are more modest, and psychological treatments are more likely to be used as adjuncts to medication treatment rather than on their own.

Substance-Use Disorders

Decades of research on the treatment of substance-use disorders support behavioral approaches, including contingency management, community reinforcement, behavioral couples and family treatments, and cognitive-behavioral approaches (Hallgren et al., 2012; Vedel & Emmelkamp, 2012). There is also considerable support for motivational interviewing, a client-centered approach for resolving ambivalence over stopping substance use. Despite evidence supporting these treatments, however, society (especially in the United States) continues to rely on methods that are not helpful, including incarceration, marginalizing those who abuse substances, and offering treatments that are neither evidence based nor cost-effective (Miller & Carroll, 2006).

Schizophrenia

Some of the earliest behavioral treatments to be developed, such as a token economy, were first used with individuals suffering from schizophrenia and related problems. Several behavioral techniques are helpful for improving the lives of patients with schizophrenia, including social-skills training, contingency management (e.g., token economy) behavioral family therapies (including communication training, problem-solving training, and other strategies), and cognitive-behavioral treatments (see Mueser & Jeste, 2008). However, unlike many of the problems for which behavior therapy alone is effective, individuals with schizophrenia typically must take antipsychotic medication as well, and the most effective approach for managing schizophrenia is a combination of pharmacological and psychological treatments.

Treatment

Behavior therapy includes a wide range of strategies. In fact, *Volume 1 (Adult Clinical Applications)* of the *Encyclopedia of Behavior Modification and Cognitive Behavior Therapy* (Hersen & Rosqvist, 2005) includes entries for 50 major techniques and 62 additional minor techniques. Although a full review of all behavioral strategies is not possible here, this section provides an overview of several commonly used techniques, including behavioral assessment, exposure-based strategies, response prevention, operant-conditioning strategies, relaxation training, stimulus-control procedures, modeling, behavioral activation for depression, social-skills training, problem-solving training, and acceptance-based behavioral therapies. Although cognitive strategies are also commonly used by behavior therapists, they are not discussed here because they are covered in depth elsewhere in this book (see Chapters 5 and 7).

Behavioral Assessment

In behavior therapy, assessment and treatment go hand in hand. Every client is assessed before treatment begins, and the assessment process continues throughout the course of treatment—and often after treatment has ended. Behavioral assessment has several functions, including identifying *target behaviors* (behaviors to be changed during therapy), determining the most appropriate course of treatment, assessing the impact of therapy over time, and assessing the final outcome of treatment. Because behavior therapists assume that a client's behavior differs across situations and contexts, behavioral assessment usually relies on *multiple methods* (e.g., interviews, direct observation of client behaviors, monitoring forms or diaries, checklists, self-report symptom measures, psychophysiological measures) and *multiple informants* (e.g., clients, family members, teachers, friends), and it occurs in *multiple situations* (e.g., home, work, school, therapist's office).

Typically, target behaviors are identified collaboratively by the therapist and client. Ideal target behaviors are those that are distressing, impairing, or dangerous to either the client or others. Target behaviors are selected with the goal of increasing flexibility in the client's behavioral repertoire. Treatment targets may include *behavioral deficits* (e.g., poor social skills, poor anger control), *behavioral excesses* (e.g., compulsive hand washing, a tendency to overmonitor one's behavior), and problems in the client's environment (e.g., restricted opportunities for dating, desirable behaviors not being followed by reinforcement).

A key component of behavioral assessment is *functional analysis*. The purpose of functional analysis is to identify the variables responsible for maintaining target behaviors. Ideally, functional analysis involves manipulating variables in the environment and measuring their impact on target behaviors. For example, if we assume that a child's tantrums are maintained by the parents' attention, we might test out our hypothesis by having the parents stop attending to the tantrums for a week or two and evaluating the impact on the child's behavior. In practice, it is often difficult to conduct experiments to confirm the causal relationships that explain behavior, and instead causal variables are inferred through methods such as interviews, questionnaires, and other tools. The abbreviation "ABC" is often used to summarize the key variables that are assessed during the process of functional analysis: A stands for the *antecedents* of the target behavior, B stands for the *behavior*, and C stands for the *consequences* of the behavior, including reinforcement or punishment from the client's environment. In practice, most behavior therapists also attend somewhat to internal variables that may contribute to the client's behavior such as biological factors (e.g., a head injury, fatigue from lack of sleep) and even personality styles.

Behavioral Interviews.   Behavioral interviews help the therapist understand both the form and function of behavior. During the interview, the therapist obtains a detailed description of the problem behavior, including information on the frequency, duration, and severity. The therapist also typically asks about the development and course of the problem over time. Another important purpose of the interview is to establish the antecedents and consequences of the target behavior. Finally, in addition to getting answers to important questions, interviews provide the therapist with direct samples of the client's behavior (e.g., style of communication, eye contact) that might not otherwise be reported by the client.

Behavioral Observation.   Behavioral observation involves observing the client in order to assess behavior as well as its antecedents and consequences. In *naturalistic observation,* the assessment occurs in the client's natural environment (for example, a teacher may record episodes of a child's disruptive behavior in the classroom). In *analog observation*, the assessment occurs in a simulated situation (for example, a client role playing a job interview). Behavioral observation can also rely on other less-direct methods such as recording (audio or video) the client's behavior, using event counters to track the number of times a behavior occurs, or measuring the by-products of a behavior (e.g., assessing self harm by looking for cut marks on the client's arm, assessing drug or alcohol use with a urine test). One of the challenges with behavioral observation (and other forms of assessment) is the problem of *reactivity*. Reactivity occurs when an individual's behavior is affected by the assessment process itself so that the assessment does not provide an accurate picture of the client's behavior under normal circumstances. For example, couples being interviewed by a therapist may communicate differently in the therapist's office than they do when they're alone. Similarly, clients asked to check a box on a diary every time they smoke a cigarette may smoke fewer cigarettes than if they were not tracking their smoking. Ways of reducing reactivity include using unobtrusive observation methods (e.g., observation through a one-way mirror) and allowing clients to habituate or adapt to the assessment context before starting to measure their behavior.

Monitoring Forms and Diaries.   Behavior therapists often ask their clients to complete diaries and monitoring forms between therapy sessions to track behaviors as they occur. Diaries can be used to establish a baseline level for problem behavior before treatment begins and to measure changes in the behavior over time. They may also help the client become more aware of a problem behavior that might otherwise not be noticed.

Diaries typically ask clients to record their overt behaviors (e.g., drinking alcohol, avoiding a feared situation) as well as thoughts, emotions, physical sensations, situations encountered, unwanted urges, and the antecedents and consequences of target behaviors.

Self-Report Scales.   Self-report scales refer to questionnaires that assess behaviors or other domains of interest (e.g., levels of depression or anxiety). They are typically completed using paper-and-pencil versions or on a computer. Unlike behavioral observation and interviews, which can be expensive and time consuming, self-report scales are typically quick and inexpensive to administer, score, and interpret. They are also often standardized and empirically supported, with evidence of both reliability and validity. The main disadvantage of self-report scales relative to other methods is that they may not provide specific information about a particular client. Rather, they typically provide little more than an overall score that offers some indication of the severity or intensity of the construct being measured (e.g., how severe a client's depression is).

Psychophysiological Assessment.   Behavioral assessment sometimes includes measurement of the client's physiological responses. For example, a man being treated for sexual dysfunction might undergo *penile plethysmography*, a process that involves fitting the penis with a device that measures changes in sexual arousal. A client undergoing behavioral treatment for hypertension might receive regular blood pressure tests to evaluate the impact of treatment. Clients being treated for sleep disorders often undergo assessments to measure their body movements, brain activity, muscle activity, or eye movements while sleeping. Finally, individuals with anxiety disorders may have their heart rate or skin conductance measured over the course of treatment as these can provide useful objective measures of the physical aspects of fear and anxiety.

Treatment Planning

Before therapy begins, the therapist and client set treatment goals. Goals should be both specific and measurable. For example, a client's goal "to stop hitting my children" is a more appropriate behavioral goal than "to become a better parent," which is both vague and difficult to quantify. Relatedly, goals should be anchored in particular behaviors or outcomes. For example, a client who wishes to be more "successful" at work must first identify exactly what it means to be successful (e.g., working more quickly, making fewer mistakes, receiving more positive feedback from supervisors, making more money). Goals should also be realistic and achievable. Finally, timelines should be set for achieving goals.

Behavior therapy encompasses a wide range of techniques, and knowing which ones to use for a particular client can be a challenge. Two main methods are used to select treatment strategies: One is based on the results of a detailed *functional analysis*, and the other is based on the client's *diagnostic profile*. In practice, both methods are often used to varying degrees.

Using the first approach, treatment strategies emerge from the results of the behavioral assessment. For example, if the assessment determines that a client's depression is a function of reduced activity, then treatment would likely involve *behavioral activation*, a strategy (discussed later in the chapter) in which clients are encouraged to increase their activity levels. Similarly, if the client's excessive alcohol use is determined to be reinforced by his or her social milieu (e.g., working in a bar, socializing with friends who drink to excess), then treatment might focus on changing patterns of reinforcement in the environment (e.g., helping the client to find a new line of work or to make new friends).

The second approach involves selecting treatment strategies based on a client's diagnosis. Increasingly, behavior therapists rely on established manualized protocols for treating individuals with particular disorders or problems. Over the years, conducting research on behavioral treatments for specific problems has necessitated the development of manualized treatments to ensure consistency in how the treatments are administered in studies. In addition, the use of evidence-based protocols in routine clinical practice increases the likelihood that treatments will be administered in the same ways in which they were originally validated. Despite the advantages of using treatment manuals, relying on standard protocols has also been criticized on the grounds that clients in clinical settings may be different than clients who participate in research studies, who are often carefully screened. Of course, the most useful manuals are often not the ones that are most heavily scripted; instead, they allow flexibility to accommodate the needs of different types of clients.

Selecting treatment strategies based on a client's diagnosis (as opposed to a detailed functional assessment) may be particularly useful in cases where clients with a particular diagnosis are relatively homogeneous, when there is a powerful treatment available for the client's disorder, and when the time and expense of completing a detailed behavioral assessment is greater than any added benefits of doing so. For example, people with specific phobias (e.g., phobias of spiders, heights, needles) almost always respond well to brief exposure-based treatments (Hood & Antony, 2012), and virtually all published treatment guidelines agree that exposure is the treatment of choice for specific phobias.

Exposure-Based Strategies

Exposure is one of the best studied and most consistently effective behavioral techniques available. It is used primarily in the treatment of anxiety disorders, but it also may be used to treat fear and anxiety in the context of other conditions (e.g., exposure to "forbidden" foods in a client who has an eating disorder). Essentially, exposure involves confronting feared stimuli directly instead of avoiding them. Most behavior therapists consider exposure to be an essential component for the treatment of fear and anxiety.

The most commonly used form of exposure is *in vivo exposure*, which involves exposure to feared situations in real life. For example, an individual who fears driving might be encouraged to practice driving. Someone who is frightened of social situations, such as public speaking or meeting strangers, might be encouraged to practice encountering these situations. In vivo exposure is often practiced in the therapy session with the therapist present as well as between sessions for homework.

A second type of exposure is *imaginal exposure*, which involves exposure to feared mental imagery. As mentioned earlier, imaginal exposure was a core component of Wolpe's systematic desensitization. However, today imaginal exposure is most likely to be recommended for individuals who tend to suppress and fear their thoughts or mental imagery rather than reduce fear of an external object or situation. For example, individuals with PTSD often suppress memories of their trauma (e.g., memories of a sexual assault), and individuals with OCD often suppress intrusive thoughts and images related to their obsessions (e.g., irrational thoughts of harming a loved one). Attempts to suppress unwanted thoughts can have the ironic effect of increasing either the distress associated with thoughts, the frequency of the thoughts, or both. In contrast, repeated exposure to unwanted, frightening thoughts leads to a reduction in fear and ultimately a reduction in the frequency of the intrusive thoughts.

A third type of exposure, called *interoceptive exposure*, involves purposely experiencing frightening physical sensations until they are no longer frightening. Interoceptive exposure is used in the treatment of individuals who become anxious or frightened when they experience physical symptoms of arousal such as a racing heart, dizziness, or breathlessness. This may include individuals with panic disorder, who typically fear experiencing panic-related sensations, as well as people with other problems who fear their physical feelings (e.g., people with height phobias who fear feeling dizzy and high places, people with social anxiety who fear shaking or sweating in front of others). Examples of interoceptive exposure exercises include hyperventilating (breathing quickly) to induce feelings of breathlessness, racing heart, and numbness or tingling, breathing through a narrow straw to induce a feeling of suffocation, and spinning in a chair to induce dizziness (Antony, Ledley, Liss, & Swinson, 2006).

Exposure is typically gradual, starting with less fear-provoking stimuli, and progressing to more frightening situations. The therapist and client together develop an *exposure hierarchy,* which is a list of feared situations rank ordered with easier items at the bottom of the list and the most difficult situations at the top. Clients start by practicing easier items, and they progress to the more difficult items as their fear improves. In addition to exposure practices involving feared objects, situations, thoughts, and feelings, practices may also involve exposure to feared stimuli in photos or on video or by using computer-generated images generated by virtual reality programs.

Several guidelines will ensure the best possible response to exposure (for reviews, see Abramowitz, Deacon, & Whiteside, 2011; Vorstenbosch, Newman, & Antony, in press). First, exposure is most effective when it is predictable (the client knows what is going to happen during the session) and controllable (the client has control over what happens during the practice). Exposure often works better when practice is frequent (e.g., daily rather than weekly). Longer practices tend to be more effective than briefer practices, although it is often not necessary for the client's fear to decrease completely before the end of the practice. Finally, some research suggests that modeling by the therapist (e.g., demonstrating how to approach the feared object or situation) can lead to better outcomes, although research findings in this area have been mixed.

Response Prevention

Response prevention involves inhibiting an unwanted behavior in order to break the association between a stimulus and response. For example, in the treatment of OCD, clients are encouraged to stop their compulsive rituals (washing, checking, counting, etc.), in combination with carrying out exposure to feared objects and situations. Without response prevention, exposure for OCD would not be particularly effective because the compulsive rituals (e.g., frequent washing) would undermine any possible benefits from exposure (e.g., touching contaminated items). Response prevention is also used in the treatment of impulse-control problems and unwanted habits (e.g., nail biting, skin picking) and for the prevention of safety behaviors across other anxiety-based problems. Instead of engaging in the behavior they are trying to change, clients are encouraged to tolerate their discomfort until it subsides. In some cases, a competing behavior may be introduced. For example, a client who is trying to quit smoking might be encouraged to chew gum instead.

Operant–Conditioning Strategies

Strategies grounded in operant-conditioning theory are based on the assumption that behaviors followed by a desirable consequence (reinforcement) will increase in frequency and behaviors followed by an undesirable consequence (punishment) will decrease in frequency. Operant-conditioning therapy (sometimes referred to by the term *applied behavior analysis*) involves changing patterns of reinforcement and punishment in the environment, which may include adding reinforcers to increase desirable behaviors (e.g., permitting a later bedtime to reward a child for completing homework), removing stimuli that reinforce undesirable behaviors (e.g., giving in to a child's tantrums), and in some cases using punishment (e.g., imposing a time-out for a child who refuses to stop hitting a younger sibling). For a detailed review of techniques based on operant conditioning, see Fisher, Piazza, and Roane (2011).

Reinforcement–Based Procedures. *Differential reinforcement* (i.e., reinforcing the absence of unwanted behaviors and the occurrence of desired alternative behaviors) has been used with success across a wide range of problems, including child behavior problems, weight-loss programs, aggression, addictions, and other problems. Examples of differential reinforcement include allowing a child to spend time on the Internet only after completing household chores and providing subsidized housing to an individual only after repeated negative drug tests. As previously mentioned, a *token economy* is another example of an operant strategy that relies on principles of reinforcement. This procedure has been used in inpatient hospital units to help manage disruptive behavior in clients. Clients participating in a token-economy environment receive tokens for desirable behaviors and can redeem the tokens for reinforcers (e.g., money, privileges) later. *Contingency management* is another reinforcement-based strategy in which the client's environment is changed so that unwanted behaviors are no longer reinforced. This method is often used in the treatment of substance-use disorders where both the social environment (e.g., spending time with friends who use substances, hanging out in places where substances are easily available) and the individual's "internal environment" (e.g., getting high, experiencing a reduction in anxiety when substances are used) reinforce the use of alcohol or other drugs. Through contingency management, an individual might be encouraged to spend more time with people who don't use substances, stay away from places where substances are easy to come by, and use more adaptive methods for managing anxiety.

Punishment–Based Strategies. Punishment involves exposing individuals to an unwanted consequence with the goal of decreasing and undesirable behavior. The term *aversive conditioning* is often used to described punishment-based procedures. An example of aversive conditioning is the use of a drug called *disulfiram* (or *Antabuse*), which is sometimes used to treat alcohol dependence. If individual drinks alcohol while taking disulfiram, various unpleasant symptoms are experienced, including nausea, vomiting, headache, breathlessness, and others. People quickly learn to stop drinking while taking disulfiram.

In general, punishment-based procedures are not considered to be effective long-term ways to change behavior. Although people often make short-term behavioral changes in response to punishment, relapse is common after the negative consequences are removed. Also, individuals sometimes find ways to avoid the negative consequences all together (compliance with punishment-based treatments is sometimes poor). For example, a person taking disulfiram may just stop the drug rather than stop drinking alcohol. For long-term behavior change, reinforcement-based strategies tend to be more effective than punishment.

Relaxation Training

Relaxation training involves using strategies for reducing the effects of anxiety and stress on the body. Methods include slow *diaphragmatic breathing* (also known as *breathing retraining*) to prevent the effects of hyperventilation (overbreathing), *guided mental imagery* to manage stress and reduce feelings of tension, and *progressive relaxation* for reducing feelings of muscle tension in the body (for a description of relaxation-based techniques and a review of relevant evidence, see Hazlett-Stevens & Bernstein, 2012).

Progressive relaxation is among the best-studied relaxation techniques, with more than 30 randomized controlled trials supporting its use for generalized anxiety disorder, headache, high blood pressure, and a range of other problems (Hazlett-Stevens & Bernstein, 2012). The treatment was first developed by Edmund Jacobson in the early 1900s (Jacobson, 1938) and then refined in the 1970s by Bernstein and Borkovec (see Bernstein, Borkovec, & Hazlett-Stevens, 2000). The process begins with a series of exercises involving alternately tensing and relaxing 16 different muscle groups, followed by several minutes of focused attention and breathing exercises. Clients are encouraged to practice the exercise (which takes about 20 minutes) daily. After a week or two of practice, the exercise is shortened from 16 muscle groups to eight muscle groups. After a few more weeks, the routine is shortened again to four muscle groups and then again by omitting the tension component of the tension–relaxation cycle. In the final stage of treatment, the client relaxes by taking a deep breath and letting go of any tension. The goal over the course of treatment is for clients to learn to relax quickly and in a variety of situations so that by the end of treatment they can apply the technique before their anxiety becomes too intense.

Stimulus-Control Procedures

The term *stimulus control* refers to a behavior being under the control of a specific cue or stimulus. In the context of behavior therapy, stimulus-control procedures aim to correct problems related to stimulus control, in particular problems in which a behavior is under the control of an inappropriate stimulus. One treatment domain in which stimulus-control procedures are used is insomnia. People who have difficulty sleeping often end up spend time in bed doing things other than sleeping such as reading, smoking, watching television, talking on the phone, and eating, to name a few. As a result, the association between the bedroom and sleep is weakened, making it more difficult to fall asleep. People with insomnia also tend to sleep at unusual times (e.g., napping to catch up on sleep, waking up late to compensate for a lack of sleep) so that evening hours are no longer a cue for sleep. An important component of the treatment of insomnia involves regaining stimulus control so that the bedroom is primarily associated with sleep and sleep only occurs during appropriate times. Clients with insomnia are encouraged to use the bedroom for only sleep and sexual intimacy, and they should leave the bedroom when they can't sleep. They are also advised to avoid napping, to get into the bed at the same time every night, and to get out of bed at the same time every morning, even if they didn't have a good night's sleep. In addition to the treatment of insomnia, stimulus-control procedures have been used in the treatment of substance dependence (for which a wide range of stimuli may take on the ability to trigger the urge to use substances) as well as other problems (for a review, see Poling & Gaynor, 2009).

Modeling

We learn how to behave, in part, from watching others behave, a process known as *modeling*. For example, we can learn to fear objects by watching others behave fearfully, and we can learn to overcome fear by watching others confront a situation without fear, especially if we see that no negative consequences occur. A therapist modeling how to approach a feared object can therefore be used to facilitate exposure therapy. Modeling is also useful for teaching complex life skills (e.g., how to make conversation with strangers, how to behave in a classroom, how to communicate effectively with one's parents or partner) or specific therapy skills (e.g., relaxation, problem solving). Modeling is rarely used alone; rather, it is typically incorporated into other strategies such as exposure or skills training (for a more detailed description of modeling, see Alden, 2005).

Behavioral Activation for Depression

Behavioral activation is based on the notion that depression is maintained by a lack of response-contingent positive reinforcement, caused by inactivity and withdrawal, which lead to reduced opportunities for contact with potential reinforcers, and therefore fewer opportunities for actions to be reinforced. Behavioral activation can be defined as "the therapeutic scheduling of specific activities for the client to complete in his or her daily life that function to increase contact with diverse, stable, and personally meaningful sources of positive reinforcement" (Kanter & Puspitasari, 2012, p. 217). As reviewed by Martell, Dimidjian, and Herman-Dunn (2010), behavioral activation was developed by Neil Jacobson in the 1990s based on previous work by researchers such as Charles Ferster, Peter Lewinsohn, Aaron Beck, and Lynn Rehm, who wrote about the role of environmental contingencies in maintaining depression and the importance of incorporating activity scheduling into its treatment.

Martell et al. (2010) described several core principles underlying behavioral activation, including the assumptions that (1) the key to changing how one feels is changing what one does; (2) although life changes can lead to depression, unhelpful short-term coping strategies can keep people stuck in their depression; and (3) figuring out what strategies are likely be helpful for a particular client lies in understanding the events that precede and follow the client's behaviors.

Activity scheduling is a core feature of behavioral activation. By becoming more active, the client begins to experience positive reinforcement and starts to become engaged in life again. In addition to increasing the client's activity, other components of behavioral activation include activity and mood monitoring, goal setting, helping clients recognize the antecedents and consequences of their behavior (i.e., functional analysis), using exercises involving attention to experience (similar to mindfulness training), problem-solving training, adopting strategies to change depressive thinking, and using strategies to prevent relapse (Martell et al., 2010).

Social-Skills Training

Being able to function effectively in our relationships and social interactions is important for ensuring success and well-being. Impairment in these areas can lead to rejection from others and ultimately to an assortment of negative consequences, including the inability to form healthy relationships and impairments in work, school, and other domains of functioning.

Social-skills training involves the use of modeling, corrective feedback, behavioral rehearsal, and other strategies to help clients to improve their abilities to communicate effectively and function better in social interactions. For example, clients who struggle with being assertive might learn ways to express their needs directly (e.g., to refuse an unreasonable request, to ask others to change their behavior) rather than allowing others to take advantage of them. Social-skills training is sometimes used in the treatment of social anxiety disorder, depression, schizophrenia, couples distress, intellectual impairment, autism spectrum disorders, and other problems that can associated with impairments in communication and social skills. Targets for social-skills training may include eye contact, body language, speech quality (e.g., volume, tone), listening skills, conversation skills, assertiveness skills, conflict skills, interview skills, dating skills, and public-speaking skills, for example. Depending on the client's level of functioning, more basic social skills (e.g., how to pay on a bus, how to order in a restaurant) may also be the target of intervention.

The process of social-skills training begins with identifying potential social-skills deficits in a supportive and nonjudgmental manner. Once the target behaviors have been identified, the next step is to identify effective ways to change the target behaviors.

The therapist models the new behaviors (e.g., improved eye contact, sitting up straight, making small talk), and clients are given an opportunity to practice the skills followed by corrective feedback. Practices can occur in the context of behavioral role plays or in real-life social interactions. Often the client's performance is videotaped and then watched together by the client and therapist. This gives clients an opportunity to observe their own behavior and make corrections as needed. For a more detailed description of social-skills training and reviews of relevant research, see Kinnaman and Bellack (2012) and Segrin (2009).

Problem–Solving Training

People often take for granted their ability to solve problems successfully. However, developing effective problem-solving skills may sometimes require both formal instruction and practice. For some people, making decisions in the face of everyday life challenges can be overwhelming and may lead to a sense of feeling paralyzed. For others, problems are solved impulsively without thinking through possible consequences. Problem-solving training is designed to help people solve problems systematically by teaching them five core steps.

Step 1: Define the Problem(s).   Here the individual is taught to describe the problem as specifically as possible: "I have to drive my children to school and the car won't start" rather than "I'm having a terrible morning." If there are several problems, then the individual is encouraged to prioritize them and identify which ones are the most important.

Step 2: Identify Possible Solutions.   This stage is often referred to as *brainstorming*. Here the individual is encouraged to come up with as many solutions as possible and without filtering them. At this step, the client should not worry about whether the proposed solutions are good or bad. For example, possible solutions to the example generated in step 1 might include "Send the children to school by taxi or bus," "Have the children stay home," "Ask a friend or neighbor to drive the children to school," "See if I can get help starting the car and then take the children to school late," and so on.

Step 3: Evaluate the Solutions.   This step involves examining the costs and benefits of each solution generated in step 2.

Step 4: Choose the Best Solution(s).   Here the individual selects the best solution based on the analysis from step 3. Sometimes this may include more than one option (e.g., sending the oldest child to school by taxi, and keeping the youngest child at home for the day).

Step 5: Implementation.   This stage involves implementing the solution that was selected. Implementation may lead to the identification of new challenges that prevent the solution from being applied, in which case the client would be encouraged to return to the list of solutions and select another one or go through the steps of problem solving to resolve the challenge in implementation.

Problem-solving training may also focus on developing other related abilities, including skills for challenging negative thinking, enhancing motivation, setting priorities, setting goals, managing time effectively, and improving organization. Problem-solving training has been used in the treatment of depression, generalized anxiety disorder, social anxiety disorder, schizophrenia, couple distress, and other problems (for a review, see Nezu & Nezu, 2012).

Acceptance-Based Behavioral Therapies

Irish playwright and author Oscar Wilde was quoted as saying, "I don't want to be at the mercy of my emotions. I want to use them, to enjoy them, and to dominate them," and it is natural to want to control unwanted emotions, thoughts, and memories. However, control-oriented behaviors such as avoidance, distraction, safety behaviors, procrastination, and compulsions are rarely helpful in the long term, especially when they are used to excess.

As reviewed previously, most behavioral strategies are designed to increase the flexibility in the client's behavioral repertoire, and part of that process involves learning to accept unwanted thoughts and emotions rather than trying to control them. *Mindfulness* is a strategy for facilitating acceptance. One of the most frequently cited definitions is that of Kabat-Zinn (1994), who defines mindfulness as "paying attention, in a particular way: on purpose, in the present moment, nonjudgmentally" (p. 4.). Individuals undergoing mindfulness training are taught to attend to their experiences (e.g., thoughts, sensations, emotions) as they occur rather than distracting, purposely ruminating about past events, or worrying about the future. They are also encouraged to accept these experiences, taking the stance that thoughts, emotions, and sensations are neither good nor bad—they just *are*. Mindfulness practices may include meditation, mindful breathing exercises, mindful scanning of the body, mindful eating, and others. The process of mindfulness is nothing new; in fact, it dates back more than 2,500 years to the earliest forms of Buddhism. What is new over the past two decades is the incorporation of mindfulness-based strategies into behavioral treatments and the systematic study of mindfulness-based treatments in well-controlled research.

A number of treatments include mindfulness as a component. One of these is *acceptance and commitment therapy* (ACT), a form of psychotherapy developed by Stephen Hayes and colleagues (2012). ACT includes two main components. The first component involves fostering acceptance. Rather than trying to control or avoid unwanted thoughts, feelings, and other private events (often referred to as *experiential avoidance*), ACT teaches clients to notice, accept, and even embrace private events. Clients are encouraged to distance themselves from their thoughts and take the perspective of an observer (rather than assuming each thought is important or meaningful). The second component of ACT involves encouraging clients to become more aware of their values and to take action so that their behaviors match their values, bringing more vitality and meaning into the client's life and ultimately increasing flexibility in the client's behavioral repertoire.

Another widely used acceptance-based behavioral treatment is *dialectical behavior therapy* (DBT), which was developed by psychologist Marsha Linehan (1993). DBT combines traditional cognitive-behavioral techniques with mindfulness-based strategies for acceptance and tolerating distress. It was first developed to treat borderline personality disorder, although it is now used for a wide range of other problems, including eating disorders, substance-use disorders, and trauma-based problems. Compared to other behavioral and cognitive-behavioral approaches, mindfulness and acceptance-based approaches are still relatively new. There is increasing support for these approaches (see Hayes, Villatte, Levin, & Hildebrandt, 2011), but there is also debate in the literature about the mechanisms underlying the effectiveness of these approaches and the extent to which they overlap with other cognitive and behavioral approaches (e.g., Arch & Craske, 2008; Hofmann & Asmundson, 2008).

Evidence

With increased pressures from managed health care to deliver effective treatments in as few sessions as possible, psychotherapists have had to examine their own practices more critically. Over the past few decades, there has been a trend toward the development of short-term treatments, and there is seemingly no end to the number of studies that have examined the effectiveness of one form of psychotherapy or another. On August 9, 2012, the American Psychological Association adopted a resolution on the effectiveness of psychotherapy (American Psychological Association, 2012), including a claim that "most valid and structured psychotherapies are roughly equivalent in effectiveness." What was not included in the resolution were definitions of the terms *valid* and *structured*. The fact is that the most validated (i.e., studied) and structured forms of psychotherapy come from the behavioral and cognitive-behavioral traditions.

Behavior Therapy as an Empirically Supported Treatment

In 1995, the Society of Clinical Psychology (Division 12 of the American Psychological Association) published one of the first attempts to define criteria for determining whether particular types of psychotherapy are effective for particular problems (Task Force on Promotion and Dissemination of Psychological Procedures, Division of Clinical Psychology—American Psychological Association, 1995). Several subsequent updates to the list (which is now maintained online at http://psychologicaltreatments.org) and extensive discussion and intense controversy were generated as a result of these efforts.

The criteria for empirically validated treatments define two levels of empirical support: *strong* (previously referred to as "well established") and *modest* (previously referred to as "probably efficacious"). The term *controversial* is used to describe treatments for which studies to have yielded conflicting results or for which a treatment is efficacious but claims regarding why it works are at odds with the research evidence. To meet criteria for *strong support*, a particular intervention has to have well-controlled studies showing that the treatment was superior to pill placebo, superior to another form of treatment, or equivalent to established treatments. Studies are also required to have used treatment manuals to ensure that therapists conducted the treatments as they were intended to be conducted, and the criteria require that the client samples be clearly described and that the benefits of the treatment had been shown by at least two different teams of investigator teams. The criteria for modest support are similar although somewhat less stringent. For example, to meet these criteria, it was not necessary to have the effects of treatment demonstrated by *two* independent teams of investigators (Chambless et al., 1998; Woody & Sanderson, 1998).

Currently, the list of empirically supported psychological treatments includes 77 treatments for particular disorders of which 60 are behavioral or cognitive-behavioral treatments and several others include behavioral elements (Society of Clinical Psychology, 2012). In other words, to the extent that this list is up-to-date and accurately reflects the research literature, the evidence supporting behavioral and cognitive-behavioral treatments for particular problems is much better developed than is the case for any other form of psychotherapy.

Although there is little doubt that clients should have the opportunity to receive treatments that work, disagreement remains among psychotherapists about what constitutes evidence. Some authors have criticized the list of empirically supported treatments, and the research on which the list is based, as being flawed or incomplete. For example, critics have argued that relying on manualized treatments turns therapists into technicians, rather than caring human beings, jeopardizes the therapeutic relationship, restricts clinical innovation, and encourages managed care companies and insurance companies to be overly restrictive about what treatments they will cover. In addition, some critics have argued that research studies often include participants who are different (e.g., less complicated, higher functioning) than those who show up for treatment in community mental-health clinics.

Proponents of manualized, empirically validated treatments challenge the issues raised and argue that many of these concerns are based on a misunderstanding of evidence-based treatments and the research on which they are based (e.g., Addis, 2002). Supporters of manualized therapies have argued that such treatments help therapists stay focused, facilitate the training and supervision of therapists, and help make clinicians more accountable for their work (Wilson, 1998). They also argue that manuals provide much more flexibility than is often assumed and that considerable evidence shows that the tradition of studying manual-based treatments has helped to spur numerous new treatments in the past few decades.

Collecting Data in the Therapist's Office

Treatment guidelines, such as the Society of Clinical Psychology's list of empirically supported treatments, provide therapists with important information about standard approaches to therapy that are likely to be effective for particular problems. However, although using evidence-based manualized treatments has many benefits, these approaches also have limitations. To start, many clients respond only partially to treatment and not at all in some cases. Large randomized controlled trials on which treatment guidelines are typically based provide only limited information about how to adapt a treatment for a particular client, especially if the client does not fully respond to the standard treatment.

Behavior therapy is historically an ideographic approach in which each client's treatment is tailored to the individual, based on a detailed functional analysis. Some behavior therapists argue that the question we should be asking is not whether a treatment works for a particular diagnosis but rather *which* treatment, by *whom*, is the most effective for a *particular individual* with a *particular problem*, and under *what circumstances*, as behavioral psychologist Gordon Paul (1967) famously asked several decades ago.

Although researchers have tried to identify ways of predicting who responds to particular types of treatment, Paul's question remains difficult to answer adequately through large-scale research studies. Therefore, in addition to being consumers of the research literature, therapists must also consider the specific circumstances that are relevant to their own particular clients. This is especially important in cases where there are no established treatments for a client's problem. Still, paying attention to the unique circumstances of one's client can be done with respect for the importance of objective data and a carefully controlled, empirical approach.

Taking an empirical approach in the therapy office includes (1) being aware of one's own biases about clients and their problems (e.g., not assuming that a client is necessarily going to respond to the exact same intervention that was effective for another client with the same problem), (2) being aware of one's biases about treatment (e.g., recognizing that not all clients respond to the same interventions; recognizing that clients change for many reasons, some of which may have nothing to do with the therapist or the therapy), (3) collecting data throughout the course of therapy to test out assumptions about the variables that maintain the client's problems, and (4) collecting data over the course of treatment to evaluate the effects of the intervention.

In some cases, behavior therapists use *single-case experimental designs* to evaluate the effects of treatment (e.g., Barlow, Nock, & Hersen, 2008). In single-case experimental designs, clients are first assessed before the intervention begins to establish a baseline for the target problem. Assessment continues throughout treatment, and beyond the final session to assess the long-term impact of therapy. Finally, aspects of the intervention are varied or manipulated to assess whether the changes observed, in fact, result from the intervention versus other variables.

An example of a single-case experimental design is the *reversal design*, which begins with a baseline phase followed by the introduction of the intervention. After a period, the intervention is withdrawn (return to baseline) and perhaps reintroduced and later withdrawn again. For example, if a therapist believes that reducing caffeine intake might improve a client's insomnia, treatment might initially include a one-week baseline data-collection phase in which there are no changes to caffeine intake, followed by a one-week treatment phase in which caffeine use is reduced. This might then be followed by a one-week return to baseline in which normal caffeine use is reintroduced followed by another week with no caffeine. If the therapist and client notice that the expected relationship between the use of caffeine and the ability to sleep is replicated during each phase of the intervention, then they can be confident that the intervention is indeed responsible for the observed changes. Replication is key: It would be much more difficult to know if the intervention was responsible for the change if the effect was just demonstrated once. There are limitations to the reversal design; for example, it is not useful for evaluating treatments for which benefits are expected to continue after treatment has been withdrawn (i.e., treatments that have *carryover effects*).

Psychotherapy in a Multicultural World

Several of the core principles (e.g., classical conditioning, reinforcement, punishment) and methods (e.g., exposure) underlying behavior therapy are assumed by behavior therapists to be universal and applicable across cultures and even across species: Much of our understanding about the principles of learning comes from research on nonhumans, including pioneering studies on animals conducted by Wolpe (who initially studied learning in dogs) and Skinner (who studied learning in rats and pigeons). Nevertheless, even if behavioral principles do apply across cultures, behavioral treatments are not clearly universally effective, even within the Western cultures where they were developed. There is much more to behavior therapy than just asking clients to practice behavioral techniques. Treatment occurs within the context of a therapeutic relationship, and there are many ways in which culture can affect the relationship between therapist and client and the acceptability of treatment, ultimately affecting the client's willingness to work within a behavioral framework.

Consider a client who has been offered exposure therapy for OCD. If the client accepts that the behavioral model for OCD makes sense and believes that exposure to feared stimuli combined with prevention of compulsive rituals will help, then the likelihood of compliance and success will be high. But what if the client is convinced that the OCD symptoms are caused by demonic possession and that the only way to control the symptoms is to distract from the intrusive thoughts and avoid the situations that trigger them? Or what if the client believes that the only acceptable way to overcome a problem is through prayer? For these individuals, it may not matter that exposure is an "effective approach" because the individual may be unwilling to try exposure.

A challenge in behavior therapy is finding ways to encourage clients to use methods that may not fit with their cultural assumptions and beliefs or to adapt behavioral methods so they are more consistent with the client's values or expectations. Increasingly, therapists are being taught to adopt a more culturally responsive approach to behavior therapy and CBT (Hays & Iwamasa, 2006), including being more aware of their own biases, learning about the cultures of their clients from a variety of sources (other than just the client), and learning about the unique ways in which one's clients have been influenced by their cultural experiences. When behavior therapists think about the effects of the environment on a client's behavior, they need to incorporate cultural influences into their definition of what constitutes the *environment*, including both positive and negative cultural influences (Hays, 2006).

Culture can influence a client's behaviors and response to treatment in many ways. Cultures in which seeking practical advice from health-care professions is a valued way of dealing with behavioral problems may be more suited for behavioral therapies than cultures where it is more acceptable to turn to prayer and counsel with one's spiritual leaders for emotional healing. Culture may also affect the client's reactions to the therapist (including the therapist's gender or manner of dressing, for example). Cultural differences between therapist and client may create language barriers that make psychotherapy difficult, or they may affect a client's trust in the therapist. For example, Native American clients are profoundly aware of their people's history of mistreatment from European Americans, and some Native American clients may find it difficult to trust therapists from a European ancestry (McDonald & Gonzalez, 2006).

For most psychotherapies, there is relatively little research on treating individuals from ethnic minority groups, and behavior therapy is no exception. Nevertheless, a handful of studies show that behavior therapy and CBT are effective for both ethnic minority groups living in Western countries, as well as individuals living in non-Western countries. For example, Hinton et al. (2005) showed that CBT could be successfully adapted for Cambodian refugees with treatment-resistant PTSD and panic attacks. Similarly, a culturally adapted course of CBT was found to be an effective addition to medication treatment for depression and anxiety symptoms in a study conducted in Pakistan comparing CBT plus antidepressants versus antidepressants alone (Naeem, Waheed, Gobbi, Ayub, & Kingdon, 2011). For a comprehensive review of the application of CBT across diverse cultural groups, see Hays and Iwamasa (2006).

CASE EXAMPLE

Background

Simon was a 40-year-old college professor who was married and had two children, ages 5 and 12. He lived in a midsized college town about a 2-hour drive from the city where he grew up. Simon was raised by his parents, along with his two older brothers, and he described his childhood as generally happy. As a child he had several close friends, despite being somewhat shy and anxious around new people. In high school, he found it more difficult to make friends and spent much of his time alone or with his family. He reported being teased regularly by his high school peers. He felt inferior to the more popular students in school, whom he perceived to be more attractive and more athletic than he was. Simon's anxiety around other people increased during his high school years and continued throughout college.

Simon met his wife when they were both completing their doctorates, and they started dating about a year after they met (after she asked him out). Simon described his relationship with his wife as supportive and close. He reported that although his wife enjoyed socializing, she had stopped spending time with many of her friends because she knew that Simon preferred her to spend time with him and their family and because he was unwilling to socialize with other couples because of his anxiety.

Problem

The main problem that brought Simon into treatment was heightened fear and avoidance in social situations, including public speaking, being the center of attention, meeting new people, casual conversations, parties, meetings, and talking on the phone. Although he reported feeling comfortable around his family and a few close friends from college, he experienced elevated anxiety when interacting with strangers or with students and colleagues at work. Being in these situations typically led to sweating, shaky hands, racing heart, and difficulty focusing. He avoided office parties whenever possible, typically ate lunch alone, and only went to meetings when absolutely necessary.

Simon completed several self-report questionnaires as part of his assessment. His score on the Social Interaction Anxiety Scale (SIAS; Mattick & Clarke, 1998) was 42, indicating a moderate level of anxiety in situations involving social interaction (e.g., parties, conversations). His score on the Social Phobia Scale (SPS; Mattick & Clarke, 1998) was 38, suggesting a moderate level of anxiety in performance-related situations (e.g., public speaking, being the center of attention). Simon also completed a behavioral approach test (BAT), involving a 10-minute simulated conversation with a stranger (an unfamiliar therapist at the clinic where he was being treated). During the BAT, Simon reported a peak anxiety level of 75 out 100, as well as several physical sensations, including sweating and racing heart.

Although Simon didn't avoid his teaching responsibilities, he used various strategies (known as *safety behaviors*) to manage his anxiety in the classroom, including lecturing with the lights dimmed, showing videos in class (instead of speaking), wearing T-shirts (to reduce the likelihood of sweating in front of the class), and avoiding eye contact with students (hoping that the lack of eye contact would make the students less likely to ask questions that he might be unable to answer). Simon's biggest fear was that he might be embarrassed or humiliated in front of others and that people would view him as boring, incompetent, or anxious.

By all accounts, Simon's teaching skills were excellent as reflected by very strong teaching evaluations. Furthermore, his colleagues seemed to enjoy his company. In the past, they had frequently invited him to join them for lunch, although the invitations had stopped over the years, presumably because he always turned them down. In social situations, Simon often avoided eye contact, and he had difficulty finding the right words to start a conversation. His goal for therapy was to feel more comfortable in social situations.

Simon received a diagnosis of *social anxiety disorder*. He had a long-standing history of shyness and social anxiety that appeared to be exacerbated during high school, perhaps as a consequence of his frequent teasing (i.e., classical conditioning). At the time of his assessment, Simon's fear appeared to be maintained by his avoidance of social situations and his reliance on safety behaviors to manage his anxiety. These behaviors were likely reinforced—by both the relief that Simon experienced when he avoided social situations and his wife's tendency to accommodate his social anxiety and avoid socializing herself (i.e., operant conditioning). Simon's fear also seemed to be related to his belief that he was likely to be negatively evaluated by others in social situations and that he might not be able to cope with negative evaluation if it did happen. Finally, Simon reported several social-skills deficits, particularly around making eye contact with others and making small talk. His difficulty in these situations was confirmed by his wife (who joined Simon for part of the interview), and it was also observed by Simon's therapist during his assessment.

Treatment

Simon's treatment included five main components: education, cognitive strategies, exposure, reduction of safety behaviors, and social-skills training. The final session focused on teaching Simon strategies to maintain his gains and prevent relapse.

Education (Session 1).   The focus of the first session was education about the nature of social anxiety and its treatment. Simon learned about the relationships among his thoughts, feelings, and behaviors, especially about the ways in which his thoughts and behaviors maintain his anxiety over time. For example, he learned that although avoidance leads to a reduction of anxiety in the short term, it helps maintain anxiety over the long term by preventing him from learning that the situations he fears are actually safe.

For homework, Simon was encouraged to read several introductory chapters from the *Shyness and Social Anxiety Workbook* (Antony & Swinson, 2008).

Cognitive Strategies (Sessions 2 and 3).   Simon was taught to identify times when his thoughts contributed to heightened anxiety, with an emphasis on *probability overestimations* (i.e., overestimating the likelihood of bad things happening—for example, assuming that others will judge him negatively) and *catastrophic thinking* (i.e., overestimating the impact of a negative event or underestimating his ability to cope—for example, assuming that it would be a disaster if his performance in class was less than perfect). Simon was taught to examine the evidence for his beliefs and to consider alternative ways of interpreting situations, with the goal of helping him to think more flexibly about the situations he feared. Although cognitive strategies were the primary focus in sessions 2 and 3, some time was also devoted to these strategies during subsequent sessions. Homework included completing thought records, conducting *behavioral experiments* (e.g., purposely making mistakes in class and evaluating the outcome), and completing readings on the use of cognitive strategies for social anxiety (Antony & Swinson, 2008).

Exposure (Sessions 4–10).   A detailed rationale for exposure therapy was introduced at session 4, including guidelines for maximizing the effectiveness of exposure (e.g., ensuring that exposure practices are frequent and prolonged, with maximum predictability and control, and minimal use of safety behaviors). At first, Simon's exposure practices consisted of behavioral role plays. For example, Simon practiced simulated exposures involving conversations with "colleagues" as role played by his therapist (during therapy sessions) and his wife (at home during homework practices). By session 6, treatment incorporated in vivo exposure practices involving speaking with colleagues, encouraging students to ask questions in class, having lunch with colleagues, socializing with other couples, and a variety of other feared situations. Homework included practicing repeated exposures to feared social situations, continuing to use the cognitive strategies, and completing readings on the use of exposure for reducing anxiety (Antony & Swinson, 2008).

Reduction of Safety Behaviors (Sessions 6–10).   At session 6, Simon was encouraged to start reducing his reliance on safety behaviors in combination with his ongoing exposure practices. For example, he purposely wore a warm shirt to class and allowed himself to sweat while lecturing. He made eye contact with students in class, kept the lights up bright while lecturing, and reduced the amount of time spent showing videos. Finally, he asked his wife to stop accommodating his anxiety behaviors. She was instead encouraged to socialize with friends, regardless of whether Simon was willing to join them, and to invite Simon to socialize as well. Homework involved continuing to practice the strategies learned up to this point.

Social–Skills Training (Sessions 9 and 10).   During the last 2 sessions of treatment, Simon practiced improving his eye contact and making small talk with others. Simon completed the number of simulated exposure practices that were videotaped to provide him with an opportunity to observe his behavior in social situations. He and his therapist then watched the video and discussed strategies that he might use for increasing his eye contact and making small talk more comfortably. Simon also integrated social-skills rehearsal into his exposure practices during the final weeks of treatment, both in session and during homework.

Relapse Prevention (Session 11).   In the final session of treatment, Simon and his therapist reviewed Simon's progress and discussed strategies for maintaining his gains, including continuing to complete thought records when feeling anxious and occasionally practicing exposure to the situations that he previously feared. Simon was encouraged to contact his therapist if he noticed his anxiety levels increasing again.

Resolution

By the end of treatment, Simon reported significant reductions in his anxiety. His score on the SIAS had decreased from 42 to 19 and was now in the mild range. His score on the SPS decreased from 38 to 22, also in the mild range. Simon also repeated the same BAT that he had completed at the start of treatment. He reported only a minimal increase in heart rate during his posttreatment BAT and a peak anxiety level of 30 out of 100 (vs. 75 out of 100 before treatment). By the end of treatment, Simon rarely avoided social situations. He and his wife socialized with other couples every few weeks, he now ate lunch with colleagues at least once per week, and he no longer relied on his safety behaviors while teaching. Despite his reduction in avoidance, he still experienced some anxiety in anticipation of social encounters, but his anxiety level typically decreased shortly after entering the situation.

Follow-Up

Simon was seen for a follow-up visit six weeks after the end of treatment. The gains he had made over the course of therapy were maintained, based on his report during the visit as well as his scores on the SIAS and SPS, which were essentially unchanged from his posttreatment assessment.

SUMMARY

Since its development in the 1950s, behavior therapy has been a thriving, evolving approach to psychotherapy, rooted in the scientific method and empirically supported principles of learning. In the past 20 years, therapists have increasingly been held accountable by their clients as well as insurance companies to offer brief, cost-effective, and efficacious treatments. This shift has led to an expansion in the role of behavior therapy and CBT for treating a wide array of psychological problems, as well as certain health conditions.

Behavior therapy differs from many other approaches in that it is brief, evidence based, directive, active, collaborative, and focused on the factors thought to maintain problem behaviors, rather than those that may have triggered a problem initially. Its roots are in early research on classical and operant conditioning, although over the years behavior therapy has expanded to incorporate cognitive strategies and, more recently, mindfulness and acceptance-based approaches.

Behavior therapy has been shown to be effective for treating a wide range of problems, including phobias, social anxiety disorder, panic disorder, generalized anxiety disorder, OCD, trauma-related disorders, depression, substance-use disorders, schizophrenia, eating disorders, sexual dysfunction, behavioral disorders of childhood, sleep disorders, borderline personality disorder, impulse-control disorders, and couple distress, as well as improving healthy lifestyle behaviors such as exercise and compliance with medical treatments.

Behavior therapy incorporates many techniques, including behavioral assessment, functional analysis, exposure-based strategies, response prevention, operant-conditioning strategies (e.g., reinforcement, aversive conditioning), relaxation training, stimulus-control procedures, modeling, behavioral activation, social-skills training, problem-solving training, acceptance-based approaches, and cognitive strategies, to name a few. Like most other psychotherapies, more research is needed on the effectiveness of behavior therapy across diverse groups, although emerging evidence generally supports the notion that behavioral treatments can be helpful across cultures, ages, and other diverse domains.

Future Directions in Behavior Therapy

For the last 60 years, a main emphasis of behavior therapy research has been on the development and evaluation of behavioral treatments. Now that behavioral treatments are well established, the focus of research is gradually shifting. The following topics are especially important emerging areas of research.

Improving Effectiveness. Although evidence-based interventions exist for most major psychological disorders, many individuals obtain only partial relief from these treatments, and some do not benefit at all. Therefore, researchers are working on finding ways to enhance our existing treatments so that more people can benefit (e.g., Antony et al., 2005). Improvements to existing treatments will first require a better understanding of the factors that contribute to outcome and effective methods of measuring the unique barriers to improvement for particular clients.

Understanding the Mechanisms Underlying Treatment. Behavior therapists have always been committed to understanding why various treatments work, and this continues to be an important area of research. With the expansion of behavior therapy to include mindfulness- and acceptance-based strategies, for example, researchers have been studying the mechanisms underlying these new approaches, trying to better understand how their goals, mechanisms, and methods are similar and different from traditional behavioral and cognitive-behavioral treatments (e.g., Arch & Craske, 2008).

Enhancing Dissemination. There is a widely recognized gap between the availability of effective behavioral treatments and the use of these treatments in clinical practice. In recent years, CBT researchers have attempted to address the gap, and several studies have begun to look at ways to increase the use of evidence-based treatments in nonresearch settings and improve access to these treatments by those who stand to most benefit from them (e.g., McHugh & Barlow, 2012).

The Role of Cognitive Enhancers Such as D–Cycloserine (DCS). Until a few years ago, DCS was mostly known for its past use as an antibiotic for treating tuberculosis. More recently, however, DCS has become better known for its ability to enhance extinction learning during exposure therapy for a range of anxiety disorders (in addition to its antibiotic effects, DCS is a partial agonist of N-methyl-D-aspartate glutamatergic receptors in the brain, which are involved in learning and memory). Taken shortly before exposure practices, DCS (compared to placebo) has been found to enhance the effects of exposure within sessions and to speed up effects of exposure across sessions so that clients can be treated more quickly (for a meta-analytic review, see Bontempo, Panza, & Bloch, 2012). Despite emerging evidence supporting DCS for augmenting the effects of exposure, questions remain, including: (1) Which learning processes are targeted by DCS during exposure therapy? (2) Can DCS enhance the effects of other behavioral or cognitive-behavioral strategies? (3) What is the optimal way to administer DCS (dosage, frequency, timing)? (4) Might DCS enhance behavioral treatments for problems other than anxiety disorders?

Adapting Behavior Therapy for Diverse Populations.   Research on behavior therapy has not paid adequate attention to the effectiveness of behavioral treatments in diverse populations, including people from varied cultural backgrounds, religious affiliations, levels of physical disability, sexual orientations, levels of education, socioeconomic status, ages, and other ways in which people differ. Although this is beginning to change (e.g., Hays & Iwamasa, 2006; Martell, Safren, & Prince, 2004), more work is needed to best understand the ways in which behavioral treatments need to be adapted for people with diverse backgrounds.

Counseling CourseMate Website:

See this text's Counseling CourseMate website at www.cengagebrain.com for learning tools such as chapter quizzing, videos, glossary flashcards, and more.

CONCLUSION

Behavior therapy (and CBT) are the most researched and best-supported approaches to psychotherapy. Behavioral treatments are here to stay, although their boundaries will likely continue to expand and shift in response to new scientific findings and societal pressures.

ANNOTATED BIBLIOGRAPHY AND WEB RESOURCES

Antony, M. M., & Roemer, L. (2011). *Behavior therapy.* Washington, DC: American Psychological Association.
This book provides an overview of both the theory and practice of behavior therapy. It reviews the history of behavior therapy, theoretical foundations, contemporary behavior therapy techniques, evidence for the effectiveness of behavior therapy, and future developments in the field.

Haynes, S. N., O'Brien, W. H., & Kaholokula, J. K. (2011). *Behavioral assessment and case formulation.* Hoboken, NJ: John Wiley & Sons.
Behavioral assessment is an integral part of the behavior therapy process. This book provides an up-to-date discussion of behavioral assessment and case formulation, including detailed information on functional analysis, as well as descriptions of the most frequently used behavioral-assessment techniques.

O'Donohue, W. T., & Fisher, J. E. (2012). *Cognitive behavior therapy: Core principles for practice.* Hoboken, NJ: John Wiley & Sons.
This contemporary guide includes chapters by leading experts covering many of the most important behavior therapy strategies, including skills training, exposure therapy, relaxation-based strategies, problem-solving training, behavioral activation, acceptance-based approaches, cognitive restructuring, and others.

Roemer, L., & Orsillo, S. M. (2009). *Mindfulness- and acceptance-based behavioral therapies in practice.* New York: Guilford Press.
This practical book provides a unified framework for integrating mindfulness- and acceptance-based behavioral strategies into clinical practice. It covers strategies from several different approaches, including mindfulness-based cognitive therapy, mindfulness-based relapse prevention, acceptance and commitment therapy, and dialectical behavior therapy.

Spiegler, M. D., & Guevremont, D. C. (2010). *Contemporary behavior therapy* (5th ed.). Belmont, CA: Wadsworth Cengage Learning.
This established text provides a comprehensive survey of contemporary behavior therapy, discussing underlying theory, relevant research, and the foundations of clinical practice and core techniques. The book takes a multidisciplinary approach, covering applications for psychology, education, social work, nursing, and rehabilitation.

CASE READINGS

Barlow, D. (1993). Covert sensitization for paraphilia. In J. R. Cautela, A. J. Kearney, L. Ascher, A. Kearney, & M. Kleinman (Eds.), *Covert conditioning casebook* (pp. 188–197). Pacific Grove, CA: Thomson Learning. [Reprinted in D. Wedding & R. J. Corsini (Eds.). (2013). *Case studies in psychotherapy* (7th ed.). Belmont, CA: Brooks/Cole-Cengage Learning.]

This detailed case illustrates the use of covert sensitization in the treatment of pedophilia in a 51-year-old minister.

Boisseau, C. L., Farchione, T. J., Fairholme, C. P., Ellard, K. K., & Barlow, D. H. (2010). The development of the unified protocol for the trans diagnostic treatment of emotional disorders: A case study. *Cognitive and Behavioral Practice, 17,* 102–113.

This case study describes the use of a cognitive-behavioral protocol for treating disorders of emotion (e.g., anxiety disorders, depression) regardless of the specific diagnosis.

Martin-Pichora, A. L., & Antony, M. M. (2011). Successful treatment of olfactory reference syndrome with cognitive behavioral therapy: A case study. *Cognitive and Behavioral Practice, 18,* 545–554.

This case describes the successful treatment of a woman suffering from olfactory reference syndrome, a problem in which individuals are convinced that they emit an offensive odor. This is the first published study on the behavioral treatment of this problem.

Peterson, B. D., Eifert, G. H., Feingold, T., & Davidson, S. (2009). Using acceptance and commitment therapy to treat distressed couples: A case study with 2 couples. *Cognitive and Behavioral Practice, 16,* 430–442.

This case study demonstrates the use of acceptance and commitment therapy (an acceptance-based behavioral treatment) for treating relationship distress.

REFERENCES

Abramowitz, J. S., Deacon, B. J., & Whiteside, S. P. H. (2011). *Exposure therapy for anxiety: Principles and practice.* New York: Guilford Press.

Addis, M. E. (2002). Methods for disseminating research products and increasing evidence-based practice: Promises, obstacles, and future directions. *Clinical Psychology: Science and Practice, 9,* 367–378.

Alden, L. (2005). Modeling. In M. Hersen & J. Rosqvist (Eds.), *Encyclopedia of behavior modification and cognitive behavior therapy: Vol. 1. Adult clinical applications* (pp. 375–379). Thousand Oaks, CA: Sage.

Allport, G. W., & Odbert, H. S. (1936). Trait names: A psycho-lexical study. *Psychological Monographs, 47,* No. 211.

American Psychological Association (2012, August 9). Resolution on the recognition of psychotherapy effectiveness—Approved August 2012. Retrieved from www.apa.org/news/press/releases/2012/08/resolution-psychotherapy.aspx.

Antony, M. M., Ledley, D. R., & Heimberg, R. G. (Eds.) (2005). *Improving outcomes and preventing relapse in cognitive behavioral therapy.* New York: Guilford Press.

Antony, M. M., Ledley, D. R., Liss, A., & Swinson, R. P. (2006). Responses to symptom induction exercises in panic disorder. *Behaviour Research and Therapy, 44,* 85–98.

Antony, M. M., & Roemer, L. (2011). *Behavior therapy.* Washington, DC: American Psychological Association.

Antony, M. M., & Stein, M. B. (Eds.) (2009). *Oxford handbook of anxiety and related disorders.* New York: Oxford University Press.

Antony, M. M., & Swinson, R. P. (2008). *Shyness and social anxiety workbook: Proven, step-by-step techniques for overcoming your fear* (2nd edition). Oakland, CA: New Harbinger Publications.

Arch, J. J., & Craske, M. G. (2008). Acceptance and commitment therapy and cognitive behavioral therapy for anxiety disorders: Different treatments, similar mechanisms? *Clinical Psychology: Science and Practice, 15,* 263–279.

Ayllon, T., & Azrin, N. H. (1968). *The token economy. A motivational system for therapy and rehabilitation.* New York: Appleton-Century-Crofts.

Bandura, A. (1969). *Principles of behavior modification.* New York: Holt, Rinehart & Winston.

Bandura, A. (1986). *Social foundations of thought and action: A social cognitive theory.* Englewood Cliffs, NJ: W. H. Freeman.

Barlow, D. (1993). Covert sensitization for paraphilia. In J. R. Cautela, A. J. Kearney, L. Ascher, A. Kearney, &

M. Kleinman (Eds.), *Covert conditioning casebook* (pp. 188–197). Pacific Grove, CA: Thomson Learning.

Barlow, D. H., Nock, M. K., & Hersen, M. (2008). *Single case experimental designs: Strategies for studying behavior change (3rd ed.).* Boston: Allyn and Bacon.

Benjamin, L. T., & Baker, D. B. (Eds.) (2000). History of psychology: The Boulder conference. *American Psychologist, 55,* 233–254.

Bernstein, D. A., Borkovec, T. D., & Hazlett-Stevens, H. (2000). *New directions in progressive relaxation training: A guidebook for helping professionals.* Westport, CT: Praeger.

Bontempo, A., Panza, K. E., & Bloch, M. H. (2012). D-cycloserine augmentation of behavioral therapy for the treatment of anxiety disorders: A meta-analysis. *Journal of Clinical Psychiatry, 73,* 533–537.

Cattell, H. B. (1989). *The 16PF: Personality in depth.* Champaign, IL: Institute for Personality and Ability Testing.

Cattell, R. B. (1943). The description of personality: Basic traits resolved into clusters. *Journal of Abnormal and Social Psychology, 38,* 476–506.

Cattell, R. B. (1946). *The description and measurement of personality.* New York: Harcourt, Brace, & World.

Chambless, D. L., Baker, M. J., Baucom, D. H., Beutler, L. E., Calhoun, K. S., Crits-Christoph, P., Crits-Christoph, P., Daiuto, A., DeRubeis, R., Detweiler, J., Haaga, D. A. F., Johnson, S. B., McCurry, S., Mueser, K. T., Pope, K. S., Sanderson, W. C., Shoham, V., Stickle, T., Williams, D. A., & Woody, S. R. (1998). Update on empirically validated therapies, II. *The Clinical Psychologist, 51*(1), 3–14.

Costa, P. T., Jr., & McCrae, R. R. (1992). *Revised NEO Personality Inventory (NEO-PI-R) and NEO Five-Factor Inventory (NEO-FFI) manual.* Odessa, FL: Psychological Assessment Resources.

Cuijpers, P., van Straten, A., Andersson, G., & van Oppen, P. (2008). Psychotherapy for depression in adults: A meta-analysis of comparative outcome studies. *Journal of Consulting and Clinical Psychology, 76,* 909–922.

Cuijpers, P., van Straten, A., E., Driessen, van Oppen, P., Bockting, C., & Andersson, G. (2012). Depression and dysthymic disorder. In P. Sturmey & M. Hersen (Eds.), *Handbook of evidence-based practice in clinical psychology: Vol. II. Adult disorders* (pp. 243–284). Hoboken, NJ: John Wiley & Sons.

Ellis, A. (2001). The rise of cognitive behavior therapy. In W. T. O'Donohue, D. A. Henderson, S. C. Hayes, J. E. Fisher, & L. J. Hayes (Eds.), *A history of the behavioral therapies: Founders' personal histories* (pp. 183–194). Reno, NV: Context Press.

Febbraro, G. A. R., Clum, G. A., Roodman, A. A., & Wright, J. H. (1999). The limits of bibliotherapy: A study of the differential effectiveness of self-administered interventions in individuals with panic attacks. *Behavior Therapy, 30,* 209–222.

Fisher, W. W., Piazza, C. C., & Roane, H. S. (Eds.) (2011). *Handbook of applied behavior analysis.* New York: Guilford Press.

Foa, E. B., Huppert, J. D., & Cahill, S. P. (2006). Emotional processing theory: An update. In B. O. Rothbaum (Ed.), *Pathological anxiety: Emotional processing in etiology and treatment.* (pp. 3–24). New York: Guilford Press.

Foa, E. B., & Kozak, M. J. (1986). Emotional processing of fear: Exposure to corrective information. *Psychological Bulletin, 99,* 20–35.

Franks, C. M. (1963). Behavior therapy, the principles of conditioning, and the treatment of the alcoholic. *Quarterly Journal of Studies on Alcohol. 24,* 511–529.

Franks, C. M. (2001). From psychodynamic to behavior therapy: Paradigm shift and personal perspectives. In W. T. O'Donohue, D. A. Henderson, S. C. Hayes, J. E. Fisher, & L. J. Hayes (Eds.), *A history of the behavioral therapies: Founders' personal histories* (pp. 195–206). Reno, NV: Context Press.

Franks, C. M., & Wilson, G. T. (1978). *Annual review of behavior therapy: Theory and practice (Vol. 5: 1977).* New York: Brunner/Mazel.

Gooding, P., & Tarrier, N. (2009). A systematic review and meta-analysis of cognitive-behavioural interventions to reduce problem gambling: Hedging our bets? *Behaviour Research and Therapy, 47,* 592–607.

Hallgren, K. A., Greenfield, B. L., Ladd, B., Glynn, L. H., & McCrady, B. S. (2012). Alcohol use disorders. In P. Sturmey & M. Hersen (Eds.), *Handbook of evidence-based practice in clinical psychology: Vol. II—Adult disorders* (pp. 133–165). Hoboken, NJ: John Wiley & Sons.

Hayes, S. C., Follette, V. M., & Linehan, M. M. (2004). *Mindfulness and acceptance: Expanding the cognitive-behavioral tradition.* New York: Guilford Press.

Hayes, S. C., Strosahl, K. D., & Wilson, K. G. (2012). *Acceptance and commitment therapy: The process and practice of mindful change* (2nd ed.). New York: Guilford Press.

Hayes, S. C., Villatte, M., Levin, M., & Hildebrandt, M. (2011). Open, aware, and active: Contextual approaches as an emerging trend in the behavioral and cognitive therapies. *Annual Review of Clinical Psychology, 7,* 141–168.

Hays, P. A. (2006). Introduction: Developing culturally responsive cognitive-behavioral therapies. In P. A. Hays & G. Y. Iwamasa (Eds.), *Culturally responsive cognitive-behavioral therapy: Assessment, practice, and supervision* (pp. 3–20). Washington, DC: American Psychological Association.

Hays, P. A., & Iwamasa, G. Y. (Eds.). (2006). *Culturally responsive cognitive-behavioral therapy: Assessment, practice, and supervision.* Washington, DC: American Psychological Association.

Hazlett-Stevens, H., & Bernstein, D. A. (2012). Relaxation. In W. T. O'Donohue & J. E. Fisher (Eds.), *Cognitive behavior therapy: Core principles for practice* (pp. 105–132). Hoboken, NJ: John Wiley & Sons.

Hersen, M., & Rosqvist, J. (Eds.) (2005). *Encyclopedia of behavior modification and cognitive behavior therapy: Vol. 1. Adult clinical applications.* Thousand Oaks, CA: Sage.

Hinton, D. E., Chhean, D., Pich, V., Hofmann, S. G., Pollack, M. H., & Safren, S. A. (2005). A randomized controlled trial of cognitive behavior therapy for Cambodian refugees with treatment resistant PTSD and panic attacks: A cross-over design. *Journal of Traumatic Stress, 18,* 617–629.

Hofmann, S. G., & Asmundson, G. J. (2008). Acceptance and mindfulness-based therapy: New wave or old hat? *Clinical Psychology Review, 28,* 1–16.

Hood, H. K., & Antony, M. M. (2012). Evidence-based assessment and treatment of specific phobias in adults. In T. E. Davis, T. H. Ollendick, & L. -G. Öst (Eds.), *Intensive one-session treatment of specific phobias* (pp. 19–42). New York: Springer.

Itard, J. -M. -G. (1962). *The wild boy of Aveyron.* New York: Meredith Company.

Jacobson, E. (1938). *Progressive relaxation.* Chicago: University of Chicago Press.

Jones, C., & Meaden, A. (2012). Schizophrenia. In P. Sturmey & M. Hersen (Eds.), *Handbook of evidence-based practice in clinical psychology: Vol. II—Adult disorders* (pp. 221–242). Hoboken, NJ: John Wiley & Sons.

Jones, M. C. (1924). A laboratory study of fear: The case of Peter. *Journal of General Psychology, 31,* 308–315.

Kabat-Zinn, J. (1994). *Wherever you go, there you are: Mindfulness meditation in everyday life.* New York: Hyperion.

Kagan, J. (1997). *Galen's prophecy: Temperament in human nature.* Boulder, CO: Westview Press.

Kanter, J. W., & Puspitasari, A. J. (2012). Behavioral activation. In W. T. O'Donohue & J. E. Fisher (Eds.), *Cognitive behavior therapy: Core principles for practice* (pp. 215–250). Hoboken, NJ: John Wiley & Sons.

Kinnaman, J. E. S., & Bellack, A. S. (2012). Social skills. In W. T. O'Donohue & J. E. Fisher (Eds.), *Cognitive behavior therapy: Core principles for practice* (pp. 251–272). Hoboken, NJ: John Wiley & Sons.

Kliem, S., Kröger, C., & Kosfelder, J. (2010). Dialectical behavior therapy for borderline personality disorder: A meta-analysis using mixed-effects modeling. *Journal of Consulting and Clinical Psychology, 78,* 936–951.

Koerner, N., Vorstenbosch, V., & Antony, M. M. (2012). Panic disorder. In P. Sturmey & M. Hersen (Eds.), *Handbook of evidence-based practice in clinical psychology: Vol. II—Adult disorders* (pp. 313–335). Hoboken, NJ: John Wiley & Sons.

Lang, P. J., Melamed, B. G., & Hart, J. (1970). A psychophysiological analysis of fear modification using an automated desensitization procedure. *Journal of Abnormal Psychology, 76,* 220–234.

Lazarus, A. A. (1958). New methods of psychotherapy: A case study. *South African Medical Journal, 33,* 660–664.

Lazarus, A. A. (2001). A brief personal account of CT (conditioning therapy), BT (behavior therapy, and CBT (cognitive-behavior therapy): Spanning three continents. In W. T. O'Donohue, D. A. Henderson, S. C. Hayes, J. E. Fisher, & L. J. Hayes (Eds.), *A history of the behavioral therapies: Founders' personal histories* (pp. 155–162). Reno, NV: Context Press.

Lindsley, O. R., Skinner, B. F., & Solomon, H. C. (1953). *Studies in behavior therapy* (Status report 1). Waltham, MA: Metropolitan State Hospital.

Linehan, M. M. (1993). *Cognitive-behavioral treatment for borderline personality disorder.* New York: Guilford Press.

Lynch, T. R., Trost, W. T., Salsman, N., & Linehan, M. M. (2007). Dialectical behavior therapy for borderline personality disorder. *Annual Review of Clinical Psychology, 3,* 181–205.

Martell, C. R., Dimidjian, S., & Herman-Dunn, R. (2010). *Behavioral activation for depression: A clinician's guide.* New York: Guilford Press.

Martell, C. R., Safren, S. A., & Prince, S. E. (2004). *Cognitive behavioral therapies with lesbian, gay, and bisexual clients.* New York: Guilford Press.

Mattick, R. P., & Clarke, J. C. (1998). Development and validation of measures of social phobia scrutiny fear and social interaction anxiety. *Behaviour Research and Therapy, 36,* 455–470.

McDonald, J. D., & Gonzalez, J. (2006). Cognitive-behavioral therapy with American Indians. In P. A. Hays & G. Y. Iwamasa (Eds.), *Culturally responsive cognitive-behavioral therapy: Assessment, practice, and supervision* (pp. 23–45). Washington, DC: American Psychological Association.

McHugh, R. K., & Barlow, D. H. (2012). *Dissemination and implementation of evidence-based psychological interventions.* New York: Oxford University Press.

Miller, W. R., & Carroll, K. M. (Eds.) (2006). *Rethinking substance abuse: What the science shows, and what we should do about it.* New York: Guilford Press.

Miller, W. R., & Rollnick, S. (2013). *Motivational interviewing: Helping people change* (3rd ed.). New York: Guilford Press.

Mischel, W. (1968). *Personality and assessment.* New York: John Wiley & Sons.

Moscovitch, D. A., Antony, M. M., & Swinson, R. P. (2009). Exposure-based treatments for anxiety disorders: Theory and process. In M. M. Antony & M. B. Stein (Eds.), *Oxford handbook of anxiety and related disorders* (pp. 461–475). New York: Oxford University Press.

Mowrer, O. H., & Mowrer, W. M. (1938). Enuresis: A method for its study and treatment. *American Journal of Orthopsychiatry, 8,* 436–459.

Mueser, K. T., & Jeste, D. V. (2008). *Clinical handbook of schizophrenia.* New York: Guilford Press.

Naeem, F., Waheed, W., Gobbi, M., Ayub, M., & Kingdon, D. (2011). Preliminary evaluation of culturally sensitive CBT for depression in Pakistan: Findings from Developing Culturally Sensitive CBT Project (DCCP). *Behavioural and Cognitive Psychotherapy, 39,* 165–173.

Nathan, P. E., & Gorman, J. M. (Eds.) (2007). *A guide to treatments that work* (3rd ed.). New York: Oxford University Press.

Nezu, A. M., & Nezu, C. M. (2012). Problem solving. In W. T. O'Donohue & J. E. Fisher (Eds.), *Cognitive behavior therapy: Core principles for practice* (pp. 159–182). Hoboken, NJ: John Wiley & Sons.

Norcross, J. C. (Ed.) (2011). *Psychotherapy relationships that work: Evidence-based responsiveness* (2nd ed.). New York: Oxford University Press.

Olatunji, B. O., Cisler, J. M., & Deacon, B. J. (2010). Efficacy of cognitive behavioral therapy for anxiety disorders: a review of meta-analytic findings. *Psychiatric Clinics of North America, 33,* 557–577.

Paul, G. L. (1967). Strategy of outcome research in psychotherapy. *Journal of Consulting Psychology, 31,* 109–118.

Pavlov, I. P. (1927). *Conditioned reflexes: An investigation of the physiological activity of the cerebral cortex.* London: Oxford University Press.

Piet, J., & Hougaard, E. (2011). The effect of mindfulness-based cognitive therapy for prevention of relapse in recurrent major depressive disorder: A systematic review and meta-analysis. *Clinical Psychology Review, 31,* 1032–1040.

Poling, A., & Gaynor, S. T. (2009). Stimulus control. In W. T. O'Donohue & J. E. Fisher (Eds.), *General principles and empirically supported principles of cognitive behavior therapy* (pp. 600–607). Hoboken, NJ: John Wiley & Sons.

Segal, Z. V., Williams, J. M. G., & Teasdale, J. D. (2013). *Mindfulness-based cognitive therapy for depression* (2nd ed.). New York: Guilford Press.

Segrin, C. (2009). Social skills training. In W. T. O'Donohue & J. E. Fisher (Eds.), *General principles and empirically supported principles of cognitive behavior therapy* (pp. 600–607). Hoboken, NJ: John Wiley & Sons.

Skinner, B. F. (1938). *The behavior of organisms.* New York: Appleton-Century.

Smith, M. T., Perlis, M. L., Park, A., Smith, M. S., Pennington, J., Giles, D. E., & Buysse, D. J. (2002). Comparative meta-analysis of pharmacotherapy and behavior therapy for persistent insomnia. *American Journal of Psychiatry, 159,* 5–11.

Society of Clinical Psychology. (2012). *Website on research-supported psychological treatments.* Retrieved August 31, 2012, from www.div12.org/PsychologicalTreatments/index.html

Sturmey, P., & Hersen, M. (Eds.) (2012), *Handbook of evidence based practice in clinical psychology: Volume II – Adult disorders.* Hoboken, NJ: John Wiley & Sons.

Task Force on Promotion and Dissemination of Psychological Procedures [Division of Clinical Psychology—American Psychological Association]. (1995). Training in and dissemination of empirically validated psychological treatments: Report and recommendations. *The Clinical Psychologist, 48*(1), 3–23.

Thorndike, E. L. (1911). *Animal intelligence: Experimental studies.* New York: Macmillan.

Touyz, S. W., Polivy, J., & Hay, P. (2008). *Eating disorders.* Göttingen, Germany: Hogrefe.

Vedel, E., & Emmelkamp, P. M. G. (2012). Illicit substance-related disorders. In P. Sturmey & M. Hersen (Eds.), *Handbook of evidence-based practice in clinical psychology: Vol. II—Adult disorders* (pp. 197–220). Hoboken, NJ: John Wiley & Sons.

Vorstenbosch, V., Newman, L., & Antony, M. M. (in press). Exposure techniques. In S. G. Hofmann (Ed.), *Cognitive behavioral therapy: A complete reference guide: Vol. 1—CBT general strategies*. Hoboken, NJ: Wiley-Blackwell.

Watson, J. B. (1913). Psychology as the behaviorist views it. *Psychological Review, 20*, 158–177.

Watson, J. B., & Rayner, R. (1920). Conditioned emotional reactions. *Journal of Experimental Psychology, 3*, 1–14.

Williams, M., Powers, M. B., & Foa, E. B. (2012). Obsessive-compulsive disorder. In P. Sturmey & M. Hersen (Eds.), *Handbook of evidence-based practice in clinical psychology: Vol. II—Adult disorders* (pp. 285–311). Hoboken, NJ: John Wiley & Sons.

Wilson, G. T. (1998). Manual-based treatment and clinical practice. *Clinical Psychology: Science and Practice, 5*, 363–375.

Wincze, J. P., & Carey, M. P. (2001). *Sexual dysfunction: A guide for assessment and treatment*. New York: Guilford Press.

Wolpe, J. (1958). *Psychotherapy by reciprocal inhibition*. Stanford, CA: Stanford University Press.

Woody, S. R., & Sanderson, W. C. (1998). Manuals for empirically supported treatments: 1998 update. *The Clinical Psychologist, 51*, 17–21.

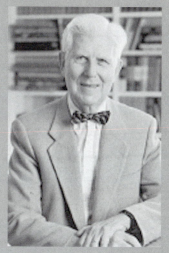

Aaron T. Beck
Courtesy of Aaron T. Beck, PhD, University of Pennsylvania

7 | COGNITIVE THERAPY

Aaron T. Beck and Marjorie E. Weishaar

OVERVIEW

Cognitive therapy is based on a theory of personality that maintains that people respond to life events through a combination of cognitive, affective, motivational, and behavioral responses. These responses are based in human evolution and individual learning history. The cognitive system deals with the way individuals perceive, interpret, and assign meanings to events. It interacts with the other affective, motivational, and physiological systems to process information from the physical and social environments and to respond accordingly. Sometimes responses are maladaptive because of misperceptions, misinterpretations, or dysfunctional, idiosyncratic interpretations of situations.

Cognitive therapy aims to adjust information processing and initiate positive change in all systems by acting through the cognitive system. In a collaborative process, the therapist and patient examine the patient's beliefs about him- or herself, other people, and the world. The patient's maladaptive conclusions are treated as testable hypotheses. Behavioral experiments and verbal procedures are used to examine alternative interpretations and generate contradictory evidence that supports more adaptive beliefs and leads to therapeutic change.

Basic Concepts

Cognitive therapy can be thought of as a theory, a system of strategies, and a series of techniques. The theory is based on the idea that the processing of information is crucial for the survival of any organism. If we did not have a functional apparatus for taking in

231

relevant information from the environment, synthesizing it, and formulating a plan of action on the basis of this synthesis, we would soon die or be killed.

Each system involved in survival—cognitive, behavioral, affective, and motivational—is composed of structures known as *schemas*. Cognitive schemas contain people's perceptions of themselves and others and of their goals and expectations, memories, fantasies, and previous learning. These greatly influence, if not control, the processing of information.

In various psychopathological conditions such as anxiety disorders, depressive disorders, mania, paranoid states, obsessive–compulsive neuroses, and others, a specific bias affects how the person incorporates new information. Thus, a depressed person has a negative bias, including a negative view of self, world, and future. In anxiety, there is a systematic bias or *cognitive shift* toward selectively interpreting themes of danger. In paranoid conditions, the dominant shift is toward indiscriminate attributions of abuse or interference, and in mania the shift is toward exaggerated interpretations of personal gain.

Contributing to these shifts are certain specific attitudes or core beliefs that predispose people under the influence of certain life situations to interpret their experiences in a biased way. These are known as *cognitive vulnerabilities*. For example, a person who has the belief that any minor loss represents a major deprivation may react catastrophically to even the smallest loss. A person who feels vulnerable to sudden death may over interpret normal body sensations as signs of impending death and have a panic attack.

Previously, cognitive theory emphasized a linear relationship between the activation of cognitive schemas and changes in the other systems; that is, cognitions (beliefs and assumptions) triggered affect, motivation, and behavior. Current cognitive theory, benefiting from recent developments in clinical, evolutionary, and cognitive psychology, views all systems as acting together as a mode. *Modes* are networks of cognitive, affective, motivational, and behavioral schemas that compose personality and interpret ongoing situations. Some modes, such as the anxiety mode, are *primal*, meaning they are universal and tied to survival. Other modes, such as conversing or studying, are minor and under conscious control. Although primal modes are thought to have been adaptive in an evolutionary sense, individuals may find them maladaptive in everyday life when they are triggered by misperceptions or overreactions. Even personality disorders may be viewed as exaggerated versions of formerly adaptive strategies. In personality disorders, primal modes are operational almost continuously.

Primal modes include primal thinking, which is rigid, absolute, automatic, and biased. Nevertheless, conscious intentions can override primal thinking and make it more flexible. Automatic and reflexive responses can be replaced by deliberate thinking, conscious goals, problem solving, and long-term planning. In cognitive therapy, a thorough understanding of the mode and all its integral systems is part of the case conceptualization. This approach to therapy teaches patients to use conscious control to recognize and override maladaptive responses.

Strategies

The overall strategies of cognitive therapy involve a collaborative enterprise between the patient and the therapist to explore dysfunctional interpretations and try to modify them, chiefly through logical examination and behavioral experiments. This *collaborative empiricism* views the patient as a practical scientist who lives by interpreting stimuli but who has been temporarily thwarted by his or her own information-gathering and -integrating apparatus (Kelly, 1955). In collaborative empiricism, the therapist asks questions to understand the patient's point of view, not solely to change the patient's mind. The patient, in turn, plays an active role in describing how he or she would like things to be different and what he or she might do to help create change (Padesky, 1993).

The second strategy, *guided discovery,* is directed toward discovering what threads run through the patient's current misperceptions and beliefs and linking them to relevant experiences in the past. Thus, the therapist and patient collaboratively weave a tapestry that tells the story of the development of the patient's disorder. Implicit in guided discovery is the notion that the therapist does not provide answers to the patient but is curious about what they will discover as they gather data, examine the data in different ways, and ask the patient what to make of new perspectives (Padesky, 1993).

Both strategies are implemented using *Socratic dialogue,* a style of questioning that helps uncover the patient's views and examines his or her adaptive and maladaptive features. The steps of Socratic dialogue are (1) asking informational questions, (2) listening, (3) summarizing, and (4) asking synthesizing or analytical questions that apply discovered information to the patient's original belief (Padesky, 1993). An example of a synthesizing or analytical question is, "How does this new information fit with your belief that you can't do anything right?"

Cognitive therapy attempts to improve reality testing through continuous evaluation of personal conclusions. The immediate goal is to reduce cognitive distortions and biased judgments, thereby shifting information processing to a more "neutral" condition so that events will be evaluated in a more balanced way.

Three major approaches are used to treat dysfunctional modes: (1) deactivate them, (2) modify their content and structure, and (3) construct more adaptive modes to neutralize them. In therapy, the first and third approaches are often accomplished simultaneously because a particular belief may be demonstrated to be dysfunctional and a new belief to be more accurate or adaptive. The deactivation of a dysfunctional mode can occur through distraction or reassurance, but lasting change is unlikely unless a person's underlying core beliefs are modified.

Techniques

Techniques used in cognitive therapy are directed primarily at correcting errors and biases in information processing and modifying the core beliefs that promote faulty conclusions. The purely cognitive techniques focus on identifying and testing the patient's beliefs, exploring their origins and basis, correcting them if they fail an empirical or logical test, and problem solving. For example, some beliefs are tied to one's culture, gender role, religion, or socioeconomic status. Therapy may be directed toward problem solving with an understanding of how these beliefs influence the patient.

Core beliefs are explored in a similar manner and are tested for their validity and adaptiveness. The patient who discovers that these beliefs are not accurate is encouraged to try out a different set of beliefs to determine whether the new beliefs are more accurate and functional.

Cognitive therapy also uses behavioral techniques such as skills training (e.g., relaxation, assertiveness training, social-skills training), role playing, behavioral rehearsal, and exposure therapy.

Other Systems

Procedures used in cognitive therapy—such as identifying common themes in a patient's emotional reactions, narratives, and imagery—are similar to the *psychoanalytic method.* However, in cognitive therapy the common thread is a meaning readily accessible to conscious interpretation, whereas in psychoanalysis the meaning is unconscious (or repressed) and must be inferred.

Psychoanalysis, psychodynamic psychotherapy, and cognitive therapy assume that behavior can be influenced by beliefs that one is not immediately aware of. However, cognitive therapy maintains that the thoughts contributing to a patient's distress are not deeply buried in the unconscious. Moreover, the cognitive therapist does not regard the patient's self-report as a screen for more deeply concealed ideas. Cognitive therapy focuses on the linkages among symptoms, conscious beliefs, and current experiences. Psychoanalytic approaches are oriented toward repressed childhood memories and motivational constructs such as libidinal needs and infantile sexuality.

Cognitive therapy is highly structured and usually short term, typically lasting from 12 to 16 weeks for the treatment of most psychiatric disorders. The therapist is actively engaged in collaboration with the patient. Psychoanalytic therapy is long term and relatively unstructured. The analyst is largely passive. Cognitive therapy attempts to shift biased information processing through the application of logic to dysfunctional ideas and the use of behavioral experiments to test dysfunctional beliefs. Psychoanalysts rely on free association and in-depth interpretations to penetrate the encapsulated unconscious residue of unresolved childhood conflicts.

Cognitive therapy and rational emotive behavior therapy (REBT) share an emphasis on the primary importance of cognition in psychological dysfunction, and both see the task of therapy as changing maladaptive assumptions and the stance of the therapist as active and directive. There are some differences, nevertheless, between these two approaches.

REBT theory states that a distressed individual has irrational beliefs that contribute to irrational thoughts and that when these are modified through direct disputation, they will disappear and the disorder will clear up. The cognitive therapist helps the patient translate interpretations and beliefs into hypotheses, which are then subjected to empirical testing. Indeed, the cognitive therapist teaches patients to question and examine their own beliefs, thus allowing patients to learn skills to help them become their own therapist. The cognitive therapist eschews the word *irrational* in favor of *dysfunctional* because problematic beliefs are nonadaptive rather than irrational. They contribute to psychological disorders because they interfere with normal cognitive processing, not because they are irrational.

A profound difference between these two approaches is that cognitive therapy maintains that each disorder has its own typical cognitive content or *cognitive specificity*. The *cognitive profiles* of depression, anxiety, and panic disorder are significantly different and require substantially different techniques. REBT, on the other hand, does not conceptualize disorders as having cognitive themes but instead focuses on the *musts*, *shoulds*, and other imperatives presumed to underlie all disorders.

The cognitive therapy model emphasizes the impact of cognitive deficits in psychopathology. Some clients experience problems because their cognitive deficits do not let them foresee delayed or long-range negative consequences. Others have trouble with concentration, directed thinking, or recall. These difficulties occur in severe anxiety, depression, and panic attacks. Cognitive deficits produce perceptual errors as well as faulty interpretations. Further, inadequate cognitive processing may interfere with the client's use of coping abilities or techniques and with interpersonal problem solving such as occurs in suicidal people. For a full comparison of cognitive therapy and rational emotive behavior therapy, see Padesky and Beck (2003).

Cognitive therapy shares many similarities with some forms of *behavior therapy* but is quite different from others. Within behavior therapy are numerous approaches that vary in their emphasis on cognitive processes. At one end of the behavioral spectrum is applied behavioral analysis, an approach that ignores "internal events," such as interpretations and inferences, as much as possible. As one moves in the other direction, cognitive mediating processes are given increasing attention until one arrives at a variety of cognitive-behavioral approaches. At this point, the distinction between the purely cognitive and the distinctly behavioral becomes unclear.

Cognitive therapy and behavior therapy share some features: They are empirical, present centered, and problem oriented, and they require explicit identification of problems and the situations in which they occur, as well as of the consequences resulting from them. In contrast to radical behaviorism, cognitive therapy applies the same kind of functional analysis to internal experiences: thoughts, attitudes, and images. Cognitions, like behaviors, can be modified by active collaboration through behavioral experiments that foster new learning. Also, in contrast to behavioral approaches based on simple conditioning paradigms, cognitive therapy sees individuals as active participants in their environments, judging and evaluating stimuli, interpreting events and sensations, and judging their own responses.

Studies of some behavioral techniques, such as exposure methods for the treatment of phobias, demonstrate that cognitive and behavioral changes work together. For example, in agoraphobia, cognitive improvement has been concomitant with behavioral improvement (Williams & Rappoport, 1983). Simple exposure to agoraphobic situations while verbalizing negative automatic thoughts may lead to improvement on cognitive measures (Gournay, 1986). Bandura (1977) has demonstrated that one of the most effective ways to change cognitions is to change performance. In real-life exposure, patients confront not only the threatening situations but also their personal expectations of danger and their assumed inability to cope with their reactions. Because the experience itself is processed cognitively, exposure can be considered a cognitive procedure.

Cognitive therapy maintains that a comprehensive approach to the treatment of anxiety and other disorders includes targeting anxiety-provoking thoughts and images. Work with depressed patients (Beck, Rush, Shaw, & Emery, 1979) demonstrates that desired cognitive changes do not necessarily follow from changes in behavior. For this reason, it is vital to know the patient's expectations, interpretations, and reactions to events. Cognitive change must be demonstrated, not assumed.

HISTORY

Precursors

Cognitive therapy's theoretical underpinnings are derived from three main sources: (1) the phenomenological approach to psychology, (2) structural theory and depth psychology, and (3) cognitive psychology. The phenomenological approach posits that the individual's view of self and the personal world are central to behavior. This concept originated in Greek Stoic philosophy and can be seen in Immanuel Kant's (1798) emphasis on conscious subjective experience. This approach is also evident in the writings of Adler (1936), Alexander (1950), Horney (1950), and Sullivan (1953).

The second major influence was the structural theory and depth psychology of Kant and Freud, particularly Freud's concept of the hierarchical structuring of cognition into primary and secondary processes.

More recent developments in cognitive psychology also have had an impact. George Kelly (1955) is credited with being the first among contemporaries to describe the cognitive model through his use of *personal constructs* and his emphasis on the role of beliefs in behavior change. Cognitive theories of emotion, such as those of Magda Arnold (1960) and Richard Lazarus (1984), which give primacy to cognition in emotional and behavioral change, have also contributed to cognitive therapy.

Beginnings

Cognitive therapy began in the early 1960s as the result of Aaron Beck's research on depression (Beck, 1963, 1964, 1967). Trained in psychoanalysis, Beck attempted to validate Freud's theory of depression as having at its core "anger turned on the self."

To substantiate this formulation, Beck made clinical observations of depressed patients and investigated their treatment under traditional psychoanalysis. Rather than finding retroflected anger in their thoughts and dreams, Beck observed a negative bias in their cognitive processing. With continued clinical observations and experimental testing, Beck developed his theory of emotional disorders and a cognitive model of depression.

The work of Albert Ellis (1962) gave major impetus to the development of cognitive-behavior therapies. Both Ellis and Beck believed that people can consciously adopt reason, and both viewed the patient's underlying assumptions as targets of intervention. Similarly, they both rejected their analytic training and replaced passive listening with active, direct dialogues with patients. Whereas Ellis confronted patients and persuaded them that the philosophies they lived by were unrealistic, Beck "turned the client into a colleague who researches verifiable reality" (Wessler, 1986, p. 5).

The work of a number of contemporary behaviorists influenced the development of cognitive therapy. Bandura's (1977) concepts of expectancy of reinforcement, self and outcome efficacies, the interaction between person and environment, modeling, and vicarious learning catalyzed a shift in behavior therapy toward the cognitive domain. Mahoney's (1974) early work on the cognitive control of behavior and his later theoretical contributions also influenced cognitive therapy. Along with cognitive therapy and rational emotive behavior therapy, Meichenbaum's (1977) cognitive-behavior modification is recognized as one of the three major self-control therapies (Mahoney & Arnkoff, 1978). Meichenbaum's combination of cognitive modification and skills training in a coping-skills paradigm is particularly useful in treating anxiety, anger, and stress. The constructivist movement in psychology and the modern movement for psychotherapy integration have been recent influences shaping contemporary cognitive therapy.

Current Status

Research: Cognitive Model and Outcome Studies

Research has tested both the theoretical aspects of the cognitive model and the efficacy of cognitive therapy for a range of clinical disorders. In terms of the cognitive model of depression, negatively biased interpretations have been found in all forms of depression: unipolar and bipolar, reactive, and endogenous (Haaga, Dyck, & Ernst, 1991). The cognitive triad, negatively biased cognitive processing of stimuli, and identifiable dysfunctional beliefs have also been found to operate in depression (Hollon, Kendall, & Lumry, 1986). The efficacy of cognitive therapy for depression has been demonstrated in numerous studies summarized by Clark, Beck, and Alford (1999). Recently, Beck (2008) has traced the evolution of the cognitive model of depression from its basis in information processing to its incorporation of the effect of early traumatic experiences on the formation of dysfunctional beliefs and sensitivity to precipitating factors in depression. He is currently interested in how genetic, neurochemical, and cognitive factors interact in depression.

For the anxiety disorders, a danger-related bias has been demonstrated in all anxiety diagnoses, including the presumed danger of physical sensations in panic attacks, the distorted perception of evaluation in social anxiety, and the negative appraisals of self and the world in posttraumatic stress disorder (PTSD). Moreover, the cognitive specificity hypothesis, which states that there is a distinct cognitive profile for each psychiatric disorder, has been supported for a range of disorders (Beck, 2005).

Controlled studies have demonstrated the efficacy of cognitive therapy in the treatment of panic disorder (Beck, Sokol, Clark, Berchick, & Wright, 1992; Clark, 1996;

Clark, Salkovskis, Hackmann, Middleton, & Gelder, 1992), social phobia (Clark, 1997; Eng, Roth, & Heimberg, 2001), generalized anxiety disorder (Butler, Fennell, Robson, & Gelder, 1991), substance abuse (Woody et al., 1983), eating disorders (Bowers, 2001; Fairburn et al., 1991; Garner et al., 1993; Pike, Walsh, Vitousek, Wilson, & Bauer, 2003; Vitousek, 1996), marital problems (Baucom, Sayers, & Sher, 1990), obsessive–compulsive disorder (Freeston et al., 1997), PTSD (Ehlers & Clark, 2000; Gillespie, Duffy, Hackmann, & Clark, 2002; Resick, 2001), and schizophrenia (Grant, Huh, Perivoliotis, Stolar, & Beck, 2011; Turkington, Dudley, Warman, & Beck, 2004; Zimmerman, Favrod, Trieu, & Pomini, 2005).

In addition, cognitive therapy appears to lead to lower rates of relapse than other treatments for anxiety and depression (Clark, 1996; Eng et al., 2001; Hollon, DeRubeis, & Evans, 1996; Hollon et al., 2005; Hollon, Stewart, & Strunk, 2006; Strunk & DeRubeis, 2001).

Suicide Research

Beck has developed key theoretical concepts regarding suicide and its prevention. Chief among his findings about suicide risk is the notion of *hopelessness.* Longitudinal studies of both inpatients and outpatients who had suicidal ideation have found that a cutoff score of 9 or more on the Beck Hopelessness Scale is predictive of eventual suicide (Beck, Brown, Berchick, Stewart, & Steer, 1990; Beck, Steer, Kovacs, & Garrison, 1985). Hopelessness has been confirmed as a predictor of eventual suicide in subsequent studies.

A recent randomized controlled trial investigated the efficacy of a brief cognitive therapy treatment for those at high risk of attempting suicide by virtue of the fact that they had previously attempted suicide and had significant psychopathology and substance abuse problems. Results indicate that cognitive therapy reduced the rate of reattempt by 50% over an 18-month period (Brown et al., 2005).

Psychotherapy Integration

Cognitive therapy has been integrated with other modalities to yield new therapeutic approaches. Schema therapy, developed by Jeffrey Young (Young, Klosko, & Weishaar, 2003), focuses on modifying maladaptive core beliefs that are developed early in life and that can underlie chronic depression and anxiety as well as personality disorders. Another approach, mindfulness-based cognitive therapy (Segal, Williams, & Teasdale, 2002), uses acceptance and meditation strategies to promote resilience and prevent recurrence of depressive episodes.

Assessment Scales

Beck's work has generated a number of assessment scales, most notably the Beck Depression Inventory (BDI; Beck, Steer, & Brown, 1996; Beck, Ward, Mendelson, Mock, & Erbaugh, 1961), the Scale for Suicide Ideation (Beck, Kovacs, & Weissman, 1979), the Suicide Intent Scale (Beck, Schuyler, & Herman, 1974), the Beck Hopelessness Scale (Beck, Weissman, Lester, & Trexler, 1974), the Beck Anxiety Inventory (Beck & Steer, 1990), the Beck Self-Concept Test (Beck, Steer, Brown, & Epstein, 1990), the Dysfunctional Attitude Scale (Weissman & Beck, 1978), the Sociotropy-Autonomy Scale (Beck, Epstein, & Harrison, 1983), the Beck Youth Inventories (Beck & Beck, 2002), the Personality Beliefs Questionnaire (Beck & Beck, 1995), and the Clark-Beck Obsessive–Compulsive Inventory (Clark & Beck, 2002). The Beck Depression Inventory is the best known of these. It has been used in hundreds of outcome studies and is routinely employed by psychologists, physicians, and social workers to monitor depression in their patients and clients.

Training

The Center for Cognitive Therapy, which is affiliated with the University of Pennsylvania Medical School, provides outpatient services and is a research institute that integrates clinical observations with empirical findings to develop theory. The Beck Institute in Bala Cynwyd, Pennsylvania, provides both outpatient services and training opportunities. In addition, clinical psychology internships and postdoctoral fellowships worldwide offer training in cognitive therapy. Research and treatment efforts in cognitive therapy are being conducted in many universities and hospitals in the United States and Europe. The *International Cognitive Therapy Newsletter* was launched in 1985 for the exchange of information among cognitive therapists. Therapists from five continents participate in the newsletter network. Founded in 1971, the European Association for Behavioural and Cognitive Therapies held its 43rd annual conference in Marrakech, Morocco, in 2013. The World Congress of Behavioural and Cognitive Therapies, composed of seven organizations from around the world, held its conference in 2013 in Lima, Peru. The International Association for Cognitive Psychotherapy will host the 8th International Congress of Cognitive Psychotherapy in Hong Kong in 2014.

The Academy of Cognitive Therapy, a nonprofit organization, was founded in 1999 by a group of leading clinicians, educators, and researchers in the field of cognitive therapy. The academy administers an objective evaluation to identify and certify clinicians skilled in cognitive therapy. In 1999, the Accreditation Council for Graduate Medical Education mandated that psychiatry residency training programs train residents to be competent in the practice of cognitive-behavior therapy.

Cognitive therapists routinely contribute to psychology, psychiatry, and behavior therapy journals. The primary journals devoted to research in cognitive therapy are *Cognitive Therapy and Research,* the *International Journal of Cognitive Psychotherapy,* and *Cognitive and Behavioral Practice.*

Cognitive therapy is represented at the annual meetings of the American Psychological Association, the American Psychiatric Association, and the American Association of Suicidology, among others. It has been such a major force in the Association for the Advancement of Behavior Therapy that the organization changed its name in 2005 to the Association for Behavioral and Cognitive Therapies (ABCT). Recent research by Norcross and Karpiak (2012) found cognitive therapy to have surpassed eclectic and integrative therapy as the leading psychotherapy delivered by psychologists.

Because of its efficacy as a short-term form of psychotherapy, cognitive therapy is achieving wider use in settings that must demonstrate cost-effectiveness or that require short-term contact with patients. It has applications in both inpatient and outpatient settings.

Many talented researchers and innovative therapists have contributed to the development of cognitive therapy. Controlled outcome studies comparing cognitive therapy with other forms of treatment are conducted with anxiety disorders, panic, drug abuse, anorexia and bulimia, geriatric depression, acute depression, and dysphoric disorder. Beck's students and associates do research on the nature and treatment of depression, anxiety, loneliness, marital conflict, eating disorders, agoraphobia, pain, personality disorders, substance abuse, bipolar disorder, and schizophrenia.

PERSONALITY

Theory of Personality

Cognitive therapy emphasizes the role of information processing in human responses and adaptation. When an individual perceives that the situation requires a response, a whole set of cognitive, emotional, motivational, and behavioral schemas are mobilized.

Previously, cognitive therapy viewed cognition as largely determining emotions and behaviors. Current thinking views all aspects of human functioning as acting simultaneously as a mode.

Cognitive therapy views personality as shaped by the interaction between innate disposition and environment (Beck, Freeman, & Davis, 2003). Personality attributes are seen as reflecting basic schemas, or interpersonal *strategies* developed in response to the environment.

Cognitive therapy maintains that psychological distress results from several factors. Although people may have biochemical predispositions to illness, they respond to specific stressors because of their learning history. The phenomena of psychopathology (but not necessarily the cause) are on the same continuum as normal emotional reactions, but they are manifested in exaggerated and persistent ways. In depression, for example, sadness and loss of interest are intensified and prolonged; in mania, there is heightened investment in self-aggrandizement; and in anxiety, there is an extreme sense of vulnerability and danger.

Individuals experience psychological distress when they perceive a situation as threatening their vital interests. At such times, their perceptions and interpretations of events are highly selective, egocentric, and rigid. This results in a functional impairment of normal cognitive activity. There is a decreased ability to turn off idiosyncratic thinking, to concentrate, to recall, or to reason. Corrective functions, which allow reality testing and refinement of global conceptualizations, are attenuated.

Cognitive Vulnerability

Each individual has a set of idiosyncratic vulnerabilities and sensitivities that predispose him or her to psychological distress. These vulnerabilities appear to be related to personality structure. Personality is shaped by temperament and cognitive schemas. Cognitive schemas are structures that contain the individual's fundamental beliefs and assumptions. Schemas develop early in life from personal experience and identification with significant others. These concepts are reinforced by further learning experiences and, in turn, influence the formation of beliefs, values, and attitudes.

Cognitive schemas may be adaptive or dysfunctional. They may be general or specific in nature. A person may have competing schemas. Cognitive schemas are generally latent but become active when stimulated by specific stressors, circumstances, or stimuli. In personality disorders, they are triggered very easily and often so that the person overresponds to a wide range of situations in a stereotyped manner.

Dimensions of Personality

The idea that certain clusters of personality attributes or cognitive structures are related to certain types of emotional response has been studied by Beck, Epstein, and Harrison (1983), who found two major personality dimensions relevant to depression and possibly to other disorders: social dependence (sociotropy) and autonomy. Beck's research revealed that dependent individuals became depressed following disruption of relationships. Autonomous people became depressed after defeat or failure to attain a desired goal. The sociotropic dimension is organized around closeness, nurturance, and dependence; the autonomous dimension is organized around independence, goal setting, self-determination, and self-imposed obligations.

Research has also established that although "pure" cases of sociotropy and autonomy do exist, most people display features of each, depending on the situation. Thus, sociotropy and autonomy are styles of behavior, not fixed personality structures. This position stands in marked contrast with psychodynamic theories of personality, which postulate fixed personality dimensions.

Thus, cognitive therapy views personality as reflecting the individual's cognitive organization and structure, which are both biologically and socially influenced. Within the constraints of one's neuroanatomy and biochemistry, personal learning experiences help determine how one develops and responds.

Variety of Concepts

Cognitive therapy emphasizes the individual's learning history, including the influence of significant life events, in the development of psychological disturbance. It is not a reductive model but recognizes that psychological distress is usually the result of many interacting factors.

Cognitive therapy's emphasis on the individual's learning history endorses social-learning theory and the importance of reinforcement. The social-learning perspective requires a thorough examination of the individual's developmental history and his or her own idiosyncratic meanings and interpretations of events. Cognitive therapy emphasizes the idiographic nature of cognition because the same event may have very different meanings for two individuals.

The conceptualization of personality as reflective of schemas and underlying assumptions is also related to social-learning theory. The way a person structures experience is based on consequences of past behavior, vicarious learning from significant others, and expectations about the future.

Theory of Causality

Psychological distress is ultimately caused by many innate, biological, developmental, and environmental factors interacting with one another, so there is no single "cause" of psychopathology. Depression, for instance, is characterized by predisposing factors such as hereditary susceptibility, diseases that cause persistent neurochemical abnormalities, developmental traumas leading to specific cognitive vulnerabilities, inadequate personal experiences that fail to provide appropriate coping skills, and counterproductive cognitive patterns such as unrealistic goals, assumptions, or imperatives. Physical disease, severe and acute stress, and chronic stress are also precipitating factors.

Cognitive Distortions

Systematic errors in reasoning called *cognitive distortions* are evident during psychological distress (Beck, 1967).

Arbitrary inference: Drawing a specific conclusion without supporting evidence or even in the face of contradictory evidence. An example is the working mother who concludes, after a particularly busy day, "I'm a terrible mother."

Selective abstraction: Conceptualizing a situation on the basis of a detail taken out of context, ignoring other information. An example is the man who becomes jealous on seeing his girlfriend tilt her head toward another man to hear him better at a noisy party.

Overgeneralization: Abstracting a general rule from one or a few isolated incidents and applying it too broadly and to unrelated situations. After a discouraging date, a woman concluded, "All men are alike. I'll always be rejected."

Magnification and minimization: Seeing something as far more significant or less significant than it actually is. A student catastrophized, "If I appear the least bit nervous in class, it will mean disaster." Another person, rather than facing the fact that his mother is terminally ill, decides that she will soon recover from her "cold."

Personalization: Attributing external events to oneself without evidence supporting a causal connection. A man waved to an acquaintance across a busy street. After not getting a greeting in return, he concluded, "I must have done something to offend him."

Dichotomous thinking: Categorizing experiences in one of two extremes—for example, as complete success or total failure. A doctoral candidate stated, "Unless I write the best exam they've ever seen, I'm a failure as a student."

Systematic Bias in Psychological Disorders

A bias in information processing characterizes most psychological disorders (see Table 7.1). This bias is generally applied to "external" information, such as communications or threats, and may start operating at early stages of information processing. A person's orienting schema identifies a situation as posing a danger or loss, for instance, and signals the appropriate mode to respond.

Cognitive Model of Depression

A *cognitive triad* characterizes depression (Beck, 1967). The depressed individual has a negative view of the self, the world, and the future and perceives the self as inadequate, deserted, and worthless. A negative view is apparent in beliefs that enormous demands exist and that immense barriers block access to goals. The world seems devoid of pleasure or gratification. The depressed person's view of the future is pessimistic, reflecting the belief that current troubles will not improve. This hopelessness may lead to suicidal ideation.

Motivational, behavioral, emotional, and physical symptoms of depression are also activated in the depressed mode. These symptoms influence a person's beliefs and assumptions, and vice versa. For example, motivational symptoms of paralysis of will are related to the belief that one lacks the ability to cope or to control an event's outcome. Consequently, there is a reluctance to commit oneself to a goal. Suicidal wishes often reflect a desire to escape unbearable problems.

The increased dependency often observed in depressed patients reflects the view of self as incompetent, an overestimation of the difficulty of normal life tasks, the expectation of failure, and the desire for someone more capable to take over. Indecisiveness similarly reflects the belief that one is incapable of making correct decisions.

TABLE 7.1   The Cognitive Profile of Psychological Disorders

Disorder	Systematic Bias in Processing Information
Depression	Negative view of self, experience, and future
Hypomania	Inflated view of self and future
Anxiety disorder	Sense of physical or psychological danger
Panic disorder	Catastrophic interpretation of bodily or mental experiences
Phobia	Sense of danger in specific, avoidable situations
Paranoid state	Attribution of bias to others
Hysteria	Concept of motor or sensory abnormality
Obsession	Repeated warning or doubts about safety
Compulsion	Rituals to ward off perceived threat
Suicidal behavior	Hopelessness and deficiencies in problem solving
Anorexia nervosa	Fear of being fat
Hypochondriasis	Attribution of serious medical disorder

The physical symptoms of depression—low energy, fatigue, and inertia—are also related to negative expectations. Work with depressed patients indicates that initiating activity actually reduces inertia and fatigue. Moreover, refuting negative expectations and demonstrating motor ability play important roles in recovery.

Cognitive Model of Anxiety Disorders

Anxiety disorders are conceptualized as excessive functioning or malfunctioning of normal survival mechanisms. Thus, the basic mechanisms for coping with threat are the same for both normal and anxious people: Physiological responses prepare the body for escape or self-defense. The same physiological responses occur in the face of psychosocial threats as in the case of physical dangers. The anxious person's perception of danger is either based on false assumptions or exaggerated, whereas the normal response is based on a more accurate assessment of risk and the magnitude of danger. In addition, normal individuals can correct their misperceptions using logic and evidence. Anxious individuals have difficulty recognizing cues of safety and other evidence that would reduce the threat of danger. Thus, in cases of anxiety, cognitive content revolves around themes of danger, and the individual tends to maximize the likelihood of harm and minimize his or her ability to cope.

Mania

The manic patient's biased thinking is the reverse of the depressive's. Such individuals selectively perceive significant gains in each life experience, blocking out negative experiences or reinterpreting them as positive, and unrealistically expecting favorable results from various enterprises. Exaggerated concepts of abilities, worth, and accomplishments lead to feelings of euphoria. The continued stimulation from inflated self-evaluations and overly optimistic expectations provides vast sources of energy and drives the manic individual into continuous goal-directed activity.

Panic Disorder

Patients with panic disorder are prone to regard any unexplained symptom or sensation as a sign of some impending catastrophe. Their cognitive processing system focuses their attention on bodily or psychological experiences and shapes these sources of internal information into the conviction that disaster is imminent. Each patient has a specific "equation." For one, distress in the chest or stomach equals heart attack; for another, shortness of breath means the cessation of all breathing; and for another, lightheadedness is a sign of impending unconsciousness.

Some patients regard a sudden surge of anger as a sign they will lose control and injure somebody. Others interpret a mental lapse, momentary confusion, or mild disorientation to mean that they are losing their mind. A crucial characteristic of people having panic attacks is the conclusion that vital systems (the cardiovascular, respiratory, or central nervous system) will collapse. Because of their fear, they tend to be overly vigilant toward internal sensations and thus to detect and magnify sensations that pass unnoticed in other people.

Patients with panic disorder show a specific cognitive deficit: an inability to view their symptoms and catastrophic interpretations realistically.

Agoraphobia

Patients who have had one or more panic attacks in a particular situation tend to avoid that situation. For example, people who have had panic attacks in supermarkets avoid going there. If they push themselves to go, they become increasingly vigilant toward their sensations and begin to anticipate having another panic attack.

The anticipation of such an attack triggers a variety of autonomic symptoms that are then misinterpreted as signs of an impending disaster (e.g., heart attack, loss of consciousness, suffocation), which can lead to a full-blown panic attack. Patients with a panic disorder that goes untreated frequently develop agoraphobia. They may eventually become housebound or so restricted in their activities that they cannot travel far from home and require a companion to venture any distance.

Phobia

In phobias, there is anticipation of physical or psychological harm in specific situations. As long as patients can avoid these situations, they do not feel threatened and may be relatively comfortable. When they enter into these situations, however, they experience the typical subjective and physiological symptoms of severe anxiety. As a result of this unpleasant reaction, their tendency to avoid the situation in the future is reinforced.

In *evaluation phobias,* there is fear of disparagement or failure in social situations, examinations, and public speaking. The behavioral and physiological reactions to the potential "danger" (rejection, devaluation, failure) may interfere with the patient's functioning to the extent that they can produce just what the patient fears will happen.

Paranoid States

The paranoid individual is biased toward attributing prejudice to others. The paranoid persists in assuming that other people are deliberately abusive, interfering, or critical. In contrast to depressed patients, who believe that supposed insults or rejections are justified, paranoid patients persevere in thinking that others treat them unjustly.

Unlike depressed patients, paranoid patients do not experience low self-esteem. They are more concerned with the *injustice* of the presumed attacks, thwarting, or intrusions than with the actual loss, and they rail against the presumed prejudice and malicious intent of others.

Obsessions and Compulsions

Patients with obsessions introduce uncertainty into the appraisal of situations that most people would consider safe. The uncertainty is generally attached to circumstances that are potentially unsafe and is manifested by continual doubts—even though there is no evidence of danger.

Obsessives continually doubt whether they have performed an act necessary for safety (for example, turning off a gas oven or locking the door at night). They may fear contamination by germs, and no amount of reassurance can alleviate the fear. A key characteristic of obsessives is this *sense of responsibility* and the belief that they are accountable for having taken an action—or having failed to take an action—that could harm them or others. Cognitive therapy views such intrusive thoughts as universal. It is the meaning assigned to the intrusive thought—that the patient has done something immoral or dangerous—that causes distress.

Compulsions are attempts to reduce excessive doubts by performing rituals designed to neutralize the anticipated disaster. A hand-washing compulsion, for instance, is based on the patient's belief that he or she has not removed all the dirt or contaminants from parts of the body. Some patients regard dirt as a source of danger, either as a cause of physical disease or as a source of offensive, unpleasant odors, and they are compelled to remove this source of physical or social danger.

Suicidal Behavior

The cognitive processing in suicidal individuals has two features. First, there is a high degree of hopelessness or belief that things cannot improve. A second feature is a cognitive deficit—a difficulty in solving problems. Although the hopelessness accentuates poor problem solving, and vice versa, the difficulties in coping with life situations can by themselves contribute to the suicidal potential. Thinking becomes more rigid, and suicide appears as the only alternative in a diminished response repertoire.

Anorexia Nervosa

Anorexia nervosa and bulimia represent a constellation of maladaptive beliefs that revolve around one central assumption: "My body weight and shape determine my worth and/or my social acceptability." Revolving around this assumption are such beliefs as "I will look ugly if I gain much more weight," "The only thing in my life that I can control is my weight," and "If I don't starve myself, I will let go completely and become enormous."

Anorexics show typical distortions in information processing. They misinterpret symptoms of fullness after meals as signs that they are getting fat. And they misperceive their image in a mirror photograph as being much fatter than it actually is.

Schizophrenia

In schizophrenia, there is a complex interaction of predisposing neurobiological, environmental, cognitive, and behavioral factors. The impaired integrative function of the brain, along with specific cognitive deficits, increases vulnerability to stressful life events and leads to dysfunctional beliefs (e.g., "I am inferior") and behaviors (e.g., social withdrawal). Excessive psychophysiological reactions occur in response to stress and repeated negative thinking. The release of corticosteroids activates the dopaminergic system, which contributes to the development of delusions and hallucinations. Cognitive disorganization is a result of neurocognitive deficits such as attentional problems, impaired executive function, and working memory. These impairments interact with heightened rejection sensitivity to produce communication deviance and intrusive, inappropriate thoughts. Delusions stem from the interplay of cognitive biases such as external attributions and the cognitive shortcut of jumping to conclusions. A tendency to distort perceptions combines with negative self-schemas to generate auditory hallucinations, which are exacerbated by beliefs that the "voice" is uncontrollable, powerful, infallible, and externally generated. Engagement in social, vocational, and pleasurable activity is compromised by neurocognitive impairment that is magnified by dysfunctional attitudes such as social indifference, low expectancies for pleasure, and defeatist beliefs regarding task performance. Low expectations for performance and success further contribute to negative symptoms.

PSYCHOTHERAPY

Theory of Psychotherapy

The goals of cognitive therapy are to correct faulty information processing and to help patients modify assumptions that maintain maladaptive behaviors and emotions. Cognitive and behavioral methods are used to challenge dysfunctional beliefs and promote more realistic adaptive thinking. Cognitive therapy initially addresses symptom relief, but its ultimate goals are to remove systematic biases in thinking and modify the core beliefs that predispose the person to future distress.

Cognitive therapy fosters change in patients' beliefs by treating beliefs as testable hypotheses to be examined through behavioral experiments jointly agreed on by patient and therapist. The cognitive therapist does not tell the client that the beliefs are irrational or wrong or that the beliefs of the therapist should be adopted. Instead, the therapist asks questions to elicit the meaning, function, usefulness, and consequences of the patient's beliefs. The patient ultimately decides whether to reject, modify, or maintain all personal beliefs, being well aware of their emotional and behavioral consequences.

Cognitive therapy is not the substitution of positive beliefs for negative ones. It is based in reality, not in wishful thinking. Similarly, cognitive therapy does not maintain that people's problems are imaginary. Patients may have serious social, financial, or health problems as well as functional deficits. In addition to real problems, however, they have biased views of themselves, their situations, and their resources that limit their range of responses and prevent them from generating solutions.

Cognitive change can promote behavioral change by allowing the patient to take risks. In turn, experience in applying new behaviors can validate the new perspective. Emotions can be moderated by enlarging perspectives to include alternative interpretations of events. Emotions play a role in cognitive change because learning is enhanced when emotions are triggered. Thus, the cognitive, behavioral, and emotional channels interact in therapeutic change, but cognitive therapy emphasizes the primacy of cognition in promoting and maintaining therapeutic change.

Cognitive change occurs at several levels: voluntary thoughts, continuous or automatic thoughts, underlying assumptions, and core beliefs. According to the cognitive model, cognitions are organized in a hierarchy, each level differing from the next in its accessibility and stability. The most accessible and least stable cognitions are voluntary thoughts. At the next level are automatic thoughts, which come to mind spontaneously when triggered by circumstances. They are the thoughts that intercede between an event or stimulus and the individual's emotional and behavioral reactions.

An example of an automatic thought experienced by a socially anxious person before going to a party is "Everyone will see I'm nervous." Automatic thoughts are accompanied by emotions and, at the time they are experienced, seem plausible, are highly salient, and are internally consistent with individual logic. They are given credibility without ever being challenged. Although automatic thoughts are more stable and less accessible than voluntary thoughts, patients can be taught to recognize and monitor them. Cognitive distortions are evident in automatic thoughts.

Automatic thoughts are generated from underlying assumptions. For example, the belief "I am responsible for other people's happiness" produces numerous negative automatic thoughts in people who perceive themselves as causing distress to others. Assumptions shape perceptions into cognitions, determine goals, and provide interpretations and meanings to events. They may be quite stable and outside the patient's awareness.

Core beliefs are contained in cognitive schemas. Therapy aims at identifying these absolute beliefs and counteracting their effects. If the beliefs themselves can be changed, the patient is less vulnerable to future distress. In schema therapy, these core beliefs are called *early maladaptive schemas* (EMSs; Young et al., 2003).

The Therapeutic Relationship

The therapeutic relationship is collaborative. The therapist assesses sources of distress and dysfunction and helps the patient clarify goals. In cases of severe depression or anxiety, patients may initially need the therapist to take a directive role. In other instances, patients may take the lead in determining goals for therapy. As part of the collaboration, the patient provides the thoughts, images, and beliefs that occur in various situations, as well as the emotions and behaviors that accompany the thoughts. The patient also shares responsibility by helping to set the agenda for each session and by doing homework between sessions. Homework helps therapy proceed more quickly and gives the patient an opportunity to practice newly learned skills and perspectives.

The therapist functions as a guide who helps the patient understand how beliefs and attitudes interact with affect and behavior. The therapist is also a catalyst who helps devise corrective experiences that lead to cognitive change and skills acquisition. Thus, cognitive therapy employs a learning model of psychotherapy. The therapist has expertise in examining and modifying beliefs and behavior but does not adopt the role of either a passive expert or the arbiter of correct thinking.

Cognitive therapists actively pursue the patient's point of view. By using warmth, accurate empathy, and genuineness (see Rogers, 1951), the cognitive therapist is curious and appreciates the patient's personal worldview. However, these qualities alone are not sufficient for therapeutic change. The cognitive therapist specifies problems, focuses on important areas, and teaches specific cognitive and behavioral techniques.

Along with having good interpersonal skills, cognitive therapists are flexible. They are sensitive to the patient's level of comfort and use self-disclosure judiciously. They provide supportive contact when necessary and operate within the goals and agenda of the cognitive approach. Flexibility in the use of therapeutic techniques depends on the targeted symptoms. For example, the inertia of depression responds best to behavioral interventions, whereas the suicidal ideation and pessimism of depression respond best to cognitive techniques. A good cognitive therapist does not use techniques arbitrarily or mechanically but applies them with sound rationale and skill—and with an understanding of each individual's needs.

To maintain collaboration, the therapist elicits feedback from the patient, usually at the end of each session. Feedback focuses on what the patient found helpful or not helpful, whether the patient has concerns about the therapist, and whether the patient has questions. The therapist may summarize the session or ask the patient to do so. Another way the therapist encourages collaboration is by providing the patient with a rationale for each procedure used. This demystifies the therapy process, increases patients' participation, and reinforces a learning paradigm in which patients gradually assume more responsibility for therapeutic change.

Definitions

Three fundamental concepts in cognitive therapy are collaborative empiricism, Socratic dialogue, and guided discovery.

Collaborative Empiricism.   The therapeutic relationship is collaborative and requires jointly determining the goals for treatment, eliciting and providing feedback, and thereby demystifying how therapeutic change occurs. The therapist and patient become co-investigators, examining the evidence to support or modify the patient's cognitions. As in scientific inquiry, interpretations or assumptions are treated as testable hypotheses.

Empirical evidence is used to determine whether particular cognitions serve any useful purpose. Prior conclusions are subjected to logical analysis. Biased thinking is exposed as the patient becomes aware of alternative sources of information. This process is conducted as a partnership between patient and therapist, with either taking a more active role as needed.

Socratic Dialogue. Questioning is a major therapeutic device in cognitive therapy, and Socratic dialogue is the preferred method. The therapist carefully designs a series of questions to promote new learning. The purposes of the therapist's questions are generally to (1) clarify or define problems; (2) assist in the identification of thoughts, images, and assumptions; (3) examine the meanings of events for the patient; and (4) assess the consequences of maintaining maladaptive thoughts and behaviors.

Socratic dialogue implies that the patient arrives at logical conclusions based on the questions posed by the therapist. Questions are not used to "trap" patients, lead them to inevitable conclusions, or attack them. Questions enable the therapist to understand the patient's point of view and are posed with sensitivity so that patients may look at their assumptions objectively and nondefensively.

Young, Rygh, Weinberger, and Beck (2008, p. 274) describe how questions change throughout the course of therapy:

> In the beginning of therapy, questions are employed to obtain a full and detailed picture of the patient's particular difficulties. They are used to obtain background and diagnostic data; to evaluate the patient's stress tolerance, capacity for introspection, coping methods and so on; to obtain information about the patient's external situation and interpersonal context; and to modify vague complaints by working with the patient to arrive at specific target problems to work on.

As therapy progresses, the therapist uses questioning to explore approaches to problems, help the patient weigh advantages and disadvantages of possible solutions, examine the consequences of staying with particular maladaptive behaviors, elicit automatic thoughts, and demonstrate EMSs and their consequences. In short, the therapist uses questioning in most cognitive therapeutic techniques.

Guided Discovery. Through guided discovery, the patient modifies maladaptive beliefs and assumptions. The therapist serves as a guide who elucidates problem behaviors and errors in logic by designing new experiences (*behavioral experiments*) that lead to the acquisition of new skills and perspectives. Guided discovery implies that the therapist does not exhort or cajole the patient to adopt a new set of beliefs. Rather, the therapist encourages the patient's use of information, facts, and probabilities to obtain a realistic perspective.

Process of Psychotherapy

Initial Sessions

The goals of the first interview are to initiate a relationship with the patient, elicit essential information, and produce symptom relief. Building a relationship with the patient may begin with questions about feelings and thoughts about beginning therapy. Discussing the patient's expectations helps put the patient at ease, yields information about the patient's expectations, and presents an opportunity to demonstrate the relationship between cognition and affect (Beck, Rush, Shaw, & Emery, 1979). The therapist also uses the initial sessions to accustom the patient to cognitive therapy, establish a collaborative framework, and deal with any misconceptions about therapy. The types of information the therapist seeks in the initial session include diagnosis, past history, current life situation, psychological problems, attitudes about treatment, and motivation for treatment.

Problem definition and symptom relief begin in the first session. Although problem definition and collection of background information may take several sessions, it is often critical to focus on a very specific problem and provide rapid relief in the first session. For example, a suicidal patient needs direct intervention to undermine hopelessness immediately. Symptom relief can come from several sources: specific problem solving, clarifying vague or general complaints into workable goals, or gaining objectivity about a disorder (e.g., making it clear that a patient's symptoms represent anxiety and nothing worse, or that difficulty concentrating is a symptom of depression and not a sign of brain disease).

Problem definition entails both functional and cognitive analyses of the problem. A functional analysis identifies elements of the problem: how it is manifested; situations in which it occurs; its frequency, intensity, and duration; and its consequences. A cognitive analysis of the problem identifies the thoughts and images a person has when emotion is triggered. It also includes investigation of the extent to which the person feels in control of thoughts and images, what the person imagines will happen in a distressing situation, and the probability of such an outcome actually occurring.

In the early sessions, then, the cognitive therapist plays a more active role than the patient. The therapist gathers information, conceptualizes the patient's problems, socializes the patient to cognitive therapy, and actively intervenes to provide symptom relief. The patient is assigned homework beginning at the first session.

Homework, at this early stage, is usually directed at recognizing the connections among thoughts, feelings, and behavior. For example, patients might be asked to record their automatic thoughts when distressed. Thus, the patient is trained from the outset to self-monitor thoughts and behaviors. In later sessions, the patient plays an increasingly active role in determining homework, and assignments focus on testing very specific assumptions.

During the initial sessions, a problem list is generated. The problem list may include specific symptoms, behaviors, or pervasive problems. These problems are assigned priorities as targets for intervention. Priorities are based on the relative magnitude of distress, the likelihood of making progress, the severity of symptoms, and the pervasiveness of a particular theme or topic.

If the therapist can help the patient solve a problem early in treatment, this success can motivate the patient to make further changes. As each problem is approached, the therapist chooses the appropriate cognitive or behavioral technique to apply and provides the patient with a rationale for the technique. Throughout therapy, the therapist elicits the patient's reactions to various techniques to ascertain whether they are being applied correctly, whether they are successful, and how they can be incorporated into homework or practical experience outside the session.

Middle and Later Sessions

As cognitive therapy proceeds, the emphasis shifts from the patient's symptoms to the patient's patterns of thinking. The connections among thoughts, emotions, and behaviors are chiefly demonstrated through the examination of automatic thoughts. Once the patient can challenge thoughts that interfere with functioning, he or she can consider the underlying assumptions that generate such thoughts.

There is usually a greater emphasis on cognitive than on behavioral techniques in later sessions, which focus on complex problems that involve several dysfunctional thoughts. Often these thoughts are more amenable to logical analysis than to behavioral experimentation. For example, the prophecy "I'll never get what I want in life" is not easily tested. However, one can question the logic of this generalization and look at the advantages and disadvantages of maintaining it as a belief.

Often such assumptions outside the patient's awareness are discovered as themes of automatic thoughts. When automatic thoughts are observed over time and across situations, assumptions appear or can be inferred. Once these assumptions and their power have been recognized, therapy aims at modifying them by examining their validity, adaptiveness, and utility for the patient.

In later sessions, the patient assumes more responsibility for identifying problems and solutions and for creating homework assignments. The therapist takes on the role of adviser rather than teacher as the patient becomes better able to use cognitive techniques to solve problems. The frequency of sessions decreases as the patient becomes more self-sufficient. Therapy is terminated when goals have been reached and the patient feels able to practice his or her new skills and perspectives independently.

Ending Treatment

Length of treatment depends primarily on the severity of the client's problems. The usual length for unipolar depression is 15 to 25 sessions at weekly intervals (Beck, Rush, Shaw, & Emery, 1979). Moderately to severely depressed patients usually require sessions twice a week for 4 to 5 weeks and then weekly sessions for 10 to 15 weeks. Most cases of anxiety are treated within a comparable period of time.

Some patients find it extremely difficult to tolerate the anxiety involved in giving up old ways of thinking. For them, therapy may last several months. Still others experience early symptom relief and leave therapy early. In these cases, little structural change has occurred, and problems are likely to recur.

From the outset, the therapist and patient share the expectation that therapy is time limited. Because cognitive therapy is present centered and time limited, there tend to be fewer problems with termination than in longer forms of therapy. As the patient develops self-reliance, therapy sessions become less frequent.

Termination is planned for, even in the first session as the rationale for cognitive therapy is presented. Patients are told that a goal of the therapy is for them to learn to be their own therapists. The problem list makes explicit what is to be accomplished in treatment. Behavioral observation, self-monitoring, self-report, and sometimes questionnaires (e.g., the Beck Depression Inventory) measure progress toward the goals on the problem list. Feedback from the patient aids the therapist in designing experiences to foster cognitive change.

Some patients have concerns about relapse or about functioning autonomously. Some of these concerns include cognitive distortions, such as dichotomous thinking ("I'm either sick or 100% cured") or negative prediction ("I'll get depressed again and won't be able to help myself"). It may be necessary to review the goal of therapy: to teach the patient ways to handle problems more effectively, not to produce a "cure" or restructure core personality (Beck, Rush, Shaw, & Emery, 1979). Education about psychological disorders, such as acknowledging the possibility of recurrent depression, is done throughout treatment so that the patient has a realistic perspective on prognosis.

During the usual course of therapy, the patient experiences both successes and setbacks. Such problems give the patient the opportunity to practice new skills. As termination approaches, the patient can be reminded that setbacks are normal and have been handled before. The therapist might ask the patient to describe how prior specific problems were handled during treatment. Therapists can also use cognitive rehearsal before termination by having patients imagine future difficulties and report how they would deal with them.

Termination is usually followed by one to two booster sessions, usually one month and two months after termination. Such sessions consolidate gains and assist the patient in employing new skills.

Mechanisms of Psychotherapy

Several common denominators cut across effective treatments. Three mechanisms of change common to all successful forms of psychotherapy are (1) a comprehensible framework, (2) the patient's emotional engagement in the problem situation, and (3) reality testing in that situation.

Cognitive therapy maintains that the modification of dysfunctional assumptions leads to effective cognitive, emotional, and behavioral change. Patients change by recognizing automatic thoughts, questioning the evidence used to support them, and modifying cognitions. Next, the patient behaves in ways congruent with new, more adaptive ways of thinking.

Change can occur only if the patient experiences a problematic situation as a real threat. According to cognitive therapy, core beliefs are linked to emotions; with affective arousal, those beliefs become accessible and modifiable. One mechanism of change, then, focuses on making accessible those cognitive constellations that produced the maladaptive behavior symptomatology. This mechanism is analogous to what psychoanalysts call "making the unconscious conscious."

Simply arousing emotions and the accompanying cognitions are not sufficient to cause lasting change. People express emotion, sometimes explosively, throughout their lives without benefit. However, the therapeutic milieu allows the patient to experience emotional arousal and reality testing simultaneously. For a variety of psychotherapies, what is therapeutic is the patient's ability to be engaged in a problem situation and yet respond to it adaptively. In terms of cognitive therapy, this means to experience the cognitions and to test them within the therapeutic framework.

APPLICATIONS

Who Can We Help?

Cognitive therapy is a present-centered, structured, active, cognitive, problem-oriented approach best suited for cases in which problems can be delineated and cognitive distortions are apparent. It was originally developed for the treatment of major psychiatric conditions but has been elaborated to treat personality disorders as well. It has wide-ranging applications to a variety of clinical and nonclinical problems. Although originally used in individual psychotherapy, it is now used with couples, families, and groups. It can be applied alone or in combination with pharmacotherapy in inpatient and outpatient settings.

Cognitive therapy is widely recognized as an effective treatment for unipolar depression. Beck, Rush, Shaw, and Emery (1979, p. 27) list criteria for using cognitive therapy alone or in combination with medication. It is the treatment of choice in cases where the patient refuses medication, prefers a psychological treatment, has unacceptable side effects to antidepressant medication, has a medical condition that precludes the use of antidepressants, or has proved to be refractory to adequate trials of antidepressants. Recent research by DeRubeis et al. (2005) indicates that cognitive therapy can be as effective as medications for the initial treatment of moderate to severe major depression.

Cognitive therapy is not recommended as the exclusive treatment in cases of bipolar affective disorder or psychotic depression. It is also not used alone for the treatment of other psychoses such as schizophrenia. Some patients with anxiety may begin treatment on medication, but cognitive therapy teaches them to function without relying on medication.

Cognitive therapy produces the best results with patients who have adequate reality testing (i.e., no hallucinations or delusions), good concentration, and sufficient memory functions. It is ideally suited to patients who can focus on their automatic thoughts, accept the therapist–patient roles, are willing to tolerate anxiety in order to do experiments, can alter assumptions permanently, take responsibility for their problems, and are willing to postpone gratification in order to complete therapy. Although these ideals are not always met, this therapy can proceed with some adjustment of outcome expectations and flexibility of structure. For example, therapy may not permanently alter schemas but may improve the patient's daily functioning.

Cognitive therapy is effective for patients with different levels of income, education, and background (Persons, Burns, & Perloff, 1988). As long as the patient can recognize the relationships among thoughts, feelings, and behaviors and takes some responsibility for self-help, cognitive therapy can be beneficial.

Treatment

Cognitive therapy consists of highly specific learning experiences designed to teach patients (1) to monitor their negative, automatic thoughts (cognitions); (2) to recognize the connections among cognition, affect, and behavior; (3) to examine the evidence for and against distorted automatic thoughts; (4) to substitute more reality-oriented interpretations for these biased cognitions; and (5) to learn to identify and alter the beliefs that predispose them to distort their experiences (Beck, Rush, Shaw, & Emery, 1979).

Both cognitive and behavioral techniques are used in cognitive therapy to reach these goals. The technique used at any given time depends on the patient's level of functioning and on the particular symptoms and problems presented.

Cognitive Techniques

Verbal techniques are used to elicit the patient's automatic thoughts, analyze the logic behind the thoughts, identify maladaptive assumptions, and examine the validity of those assumptions. Automatic thoughts are elicited by questioning the patient about those thoughts that occur during upsetting situations. If the patient has difficulty recalling thoughts, then imagery or role playing can be used. Automatic thoughts are most accurately reported when they occur in real-life situations. Such "hot" cognitions are accessible, powerful, and habitual. The patient is taught to recognize and identify thoughts and to record them when upset.

Cognitive therapists do not interpret patients' automatic thoughts but instead explore their meanings, particularly when a patient reports fairly neutral thoughts yet displays strong emotions. In such cases, the therapist asks what those thoughts mean to the patient. For example, after an initial visit, an anxious patient called his therapist in great distress. He had just read an article about drug treatments for anxiety. His automatic thought was "Drug therapy is helpful for anxiety." The meaning he ascribed to this was "Cognitive therapy can't possibly help me. I am doomed to failure again."

Automatic thoughts are tested by direct evidence or by logical analysis. Evidence can be derived from past and present circumstances, but, true to scientific inquiry, it must be as close to the facts as possible. Data can also be gathered in behavioral experiments. For example, if a man believes he cannot carry on a conversation, he might try to initiate brief exchanges with three people. The empirical nature of behavioral experiments allows patients to think in a more objective way.

Examination of the patient's thoughts can also lead to cognitive change. Questioning may uncover logical inconsistencies, contradictions, and other errors in thinking. Identifying cognitive distortions is in itself helpful because patients then have specific errors to correct.

Maladaptive assumptions are usually much less accessible to patients than automatic thoughts. Some patients are able to articulate their assumptions, but most find it difficult. Assumptions appear as themes in automatic thoughts. The therapist may ask the patient to abstract rules underlying specific thoughts. The therapist might also infer assumptions from these data and present these assumptions to the patient for verification. A patient who had trouble identifying her assumptions broke into tears on reading an assumption inferred by her therapist—an indication of the salience of that assumption. Patients always have the right to disagree with the therapist and find more accurate statements of their beliefs.

Once an assumption has been identified, it is open to modification. This can occur in several ways: by asking the patient whether the assumption seems reasonable, by having the patient generate reasons for and against maintaining the assumption, and by presenting evidence contrary to the assumption. Even though a particular assumption may seem reasonable in a specific situation, it may appear dysfunctional when universally applied. For example, being highly productive at work is generally reasonable, but being highly productive during recreational time may be unreasonable. A physician who believed he should work to his top capacity throughout his career may not have considered the prospect of early burnout. Thus, what may have made him successful in the short run could lead to problems in the long run. Specific cognitive techniques include decatastrophizing, reattribution, redefining, and decentering.

Decatastrophizing, also known as the *what-if technique* (Beck & Emery, 1985), helps patients prepare for feared consequences. This is helpful in decreasing avoidance, particularly when combined with coping plans (Beck & Emery, 1985). If anticipated consequences are likely to happen, these techniques help identify problem-solving strategies. Decatastrophizing is often used with a time-projection technique to widen the range of information and broaden the patient's time perspective.

Reattribution techniques test automatic thoughts and assumptions by considering alternative causes of events. This is especially helpful when patients personalize or perceive themselves as the cause of events. It is unreasonable to conclude, in the absence of evidence, that another person or single factor is the sole cause of an event. Reattribution techniques encourage reality testing and appropriate assignment of responsibility by requiring examination of all the factors that impinge on a situation.

Redefining is a way to mobilize a patient who believes a problem to be beyond personal control. Burns (1985) recommends that lonely people who think, "Nobody pays any attention to me" redefine the problem as "I need to reach out to other people and be caring." Redefining a problem may include making it more concrete and specific and stating it in terms of the patient's own behavior.

Decentering is used primarily in treating anxious patients who wrongly believe they are the focus of everyone's attention. After they examine the logic behind the conviction that others would stare at them and be able to read their minds, behavioral experiments are designed to test these particular beliefs. For example, one student who was reluctant to speak in class believed his classmates watched him constantly and noticed his anxiety. By observing them instead of focusing on his own discomfort, he saw some students taking notes, some looking at the professor, and some daydreaming. He concluded that his classmates had other concerns.

The cognitive domain comprises thoughts and images. For some patients, pictorial images are more accessible and easier to report than thoughts. This is often the case with anxious patients. Ninety percent of anxious patients in one study reported visual images before and during episodes of anxiety (Beck, Laude, & Bohnert, 1974). Gathering information about imagery, then, is another way to understand conceptual systems. Spontaneous images provide data on the patient's perceptions and interpretations of events. Other specific imagery procedures used to modify distorted cognitions are discussed by Beck and Emery (1985) and Judith Beck (1995).

In some cases, imagery is modified for its own sake. *Intrusive imagery,* such as imagery related to trauma, can be directly modified to reduce its impact. Patients can change aspects of an image by "rewriting the script" of what happened, making an attacker shrink in size to the point of powerlessness or empowering themselves in the image. The point of restructuring such images is not to deny what actually happened but to reduce the ability of the image to disrupt daily functioning.

Imagery is also used in role plays because of its ability to access emotions. Experiential techniques, such as dialogues between one's healthy self and one's negative thoughts, are used to mobilize affect and help patients both believe and feel that they have the right to be free of harmful and self-defeating patterns.

Behavioral Techniques

Cognitive therapy uses behavioral techniques to modify automatic thoughts and assumptions. It uses behavioral experiments designed to challenge specific maladaptive beliefs and promote new learning. In a behavioral experiment, for example, a patient may predict an outcome based on personal automatic thoughts, carry out the agreed-upon behavior, and then evaluate the evidence in light of the new experience.

Behavioral techniques are also used to expand patients' response repertories (skills training), relax them (progressive muscle relaxation) or make them active (activity scheduling), prepare them for avoided situations (behavioral rehearsal), or expose them to feared stimuli (exposure therapy). Because behavioral techniques are used to foster cognitive change, it is crucial to know the patient's perceptions, thoughts, and conclusions after each behavioral experiment.

Homework gives patients the opportunity to apply cognitive principles between sessions. Typical homework assignments focus on self-observation and self-monitoring, structuring time effectively, and implementing procedures for dealing with concrete situations. Self-monitoring is applied to the patient's automatic thoughts and reactions in various situations. New skills, such as challenging automatic thoughts, are also practiced as homework.

Hypothesis testing has both cognitive and behavioral components. In framing a "hypothesis," it is necessary to make it specific and concrete. A resident who insisted, "I am not a good doctor" was asked to list what was needed to arrive at that conclusion. The therapist contributed other criteria as well because the physician had overlooked such factors as rapport with patients and the ability to make decisions under pressure. The resident then monitored his behavior and sought feedback from colleagues and supervisors to test his hypothesis, coming to the conclusion "I am a good doctor *for my level of training and experience.*"

Exposure therapy serves to provide data on the thoughts, images, physiological symptoms, and self-reported level of tension experienced by the anxious patient. Specific thoughts and images can be examined for distortions, and specific coping skills can be taught. By dealing directly with a patient's idiosyncratic thoughts, cognitive therapy is able to focus on that patient's particular needs. Patients learn that their predictions are not always accurate, and they then have the data to challenge anxious thoughts in the future.

Behavioral rehearsal and *role playing* are used to practice skills or techniques that are later applied in real life. Modeling is also used in skills training. Often role playing is videotaped so that an objective source of information is available with which to evaluate performance.

Diversion techniques, which are used to reduce strong emotions and decrease negative thinking, include physical activity, social contact, work, play, and visual imagery.

Activity scheduling provides structure and encourages involvement. Rating (on a scale of 0 to 10) the degree of mastery and pleasure experienced during each activity of the day achieves several things: Patients who believe their depression is at a constant level see mood fluctuations; those who believe they cannot accomplish or enjoy anything are contradicted by the evidence; and those who believe they are inactive because of an inherent defect are shown that activity involves some planning and is reinforcing in itself.

Graded-task assignment calls for the patient to initiate an activity at a nonthreatening level while the therapist gradually increases the difficulty of assigned tasks. For example, someone who has difficulty socializing might begin interacting with one other person, interact with a small group of acquaintances, or socialize with people for just a brief period of time. Step by step, the patient comes to increase the time spent with others.

Cognitive therapists work in a variety of settings. Patients are referred by physicians, schools and universities, and other therapists who believe that cognitive therapy would be especially helpful. Many patients are self-referred. The Academy of Cognitive Therapy maintains an international referral list of therapists on its Web site (www .academyofct.org).

Cognitive therapists generally adhere to 45-minute sessions. Because of the structure of cognitive therapy, much can be accomplished in this time. Patients are frequently asked to complete questionnaires, such as the BDI, before the start of each session. Most sessions take place in the therapist's office. However, real-life work with anxious patients occurs outside the therapist's office. A therapist might take public transportation with an agoraphobic, go to a pet store with a rodent phobic, or travel in an airplane with someone afraid of flying.

Confidentiality is always maintained, and the therapist obtains informed consent for audiotaping and videotaping. Such recording is used in skills training or as a way to present evidence contradicting the patient's assumptions. For example, a patient who believes she looks nervous whenever she converses might be videotaped in conversation to test this assumption. Her appearance on camera may convince her that her assumption was in error and help her identify specific behaviors to improve. Occasionally, patients take audiotaped sessions home to review content material between sessions.

Sessions are usually conducted on a weekly basis, with severely disturbed patients seen more frequently in the beginning. Cognitive therapists give their patients phone numbers at which they can be reached in the event of an emergency.

Whenever possible, and with the patient's permission, significant others such as friends and family members are included in a therapy session to review the treatment goals and explore ways in which the significant others might be helpful. This is especially important when family members misunderstand the nature of the illness, are overly solicitous, or are behaving in counterproductive ways. Significant others can be of great assistance in therapy, helping to sustain behavioral improvements by encouraging homework and assisting the patient with reality testing.

Problems may arise in the practice of cognitive therapy. For example, patients may misunderstand what the therapist says, and this may result in anger, dissatisfaction, or hopelessness. When the therapist perceives such a reaction, he or she elicits the patient's thoughts, just as with any other automatic thoughts. Together the therapist and client look for alternative interpretations. The therapist who has made an error accepts responsibility and corrects the mistake.

Problems sometimes result from unrealistic expectations about how quickly behaviors should change, from the incorrect or inflexible application of a technique, or from lack of attention to central issues. Problems in therapy require that the therapist attend to his or her own automatic thoughts and look for distortions in logic that create strong affect or prevent adequate problem solving.

Beck, Rush, Shaw, and Emery (1979) provide guidelines for working with difficult patients and those who have histories of unsuccessful therapy: (1) Avoid stereotyping the patient as *being* the problem rather than *having* the problem, (2) remain optimistic, (3) identify and deal with your own dysfunctional cognitions, (4) remain focused on the task instead of blaming the patient, and (5) maintain a problem-solving attitude. By following these guidelines, the therapist is able to be more resourceful with difficult patients. The therapist also can serve as a model for the patient, demonstrating that frustration does not automatically lead to anger and despair.

Evidence

Evidence-based practice in psychology (EBPP) advocates the application of empirically supported principles of psychological assessment, case formulation, therapeutic relationship, and intervention in the delivery of effective psychological care (APA Presidential Task Force on Evidence-Based Practice, 2006). The evidence base for any psychological treatment is evaluated in terms of its efficacy, or demonstrated causal relationship to outcome, and its utility or generalizability and feasibility—in other words, its internal and external validity. The best available research is then combined with clinical expertise in the context of patient characteristics, culture, and preferences to promote the effective practice of psychology and public health.

A fundamental component of evidence-based practice is empirically supported treatments, those demonstrated to work for a certain disorder or problem under specified circumstances. Randomized controlled trials (RCTs) in psychology, as in other health fields, are the standard for drawing causal inferences and provide the most direct and internally valid demonstration of treatment efficacy. Meta-analysis, a systematic way to synthesize results from multiple studies, is used to quantitatively measure treatment outcome and effect sizes. Other research designs, such as qualitative research and single-case experimental designs, are used to describe experiences, generate new hypotheses, and examine causal relationships for an individual, but RCTs and meta-analysis are best suited for examining whether a treatment works for a number of people.

Cognitive therapy (CT) and cognitive-behavioral therapies (CBT, the atheoretical combination of cognitive and behavioral strategies) are based on empirical studies. Individual RCTs, reviews of the literature of outcome studies for a range of disorders, and meta-analyses all document the success of CT and CBT in the treatment of depression and anxiety disorders in particular (Beck, 2005; Butler, Chapman, Forman, & Beck, 2006; DeRubeis & Crits-Christoph, 1998; Gloaguen, Cottraux, Cucherat, & Blackburn, 1998; Gould, Otto, & Pollack, 1995; Wampold, Minami, Baskin, & Callen Tierney, 2002). The review of 16 methodologically rigorous meta-analyses by Butler et al. (2006) found large effect sizes for unipolar depression, generalized anxiety disorder, panic disorder with or without agoraphobia, social phobia, and childhood depressive and anxiety disorders. Moderate effect sizes were found for marital distress, anger, childhood somatic disorders, and chronic pain. Relatively small effect sizes were found for adjunctive CBT for schizophrenia and for bulimia nervosa. Other studies have found that CT–CBT yield lower relapse rates than antidepressant medications (Hollon et al., 2005) and reduce the risk of symptoms returning following treatment termination for depression and anxiety disorders (Hollon et al., 2006).

One criticism of the reliance on RCTs in psychotherapy research is that the samples studied are so carefully screened to eliminate comorbidity or other threats to experimental control that they do not represent real groups in the community, who often have multiple problems. However, a landmark study by Brown et al. (2005) showed success for cognitive therapy for the prevention of suicide attempts among people at high risk for suicide. The participants in this study had more than one psychiatric diagnosis, and 68% had substance abuse problems. A study by DeRubeis et al. (2005) similarly included participants with comorbidity.

In addition to best available research, another component of evidence-based practice is clinical expertise—the advanced clinical skills to assess, diagnose, and treat disorders. The importance of clinical expertise is demonstrated in the study by DeRubeis et al. (2005), which concluded that CT can be as effective as medications for the initial treatment of depression, but the degree of effectiveness may depend on a high level of therapist experience or expertise.

The generalizability of CT–CBT has been examined in a few studies. Stirman and colleagues (Stirman, DeRubeis, Crits-Cristoph & Rothman, 2005) found that clinical characteristics of subjects in RCTs matched those of patients in clinical settings. Similarly, Persons and associates (Persons, Bostrom, & Bertagnolli, 1999) found that clinic patients treated with CT for depression improved comparably to those in RTCs. In addition, studies of schizophrenic patients at National Health Service clinics in the United Kingdom found improved symptoms using CT as an adjunct to pharmacotherapy (Tarrier, 2008).

Because training in evidence-based therapies has been mandated by the Accreditation Council for Graduate Medical Education, CT–CBT is being taught in psychiatry residency programs in the United States. As the number of professionals with expertise in cognitive therapy increases, research may be further directed both toward refining the therapy for more populations in need and toward exploring ways to make it cost-effective and available in community settings.

Psychotherapy in a Multicultural World

Cognitive therapy begins with an understanding of the patient's beliefs, values, and attitudes. These exist within a cultural context, and the therapist must understand that context. Cognitive therapy focuses on whether these beliefs are adaptive for the patient and whether they pose difficulties or lead to dysfunctional behavior. Cognitive therapy does not work on changing beliefs in an arbitrary way, nor is it an attempt to impose the therapist's beliefs on the patient. Rather, it helps the individual examine his or her own beliefs and whether they foster emotional well-being. Sometimes people's personal beliefs are at odds with the cultural values around them. Other times, a person's beliefs may be changing with cultural changes, as in rapid modernization or migration to a new country, and discrepancies may cause distress. In these cases, cognitive therapy may help patients think flexibly in order to reconcile their beliefs with environmental constraints or empower them to find solutions.

Beck's work has been translated into more than a dozen languages, and cognitive therapists are represented by organizations worldwide. Research in cognitive therapy has been conducted in many countries, primarily industrial economies. There is a need to expand cognitive therapy research further into developing nations.

CASE EXAMPLE

This case example of the course of treatment for an anxious patient illustrates the use of both behavioral and cognitive techniques.

Presenting Problem

The patient was a 21-year-old male college student who complained of sleep-onset insomnia and frequent awakenings, halting speech and stuttering, shakiness, feelings of nervousness, dizziness, and worrying. His sleep difficulties were particularly acute before exams or athletic competitions. He attributed his speech problems to his search for the "perfect word."

The patient was raised in a family that valued competition. As the eldest child, he was expected to win all the contests. His parents were determined that their children should surpass them in achievements and successes. They so strongly identified with the patient's achievements that he believed, "My success is their success."

The patient was taught to compete with other children outside the family as well. His father reminded him, "Never let anyone get the best of you." As a consequence of viewing others as adversaries, he developed few friends. Feeling lonely, he tried desperately to attract friends by becoming a prankster and by telling lies to enhance his image and make his family appear more attractive. Although he had acquaintances in college, he had few friends because he was unable to self-disclose, fearing that others would discover he was not all that he would like to be.

Early Sessions

After gathering initial data regarding diagnosis, context, and history, the therapist attempted to define how the patient's cognitions contributed to his distress (T = therapist; P = patient).

T: What types of situations are most upsetting to you?

P: When I do poorly in sports, particularly swimming. I'm on the swim team. Also, if I make a mistake, even when I play cards with my roommates. I feel really upset if I get rejected by a girl.

T: What thoughts go through your mind, let's say, when you don't do so well at swimming?

P: I think people think much less of me if I'm not on top, a winner.

T: And how about if you make a mistake playing cards?

P: I doubt my own intelligence.

T: And if a girl rejects you?

P: It means I'm not special. I lose value as a person.

T: Do you see any connections here, among these thoughts?

P: Well, I guess my mood depends on what other people think of me. But that's important. I don't want to be lonely.

T: What would that mean to you, to be lonely?

P: It would mean there's something wrong with me, that I'm a loser.

At this point, the therapist began to hypothesize about the patient's organizing beliefs: that his worth is determined by others, that he is unattractive because there is something inherently wrong with him, that he is a loser. The therapist looked for evidence to support the centrality of these beliefs and remained open to other possibilities.

The therapist assisted the patient in generating a list of goals to work on in therapy. These goals included (1) decreasing perfectionism, (2) decreasing anxiety symptoms, (3) decreasing sleep difficulties, (4) increasing closeness in friendships, and (5) developing his own values apart from those of his parents. The first problem addressed was anxiety. An upcoming exam was chosen as a target situation. This student typically studied far beyond what was necessary, went to bed worried, finally fell asleep, woke during the night thinking about details or possible consequences of his performance, and went to exams exhausted. To reduce ruminations about his performance, the therapist asked him to name the advantages of dwelling on thoughts of the exam.

P: Well, if I don't think about the exam all the time I might forget something. If I think about the exam constantly, I think I'll do better. I'll be more prepared.

T: Have you ever gone into a situation less "prepared"?

P: Not an exam, but once I was in a big swim meet and the night before I went out with friends and didn't think about it. I came home, went to sleep, got up, and swam.

T: And how did it work out?

P: Fine. I felt great and swam pretty well.

T: Based on that experience, do you think there's any reason to try to worry less about your performance?

P: I guess so. It didn't hurt me not to worry. Actually, worrying can be pretty distracting. I end up focusing more on how I'm doing than on what I'm doing.

The patient came up with his own rationale for decreasing his ruminations. He was then ready to consider giving up his maladaptive behavior and risk trying something new. The therapist taught the patient progressive relaxation, and the patient began to use physical exercise as a way to relieve anxiety.

The patient was also instructed in how cognitions affect behavior and mood. Picking up on the patient's statement that worries can be distracting, the therapist proceeded.

T: You mentioned that when you worry about your exams, you feel anxious. What I'd like you to do now is imagine lying in your bed the night before an exam.

P: Okay, I can picture it.

T: Imagine that you are thinking about the exam and you decide that you haven't done enough to prepare.

P: Yeah, OK.

T: How are you feeling?

P: I'm feeling nervous. My heart is beginning to race. I think I need to get up and study some more.

T: Good. When you think you're not prepared, you get anxious and want to get up out of bed. Now, I want you to imagine that you are in bed the night before the exam. You have prepared in your usual way and are ready. You remind yourself of what you have done. You think that you are prepared and know the material.

P: OK. Now I feel confident.

T: What do you notice about these two scenarios?

P: I see how my mind-set affects my anxiety. I guess if I really have studied, I can let myself rest.

Over the next few weeks, the patient was taught how to record automatic thoughts, recognize cognitive distortions, and respond to them. For homework, he was asked to record his automatic thoughts if he had trouble falling asleep before an exam. One automatic thought he had while lying in bed was "I should be thinking about the exam." His response was "Thinking about the exam is not going to help me sleep. I did study." Another thought was "I must go to sleep now! I must get eight hours of sleep!" His response was "I have left leeway, so I have time. Sleep is not so crucial that I have to worry about it." He was able to shift his thinking to a positive image of himself floating in clear blue water.

By observing his automatic thoughts across a variety of situations—academic, athletic, and social—the patient identified dichotomous thinking (e.g., "I'm either a winner or a loser") as a frequent cognitive distortion. Perceiving the consequences of his behavior as either totally good or completely bad resulted in major shifts in mood. Two techniques that helped with his dichotomous thinking were reframing the problem and building a continuum between his dichotomous categories.

Here the problem is reframed:

T: Can you think of reasons for someone not to respond to you other than because you're a loser?

P: No. Unless I really convince them I'm great, they won't be attracted.

T: How would you convince them of that?

P: To tell you the truth, I'd exaggerate what I've done. I'd lie about my grade point average or tell someone I placed first in a race.

T: How does that work out?

P: Actually, not too well. I get uncomfortable and they get confused by my stories. Sometimes they don't seem to care. Other times they walk away after I've been talking a lot about myself.

T: So in some cases, they don't respond to you when you focus the conversation on yourself.

P: Right.

T: Does this have anything to do with whether you're a winner or a loser?

P: No, they don't even know who I am deep down. They're just turned off because I talk too much.

T: I see. It sounds like they're responding to your conversational style.

The therapist reframed the problem from a situation in which something was inherently wrong with the patient to one characterized by a problem of social skills. Moreover, the theme "I am a loser" appeared so powerful to the patient that he labeled it as his "main belief." This assumption was traced historically to the constant criticism from his parents for mistakes and perceived shortcomings. By reviewing his history, he was able to see that his lies prevented people from getting closer, reinforcing his belief that they didn't want to be close. In addition, he believed that his parents made him whatever success he was and that no achievement was his alone. This had made him angry and lacking in self-confidence.

Later Sessions

As therapy progressed, the patient's homework increasingly focused on social interaction. He practiced initiating conversations and asking questions in order to learn more about other people. He also practiced "biting his tongue" instead of telling small lies about himself. He monitored people's reactions to him and saw that they were varied but generally positive. By listening to others, he found that he admired people who could openly admit shortcomings and joke about their mistakes. This experience helped him understand that it was useless to categorize people, including himself, as winners and losers.

In later sessions, the patient described his belief that his behavior reflected on his parents and vice versa. He said, "If they look good, it says something about me and if I look good, they get the credit." One assignment required him to list the ways in which he was different from his parents. He remarked, "Realizing that my parents and I are separate made me realize I could stop telling lies." Recognizing how he was different from his parents freed him from their absolute standards and allowed him to be less self-conscious when interacting with others.

Subsequently, the patient was able to pursue interests and hobbies that had nothing to do with achievement. He was able to set moderate and realistic goals for schoolwork, and he began to date.

SUMMARY

Cognitive therapy has grown quickly because of its empirical basis and demonstrated efficacy. Borrowing some of its concepts from cognitive theorists and several techniques from behavior therapy and client-oriented psychotherapy, cognitive therapy consists of a broad theoretical structure of personality and psychopathology, a set of well-defined therapeutic strategies, and a wide variety of therapeutic techniques. Similar in many ways to rational emotive behavior therapy, which preceded but developed parallel to cognitive therapy, this system of psychotherapy has acquired strong empirical support for its theoretical foundations. Many outcome studies have demonstrated its efficacy, especially in the treatment of depression. The related theoretical formulations of depression have been supported by more than 100 empirical studies. Other concepts—such as the cognitive triad in depression, the concept of specific cognitive profiles for specific disorders, cognitive processing, and the relationship of hopelessness to suicide—have also received strong support.

Outcome studies have investigated cognitive therapy with major depressive disorders, generalized anxiety disorder, dysthymic disorder, drug abuse, alcoholism, panic disorder, anorexia, and bulimia. In addition, cognitive therapy has been applied successfully to the treatment of obsessive–compulsive disorder, hypochondriasis, and various personality disorders. In conjunction with psychotropic medication, it has been used to treat delusional disorders and bipolar disorder.

Much of the popularity of cognitive therapy is attributable to strong empirical support for its theoretical framework and to the large number of outcome studies with clinical populations. In addition, there is no doubt that the intellectual atmosphere of the "cognitive revolution" has made the field of psychotherapy more receptive to this new therapy. A further attractive feature of cognitive therapy is that it is readily teachable. The various therapeutic strategies and techniques have been described and defined in such a way that one year's training is usually sufficient for a psychotherapist to attain a reasonable level of competence as a cognitive therapist.

Although cognitive therapy focuses on understanding the patient's problems and applying appropriate techniques, it also attends to the nonspecific therapeutic characteristics of the therapist. Consequently, the basic qualities of empathy, acceptance, and personal regard are highly valued.

Because therapy is not conducted in a vacuum, cognitive therapists pay close attention to patients' interpersonal relations and confront them continuously with problems they may be avoiding. Further, therapeutic change can take place only when patients are emotionally engaged with their problems. Therefore, the experience of emotion during therapy is a crucial feature. The patient's reactions to the therapist and vice versa are also important. Excessive and distorted responses to the therapist are elicited and evaluated just like any other type of ideational material. In the presence of the therapist, patients learn to correct their misconceptions, which were often derived from early experiences.

Cognitive therapy may offer an opportunity for a rapprochement between psychodynamic therapy and behavior therapy. In many ways, it provides a common ground for these two disciplines. Currently, the number of cognitive therapists within the behavior therapy movement is growing. In fact, many behavior therapists view themselves as cognitive-behavior therapists.

Looking to the future, the boundaries of the theoretical background of cognitive therapy are expected to gradually expand to encompass or penetrate the fields of cognitive psychology and social psychology. There is already an enormous amount of interest in social psychology, which provides the theoretical background of cognitive therapy.

In an era of cost containment, this short-term approach will prove to be increasingly attractive to third-party payers as well as to patients. Future empirical studies of its processes and effectiveness will undoubtedly be conducted to determine whether cognitive therapy can fulfill its promise.

Counseling CourseMate Website:

See this text's Counseling CourseMate website at www.cengagebrain.com for learning tools such as chapter quizzing, videos, glossary flashcards, and more.

ANNOTATED BIBLIOGRAPHY

Beck, A. T., Freeman, A., Davis, D., & Associates. (2004). *Cognitive therapy of personality disorders* (2nd edition). New York: Guilford Press.
This book presents the research and theory behind the cognitive conceptualization of personality disorders. Specific beliefs and attitudes for each personality disorder are presented along with intervention techniques.

Beck, A. T., Rush, A. J., Shaw, B. F., & Emery, G. (1979). *Cognitive therapy of depression.* New York: Guilford Press.

Perhaps Beck's most influential book, this work presents the cognitive model of depression and treatment interventions. This book codified what actually happens in cognitive therapy and thus set a standard for other psychotherapies to follow.

Beck, J. S. (1995). *Cognitive therapy: Basics and beyond.* New York: Guilford Press.
Dr. Judith Beck presents an updated manual for cognitive therapy. She begins with how to develop a cognitive case

conceptualization and instructs the reader in how to identify deeper-level cognitions, prepare for termination, and anticipate problems.

Clark, D. A., & Beck, A. T. (2010). *Cognitive therapy of anxiety disorders: Science and practice.* New York: Guilford Press.

This book fully describes the cognitive theory of anxiety disorders, backed by research. It then presents the treatment of specific anxiety disorders, including panic disorder, social phobia, PTSD, obsessive–compulsive disorder, and generalized anxiety disorder.

Ellis, T. E., & Newman, C. F. (1996). *Choosing to live: How to defeat suicide through cognitive therapy.* Oakland, CA: New Harbinger Publications.

This book is for clients and clinicians alike. The strategies presented are well grounded in research and aimed at reducing hopelessness and increasing problem solving. This book has been used as a treatment manual in clinical research.

Kingdon, D. G., & Turkington, D. (2005). *Cognitive therapy of schizophrenia.* New York; Guilford Press.

This book describes how schizophrenia, long thought to be an illness not amenable to psychological interventions, can be treated with a combination of medication and cognitive techniques that work directly with hallucinations and delusions.

CASE READINGS

Beck, A. T., Rush, J., Shaw, B., & Emery, G. (1979). Interview with a depressed and suicidal patient. In *Cognitive therapy of depression* (pp. 225–243). New York: Guilford Press. [Reprinted in D. Wedding & R. J. Corsini (Eds.). (2013). *Case studies in psychotherapy.* Belmont, CA: Brooks/Cole.]

This interview with a suicidal patient features an outline of the types of assessments and interventions made by cognitive therapists in an initial session. Substantial change occurs in one session, as demonstrated in the verbatim transcript of the interview.

Bennett-Levy, J., Butler, G., Fennell, M., Hackmann, A., Mueller, M., & Westbrook, D. (Eds.). (2004). *Oxford guide to behavioral experiments in cognitive therapy.* Oxford, UK: Oxford University Press.

The numerous case descriptions in this text amply demonstrate the utility of behavioral experiments. The creativity and variety of the experiments inspires clinicians to

use behavioral experiments to challenge clients' maladaptive beliefs.

Greenberger, D., & Padesky, C. A. (1995). *Mind over mood: A cognitive therapy treatment manual for clients.* New York: Guilford Press.

This is a workbook for clients that teaches cognitive techniques. It can stand alone but is most helpful when used within therapy. It is an excellent resource for cognitive therapists in training because it uses three case studies to teach cognitive techniques.

Wright, J. H., Basco, M. R., & Thase, M. E. (2006). *Learning cognitive-behavior therapy: An illustrated guide.* Washington, D. C. : American Psychiatric Publishing.

Accompanied by a DVD demonstrating cognitive techniques with clients, this text takes the reader step by step from case formulation to the treatment of complex cases.

REFERENCES

Adler, A. (1936). The neurotic's picture of the world. *International Journal of Individual Psychology, 2,* 3–10.

Alexander, E. (1950). *Psychosomatic medicine: Its principles and applications.* New York: Norton.

APA Presidential Task Force on Evidence-Based Practice. (2006). Evidence-based practice in psychology. *American Psychologist, 61,* 271–285.

Arnold, M. (1960). *Emotion and personality* (Vol. 1). New York: Columbia University Press.

Bandura, A. (1977). *Social learning theory.* Englewood Cliffs, NJ: Prentice-Hall.

Baucom, D., Sayers, S., & Sher, T. (1990). Supplementary behavioral marital therapy with cognitive restructuring and emotional expressiveness training: An outcome investigation. *Journal of Consulting & Clinical Psychology, 58,* 636–645.

Beck, A. T. (1963). Thinking and depression. 1. Idiosyncratic content and cognitive distortions. *Archives of General Psychiatry, 9,* 324–333.

Beck, A. T. (1964). Thinking and depression. 2. Theory and therapy. *Archives of General Psychiatry, 10,* 561–571.

Beck, A. T. (1967). *Depression: Clinical, experimental, and theoretical aspects.* New York: Hoeber. [Republished as *Depression: Causes and treatment.* Philadelphia: University of Pennsylvania Press, 1972.]

Beck, A. T. (2005). The current state of cognitive therapy. *Archives of General Psychiatry, 62,* 953–959.

Beck, A. T. (2008). The evolution of the cognitive model of depression and its neurobiological correlates. *American Journal of Psychiatry, 165*(8), 969–977.

Beck, A. T., & Beck, J. S. (1995). *The Personality Belief Questionnaire.* Bala Cynwyd, PA: Beck Institute for Cognitive Therapy and Research.

Beck, J. S., & Beck, A. T. (2002). *Beck Youth Inventories of Emotional and Social Impairment.* San Antonio, TX: The Psychological Corporation.

Beck, A. T., Brown, G., Berchick, R. J., Stewart, B. L., & Steer, R. A. (1990). Relationship between hopelessness and ultimate suicide: A replication with psychiatric outpatients. *American Journal of Psychiatry, 147*(2), 190–195.

Beck, A. T., & Emery, G. (1985). *Anxiety disorders and phobias: A cognitive perspective.* New York: Basic Books.

Beck, A. T., Epstein, N., & Harrison, R. (1983). Cognitions, attitudes and personality dimensions in depression. *British Journal of Cognitive Psychotherapy, 1*(1), 1–16.

Beck, A. T., Freeman, A., & Davis, D. D. (2003). *Cognitive therapy of personality disorders.* New York: Plenum.

Beck, A. T., Kovacs, M., & Weissman, A. (1979). Assessment of suicidal intention: The scale for suicidal ideation. *Journal of Consulting and Clinical Psychology, 47,* 343–352.

Beck, A. T., Laude, R., & Bohnert, M. (1974). Ideational components of anxiety neurosis. *Archives of General Psychiatry, 31,* 319–325.

Beck, A. T., Rush, A. J., Shaw, B. F., & Emery, G. (1979). *Cognitive therapy of depression.* New York: Guilford Press.

Beck, A. T., Schuyler, D., & Herman, I. (1974). Development of the suicidal intent scales. In A. T. Beck, H. L. P. Resnik, & D. J. Lettieri (Eds.), *The prediction of suicide* (pp. 45–56). Bowie, MD: Charles Press.

Beck, A. T., Sokol, L., Clark, D. A., Berchick, R. J., & Wright, F. D. (1992). A crossover study of focused cognitive therapy for panic disorder. *American Journal of Psychiatry, 149,* 778–783.

Beck, A. T., & Steer, R. A. (1990). *Beck Anxiety Inventory manual.* San Antonio, TX: The Psychological Corporation.

Beck, A. T., Steer, R. A., & Brown, G. K. (1996). *The Beck Depression Inventory manual* (2nd ed.). San Antonio, TX: The Psychological Corporation.

Beck, A. T., Steer, R. A., Brown, G., & Epstein, N. (1990). The Beck Self-concept Test. *Psychological Assessment: A Journal of Consulting and Clinical Psychology, 2,* 191–197.

Beck, A. T., Steer, R. A., Kovacs, M., & Garrison, B. (1985). Hopelessness and eventual suicide: A 10-year study of patients hospitalized with suicidal ideation. *American Journal of Psychiatry, 412,* 559–563.

Beck, A. T., Ward, C. H., Mendelson, M., Mock, J. E., & Erbaugh, J. K. (1961). An inventory for measuring depression. *Archives of General Psychiatry, 4,* 561–571.

Beck, A. T., Weissman, A., Lester, D., & Trexler, L. (1974). The measurement of pessimism: The hopelessness scale. *Journal of Consulting and Clinical Psychology, 42,* 861–865.

Beck, J. S. (1995). *Cognitive therapy: Basics and beyond.* New York: Guilford Press.

Bennett-Levy, J., Butler, G., Fennell, M., Hackmann, A., Mueller, M., & Westbrook, D. (Eds.). (2004). *Oxford guide to behavioral experiments in cognitive therapy.* Oxford, UK: Oxford University Press.

Bowers, W. A. (2001). Cognitive model of eating disorders. *Journal of Cognitive Psychotherapy: An International Quarterly, 15,* 331–340.

Brown, G. K., Ten Have, T., Henriques, G. R., Xie, S. X., Hollander, J. E., & Beck, A. T. (2005). Cognitive therapy for the prevention of suicide attempts: A randomized controlled trial. *Journal of the American Medical Association, 294*(5), 563–570.

Burns, D. D. (1985). *Intimate connections.* New York: Morrow.

Butler, A. C., Chapman, J. E., Forman, E. M., & Beck, A. T. (2006). The empirical status of cognitive-behavioral therapy: A review of meta-analyses. *Clinical Psychology Review, 26,* 17–31.

Butler, G., Fennell, M., Robson, D., & Gelder, M. (1991). Comparison of behavior therapy and cognitive behavior therapy in the treatment of generalized anxiety disorder. *Journal of Consulting & Clinical Psychology, 59,* 167–175.

Clark, D. A., & Beck, A. T. (2010). *Cognitive therapy of anxiety disorders: Science and practice.* New York: Guilford Press.

Clark, D. A., & Beck, A. T. (2002). *Clark-Beck Obsessive Compulsive Inventory.* San Antonio, TX: The Psychological Corporation.

Clark, D. A., Beck, A. T., & Alford, B. A. (1999). *Scientific foundations of cognitive theory and therapy of depression.* New York: John Wiley.

Clark, D. M. (1996). Panic disorder: From theory to therapy. In P. Salkovskis (Ed.), *Frontiers of cognitive therapy* (pp. 318–344). New York: Guilford Press.

Clark, D. M. (1997). Panic disorder and social phobia. In D. M. Clark & C. G. Fairburn (Eds.), *Science and practice of cognitive behavior therapy* (pp. 122–153). New York: Oxford University Press.

Clark, D. M., Salkovskis, P. M., Hackmann, A., Middleton, H., & Gelder, M. (1992). A comparison of cognitive therapy, applied relaxation, and imipramine in the treatment of panic disorder. *British Journal of Psychiatry, 164,* 759–769.

DeRubeis, R. J., and Crits-Cristoph, P. (1998). Empirically supported individual and group psychological treatments for adult mental disorders. *Journal of Consulting and Clinical Psychology, 66,* 37–52.

DeRubeis, R. J., Hollon, S. D., Amsterdam, J. D., Shelton, R. C., Young, P. R., Salomon, R. M., O'Reardon, J. P., Lovett, M. L., Gladis, M. M., Brown, L. L., & Gallup, R. (2005). Cognitive therapy vs. medication in the treatment of moderate to severe depression. *Archives of General Psychiatry, 62,* 409–416.

Ehlers, A., & Clark, D. M. (2000). A cognitive model of posttraumatic stress disorder. *Behaviour Research and Therapy, 38,* 319–345.

Ellis, A. (1962). *Reason and emotion in psychotherapy.* New York: Lyle Stuart.

Ellis, T. E., & Newman, C. F. (1996). *Choosing to live: How to defeat suicide through cognitive therapy.* Oakland, CA: New Harbinger Publications.

Eng, W., Roth, D. A., & Heimberg, R. G. (2001). Cognitive behavioral therapy for social anxiety. *Journal of Cognitive Psychotherapy: An International Quarterly, 15,* 311–319.

Fairburn, C. C., Jones, R., Peveler, R. C., Hope, R. A., Carr, S. J., Solomon, R. A., et al. (1991). Three psychological treatments for bulimia nervosa: A comparative trial. *Archives of General Psychiatry, 48,* 463–469.

Freeston, M. H., Ladouceur, R., Gagnon, F., Thibodeau, N., Rheaume, J., Letarte, H., et al. (1997). Cognitive behavioral treatment of obsessive thoughts: A controlled study. *Journal of Consulting and Clinical Psychology, 65,* 405–413.

Garner, D. M., Rockert, W., Davis, R., Garner, M. V., Olmsted, M. P., & Eagle, M. (1993). Comparison of cognitive-behavioral and supportive–expressive therapy for bulimia nervosa. *American Journal of Psychiatry, 150,* 37–46.

Gillespie, K., Duffy, M., Hackmann, A., & Clark, D. M. (2002). Community-based cognitive therapy in the treatment of posttraumatic stress disorder following the Omagh bomb. *Behaviour Research and Therapy, 40,* 345–357.

Gloaguen, V., Cottraux, J., Cucherat, M., & Blackburn, I. M. (1998). A meta-analysis of the effects of cognitive therapy in depressed patients. *Journal of Affective Disorders, 49,* 59–72.

Gould, R. A., Otto, M. W., & Pollack, M. H. (1995). A meta-analysis of treatment outcome for panic disorder. *Clinical Psychology Review, 15,* 819–844.

Gournay, K. (1986, September). *Cognitive change during the behavioral treatment of agoraphobia.* Paper presented at Congress of the 16th European Association for Behavior Therapy, Lucerne, Switzerland.

Grant, P. M., Huh, G. A., Periviolitis, D., Stolar, N. M., & Beck, A. T. (2011). Randomized trial to evaluate the efficacy of cognitive therapy for low-functioning patients with schizophrenia. *Archives of General Psychiatry, 69,* 121–127.

Greenberger, D., & Padesky, C. A. (1995). *Mind over mood: A cognitive therapy treatment manual for clients.* New York: Guilford Press.

Haaga, D. A. E., Dyck, M. J., & Ernst, D. (1991). Empirical status of cognitive theory of depression. *Psychological Bulletin, 110*(2), 215–236.

Hollon, S. D., DeRubeis, R. J., & Evans, M. D. (1996). Cognitive therapy in the treatment and prevention of depression. In P. Salkovskis (Ed.), *Frontiers of cognitive therapy* (pp. 293–317). New York: Guilford.

Hollon, S. D., DeRubeis, R. J., Shelton, R. C., Amsterdam, J. D., Salomon, R. M., O'Reardon, J. P., Lovett, M. L., Young, P. R., Haman, K. L., Freeman, B. B., & Gallop, R. (2005). Prevention of relapse following cognitive therapy vs. medication in moderate to severe depression. *Archives of General Psychiatry, 62,* 417–422.

Hollon, S. D., Kendall, P. C., & Lumry, A. (1986). Specificity of depressotypic cognitions in clinical depression. *Journal of Abnormal Psychology, 95,* 52–59.

Hollon, S. D., Stewart, M. O., & Strunk, D. (2006) Enduring effects for cognitive behavior therapy in the treatment of depression and anxiety. *Annual Review of Psychology, 57,* 285–315.

Horney, K. (1950). *Neurosis and human growth: The struggle toward self-realization.* New York: Norton.

Kant, I. (1798). *The classification of mental disorders.* Konigsberg, Germany: Nicolovius.

Kelly, G. (1955). *The psychology of personal constructs.* New York: Norton.

Kingdon, D. G., & Turkington, D. (2005). *Cognitive therapy of schizophrenia.* New York; Guilford Press.

Lazarus, R. (1984). On the primacy of cognition. *American Psychologist, 39,* 124–129.

Mahoney, M. J. (1974). *Cognition and behavior modification.* Cambridge, MA: Ballinger.

Mahoney, M. J., & Arnkoff, D. (1978). Cognitive and self-control therapies. In S. L. Garfield & A. E. Bergin (Eds.), *Handbook of psychotherapy and behavior change: An empirical analysis* (pp. 689–722). New York: Wiley.

Meichenbaum, D. (1977). *Cognitive-behavior modification: An integrative approach.* New York: Plenum.

Norcross, J., & Karpiak, C. (2012). Clinical psychologists in the 2010s: 50 years of the APA Division of Clinical Psychology. *Clinical Psychology: Science and Practice*, 9, 1–12.

Padesky, C. A. (1993). Socratic questioning: Changing minds or guiding discovery? Keynote address delivered at the European Congress of Behavioural and Cognitive Therapies, London. Retrieved from www.padesky.com.

Padesky, C. A., & Beck, A. T. (2003). Science and philosophy: Comparison of cognitive therapy and rational emotive behavior therapy. *Journal of Cognitive Psychotherapy; An International Quarterly, 17,* 211–224.

Persons, J. B., Bostrom, A., & Bertagnolli, A. (1999). Results of randomized controlled trials of cognitive therapy for depression generalize to private practice. *Cognitive Therapy and Research, 23,* 535–548.

Persons, J. B., Burns, D. D., & Perloff, J. M. (1988). Predictors of dropout and outcome in cognitive therapy for depression in a private practice setting. *Cognitive Therapy and Research, 12,* 557–575.

Pike, K. M., Walsh, B. T., Vitousek, K., Wilson, G. T., & Bauer, J. (2003). Cognitive behavior therapy in the post hospitalization treatment of anorexia nervosa. *American Journal of Psychiatry, 160,* 2046–2049.

Resick, P. A. (2001). Cognitive therapy for posttraumatic stress disorder. *Journal of Cognitive Psychotherapy: An International Quarterly, 15,* 321–329.

Rogers, C. (1951). *Client-centered therapy.* Boston: Houghton Mifflin.

Segal, Z. V., Williams, J. M. G., & Teasdale, J. D. (2002). *Mindfulness-based cognitive therapy for depression.* New York: Guilford Press.

Stirman, S. W., DeRubeis, R. J., Crits-Cristoph, P., & Rothman, A. (2005). Can the randomized controlled trial literature generalize to nonrandomized patients? *Journal of Consulting and Clinical Psychology, 73,* 127–135.

Strunk, D. R., & DeRubeis, R. J. (2001). Cognitive therapy for depression: A review of its efficacy. *Journal of Cognitive Psychotherapy: An International Quarterly, 15,* 289–297.

Sullivan, H. S. (1953). *The interpersonal theory of psychiatry.* New York: Norton.

Tarrier, N. (2008). Schizophrenia and other psychotic disorders. In D. H. Barlow (Ed.), *Clinical handbook for psychological disorders: A step-by-step treatment manual* (4th ed., pp. 463–491). New York: Guilford Press.

Turkington, D., Dudley, R., Warman, D. M., & Beck, A. T. (2004). Cognitive-behavioral therapy for schizophrenia: A review. *Journal of Psychiatric Practice, 10,* 5–16.

Vitousek, K. M. (1996). The current status of cognitive behavioral models of anorexia nervosa and bulimia nervosa. In P. Salkovskis (Ed.), *Frontiers of cognitive therapy* (pp. 383–418). New York: Guilford.

Wampold, B. E., Minami, T., Baskin, T. W., & Callen Tierney, S. (2002). A meta-(re)analysis of the effects of cognitive therapy versus other therapies for depression. *Journal of Affective Disorders, 68,* 159–165.

Weissman, A., & Beck, A. T. (1978). *Development and validation of the Dysfunctional Attitude Scale.* Paper presented at the 12th annual meeting of the Association for Advancement of Behavior Therapy, Chicago.

Wessler, R. L. (1986). Conceptualizing cognitions in the cognitive-behavioral therapies. In W. Dryden & W. Golden (Eds.), *Cognitive-behavioural approaches to psychotherapy* (pp. 1–30). London: Harper & Row.

Williams, S. L., & Rappoport, A. (1983). Cognitive treatment in the natural environment for agoraphobics. *Behavior Therapy, 14,* 299–313.

Woody, G. E., Luborsky, L., McClellan, A. T., O'Brien, C. P., Beck, A. T., Blaine, J., et al. (1983). Psychotherapy for opiate addicts: Does it help? *Archives of General Psychiatry, 40,* 639–645.

Wright, J. H., Basco, M. R., & Thase, M. E. (2006). *Learning cognitive-behavior therapy: An illustrated guide.* Washington, D. C. : American Psychiatric Publishing.

Young, J. E., Rygh, J. L., Weinberger, A. D., & Beck, A. T. (2008). Cognitive therapy for depression. In D. H. Barlow (Ed.), *Clinical handbook of psychological disorders: A step-by-step treatment manual* (4th ed., pp. 250–305). New York: Guilford Press.

Young, J. E., Klosko, J. S., & Weishaar, M. E. (2003). *Schema therapy: A practitioner's guide.* New York: Guilford Press.

Zimmerman, G., Favrod, J., Trieu, V. H., & Pomini, V. (2005). The effect of cognitive behavioural treatment on the positive symptoms of schizophrenia spectrum disorders: A meta-analysis. *Schizophrenia Research, 77,* 1–9.

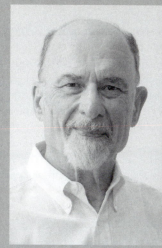

Irvin Yalom
Courtesy of Irvin Yalom

Rollo May (1909–1994)
Courtesy of Kirk Schneider

8 | EXISTENTIAL PSYCHOTHERAPY[1]

Irvin D. Yalom and Ruthellen Josselson

OVERVIEW

Existential psychotherapy is a form of therapy that can be integrated with other approaches, not an independent "school" of therapy like cognitive behaviorism or psychoanalysis. Rather than being a technical approach that offers a new set of rules for psychotherapy, it represents a way of thinking about human experience that can be—or perhaps should be—a part of all therapies.

Everyone must confront the timeless and intractable issues of the *ultimate concerns:* death, freedom, isolation, and meaning. An existential approach to therapy involves someone, a therapist, willing to walk unflinchingly with patients through life's deepest and most vexing problems. Existential psychotherapy is an attitude toward human suffering and has no manual. It asks deep questions about the nature of the human being and the nature of anxiety, despair, grief, loneliness, isolation, and anomie. It also deals centrally with the questions of meaning, creativity, and love. Out of reflection on these human experiences, existential psychotherapists have devised attitudes toward therapy that do not distort human beings in the very effort of trying to help them.

Many therapists, in fact, practice existential psychotherapy without labeling it as such. In his seminal work, *Existential Psychotherapy,* Yalom (1980) tells of taking part in an Armenian cooking class where the teacher, who did not speak English well, taught

[1] This chapter includes material from an earlier chapter in *Current Psychotherapies* by Rollo May and Irvin Yalom.

mainly by demonstration. But as hard as Yalom tried, he could never quite make his dishes taste as good as hers. He decided to observe his teacher more carefully, and in one lesson noted that when she finished her preparation she handed her dish to her assistant, who took it into the kitchen to place into the oven. He observed the assistant and was astounded, and edified, to note that that before throwing the dish in the oven, she threw in handfuls of various spices that struck her fancy. These "throw-ins" he likened to the interactions that therapists have with their patients, which, because they are not conceptualized within their theoretical "recipe," go unnoticed. Perhaps, however, these off-the-record extras are the critical ingredients. And perhaps these throw-ins refer to the shared issues of human existence—in short, to existential psychotherapy.

Basic Concepts

Existentialists regard people as meaning-making beings who are both subjects of experience and objects of self-reflection. We are mortal creatures who, because we are self-aware, know that we are mortal. Yet it is only in reflecting on our mortality that we can learn how to live. People ask themselves questions concerning their being: Who am I? Is life worth living? Does it have a meaning? How can I realize my humanity? Existentialists hold that, ultimately, each of us must come to terms with these questions, and each of us is responsible for who we are and what we become.

Because existentialists are sensitive to the ways in which theories may dehumanize people and render them as objects, authentic experience takes precedence over artificial explanations. When experiences are molded into some preexisting theoretical model, they lose their authenticity and become disconnected from the individual who experienced them. Existential psychotherapists, then, focus on the subjectivity of experience rather than "objective" diagnostic categories.

The Ultimate Concerns

Issues such as choice, responsibility, mortality, or purpose in life are ones that all therapists suspect are central concerns of patients. More and more, patients come to therapy with vague complaints about loss of purpose or meaning. But it is often more comfortable for the therapist to reframe these concerns into symptoms and talk with patients about medication or prescribe manualized exercises than to engage genuinely with them as they search for meaning in life. Many diagnosable presenting "symptoms" may mask existential crises.

The existential dilemma ensues from the existential reality that, although we crave to persist in our being, we are finite creatures; that we are thrown alone into existence without a predestined life structure and destiny; that each of us must decide how to live as fully, happily, ethically, and meaningfully as possible. Yalom defines four categories of "ultimate concerns" that encompass these fundamental challenges of the human condition: freedom, isolation, meaning, and death.

Freedom

The term *freedom* in the existential sense does not refer to political liberty or to the greater range of possibilities in life that come from increasing one's psychological awareness. Instead, it refers to the idea that we all live in a universe without inherent design in which we are the authors of our own lives. Life is groundless, and we alone are responsible for our choices. This existential freedom carries with it terrifying responsibility and is always connected to dread. It is the kind of freedom people fear so much that they enlist dictators, masters, and gods to remove the burden from them. Erich Fromm

(1941) described "the lust for submission" that accompanies the effort to escape from that freedom.

Ultimately, we are responsible for what we experience in and of the world. Responsibility is inextricably linked to freedom because we are responsible for the sense we make of our world and for all of our actions and our failures to act. An appreciation of responsibility in this sense is very unsettling. If we are, in Sartre's terms, "the uncontested author" of everything that we have experienced, then our most cherished ideas, our most noble truths, the very bedrock of our convictions are all undermined by the awareness that everything in the universe is contingent. We bear the burden of *knowing* that we are responsible for all of our experience.

The complement to responsibility is our *will*. Although this concept has waned lately in the social sciences, replaced by terms such as *motivation,* people are still ultimately responsible for the decisions they make. To claim that a person's behavior is explained (i.e., caused) by a certain motivation is to deny that person's responsibility for his or her actions. To abrogate such responsibility is to live inauthentically in what Sartre has called *bad faith.* Because of the dread of our ultimate freedom, people erect a plethora of defenses, some of which give rise to psychopathology. The work of therapy is very much about the assumption or reassumption of responsibility for one's experience. Indeed, the therapeutic enterprise can be conceived of as one in which the client actively increases and embraces his or her freedom: freedom from destructive habits, self-imposed paralysis of the will, or self-limiting beliefs, just to name a few.

Isolation

Individuals may be isolated from others (*interpersonal isolation*) or from parts of themselves (*intrapersonal isolation*). But there is a more basic form of isolation, *existential isolation,* that pertains to our aloneness in the universe. Though we are comforted by connections to other human beings, we nonetheless enter and leave the world alone and must always manage the tension between our wish for contact with others and our knowledge of our aloneness. Erich Fromm believed that isolation is the primary source of anxiety.

Aloneness is different from loneliness, which is also a ubiquitous issue in therapy. Loneliness results from social, geographic, and cultural factors that support the breakdown of intimacy. Or people may lack the social skills or have personality styles inimical to intimacy. But *existential* isolation cuts even deeper; it is a more basic isolation that is riveted to existence and refers *to an unbridgeable gulf between oneself and others*. It is most commonly experienced in the recognition that one's death is always solitary, a common theme among poets and writers. But many people are in touch with their dread of existential isolation when they recognize the terror of feeling that there may be moments when no one in the world is thinking of them. Or walking alone on a deserted beach in another country, one may be struck with a dreadful thought: "Right at this moment, no one knows where I am." If one is not being thought about by someone else, is one still real?

In working with people who have lost a spouse, Yalom was struck not only by their loneliness but also by the accompanying despair at living an unobserved life—of having no one who knows what time they come home, go to bed, or wake up. Many individuals continue a highly unsatisfying relationship precisely because they crave a life witness, a buffer against the experience of existential isolation.

The professional literature regarding the therapist–patient relationship abounds with discussions of encounter, genuineness, accurate empathy, positive unconditional regard, and "I–Thou" relating. A deep sense of connection does not "solve" the problem of existential isolation, but it provides solace. Yalom recalls one of the members of his cancer group who said, "I know we are each ships passing in the dark and each of us is a lonely ship, but still it is mighty comforting to see the bobbing lights of the other nearby boats." Still, we are ultimately alone. Even a therapist cannot change that. Yalom comments that an important milestone in therapy is the patient's realization that, "there is a point beyond which [the therapist] can offer nothing more. In therapy, as in life, there is an inescapable substrate of lonely work and lonely existence" (1980, p. 137).

To the extent that one takes full responsibility for one's life, one also encounters the sense of existential isolation. To forgo the sense that one is created or guarded by another is to confront the cosmic indifference of the universe and one's fundamental aloneness within it.

Meaning

All humans must find some meaning in life, although none is absolute and none is given to us. We create our own world and have to answer for ourselves why we live and how we shall live. One of our major life tasks is to invent a purpose sturdy enough to support a life; often we have a sense of discovering a meaning, and then it may seem to us that it was out there waiting for us. Our ongoing search for substantial purpose-providing life structures often throws us into a crisis. More individuals seek therapy because of concerns about purpose in life than therapists often realize. The complaints take many different forms: "I have no passion for anything." "Why am I living? Surely life must have some deeper significance." "I feel so empty—just trying to get ahead makes me feel so pointless, so useless." "Even now, at the age of 50, I still don't know what I want to do when I grow up."

In his memoir of being an existential psychotherapist, *The Listener*, Allen Wheelis (1999) tells about a moment with his dog, Monty:

> If then I bend over and pick up a stick, he is instantly before me. The great thing has now happened. He has a mission. . . . It never occurs to him to evaluate the mission. His dedication is solely to its fulfillment. He runs or swims any distance, over or through any obstacle, to get that stick.
>
> And, having got it, he brings it back: for his mission is not simply to get it but to return it. Yet, as he approaches me, he moves more slowly. He wants to give it to me and give closure to his task, yet he hates to have done with his mission, to again be in the position of waiting.
>
> For him as for me, it is necessary to be in the service of something beyond the self. Until I am ready he must wait. *He is lucky to have me to throw his stick.* I am waiting for God to throw mine. Have been waiting a long time. Who knows when, if ever, he will again turn his attention to me, and allow me, as I allow Monty, my mood of mission? (as cited at www.yalom.com/lec/pfister)

If only someone would throw me my *stick.* Who among us has not had that wish? How reassuring it would be to know that somewhere there exists a true purpose in life rather than only the *sense* of purpose in life. If all purpose is self-authored, then one must confront the ultimate groundlessness of existence. We throw our own sticks.

A sense of meaning emerges from plunging into an enlarging, fulfilling, self-transcending endeavor. The work of the therapist is to identify and help remove the obstacles to such engagement. If one is authentically immersed in the river of life, then the question of meaning drifts away.

Death

Overshadowing all these ultimate concerns, the awareness of our inevitable demise is the most painful and difficult. We strive to find meaning in the context of our existential aloneness and take responsibility for the choices we make within our free-dom to choose, yet one day we will cease to be. And we live our lives with that aware-ness in the shadow. Death is always the distant thunder at our picnic, however much we may wish to deny it.

Of course, we cannot live every moment wholly aware of death. This would be, in Yalom's phrase, like staring at the sun. Because we cannot live frozen in fear, we gen-erate methods to soften death's terror. We assuage it by projecting ourselves into the future through our children, trying to grow rich and famous, developing compulsive behaviors, or fostering an impregnable belief in an ultimate rescuer. Our fear of death is a profound dread of nonbeing, the impossibility of further possibility, as Hegel put it. And fears of death can lurk disguised behind many symptoms as well. Yet confronting death allows us to live fuller, richer, and more compassionate lives.

Everything fades. This is the sad existential truth. Life is truly linear and irrevers-ible. This knowledge can lead us to take stock of ourselves and ask how we can live our lives as fully as possible. Existential psychotherapy emphasizes the importance of living mindfully and purposefully, aware of one's possibilities and limits in a context of abso-lute freedom and choice. Death, in this view, enriches life.

The Therapeutic Stance: The Fellow Traveler

Awareness of the ultimate concerns as givens of existence fundamentally changes the relationship between therapist and patient to that of *fellow travelers*. From this van-tage point, even labels of *patient* or *therapist, client* or *counselor, analysand* or *analyst* become inappropriate to the nature of the relationship because they suggest distinc-tions between "them" (the afflicted) and "us" (the healers). However, *we are all in this together,* and there is no therapist and no person immune to the inherent tragedies of existence. Sharing the essence of the human condition becomes the bedrock of the work of existential psychotherapy.

Other Systems

Many other systems of psychotherapy make use of some of the basic tenets of existen-tial psychotherapy. Most recently, the increasing interest in the here and now and the awareness of the present moment in many schools of psychotherapy reflect the focus on genuineness and authentic encounter that characterizes the approach of the existential psychotherapist. Like Gestalt, expressive, dynamic, and systemic therapies, the experi-ence of the therapeutic relationship is of great interest given the assumption that change is based on lived experience. The stance of the existential therapist is aligned with other therapies that are phenomenological, holistic, and goal-directed such as Adlerian, Rogerian, neo-Freudian, and relational psychoanalytic therapies. Like the analytic thera-pies, existential therapy encourages work with dreams and analyzes them in relation to their existential as well as autobiographical themes. Like the cognitive therapies, it encourages reflection on belief systems and examination of meaning making with an aim of taking responsibility for one's choices and grappling with freedom. Cognitive restructuring techniques that aim at replacing maladaptive beliefs with personally mean-ingful values are fully consistent with an existential approach. Existential therapy parts company with those therapies aimed solely at the behavioral reduction or elimination of symptoms or that rely on manualized treatments. Existential therapy regards symptoms as signals that may mark existential crises and necessitate exploration of a person's ex-periences of self in the world and therefore necessitates a unique approach for each in-dividual. The existential approach to psychotherapy shines a light on aspects of practice that are probably present in all therapies but puts existential issues in the foreground in order to sensitize the therapist to their importance and prepare therapists to discuss them forthrightly with their patients. It encourages therapists who work in a range of theoretical systems to regard themselves as fellow travelers on the rutted road of existence rather than as all-knowing experts; this distinction, though, may pertain more to individual practitioners than to schools of therapy.

HISTORY

Precursors

These major existential concerns are not new, of course. An unbroken stream of philosophers, theologians, and poets since the beginning of recorded history has wrestled with these issues. Down through history, these questions have occupied many thinkers.

The Greek philosopher Epicurus anticipated the contemporary idea of the unconscious when he emphasized that death concerns may not be conscious to the individual but might be inferred by disguised manifestations. He constructed a number of arguments to alleviate death anxiety, which he taught his students. Epicurus believed that the soul was mortal and perishes with the body; hence, there is nothing to fear in the afterlife. And why fear death, he wondered, when we can never perceive it? Another argument he advanced was that of symmetry: Our state of nonbeing after death is the same as before our birth. As Vladimir Nabokov, the great Russian novelist later wrote, "our life is a crack of light between two eternities of darkness" (1967, p. 17). St. Augustine believed that only in the face of death is a person's self born. And many philosophers since the dawn of philosophy have concluded that the idea of death enriches life.

Beginnings

The contemporary term *existentialism* is most often associated with French philosophers Jean Paul Sartre and Gabriel Marcel, who developed this philosophy in the 1940s. Existential therapists have also been influenced by the work of such philosophers as Martin Heidegger, Edmund Husserl, Emmanuel Levinas, and Martin Buber.

The central foundational philosophers of existential psychotherapy are two 19th-century intellectual giants: Søren Kierkegaard and Friedrich Nietzsche. Both were reacting to the mechanistic dehumanization of people in a technological world, and both can be counted among the most remarkable psychologists of all time. When one reads Kierkegaard's profound analyses of anxiety and despair or Nietzsche's acute insights into the dynamics of resentment and the guilt and hostility that accompany repressed emotional powers, it is difficult to realize that one is reading works written more than 150 years ago and not a contemporary psychological analysis.

Swiss psychiatrist Ludwig Binswanger (1881–1966), a colleague and friend of Sigmund Freud, was the first physician to combine psychotherapy with existentialism. His famous and now classic case of Ellen West published in 1944 (see Binswanger, 1958), in which a patient with anorexia nervosa decides to commit suicide, provoked much debate within psychotherapeutic circles. Binswanger's work was part of a broader phenomenological–existential psychotherapeutic orientation that developed in central Europe in response to dissatisfaction with the theoretical frameworks of psychiatry and psychoanalysis. The members of this movement—among them Medard Boss, Eugene Minkowski, Erwin Straus, and Roland Kuhn—thought that the effort to detail human existence by means of an objective–descriptive scientific theory distracted attention from the authentic encounter that formed the basis of therapy. In 1988, a Society for Existential Analysis was formed in the United Kingdom that publishes a journal, *Existential Analysis*.

Existential psychotherapy was introduced to the United States in 1958 with the publication of *Existence: A New Dimension in Psychiatry and Psychology,* edited by Rollo May, Ernest Angel, and Henri Ellenberger. The main presentation and summary of existential therapy were in the first two chapters, which were written by May: "The Origins of the Existential Movement in Psychology" and "Contributions of Existential Psychology." The remainder of the book is made up of essays and case studies by European existentialists (Henri Ellenberger, Eugene Minkowski, Erwin Straus, V E. von Gebsattel, Ludwig Binswanger, and Ronald Kuhn).

Rollo May was trained as a psychoanalyst in the William Alanson White Institute, a neo-Freudian institute in New York, and he was already a practicing analyst when he read in the early 1950s about existential therapies in Europe. His books, which sought to reconcile existential ideas with psychoanalysis, became important texts of existential psychotherapy, especially in the United States. He wrote, among other books, *Man's Search for Himself* (1953), *Freedom and Destiny* (1981), and *The Cry for Myth* (1991).

Erich Fromm, a founder (in 1946) of the William Alanson White Institute, also wrote many books that explored existential issues. *Escape from Freedom* (1941) focuses on the human tendency to submit to authority as a way of defending against the existential terrors of free choice. *The Art of Loving* (1956) addressed the dilemmas of existential isolation.

The first comprehensive textbook in existential psychotherapy was written by Irvin Yalom (1980) and titled *Existential Psychotherapy.* In this work and in his subsequent books of case studies, *Love's Executioner* (1989) and *Momma and the Meaning of Life* (1999), as well as in his novels—*When Nietzsche Wept* (1992), *Lying on the Couch* (1996), *The Schopenhauer Cure* (2005), and *The Spinoza Problem* (2012)—Yalom attempted to detail what an existential psychotherapist actually *does* in the therapeutic session. His book *Staring at the Sun: Overcoming the Terror of Death* (2008) focuses on the experience and the treatment of high levels of death anxiety.

Other writers who have offered existential approaches to psychotherapy have also furthered its popularity in the United States. Viktor Frankl wrote *Man's Search For Meaning* (1956), a widely read and highly influential text that sets out an approach to *logotherapy,* a form of psychotherapy focused on will, freedom, meaning, and responsibility. Allen Wheelis (1973), a San Francisco existential psychoanalyst, wrote eloquently about his therapeutic encounters in which the specter of death and the search for meaning play central roles. Of his 14 books, *How People Change* is the best known. He wrote the following of psychotherapy:

> If . . . the determining causes of which we gain awareness lie within, or are brought within, our experience, and if we use this gain in understanding to create present options, freedom will be increased, and with it greater responsibility for what we have been, are, and will become. (1973, p. 117)

Current Status

The spirit of existential psychotherapy has never supported the formation of specific institutes because it deals with the *presuppositions underlying therapy of any kind.* Its concern was with concepts about human beings and not with specific techniques. This leads to the dilemma that existential therapy has been quite influential, but there are very few adequate training courses in this kind of therapy simply because it is not training in a specific technique. Existentially oriented psychotherapists tend to further their knowledge through their own personal therapy and supervision and by reading philosophy and great literature.

Therapists trained in different schools can legitimately call themselves existential if their assumptions are similar to those described in this chapter. Irvin Yalom was trained in a neo-Freudian tradition. Even such an erstwhile behavior therapist as Arnold Lazarus uses some existential presuppositions in his multimodal psychotherapy. Fritz Perls and Gestalt therapy rest on existential grounds. All of this is possible because existential psychotherapy is a way of conceiving the human being.

Existential therapists are centrally concerned with rediscovering the living person amid the dehumanization of modern culture. To do this, they engage in in-depth psychological analysis. Their focus is less on alleviating symptoms and more on greater awareness and freedom in relation to living.

Summing up the existential therapeutic position 25 years after he wrote his classic influential text, Yalom (2008) describes the need for an inclusive perspective in psychotherapy in these words:

> Psychological distress issues *not only* from our biological genetic substrate (a psycho–pharmacologic model), *not only* from our struggle with suppressed instinctual strivings (a Freudian position), *not only* from our internalized significant adults who may be uncaring, unloving, neurotic (an object relations position), *not only* from disordered forms of thinking (a cognitive-behavioral position), *not only* from shards of forgotten traumatic memories, nor from current life crises involving one's career and relationship with significant others, *but also—but also*—from a confrontation with our existence. (2008, p. 180)

In the contemporary climate of focus on brief, manualized treatments oriented to symptom reduction, driven by market forces rather than human need, all the human-focused approaches to psychotherapy suffer (McWilliams, 2005). In most training programs, across professions, psychotherapy that focuses on the subtleties of human experience is being taught less and less in favor of technological expedience and compliance with the dictates of managed care companies. Chagrined at seeing the life being squeezed out of psychotherapy as it was becoming more mechanized and less human and intimate, Yalom wrote a highly accessible guide for therapists, both novice and seasoned, titled *The Gift of Therapy* (2002). Judging from its enormous sales, there is a massive wish among psychotherapists to engage the issues of existence and presence with their patients. The tenets of existential psychotherapy will perhaps serve future generations when deeper forms of healing again become more, or more widely, possible.

PERSONALITY

Theory of Personality

In Tolstoy's *The Death of Ivan Illych,* the central character, Ivan Illych, a self-involved, self-satisfied, pompous bureaucrat, is dying in pain and suddenly realizes that he is dying badly because he has lived badly. "'Maybe I did not live as I ought to have done,' it suddenly occurred to him. 'But how could that be, when I did everything properly?'" (1980, p. 145). Ivan Illych's realization of the impoverishment of his life leads him, in the last days of his life, to relate more authentically and empathically to his family, thus redeeming his life at the very end. The existential focus of a theory of personality concerns whether people are living as authentically and meaningfully as possible.

Existential psychotherapy is a *dynamic psychotherapy*. It takes from Freud the model of personality as a system of forces in conflict with one another. The emotions and behavior (both adaptive and pathological) that constitute personality may exist at different levels of consciousness, some entirely out of awareness, and they may conflict. Thus, when we speak of the "psychodynamics" of an individual, we refer to that individual's conflicting conscious and unconscious motives and fears. Dynamic psychotherapy is psychotherapy based on this internal conflict model of personality structure.

Existential Psychodynamics

In contrast to the Freudian model, which posits conflict between instincts and the demands of the environment (or the superego, which is the environment internalized), and in contrast to the interpersonal and object relational models that posit conflict stemming from interactions with significant powerful others in childhood, the existential model of personality postulates that the basic conflict is between the individual and the "givens," the ultimate concerns of existence. Thus, the existential system replaces the Freudian system of

$$\text{Drive} \rightarrow \text{Anxiety} \rightarrow \text{Defense Mechanism}$$
$$\text{with}$$
$$\text{Awareness of Ultimate Concern} \rightarrow \text{Anxiety} \rightarrow \text{Defense Mechanism}$$

If we "bracket" the outside world, if we put aside the everyday concerns with which we ordinarily fill our lives and reflect deeply on our situations in the world, then we must confront the dilemmas of the ultimate concerns (detailed previously) that are an inescapable part of the human being's existence in the world. The individual's confrontation with each of these constitutes the content of the inner conflict from the existential frame of reference.

As people, we are influenced by the physical environment, the presence or absence of other people, genetics, and social or cultural variables. In other words, we are influenced by our destiny. Because we are stimulated in certain ways, we respond in certain ways. As subjects, however, we are aware of the fact that these things are happening to us. We perceive, ponder, and act on this information. We determine which experiences are valuable and which are not and then act according to these personal formulations. What is crucial is "man's capacity to stand outside himself, to know he is the subject as well as the object of experience, to see himself as the entity who is acting in the world of objects" (May, 1967, p. 75). As humans, we view the world, and we can view ourselves viewing it. It is this consciousness of self that allows people to escape determinism and personally influence what they do.

> Consciousness of self gives us the power to stand outside the rigid chain of stimulus and response, to pause, and by this pause to throw some weight on either side, to cast some decision about what the response will be. (May, 1953, p. 161)

A full understanding of a person involves both knowledge of that person's circumstances (the objective part) and how that person subjectively structures and values those circumstances (the subjective part).

Existential psychotherapy does not offer a theory of individual differences, but it attends carefully to how each individual deals with the ultimate concerns. Therefore, the existential understanding of personality is inherently tied to its approach to psychotherapy.

Variety of Concepts

May attributes anxiety to the fundamental clash between being and the threat of nonbeing. A certain amount of anxiety is therefore a normal and inevitable aspect of every personality. Anxiety confronts each of us with a major challenge. This unpleasant emotion intensifies whenever we choose to boldly assert our innate potentials. Emphatically affirming that we exist also brings a reminder that someday we will not. It is all too tempting to repress or intellectualize our understanding of death, deny our being-in-the-world (*Dasein*), and opt for the apparent safety of social conformity and apathy. The healthy course is to accept nonbeing as an inseparable part of being. This will enable us to live what life we have to the fullest:

> To grasp what it means to exist, one needs to grasp the fact that he might not exist, that he treads at every moment on the sharp edge of possible annihilation and can never escape the fact that death will arrive at some unknown moment . . . [Thus] the confronting of death gives the most positive reality to life itself. (May, 1958, p. 47)

Freedom

Ordinarily we do not think of freedom as a source of anxiety or conflict. Quite the contrary—freedom is generally viewed as an unequivocally positive concept. The history of Western civilization is punctuated by a yearning and striving toward freedom. Yet freedom in the existential frame of reference is riveted to dread.

From an existential viewpoint, conflicts over freedom ensue from the reality that the human being enters and ultimately departs an unstructured universe without a coherent grand design. *Freedom* refers to the fact that the human being is responsible for and the author of his or her own world, own life design, and own choices and actions. The human being, as Sartre puts it, is "condemned to freedom" (1956, p. 631). Rollo May (1981) holds that freedom, to be authentic, requires the individual to confront the limits of his or her destiny. He defined destiny "as the pattern of limits and talents that constitutes the 'givens' in life. . . . Our destiny cannot be cancelled out . . . but we can choose how we shall respond, how we shall live out our talents" (p. 89).

If it is true that we create our self and our world, then it also means that there is no ground beneath us: There is only an abyss, a void, nothingness. This has terrifying implications. Such awareness of freedom and groundlessness conflicts with our deep need and wish for ground and structure, creates anxiety, and invokes a variety of defense mechanisms.

Awareness of freedom implies responsibility for one's life. Individuals differ enormously in the degree of responsibility they are willing to accept for their life situations and in their modes of denying responsibility. For example, some individuals displace responsibility for their situations onto other people, onto life circumstances, onto bosses and spouses, and, when they enter treatment, they transfer responsibility for their therapy to their psychotherapist. Other individuals deny responsibility by experiencing themselves as innocent victims who suffer from external events (and remain unaware that they themselves have set these events into motion). Still others shirk responsibility by temporarily being "out of their minds"—they enter a temporary irrational state in which they are not accountable even to themselves for their behavior.

Another aspect of freedom is *willing*. To be aware of responsibility for one's situation is to enter the vestibule of action or, in a therapy situation, of change. Willing represents the passage from responsibility to action, moving from wishing to deciding (May, 1969). Many individuals have enormous difficulties in experiencing or expressing a wish. Wishing is closely aligned to feeling, and affect-blocked individuals cannot act spontaneously because they cannot feel and thus cannot wish. *Impulsivity* avoids wishing by failing to discriminate among wishes. Instead, individuals act impulsively and promptly on all wishes. *Compulsivity,* another disorder of wishing, is characterized by individuals driven by unconscious inner demands that often run counter to their consciously held desires.

Once an individual fully experiences a wish, he or she is faced with *decision*. Many individuals can be extremely clear about what they wish but still not be able to decide or to choose. Often they experience a decisional panic; they may attempt to delegate the decision to someone else, or they act in such a way that the decision is made for them by circumstances that they unconsciously have brought to pass.

Thus, personality is informed by how people deal with the dilemmas of freedom. From the duty-bound to the capricious to the dependent, people have an array of mechanisms to deny or displace their freedom.

Isolation

Coming to terms with existential isolation, our inherent aloneness in the universe, is a second dynamic conflict that structures the personality. Each individual in the dawn of consciousness creates a primary self by permitting consciousness to curl back on itself and differentiate a self from the remainder of the world. Only after the individual becomes "self-conscious" can he or she begin to constitute other selves. Yet the individual cannot escape the knowledge that (1) he or she constitutes others and (2) he or she can never fully share his or her consciousness with others. There is no stronger reminder of existential isolation than a confrontation with death. The individual who faces death invariably becomes acutely aware of existential isolation.

Awareness of our fundamental isolation may invoke an unfulfillable wish to be protected, to merge, and to be part of a larger whole. Bugental (1976) points out that all relationships are poised on the poles of being *a part of* and *apart from,* the twin perils of merger and isolation. Fear of existential isolation (and the defenses against it) underlies a great deal of interpersonal psychopathology. Often relationships are troubled by the effort of one person to *use* another for some function rather than to *relate* to the other out of caring for that person's being. If one is overcome with dread in the face of isolation, one will not be able to turn toward others but instead will use others as a shield against isolation. In such instances, relationships will be distortions of what might have been authentic relationships.

Some individuals experience panic when they are alone. These individuals begin to doubt their own existence and believe that they exist only in the presence of another, that they exist only so long as they are responded to or are thought about by another individual.

Many attempt to deal with isolation through *fusion:* They soften their ego boundaries and become part of another individual. They avoid personal growth and the sense of isolation that accompanies growth. Fusion underlies the experience of being in love. The wonderful thing about romantic love is that the lonely "I" disappears into the "we." Others may fuse with a group, a cause, a country, or a project. To be like everyone else—to conform in dress, speech, and customs, to have no thoughts or feelings that are different—saves one from the isolation of the lonely self.

Compulsive sexuality is also a common response to terrifying isolation. Promiscuous sexual coupling offers a powerful but temporary respite for the lonely individual. It is temporary because it is only a caricature of a relationship. The sexually compulsive individual does not relate to the whole being of the other but relates only to the part of that individual that meets his or her need. Sexually compulsive individuals do not know their partners; they show and see only those parts that facilitate seduction and the sexual act.

Meaninglessness

The third existential influence on personality is meaninglessness. If each person must die, and if each person constitutes his or her own world, and if each is alone in an indifferent universe, then what possible meaning can life have? Why do we live? How shall we live? If there is no preordained design in life, then we must construct our own meaning in life. The fundamental question then becomes, "Is it possible that a self-created meaning is sturdy enough to bear one's life?" The third internal conflict stems from this dilemma: *How does a being who requires meaning find meaning in a universe that has no meaning?*

The human being appears to require meaning. Our perceptual neuropsychological organization is such that we instantaneously pattern random stimuli. We organize them automatically into figure and ground and may even create a story about them. When confronted with a broken circle, we automatically perceive it as complete. When any situation or set of stimuli defies patterning, we fit the situation into a recognizable pattern.

In the same way that individuals organize random stimuli, so they also face existential situations: In an unpatterned world, an individual is acutely unsettled and searches for a pattern, an explanation, a meaning for existence.

A sense of meaning of life is necessary for still another reason: From a meaning schema, we generate a hierarchy of values. Values provide us with a blueprint for life conduct; values tell us not only *why* we live but also *how* to live.

To grow as a person, one must constantly challenge one's structure of meaning, which is the core of one's existence, and this necessarily causes anxiety. Thus, to be human is to have the urge to expand one's awareness, but to do so causes anxiety. Growth, and with it normal anxiety, consists of the giving up of immediate security for the sake of more extensive goals (May, 1967). The authentic person recognizes the hazards of exploring uncharted territory and does so nonetheless. The anxiety associated with moving forward into the unknown is an unfortunate concomitant of exercising one's freedom and realizing a quest for meaning.

As people tell the stories of their lives, their meanings are implicit. Their personal narratives are structured around their purposes and values, and the ways they narrate their lives reflect how they understand themselves as unique individuals and socially located beings. Narrative, then, becomes another dimension or level of personality (McAdams & Pals, 2006) and discloses the sense of personal unity and identity that construct meaning in life.

Death

The fourth and perhaps most central conflict is the confrontation with death. Death is the ultimate existential concern. It is apparent to all that death will come and that there is no escape. It is a terrible truth, and at the deepest levels we respond to it with mortal terror. "Everything," as Spinoza states, "wishes to persist in its own being" (1954, p. 6). From the existential point of view, a core inner conflict is between awareness of inevitable death and the simultaneous wish to continue to live.

Death plays a major role in one's internal experience. It haunts the individual like nothing else does. It rumbles continuously under the membrane of life. The child at an early age is pervasively concerned with death, and one of the child's major developmental tasks is to deal with the terror of obliteration. To cope with this terror, we erect defenses against death awareness. These defenses are denial based; they shape character structure and, if maladaptive, result in clinical maladjustment.

Psychopathology, to a very great extent, is the result of failed death transcendence; that is, symptoms and maladaptive character structure have their origin in the individual terror of death. Many defense mechanisms might be employed for dealing with the anxiety emerging from awareness of death, among them an irrational belief in personal "specialness" and an irrational belief in the existence of an "ultimate rescuer" (Yalom, 1980).

Specialness.   Individuals have deep, powerful beliefs in personal inviolability, invulnerability, and immortality. Although at a rational level we recognize the foolishness of these beliefs, we nonetheless believe, at a deeply unconscious level, that the ordinary laws of biology do not apply to us. People can camouflage their fears of death behind a belief that one's specialness will somehow override the dread decree. Again, Tolstoy's Ivan Illych offers an apt example:

> In the depth of his heart he knew he was dying, but not only was he not accustomed to the thought, he simply did not and could not grasp it.

The syllogism he had learnt from Kiezewetter's Logic, "Caius is a man, men are mortal, therefore Caius is mortal," had always seemed to him correct as applied to Caius, but certainly not as applied to himself. That Caius—man in the abstract—was mortal, was perfectly correct, but he was not Caius, not an abstract man, but a creature quite, quite separate from all others. He had been little Vanya, with a mamma and a papa . . . What did Caius know of the smell of that striped leather ball Vanya had been so fond of? Had Caius kissed his mother's hand like that . . . ? Had Caius been in love like that? Could Caius preside at a session as he did? Caius really was mortal, and it was right for him to die, but for me, little Vanya, Ivan Illych, with all my thoughts and emotions, it's altogether a different matter. It cannot be that I ought to die. That would be too terrible. (pp. 131–132)

What psychotherapists might simply label *narcissism* or *entitlement* may actually be subterfuge for the belief that specialness is an antidote to death. Similarly, workaholism or preoccupation with getting ahead, preparing for the future, amassing material goods, or becoming more powerful or more eminent can be compulsive ways of unconsciously trying to ensure immortality.

Where the defense of specialness operates satisfactorily for a time, a crisis in the lives of these individuals occurs when their belief system is shattered and a sense of unprotected ordinariness intrudes. They frequently seek therapy when the defense of specialness is no longer able to ward off anxiety—for example, at times of severe illness or at the interruption of what had always appeared to be an eternal, upward spiral. In cases of trauma, it is sometimes the "Why me?" question that haunts the trauma survivor. To ask, "Why not me?" is to undermine the defensive sense of specialness, a specialness that ultimately (and irrationally) seems to protect against death.

The Belief in the Existence of an Ultimate Rescuer.   A second denial system is belief in an ultimate rescuer. People may imagine their rescuer to be human or divine, but the belief is in someone who is watching over them in an indifferent world. To keep the specter of death at bay, people may unconsciously create a belief in a personal omnipotent savior who eternally guards and protects their welfare, who may let them get to the edge of the abyss but who will always bring them back. An excess of this particular defense mechanism results in a character structure displaying passivity, dependency, and obsequiousness. Often such individuals dedicate their lives to locating and appeasing an ultimate rescuer.

One of Yalom's patients, Elva, an elderly woman, came to therapy because she was traumatized by having her purse snatched. Located within and beneath the resulting panic was her inability to let go of her departed husband who, at a very deep level, she believed would continue to protect her. The purse snatching and ensuing sense of vulnerability challenged this belief in her husband as an ultimate rescuer. In this case, we see how such beliefs may be camouflaged by seemingly unrelated experiences.

PSYCHOTHERAPY

Theory of Psychotherapy

A substantial proportion of practicing psychotherapists consider themselves existentially (or humanistically) oriented. Yet few, if any, have received any systematic training in existential therapy. One can be reasonably certain of this because there are few comprehensive training programs in existential therapy. Although many excellent books illuminate some aspect of the existential frame of reference (Becker, 1973; Bugental, 1976; Koestenbaum, 1978; May, 1953, 1967, 1969; May, Angel, & Ellenberger, 1958), Yalom's book (1980) is the only one to present a systematic, comprehensive view of the existential therapeutic approach.

Existential therapy is *not* a comprehensive psychotherapeutic system; it is a frame of reference—a paradigm by which one views and understands a patient's suffering in a particular manner. Existential therapists begin with presuppositions about the sources of a patient's anguish and view the patient in human rather than behavioral or mechanistic terms. They may employ any of a large variety of techniques used in other approaches insofar as they are consistent with basic existential presuppositions and a human, authentic therapist–patient encounter.

The vast majority of experienced therapists, regardless of adherence to some particular ideological school, employ many existential insights and approaches. All competent therapists realize, for example, that an apprehension of one's finiteness can often catalyze a major inner shift of perspective, that it is the relationship that heals, that patients are tormented by choice, that a therapist must catalyze a patient's will to act, and that the majority of patients are bedeviled by a lack of meaning in their lives.

It is also true that the therapist's belief system determines the type of clinical data that he or she encounters. Therapists subtly or unconsciously cue patients to provide them with certain material. Jungian patients have Jungian dreams. Freudian patients discover themes of oedipal competition. Cognitive therapists are attuned to "irrational" beliefs. The therapist's perceptual system is affected by her or his ideological system. Thus, the therapist tunes in to the material that she or he wishes to obtain. So, too, with the existential approach. If therapists tune their mental apparatus to the right channel, it is astounding how frequently patients discuss concerns emanating from existential conflicts. Moreover, there are patients who have had a long-term enduring interest in existential issues. These people connect deeply to a therapist who can speak with them about their existential dilemmas and who places importance on the issues that concern them.

An existential therapist is someone with a sensibility to existential issues. No therapist focuses on existential issues all the time. These issues are important to some patients at some but not all stages of therapy.

The basic approach in existential therapy is strategically similar to other dynamic therapies. The therapist assumes that the patient experiences anxiety that issues from some existential conflict that is at least partially unconscious and that suffering ensues from "problems in being" (Wheelis, 1973). The patient handles anxiety by a number of ineffective, maladaptive defense mechanisms that may provide temporary respite from anxiety but ultimately so cripple the individual's ability to live fully and creatively that these defenses merely result in still further secondary anxiety. The therapist helps the patient embark on a course of self-investigation in which the goals are to understand the unconscious conflict, identify the maladaptive defense mechanisms, discover their destructive influence, diminish secondary anxiety by correcting these heretofore restrictive modes of dealing with self and others, and develop other ways of coping with primary anxiety.

Although the basic strategy in existential therapy is similar to other dynamic therapies, the content is radically different. In many respects, the process differs as well; the existential therapist's different mode of understanding the patient's basic dilemma results in many differences in the strategy of psychotherapy. For example, because the existential view of personality structure emphasizes the depth of experience at any given moment, the existential therapist does not spend a great deal of time helping the patient to recover the past. The existential therapist strives for an understanding of the patient's *current* life situation and *current* enveloping unconscious fears. The existential therapist believes, as do other dynamic therapists, that the nature of the therapist–client relationship is fundamental in good psychotherapeutic work. However, the accent is not on transference but on the relationship as fundamentally important in itself, especially in regard to engagement and connection. The existential therapist works in the present tense. The individual is to be understood and helped to understand him- or herself from the perspective of a here-and-now *cross section,* not from the perspective of a historical *longitudinal section.*

Consider the use of the word *deep.* Freud defines *deep* as "early," and so the deepest conflict meant the earliest conflict in the individual's life. Freud's psychodynamics are developmentally based. *Fundamental* and *primary* are to be grasped chronologically: Each is synonymous with "first." Thus, the fundamental sources of anxiety, for example, are considered to be the earliest calamities: separation and castration.

From the existential perspective, *deep* means the most fundamental concerns facing the individual at that moment. The past (i.e., one's memory of the past) is important only insofar as it is part of one's current existence and has contributed to one's current mode of facing ultimate concerns. The immediate, currently existing ground beneath all other ground is important from the existential perspective. Thus, the existential conception of personality is in the awareness of the depths of one's immediate experiences. Existential therapy does not attempt to excavate and understand the past; instead, it is directed toward the future's becoming the present and explores the past only as it throws light on the present. The therapist must continually keep in mind that we create our past and that our present mode of existence dictates what we choose to remember of the past. The therapeutic focus is on the self-experience of the patient and attends to the patient's capacity for self-actualization, even self-transcendence, through engagement in life.

Process of Psychotherapy

In the existential framework, anxiety is so riveted to existence that it has a different connotation from the way anxiety is regarded in other frames of reference. The existential therapist hopes to alleviate crippling levels of anxiety but not to eliminate it. Life cannot be lived (nor can death be faced) without anxiety. The therapist's task, as May reminds us (1977, p. 374), is to reduce anxiety to tolerable levels and then to use it constructively.

We can best understand the process of psychotherapy in the existential approach by considering the therapeutic leverage inherent in some of the ultimate concerns. Each of the ultimate human concerns (death, freedom, isolation, and meaninglessness) has implications for the process of therapy.

Existential Psychotherapy and Freedom

A major component of freedom is *responsibility*—a concept that deeply influences the existential therapist's therapeutic approach. Sartre equates responsibility with *authorship:* To be responsible means to be the author of one's own life design. The existential therapist continually focuses on each patient's responsibility for his or her own distress. Bad genes or bad luck do not cause a patient to be lonely or chronically abused or neglected by others. Until patients realize that they are responsible for their own conditions, there is little motivation to change.

The therapist must identify methods and instances of responsibility avoidance and then make these known to the patient. Therapists may use a wide variety of techniques to focus the patient's attention on responsibility. Many therapists interrupt the patient whenever they hear the patient avoiding responsibility. When patients say they "can't" do something, the therapist immediately comments, "You mean you 'won't' do it." As long as one believes in "can't," one remains unaware of one's active contribution to one's situation. Such therapists encourage patients to *own* their feelings, statements, and actions. If a patient comments that he or she did something "unconsciously," the therapist might inquire, "Whose unconscious is it?" The general principle is obvious: Whenever the patient laments about his or her life situation, the therapist inquires how the patient created that situation.

Often it is helpful to keep the patient's initial complaints in mind and then, at appropriate points in therapy, juxtapose these initial complaints with the patient's in-therapy behavior. For example, consider a patient who sought therapy because of feelings of isolation and loneliness. During the course of therapy, the patient expressed at great length his sense of superiority and his scorn and disdain of others. These attitudes were rigidly maintained; the patient manifested great resistance to examining, much less changing, these opinions. The therapist helped this patient understand his responsibility for his personal predicament by reminding the patient, whenever he discussed his scorn of others, "And you are lonely."

Responsibility is one component of freedom. Earlier we described another, *willing*, which may be further subdivided into *wishing* and *deciding*. Consider the role of *wishing*. How often does the therapist participate with a patient in some such sequence as this:

"What shall I do? What shall I do?"
"What is it that stops you from doing what you want to do?"
"But I don't *know* what I want to do! If I knew that, I wouldn't need to see you!"

These patients know what they should do, ought to do, or must do, but they do not experience what they *want* to do. Many therapists, in working with patients who have a profound incapacity to wish, have shared May's inclination to shout, "Don't you ever *want* anything?" (1969, p. 165). These patients have enormous social difficulties because they have no opinions, no inclinations, and no desires of their own.

Often the inability to wish is embedded in a more global disorder—the inability to feel. In many cases, the bulk of psychotherapy consists of helping patients to dissolve their affect blocks. This therapy is slow and grinding. Above all, the therapist must persevere and, time after time, must continue to press the patient with, "What do you feel? What do you want?" Repeatedly, the therapist will need to explore the source and nature of the block and of the stifled feelings behind it. The inability to feel and to wish is a pervasive characterological trait, and considerable time and therapeutic perseverance are required to effect enduring change.

There are other modes of avoiding wishing in addition to blocking of affect. Some individuals avoid wishing by not discriminating among wishes, by acting impulsively on all wishes. In such instances, the therapist must help the patient make some internal discrimination among wishes and assign priorities to each. The patient must learn that two wishes that are mutually exclusive demand that one be relinquished. If, for example, a meaningful, loving relationship is a wish, then a host of conflicting interpersonal wishes—such as the wish for conquest or power or seduction or subjugation—must be denied.

Decision is the bridge between wishing and action. Some patients, even though they are able to wish, are still unable to act because they cannot *decide*. One of the more common reasons that deciding is difficult is that every *yes* involves a *no*. Renunciation invariably accompanies decision, and a decision requires a relinquishment of other options—often options that may never come again. The patient must come to terms with the unalterable fact that *alternatives exclude*.

The therapist must help patients make choices. Patients must recognize that they themselves, not the therapist, must generate and choose among options. In helping patients communicate effectively, therapists teach that one must *own* one's feelings. It is equally important that one owns one's decisions. Some patients are panicked by the various implications of each decision. The "what ifs" torment them. *What if I leave my job and can't find another? What if I leave my children alone and they get hurt?* It is often useful to ask the patient to consider the entire scenario of each what if in turn, to fantasize it happening with all the possible ramifications, and then to experience and analyze emerging feelings.

Patients may also feel paralyzed by an inability to tolerate uncertainty. A young woman scientist came to therapy because she was unable to decide whether to move back to her hometown to be near her family, which she very much wanted to do, or stay in her current city and job, neither of which she liked. Most of all, she hoped to meet a man who could be a life partner, something she had been unable to do in any of the cities she had recently lived in while she was studying and pursuing her career goals. In scientific fashion, she had researched all possibilities, exhaustively checking, for example, dating Web sites to see which men were looking for partners in her hometown. None of them seemed suitable. What if she gave up her prestigious job for a lesser one in her hometown and *still* didn't meet anyone? She would then still be lonely and now full of regret and remorse. What she wanted was for someone to tell her the right decision. The therapeutic task with her was to help her face the inevitability of uncertainty in life: There are never guarantees, no matter how scientifically one approaches one's decisions.

A general posture toward decision making is to assume that the therapist's task is not to *create* will but instead to *disencumber* it. The therapist cannot flick the decision switch or inspire the patient with resoluteness. It is the therapist's task to help remove the obstacles to decision making. Once that is done, the individual will naturally move into a more autonomous position in just the way, as Karen Horney (1950) put it, that an acorn develops into an oak tree.

The therapist must help patients understand that decisions are unavoidable. One makes decisions all the time and often conceals from oneself the fact that one is deciding. It is important to help patients understand the inevitability of decisions and identify how they make decisions. Many patients decide *passively* by, for example, letting another person decide for them. They may terminate an unsatisfactory relationship by unconsciously acting in such a way that the partner makes the decision to leave. In such instances, the final outcome is achieved, but the patient may be left with many negative repercussions. The patient's sense of powerlessness is merely reinforced, and he or she continues to experience him- or herself as one to whom things happen rather than as the author of his or her own life situation. The *way* one makes a decision is often as important as the content of the decision. An active decision reinforces the individual's active acceptance of his or her own power and resources.

Existential Isolation and Psychotherapy

No relationship can eliminate existential isolation, but aloneness can be shared in such a way that love compensates for its pain. The experience of existential isolation is so anguishing that defenses are fairly quickly and firmly instituted against it. Yet the capacity to acknowledge deeply our isolated situation in existence also makes it possible to move toward authentic relationships with other (similarly isolated) beings. Patients who grow in psychotherapy learn not only the rewards of intimacy but also its limits: They learn what they *cannot* get from others.

An important step in treatment consists of helping patients address existential isolation directly. Those who lack sufficient experiences of closeness and true relatedness in their lives are particularly incapable of tolerating isolation. Adolescents from loving, supportive families are able to grow away from their families with relative ease and to tolerate the separation and loneliness of young adulthood. On the other hand, those who grow up in tormented, highly conflicted families find it extremely difficult to leave the family. The more disturbed the family, the harder it is for children to leave: They are ill equipped to separate and therefore cling to the family for shelter against isolation and anxiety.

Many patients have enormous difficulty spending time alone. Some may feel they exist only in the eyes of others. Consequently, they construct their lives in such a way that they eliminate time alone. Two of the major problems that result from this are the desperation with which they seek certain kinds of relationships and the use of others to assuage the pain accompanying isolation. The therapist must find a way to help the patient confront isolation in a dosage and with a support system suited to that patient. Some therapists, at an advanced stage of therapy, advise periods of self-enforced isolation during which the patient is asked to monitor and record thoughts and feelings.

The anxiety of existential isolation is best assuaged through the creation of meaningful and mutual relationships with others. Many patients who feel unloved actually suffer from difficulties in the capacity to love. Too occupied with what they need from others, they cannot give to others and cannot participate in reciprocity and mutuality. To love means to be actively concerned with the welfare and growth of another. In *The Art of Loving*, Erich Fromm (1956) wrote "the ability to be alone is the condition for the ability to love (p. 94)." Two partners unable to tolerate aloneness create an A-frame that holds them both up but is a poor basis for marriage.

The authentic human encounter must be modeled by the therapist, who is available to meet the patient in the space between "I" and "Thou." It is the therapeutic relationship that heals. Presence, genuineness, and receptiveness on the part of the therapist form the attitude that invites true *meeting* in a real relationship with the patient. The aim of the therapist is to bring something to life in the patient rather than impose something. The therapist stays with this task selflessly, attempting to enter the patient's world and experience it as the patient experiences it. The existential therapist tries to do this from a position of being a fellow traveler—not as a technique of psychotherapy.

Meaninglessness and Psychotherapy

To deal effectively with meaninglessness, therapists must first increase their sensitivity to the topic, listen differently, and become aware of the importance of meaning in the lives of individuals. For some patients, the issue of meaninglessness is profound and pervasive. Carl Jung once estimated that more than 30% of his patients sought therapy because of a sense of personal meaninglessness (1966, p. 83).

The therapist must be attuned to the overall focus and direction of the patient's life. Is the patient reaching beyond him- or herself? Or is he or she entirely immersed in the daily routine of staying alive? Yalom (1980) reported that his therapy was rarely successful unless he was able to help patients focus on something beyond these pursuits. Simply by increasing their sensitivity to these issues, the therapist can help them focus on values outside themselves. Therapists, for example, can begin to wonder about the patient's belief systems, inquire deeply into the loving of another, ask about long-range hopes and goals, and explore creative interests and pursuits.

Viktor Frankl, who placed great emphasis on the importance of meaninglessness in contemporary psychopathology, stated that "happiness cannot be pursued, it can only ensue" (1963, p. 165). The more we deliberately search for self-satisfaction, the more it eludes us, whereas the more we fulfill some self-transcendent meaning, the more happiness will ensue.

Therapists must find a way to help self-centered patients develop curiosity and concern for others. The therapy group is especially well suited for this endeavor: The pattern in which self-absorbed, narcissistic patients take without giving often becomes highly evident in the therapy group. In such instances, therapists may attempt to increase an individual's ability and inclination to empathize with others by periodically requesting that patients guess how others are feeling at various junctures of the group.

But the major solution to the problem of meaninglessness is engagement. Wholehearted engagement in any of the infinite array of life's activities enhances the possibility of one's patterning the events of one's life in some coherent fashion. To fashion a home, to care about other individuals and about ideas or projects, to search, to create, to build—all forms of engagement are twice rewarding: They are intrinsically enriching, and they alleviate the dysphoria that stems from being bombarded with the unassembled brute data of existence.

The therapist must approach engagement with the same attitudinal set used with wishing. The desire to engage life is always there with the patient, and therefore the therapist's activity should be directed toward the removal of obstacles in the patient's way. The therapist begins to explore what prevents the patient from loving another individual. Why is there so little satisfaction from his or her relationships with others? Why is there so little satisfaction from work? What blocks the patient from finding work commensurate with his or her talents and interests or finding some pleasurable aspects of current work? Why has the patient neglected creative or spiritual or self-transcendent strivings?

Death and Psychotherapy

An increased awareness of one's finiteness stemming from a personal confrontation with death may cause a radical shift in life perspective and lead to personal change. A patient named Carlos, dying of cancer, had increased his preoccupation with having sex with as many women as possible. But as Yalom, his therapist, insisted that he reflect on how he had been living his life, Carlos made astonishing change in his last months. As he lay dying, he thanked his therapist for having saved his life.

Death as an Awakening Experience

An *awakening experience* is a type of urgent experience that propels the individual into a confrontation with an existential situation. The most powerful awakening experience is confrontation with one's personal death. Such a confrontation has the power to provide a massive shift in the way one lives in the world. Some patients report that they learn simply that "existence cannot be postponed." They no longer put off living until some time in the future; they realize that one can really live only in the present. The neurotic individual rarely lives in the present but is either continuously obsessed with events from the past or fearful of anticipated events in the future.

A confrontation with an awakening experience persuades individuals to count their blessings, to become aware of their natural surroundings: the elemental facts of life, changing seasons, seeing, listening, touching, and loving. Ordinarily what we *can* experience is diminished by petty concerns, by thoughts of what we cannot do or what we lack, or by threats to our prestige.

Many terminally ill patients, when reporting personal growth emanating from their confrontation with death, have lamented, "What a tragedy that we had to wait till now, till our bodies were riddled with cancer, to learn these truths." This is an exceedingly important message for therapists. The therapist can obtain considerable leverage to help "everyday" patients (i.e., patients who are not physically ill) increase their awareness of death earlier in their life cycle. With this aim in mind, some therapists have employed structured exercises to confront the individual with personal death. Some group leaders begin a brief group experience by asking members to write their own epitaph or obituary, or they provide guided fantasies in which group members imagine their own death and funeral.

Many existential therapists do not believe that artificially introduced death confrontations are necessary or advisable. Instead, they attempt to help the patient recognize the signs of mortality that are part of the fabric of everyday life. If the therapist and the patient are tuned in, there is considerable evidence of death anxiety in every psychotherapy. Every patient suffers losses through death of parents, friends, and associates. Dreams are haunted with death anxiety. Every nightmare is a dream of raw death anxiety. Everywhere around us are reminders of aging: Our bones begin to creak, age spots appear on our skin, we go to reunions and note with dismay how everyone *else* has aged. Our children grow up. The cycle of life envelops us.

An important opportunity for confrontation with death arises when patients experience the death of someone close to them. The traditional literature on grief primarily focuses on two aspects of grief work: loss and the resolution of ambivalence that so strongly accentuates the dysphoria of grief. But a third dimension must be considered: The death of someone close to us confronts us with our own death.

Often grief has a very different tone, depending on the individual's relationship with the person who has died. The loss of a parent confronts us with our vulnerability: If our parents could not save themselves, then who will save us? When parents die, nothing remains between ourselves and the grave. At the moment of our parents' deaths, we ourselves constitute the barrier between our children and their death.

The death of a spouse often evokes the fear of existential isolation. The loss of the significant other increases our awareness that, try as hard as we can to go through the world two by two, there is nonetheless a basic aloneness we must bear. Yalom reports a patient's dream the night after learning that his wife had inoperable cancer.

> I was living in my old house in [a house that had been in the family for three generations]. A Frankenstein monster was chasing me through the house. I was terrified. The house was deteriorating, decaying. The tiles were crumbling and the roof leaking. Water leaked all over my mother. [His mother had died six months earlier.] I fought with him. I had a choice of weapons. One had a curved blade with a handle, like a scythe. I slashed him and tossed him off the roof. He lay stretched out on the pavement below. But he got up and once again started chasing me through the house. (1980, p. 168)

The patient's first association to this dream was "I know I've got a hundred thousand miles on me." Obviously his wife's impending death reminded him that his life and his body (symbolized in the dream by the deteriorating house) were also finite. As a child, this patient was often haunted by the monster who returned in this nightmare.

Children try many methods of dealing with death anxiety. One of the most common is the personification of death: imagining death as some finite creature—a monster, a sandman, a bogeyman, and so on. This is very frightening to children but nonetheless far less frightening than the truth—that they carry the spores of their own death within them. If death is "out there" in some physical form, then possibly it may be eluded, tricked, or pacified.

Milestones provide another opportunity for the therapist to focus the patient on existential facts of life. Even simple milestones such as birthdays and anniversaries are useful levers. These signs of passage are often capable of eliciting pain (consequently, we often deal with such milestones by reaction formation in the form of a joyous celebration).

Major life events such as a threat to one's career, a severe illness, retirement, commitment to a relationship, and separation from a relationship can be important awakening experiences that offer opportunities for an increased awareness of death anxiety. Often these experiences are painful, and therapists feel compelled to focus entirely on pain alleviation. In so doing, however, they miss rich opportunities for deep therapeutic work that reveal themselves at those moments.

Birthdays, grief, reunions, dreams, or the empty nest prime the individual for awakening. These become occasions for reflection on how one has lived one's life. In *Thus Spake Zarathustra,* Nietzsche (1954) poses a challenge: What if you are to live the identical life again and again throughout eternity—how would that change you? The idea of living your identical life again and again for all eternity can be jarring, a sort of *petite* existential shock therapy. It often serves as a sobering thought experiment, leading one to consider seriously how one is really living.

Properly used, regret is a tool that can jar patients into taking actions to prevent its further accumulation. One can examine regret both by looking behind and by looking ahead. If regret reflects what has not been fulfilled, then one can choose either to amass more regret or to plan one's life to make the changes that will avoid regret. The therapeutic question becomes, "How can you live now without building new regrets? What do you have to do to change your life?"

Death as a Primary Source of Anxiety   The fear of death constitutes a primary fount of anxiety: It is present early in life, it is instrumental in shaping character structure, and it continues throughout life to generate anxiety that results in manifest distress and the erection of psychological defenses. However, it is important to keep in mind that death anxiety exists at the very deepest levels of being, is heavily repressed, and is rarely experienced in its full sense. Often, death anxiety per se is not easily visible in the clinical picture.

Even though death anxiety may not explicitly enter the therapeutic dialogue, a theory of anxiety based on death awareness may provide therapists with a frame of reference that greatly enhances their effectiveness. Death anxiety is directly proportional to the amount of each person's "unlived life." Those individuals who feel they have lived their lives richly, have fulfilled their potential and their destiny, experience less panic in the face of death.

There are patients, however, who are suffused with overt death anxiety at the very onset of therapy. Sometimes, there are life situations in which the patient has such a rush of death anxiety that the therapist cannot evade the issue. In long-term, intensive therapy, explicit death anxiety is always to be found and must be considered in the therapeutic work.

Mechanisms of Psychotherapy

Existential psychotherapy is not limited to and may not even be focused on a discussion of these ultimate concerns, although the alert therapist aims not to shy away from them or change the subject. Still, the mechanisms of existential psychotherapy maximize the possibility of a clear view of these fundamental human experiences by fostering engagement with the anxieties of existence and being. Through authenticity and presence, the therapist strives to counter avoidance and withdrawal. The mechanisms of existential psychotherapy involve a focus on the here and now and a view of the therapist–patient relationship as one of fellow travelers. The therapeutic stance is founded on empathy and may also include the use of dreams.

Empathy

Empathy is the most powerful tool we have in our efforts to connect with other people: It is the glue of human connectedness and permits one to feel, at a deep level, what someone else is feeling. The existential therapist attempts to see the world from the point of view of the patient. *Patients view the therapy hours in very different ways from therapists.* Again and again, therapists, even highly experienced ones, are surprised to rediscover this phenomenon when their patients describe an intense emotional reaction about the previous hour that the therapist cannot recall. It is extraordinarily difficult to really know what the other feels; far too often we, as therapists, project our own feelings onto the other.

Therapists don't have to have had the same experience as patients to be empathetic. They might try to follow the maxim that "I am human and let nothing human be alien to me." This requires that therapists be open to that part of themselves that corresponds to any deed or fantasy offered by patients, no matter how heinous, violent, lustful, or sadistic.

The Here and Now

The nitty-gritty of *doing* therapy involves intense focus on the here and now. What is happening in the interpersonal space between patient and therapist right here, right now? Therapy is a social microcosm in the sense that sooner or later, if the therapy is not highly structured, the interpersonal and existential problems of the patient will manifest themselves in the here and now of the therapy relationship. If, in life, the patient is demanding or fearful or arrogant or self-effacing or seductive or controlling or judgmental or maladaptive interpersonally in any other way, then these traits will be displayed in living color in the here and now of the therapy hour. The therapist need only be alert to what is happening in the interaction with the patient and to try to find the analogues to what the patient reports to be his or her difficulties in outside relationships. To fully access the here and now, therapists have to access their own feelings and use these as a barometer of what is happening in the interaction. If the therapist is bored, there is something the patient is doing to induce that boredom. Perhaps the patient fears intimacy or is silently rageful toward the therapist. Only by acknowledging his or her feelings in the immediacy of the interaction can the therapist access what is being enacted by the patient. To do this well, the therapist must both have deep self-knowledge and the skill to give feedback tactfully and kindly, to avoid accusation of the patient, and above all be ready when necessary to acknowledge his or her own contribution to the problematic interaction.

Attention to the here and now invites attention to the *immediacy* of the interaction in the moment in which it occurs. Patients may find this unfamiliar or resist the intimacy that here-and-now processing engages. Yet it is here that the greatest vitality in the therapy hour will be manifest as a fully present therapist forges an authentic connection with a fully present patient, both sharing the phenomenology of their experiences.

It is the task of the therapist to maintain focus on what is transpiring in the relationship as it develops. A simple check-in brings this relationship to the center of attention, asking, for example, such questions as: "How are you and I doing today?" "Are there feelings about me you took home from the last session?" "I've noticed a real shift in the session today. At first it seemed we were very distant and in the past 20 minutes, I felt much closer. Was your experience the same? What enabled us to get closer then?" *Therapy is always an alternating sequence of interaction and reflection on that interaction.*

What occurs in the here and now will always have analogues in the patient's life. As patients take risks with self-experience in the present of the therapy hour, they will become more courageous in taking such risks in their outside lives. As patients come to recognize their blocks to full engagement, their constriction, their flights from responsibility, their difficulties in relating to others, they will better understand what impedes their life projects and relationships. Patients develop a new internal standard for the quality of a genuine relationship. Having achieved it with the therapist, they may well have the confidence and willingness to form similarly good relationships in the future.

The therapist never makes decisions for patients and is alert to any internal convictions that she or he knows what is best for the patient. The role of the therapist is "catalytic" (Wheelis, 1973). Therapy is aimed toward removing roadblocks to purposeful living and helping patients assume responsibility for their actions, not providing solutions.

Dreams

Dreams are a very important access road to the inner life of patients. They comment on the therapy relationship, existential experiences, and unconscious fantasies, and they contain metaphors for the deepest aspects of the person. Yalom (2002) recounts the following story in *The Gift of Therapy* to demonstrate how dreams can enliven and direct the therapy. One of his patients had the following dream:

> I was on the porch of my home looking through the window at my father sitting at his desk. I went inside and asked him for gas money for my car. He reached into his pocket and as he handed me a lot of bills he pointed to my purse. I opened my wallet and it already was crammed with money. Then I said that my gas tank was empty and he went outside to my car and pointed to the gas gauge, which said, "full." (p. 232)

In his analysis of this dream, Yalom points out the following:

> The major theme in this dream was emptiness versus fullness. The patient wanted something from her father (and from me since the room in the dream closely resembled the configuration of my office) but she couldn't figure out what she wanted. She asked for money and gasoline but her wallet was already stuffed with money and her gas tank was full. The dream depicted her pervasive sense of emptiness, as well as her belief that I had the power to fill her up if she could only discover the right question to ask. Hence she persisted in craving something from me—compliments, doting, special treatment, birthday presents—all the while knowing she was off the mark. My task in therapy was to redirect her attention—away from gaining supplies from another and towards the richness of her own inner resources. (p. 233)

Fellow Travelers

Sometimes many hours go by without the voicing of any existential content, but the therapist–patient relationship is influenced by the existential perspective in every single session. Existential therapists experience and present themselves as real, self-revealing *fellow travelers*.

We all, whether in the role of patients or therapists or just human beings, must come to terms with our eventual death, with our aloneness in the universe, with finding meaning in life, and with recognizing our freedom and taking responsibility for the lives we lead. The wise therapist recognizes that these are issues with which we must struggle together; the therapist is only privileged in the sense of being able, one hopes, to talk honestly about what these concerns entail.

Working with people from an existential approach goes far beyond taking up a professional role, using techniques, manuals, or clinical protocols. Rather, one is providing a sanctuary and a relationship for the exploration of being and becoming and the confrontation with existential givens of life (Craig, 2012).

Such a stark confrontation with the ultimate concerns of life leads to a recognition of the primacy of connectedness in human life. What is central to existential psychotherapy is the relationship between therapist and patient. But there are no prescribed formulas for this relationship. The therapeutic venture is always spontaneous, creative, and uncertain. Indeed, the therapist creates a new therapy for each patient. The therapist gropes toward the patient with improvisation and intuition. The heart of psychotherapy is a caring, deeply human meeting between two people, one more troubled than the other (generally, but not always, the patient). Both are exposed to the same existential issues of meaning, isolation, freedom, and death. There is no distinction between "them" (the afflicted) and "us" (the healers).

Genuineness, so crucial to effective therapy, takes on a new dimension when a therapist deals honestly with existential issues. We have to abandon all vestiges of a medical model that posits that a patient suffering from a strange affliction needs a dispassionate, immaculate, expert healer. We all face the same terror: the wound of mortality, the worm at the core of existence. To be truly present with patients dealing with death anxiety, the therapist must be open to his or her own death anxiety, not in a glib or superficial way but with a profound awareness. This is no easy task, and no training program prepares therapists for this type of work.

Fellow travelers focusing on the here and now, on the relational space between them, explore together the dilemmas of human interaction that often underlie the blocks to finding the meaning and connection in life that soften the terrors of death. Focus on the dynamics of the therapeutic relationship as it unfolds enables vitality and engagement. The therapist's most valuable instrument is his or her own self, and therefore the personal exploration that can only be conducted in one's own therapy is a necessary part of the training of a therapist. Psychotherapy is a psychologically demanding enterprise, and therapists must develop the awareness and inner strength to cope with the many occupational hazards of psychotherapy. Only through personal therapy can therapists become aware of their own blind spots and dark sides and thus become able to empathize with the extensive range of human wishes and impulses. A personal therapy experience also permits the student therapist to experience the therapeutic process from the patient's seat: the tendency to idealize the therapist, the yearning for dependency, the gratitude toward a caring and attentive listener, the power granted to the therapist. Self-knowledge is not achieved once and for all; therapists can only benefit from reentering therapy at many stages of life.

Therapist Transparency

As a fellow traveler along the same road as the patient, the therapist tries to be as authentic and genuine as possible. The therapist must be willing to disclose his or her feelings in the here and now, fully open to what is being engendered in his or her inner experience by the interaction with the patient. From an existential psychotherapy standpoint, it is the *examined* therapeutic relationship that heals.

Existential therapists are willing to let patients matter to them and also to acknowledge their errors. Disclosure by the therapist always facilitates therapy. Still, the reflective therapist must also be mindful of the boundaries and the meanings of the boundaries on such disclosure and resist temptations to engage in various forms of exploitation of the patient. Therapists reveal themselves when it enhances therapy, not because of their own needs or rules. This is why personal therapy is so important for doing this kind of work.

Therapist disclosure should be primarily about feelings in the here and now in the relationship with the patient. Such disclosure must be well processed and tactful, never impulsive. For example, the therapist might tell the patient when she or he feels closer to the patient as a result of the patient's sharing, or more distant as a result of the patient's reluctance to confront some more emotionally charged issues. "I find myself afraid of your criticism, probably like others in your life." "I feel that your putting me on a pedestal makes me feel farther away from you." "I feel I have to be very careful about what I say because you seem to scan everything I say for signs of my approval or disapproval." The therapist uses disclosure in the service of the welfare of the patient, not as an end in itself. Therapists must take care not to disclose what might be (or feel) destructive to the patient. They must respect the pace of therapy and what patients are or are not ready to hear.

APPLICATIONS

Who Can We Help?

The clinical setting often determines the applicability of the existential approach. In each course of therapy, the therapist must consider the goals appropriate to the clinical setting. To take one example, in an acute inpatient setting in which the patient will be hospitalized for as brief a time as possible, the goal of therapy is crisis intervention. The therapist hopes to alleviate symptoms and restore the patient to a precrisis level of functioning. Deeper, more ambitious goals are unrealistic and inappropriate to that situation.

In situations in which patients not only desire symptomatic relief but also hope to attain greater personal growth, the existential approach is generally useful. A thorough existential approach with ambitious goals is most appropriate in long-term therapy, but even in briefer approaches, some aspect of the existential mode (e.g., an emphasis on responsibility, deciding, an authentic therapist–patient encounter, grief work) is often incorporated into the therapy.

An existential approach to therapy is appropriate with patients who confront some boundary situation—that is, a confrontation with death, the facing of some important irreversible decision, a sudden thrust into isolation, or milestones that mark passages from one life era into another. But therapy need not be limited to these explicit existential crises. Existential psychotherapy can be applied to a diverse range of patients in different modalities (Schneider, 2007). In every course of therapy, there is abundant evidence of patients' anguish stemming from existential conflicts. The availability of such data is entirely a function of the therapist's attitudinal set and perceptivity. The decision to work on these levels should be a joint patient–therapist decision.

Treatment

Existential therapy has its primary applications in an individual therapy setting. However, various existential themes and insights may be successfully applied in a variety of other settings, including group therapy, family therapy, and couples therapy.

The concept of responsibility has particularly widespread applicability. It is a keystone of the group therapeutic process, in which patients learn how their behavior is viewed by others, how their behavior makes others feel, how they create the opinions others have of them, and how others' opinions shapes their views of themselves. Group members begin to understand that they are responsible for how others treat them and for the way in which they regard themselves (Yalom & Lecsz, 2005). Indeed, patients can see how they create in others the very reactions that trouble them in their outside lives (Josselson, 2007).

In group therapy, all members are "born" simultaneously. Each starts out on an equal footing. Each gradually scoops out and shapes a particular life space in the group. Thus, each person is responsible for the interpersonal position he or she creates in the group (and in life). The therapeutic work in the group then not only allows individuals to change their way of relating to one another but also brings home to them in a powerful way the extent to which they have created their own life predicaments—clearly an existential therapeutic mechanism.

Often the therapist uses his or her own feelings to identify the patient's contribution to his or her life predicament. For example, a depressed 48-year-old woman complained bitterly about the way her children treated her: They dismissed her opinions, were impatient with her, and, when some serious issue was at stake, addressed their comments to their father. When the therapist tuned in to his feelings about this patient, he became aware of a whining quality in her voice that tempted *him* not to take her seriously and to regard her somewhat as a child. He shared his feelings with the patient, and it proved enormously useful to her. She became aware of her childlike behavior in many areas and began to realize that her children treated her precisely as she "asked" to be treated.

Not infrequently, therapists must treat patients who are panicked by a decisional crisis. Yalom (1980) describes one therapeutic approach in such a situation. The therapist's basic strategy consisted of helping the patient uncover and appreciate the existential implications of the decision. The patient was a 66-year-old widow who sought therapy because of her anguish about a decision to sell a summer home. The house required constant attention to gardening, maintenance, and protection and seemed a considerable burden to a frail aging woman in poor health. Finances affected the decision as well, and she asked many financial and realty consultants to assist her in making the decision.

The therapist and the patient explored many factors involved in the decision and then gradually began to explore more deeply. Soon a number of painful issues emerged. For example, her husband had died a year earlier and she mourned him still. The house was still rich with his presence, and drawers and closets brimmed with his personal effects. A decision to sell the house also required a decision to come to terms with the fact that her husband would never return. She considered her house her "drawing card" and harbored serious doubts whether anyone would visit her without the enticement of her lovely estate. Thus, a decision to sell the house meant testing the loyalty of her friends and risking loneliness and isolation. Yet another reason concerned the great tragedy of her life—her childlessness. She had always envisioned the estate passing on to her children and to her children's children. The decision to sell the house thus was a decision to acknowledge the failure of her major symbolic immortality project. The therapist used the house-selling decision as a springboard to these deeper issues and eventually helped the patient mourn her husband, herself, and her unborn children.

Once the deeper meanings of a decision are worked through, the decision generally glides easily into place. In this case, after approximately a dozen sessions, the patient effortlessly made the decision to sell the house.

Questions of meaning are often most accessible to therapists who use an existential approach, and subschools of therapy have developed to highlight the focus on meaning (Wong, 2010). A conscious appraisal of meanings as well as exploration of the unconscious meanings being lived can enable patients to live more fully and zestfully.

Existentially oriented therapists strive toward honest, mutually open relationships with their patients. The patient–therapist relationship helps the patient clarify other relationships. Patients almost invariably distort some aspect of their relationship to the therapist. The therapist, drawing from self-knowledge and experience of how others view him or her, is able to help the patient distinguish distortion from reality.

The experience of an intimate encounter with a therapist has implications that extend beyond relationships with other people. For one thing, the therapist is generally someone whom the patient particularly respects. But even more important, the therapist is someone, often the only one, who *really* knows the patient. To tell someone else all one's darkest secrets and still be fully accepted by that person is enormously affirmative.

Existential thinkers such as Erich Fromm, Abraham Maslow, and Martin Buber all stress that true caring for another means to care about the other's growth and to want to bring something to life in the other. Buber (1965) uses the term *unfolding,* which he suggests should be the way of the educator and the therapist: One uncovers what was there all along. The term *unfolding* has rich connotations and stands in sharp contrast to the goals of other therapeutic systems. One helps the patient unfold by *meeting,* by existential communication. Perhaps the most important concept of all in describing the patient–therapist relationship is what May et al. term *presence* (1958, p. 80). The therapist must be fully present, striving for an authentic encounter with the patient.

Evidence

Psychotherapy evaluation is always a difficult task. The more focused and specific the approach and the goals, the easier it is to measure outcome. Symptomatic relief or behavioral change may be quantified with reasonable precision. But more ambitious therapies, which seek to affect deeper layers of the individual's mode of being in the world, defy quantification. These problems of evaluation are illustrated by the following vignettes reported by Yalom (1980).

> A 46-year-old mother accompanied the youngest of her four children to the airport, from which he departed for college. She had spent the last 26 years rearing her children and longing for this day. No more impositions, no more incessantly living for others, no more cooking dinners and picking up clothes. Finally she was free.
>
> Yet as she said good-bye she unexpectedly began sobbing loudly, and on the way home from the airport a deep shudder passed through her body. "It is only natural," she thought. It was only the sadness of saying good-bye to someone she loved very much. But it was much more than that, and the shudder soon turned into raw anxiety. The therapist whom she consulted identified it as a common problem: the empty nest syndrome. (p. 336)

Of course she was anxious. How could it be otherwise? For years she had based her self-esteem on her performance as a mother, and suddenly she found no way to validate herself. The whole routine and structure of her life had been altered. Gradually, with the help of Valium, supportive psychotherapy, an assertiveness training group, several adult education courses, a lover or two, and a part-time volunteer job, the shudder shrank to a tremble and then vanished. She returned to her premorbid level of comfort and adaptation.

This patient happened to be part of a psychotherapy research project, and there were outcome measures of her psychotherapy. Her treatment results could be described as excellent on each of the measures used—symptom checklists, target problem evaluation, and self-esteem. Obviously, she had made considerable improvement. Yet, despite this, it is entirely possible to consider this case as one of missed therapeutic opportunities.

Consider another patient in almost precisely the same life situation. In the treatment of this second patient, the therapist, who was existentially oriented, attempted to nurse the shudder rather than anesthetize it. This patient experienced what Kierkegaard called "creative anxiety." The therapist and the patient allowed the anxiety to lead them into important areas for investigation. True, the patient suffered from the empty nest syndrome; she had problems of self-esteem; she loved her child but also envied him for the chances in life she had never had; and, of course, she felt guilty because of these "ignoble" sentiments.

The therapist did not simply allow her to find ways to fill her time but also plunged into an exploration of the *meaning* of the fear of the empty nest. She had always desired freedom but now seemed terrified of it. Why?

A dream illuminated the meaning of the shudder. The dream consisted simply of holding in her hand a 35-mm photographic slide of her son juggling and tumbling. The slide was peculiar, however, in that it showed movement; she saw her son in a multitude of positions all at the same time. In the analysis of the dream, her associations revolved around the theme of time. The slide captured and framed time and movement. It kept everything alive but made everything stand still. It froze life. "Time moves on," she said, "and there's no way I can stop it. I didn't want John to grow up . . . whether I like it or not time moves on. It moves on for John and it moves on for me as well."

This dream brought her own finiteness into clear focus and, rather than rush to fill time with various distractions, she learned to appreciate time in richer ways than previously. She moved into the realm that Heidegger described as *authentic being:* She wondered not so much at the *way* things are but *that* things are. She recognized that life is seriously linear and irreversible, that everything fades, and that she still had time to live purposefully and meaningfully. Although one could argue that therapy helped the second patient more than the first, it would not be possible to demonstrate this conclusion on any standard outcome measures. In fact, the second patient probably continued to experience more anxiety than the first did; but anxiety is a part of existence, and no individual who continues to grow and create will ever be free of it.

These gains continue to elude randomized-control objective forms of research. Yet nearly all psychotherapy research, especially research on common factors, has substantiated a central premise of existential psychotherapy—that it is the relationship that heals (Frank & Frank, 1991; Gelso & Hayes, 1998; Norcross, 2002; Safran & Muran, 1996; Wampold, 2001). Logotherapy, derived from the work of Victor Frankl, highlights meaning as an existential concern and has developed several instruments to assess the experience of purpose in living (Schulenberg, Hutzell, Nassif, & Rogina, 2008). Issues of meaning are perhaps the most researched of the ultimate concerns by psychotherapy researchers.

Psychotherapy in a Multicultural World

Existential psychotherapy considers the situation of the whole person located in society and culture. Cultural, racial, or national identities are not add-ons: They are essential aspects of the phenomenology of the client and intrinsic to the treatment. Existential psychotherapy is oriented to all aspects of human uniqueness and difference and takes into account and investigates the meanings of age, sexual orientation, ethnicity, and so on. For multicultural or multiracial people, or for people moving between phenomenological worlds, the recognition and embrace of freedom to act may be at the forefront (Taylor & Nanney, 2011).

All humans, regardless of cultural background, share in the dilemmas of existence and must come to terms with the ultimate concerns of freedom, isolation, meaninglessness, and death. The potential difficulties come in treating people who have adopted wholesale formulas for managing these concerns that were provided by their cultural, often religious, systems.

Yalom had such a struggle with a young orthodox rabbi who requested a consultation with him. The rabbi said he was in training to become an existential therapist but was experiencing some dissonance between his religious background and the psychological formulations of existential psychotherapy. At first deferential during the session, the rabbi's demeanor slowly changed, and he began to voice his beliefs with such zeal as to make Yalom suspect that the real purpose of his visit was to convert him to the religious life.

Yalom acknowledged the fundamental antagonism between their views. The rabbi's belief in an omnipresent, omniscient personal God watching him, protecting him, and providing him a life design was indeed incompatible with the core of the existential stance that we are free, alone, thrown randomly into an uncaring universe, and mortal.

"But you," the rabbi responded with intense concern on his face, "how can you live with only these beliefs? And without meaning? How can you live without belief in something greater than yourself? What meaning would there be if everything is destined to fade? My religion provides me with meaning, wisdom, morality, with divine comfort, with a way to live."

To this, Yalom responded, "I don't consider that a rational response, Rabbi. Those commodities—meaning, wisdom, morality, living well—are *not* dependent on a belief in God. And, yes, *of course,* religious belief makes you feel good, comforted, virtuous—that is exactly what religions are invented to do. You ask how I can live. I believe I live well. I'm guided by human-generated doctrines. I believe in the Hippocratic oath I took as a physician and dedicate myself to helping others heal and grow. I live a moral life. I feel compassion for those about me. I live in a loving relationship with my family and friends. I don't need religion to supply a moral compass."

Yalom has never had a desire to undermine anyone's religious faith, but strong religious belief that overshadows personal struggle with the ultimate concerns may preclude exploration of existential issues. Most, perhaps all, cultures create belief systems that defend against the terrors of stark confrontation with existential concerns. The dilemma for the existential therapist is to recognize the way in which these belief systems provide a sense of meaning for the patient, to stay authentic with regard to his or her own beliefs, and still find ways to increase the patient's engagement with purpose and meaning in life.

A depressed patient whose cultural background dictates unquestioning filial obedience found it difficult to pursue her own life goals. Efforts to engage her in addressing her own responsibility for her choices in life were met with her declaring that she must do what her father requires of her. The existential therapist must then help this patient see herself as making a deliberate choice in this regard—to obey her father rather than to follow her own desires. Obedience itself can be an existential choice for which one can take full responsibility.

CASE EXAMPLE

A Simple Case of Divorce

David, a 50-year-old scientist, had been married for 27 years and had recently decided to separate from his wife. He sought therapy because of the degree of anxiety he was experiencing in anticipation of confronting his wife with his decision.

The situation was in many ways a typical midlife scenario. The patient had two children; the youngest had just graduated from college. In David's mind, the children had always been the main element binding him and his wife together. Now that the children were self-supporting and fully adult, David felt there was no reasonable point in continuing the marriage. He reported that he had been dissatisfied with his marriage for many years and on three previous occasions had separated from his wife, but, after only a few days, had become anxious and returned, crestfallen, to his home. Bad as the marriage was, David concluded that it was less unsatisfactory than the loneliness of being single.

The reason for his dissatisfaction with his marriage was primarily boredom. He had met his wife when he was 17, a time when he had been extremely insecure, especially in his relationships with women. She was the first woman who had ever expressed interest in him. David came from a blue-collar family (as had his wife). He was exceptionally intellectually gifted and was the first member of his family to attend college. He won a scholarship to an Ivy League school, obtained two graduate degrees, and embarked on an outstanding academic research career. His wife was not gifted intellectually, chose not to go to college, and during the early years of their marriage worked to support David in graduate school.

For most of their married life, his wife immersed herself in the task of caring for the children while David ferociously pursued his professional career. He had always experienced his relationship to his wife as empty and had always felt bored with her company. In his view, she had an extremely mediocre mind and was so restricted characterologically that he found it constraining to be alone with her and embarrassing to share her with friends. He experienced himself as continually changing and growing, whereas his wife, in his opinion, had become increasingly rigid and unreceptive to new ideas. The prototypic scenario of the male in midlife crisis seeking a divorce was made complete by the presence of the "other woman"—an intelligent, vivacious, attractive woman 15 years younger than himself.

David's therapy was long and complex, and several existential themes emerged during the course of therapy. Responsibility was an important issue in his decision to leave his wife. First, there is the moral sense of responsibility. After all, his wife gave birth to and raised his children and had supported him through graduate school. He and his wife were at an age where he was far more "marketable" than she; that is, he had significantly higher earning power and was biologically able to father children. What moral responsibility, then, did he have to his wife?

David had a high moral sense and would, for the rest of his life, torment himself with this question. It had to be explored in therapy, and, consequently, the therapist confronted him explicitly with the issue of moral responsibility during David's decision-making process. The most effective mode of dealing with this anticipatory dysphoria was to leave no stone unturned in his effort to improve the marriage.

The therapist helped David examine the question of his responsibility for the failure of the marriage. To what degree was he responsible for his wife's mode of being with him? For example, the therapist noted that he himself felt somewhat intimidated by David's quick, facile mind: The therapist also was aware of a concern about being criticized or judged by David. How judgmental was David? Was it not possible that he squelched his wife? Had he engaged differently with her, might he have helped her develop greater flexibility, spontaneity, and self-awareness?

The therapist also helped David consider whether he was displacing onto the marriage dissatisfaction that belonged elsewhere in his life. A dream pointed the way toward some important dynamics:

> I had a problem with liquefaction of earth near my pool. John [a friend who was dying from cancer] sinks into the ground. It was like quicksand. I used a giant power auger to drill down into the quicksand. I expect to find some kind of void under the ground but instead I found a concrete slab five to six feet down. On the slab I found a receipt of money someone had paid me for $501. I was very anxious in the dream about that receipt since it was greater than it should have been.

One of the major themes of this dream had to do with death and aging. First, there was the theme of his friend who had cancer. David attempted to find his friend by using a giant auger. In the dream, David experienced a great sense of mastery and power during the drilling. The symbol of the auger seemed clearly phallic and initiated a profitable exploration of sexuality—David had always been sexually driven, and the dream illuminated how he used sex (and especially sex with a young woman) as a mode of gaining mastery over aging and death. Finally, he is surprised to find a concrete slab (which elicited associations of morgues, tombs, and tombstones).

He was intrigued by the numerical figures in the dream (the slab was "five to six feet" down, and the receipt was for precisely $501). In his associations, David made the interesting observation that he was 50 years old and the night of the dream was his 51st birthday. Though he did not consciously dwell on his age, the dream made it clear that at an unconscious level, he had considerable concern about being over 50. Along with the slab that was between five and six feet deep and the receipt that was just over $500, there was his considerable concern in the dream about the amount cited in the receipt being too great. On a conscious level, he denied his aging.

If David's major distress stemmed from his growing awareness of his aging and diminishment, then a precipitous separation from his wife might have represented an attempt to solve the wrong problem. Consequently, the therapist helped David plunge into a thorough exploration of his feelings about his aging and his mortality. The therapist's view was that only by fully dealing with these issues would he be more able to ascertain the true extent of the marital difficulties. The therapist and David explored these issues over several months. He attempted to deal more honestly with his wife than before, and soon he and his wife made arrangements to see a marital therapist for several months.

After these steps were taken, David and his wife ultimately decided that there was nothing salvageable in the marriage, and they separated. The months following his separation were exceedingly difficult. The therapist provided support during this time but did not try to help David eliminate his anxiety; instead, he attempted to help David use his anxiety in a constructive fashion. David's inclination was to rush into an immediate second marriage, whereas the therapist persistently urged him to look at the fear of isolation that on each previous separation had sent him back to his wife. It was important now to be certain that fear did not propel him into an immediate second marriage.

David found it difficult to heed this advice because he felt so much in love with the new woman in his life. The state of being in love is one of the great experiences in life. In therapy, however, being in love raises many problems; the pull of romantic love is so great that it engulfs even the most well-directed therapeutic endeavors. David found his new partner to be the ideal woman, no other woman existed for him, and he attempted to spend all his time with her. When with her, he experienced a state of continual bliss: All aspects of the lonely "I" vanished, leaving only a very blissful state of "we-ness."

What finally made it possible for David to work in therapy was that his new friend became somewhat frightened by the power of his embrace. Only then was he willing to look at his extreme fear of being alone and his reflex desire to merge with a woman. Gradually, he became desensitized to being alone. He observed his feelings, kept a journal of them, and worked hard on them in therapy. He noted, for example, that Sundays were the worst time. He had an extremely demanding professional schedule and had no difficulties during the week. Sundays were times of extreme anxiety. He became aware that part of that anxiety was that he had to take care of himself on Sunday. If he wanted to do something, he himself had to schedule the activity. He could no longer rely on that being done for him by his wife. He discovered that an important function of ritual in culture and the heavy scheduling in his own life was to conceal the void, the total lack of structure beneath him.

These observations led him, in therapy, to face his need to be cared for and shielded. The fears of isolation and freedom buffeted him for several months, but gradually he learned how to be alone in the world and what it meant to be responsible for his own being. In short, he learned how to be his own mother and father—always a major therapeutic objective of psychotherapy.

SUMMARY

Existential psychotherapy views the patient as a full person, not as a composite of drives, archetypes, conditioning, or irrational beliefs or as a "case." People are regarded as struggling, feeling, thinking, and suffering beings who have hopes, fears, and relationships, who wrestle to create meaningful lives. It takes a life-affirming approach to an essentially tragic view of life. Anxiety will always be present but can be channeled into creative, life-enhancing pursuits. Awareness of the inevitability of death can enrich life.

The original criticism of existential therapy as "too philosophical" has lessened as people recognize that all effective psychotherapy has philosophical implications. The genuine human encounter between patient and therapist engenders possibility of new meanings, new forms of relationship, and a possibility of self-actualization. The central aim of the founders of existential psychotherapy was that its emphases would influence therapy of all schools. That this has been occurring is quite clear. Existential therapy is not a technique. It is "an encounter with one's own existence in an immediate and quintessential form" (May, 1967, p. 134) in the company of a therapist who is fully present.

Our present age is one of disintegration of cultural and historical mores, of love and marriage, the family, inherited religions, and so forth. Given these realities, the existential emphasis on meaning, responsibility, and living a finite life fully will become increasingly important.

 Counseling CourseMate Website:

See this text's Counseling CourseMate website at www.cengagebrain.com for learning tools such as chapter quizzing, videos, glossary flashcards, and more.

ANNOTATED BIBLIOGRAPHY

Becker, E. (1973). *Denial of death*. New York: Free Press.
    In this Pulitzer Prize–winning book, Becker's thesis is that human behavior and mental disorder have their deepest roots in our denying our deaths. The book is a useful resource, particularly for therapists, for reflecting on and coming to terms with death anxiety. Among its topics are meditations on the need for illusions and "immortality projects."

Wheelis, A. (1973). *How people change*. New York: Harper & Row.
    This is a short, lyrical, highly readable and accessible book that demonstrates the *attitude* of existential psychotherapy. Wheelis dramatizes the difficulty of intentional change and discusses the need for will, courage, and action in the effort to change.

Yalom, I. (1980). *Existential psychotherapy*. New York: Basic Books.

This is the textbook of existential psychotherapy that elucidates in more detail the ideas presented in this chapter. A major task of the book is to build a bridge between theory and clinical application. It includes many case examples as well as the philosophical foundations of this approach. (See also the DVD *Confronting Death and Other Existential Issues in Psychotherapy* in which Yalom illuminates the existential perspective and how it can be skillfully utilized to enliven the psychotherapeutic encounter. Available from www.psychotherapy.net)

Yalom, I. D. (2002). *The gift of therapy*. New York: HarperCollins.
    This book includes the wisdom of existential psychotherapy in 85 one- to two-page "lessons." Each lesson is illustrated with a brief case example.

CASE READINGS

Lindner, R. (1987). The jet-propelled couch. In *The Fifty-Minute Hour*. New York: Dell.

A great classic in the psychotherapy literature that, although not directly existential in its thinking, demonstrates that we are all more human than otherwise, that

we are quite literally "fellow travelers." No student of psychotherapy should miss this story.

Schneider, K. J., & Krug, O. T. (2010). *Existential-humanistic therapy: Theories of psychotherapy*. Washington, DC: American Psychological Association.

This book includes numerous cases that help readers understand the practical applications of existential psychotherapy, and it illustrates how existential and humanistic theories can be integrated with strategies and techniques derived from other approaches to therapy.

Yalom, I. D. (1989). *Love's executioner and other tales of psychotherapy*. New York: Basic Books. [A case study from this book, "If Rape Were Legal . . .," is reprinted in D. Wedding & R. J. Corsini (Eds.). (2013). *Case studies in psychotherapy*. Belmont, CA: Brooks/Cole.]

The actual practice of existential psychotherapy is best illustrated in these longer tales of the therapist–patient encounter. Of note are the examples of how therapist genuineness and self-disclosure foster healing.

Yalom, I. D. (1999). *Momma and the meaning of life*. New York: Basic Books.

This work offers more tales of psychotherapy. See especially a story entitled "Seven Lessons in the Therapy of Grief," which demonstrates the slowness and complexity of grief resolution in the face of death anxiety.

Yalom, I. D., & Elkins, G. (1974). *Everyday gets a little closer*. New York: Basic Books.

In this illuminating work, Yalom and his patient, Ginny Elkins, each keep notes and write a record of their therapy sessions. The final product allows an extraordinary look at how differently patient and therapist experience the therapeutic encounter.

REFERENCES

Becker, E. (1973). *Denial of death*. New York: Free Press.

Binswanger, L. (1958). The case of Ellen West. In R. May, E. Angel, & H. Ellenberger (Eds.), *Existence: A new dimension in psychology and psychiatry* (pp. 237–364). New York: Basic Books.

Buber, M. (1965). *The knowledge of man*. New York: HarperCollins.

Bugental, J. (1976). *The search for existential identity*. San Francisco: Jossey-Bass.

Craig, E. (2012). Human existence (Cún Zài): What is it? What's in it for us as existential psychotherapists? *The Humanistic Psychologist, 40*(1), 1–22.

Frank, J. D., & Frank, J. B. (1991). *Persuasion and healing: A comparative study of psychotherapy* (3rd ed.). Baltimore: Johns Hopkins University Press.

Frankl, V. (1963). *Man's search for meaning: An introduction to logotherapy*. New York: Pocket Books.

Fromm, E. (1941). *Escape from freedom*. New York: Holt.

Fromm, E. (1956). *The art of loving*. New York: Holt.

Gelso, C. J., & Hayes, J. A. (1998). *The psychotherapy relationship: Theory, research, and practice*. New York: Wiley.

Horney, K. (1950). *Neurosis and human growth: The struggle toward self-realization*. New York: W.W. Norton.

Josselson, R. (2007). *Playing Pygmalion: How people create one another*. New York: Rowman & Littlefield.

Jung, C. G. (1966). *Collected works: The practice of psychotherapy* (Vol. 16). New York: Pantheon, Bollingen Series.

Koestenbaum, P. (1978). *The new image of man*. Westport, CT: Greenwood Press.

May, R. (1953). *Man's search for himself*. New York: Norton.

May, R. (1958). Contributions of existential psychotherapy. In R. May, E. Angel, & H. F. Ellenberger (Eds.), *Existence: A new dimension in psychiatry and psychology* (pp. 37–91). New York: Basic Books.

May, R. (1967). *Psychology and the human dilemma*. Princeton, NJ: Van Nostrand.

May, R. (1969). *Love and will*. New York: Norton.

May, R. (1977). *The meaning of anxiety* (rev. ed.). New York: Norton.

May, R. (1981). *Freedom and destiny*. New York: Norton.

May, R. (1991). *The cry for myth*. New York: Norton.

May, R., Angel, E., & Ellenberger, H. F. (Eds.). (1958). *Existence: A new dimension in psychiatry and psychology*. New York: Basic Books.

McAdams, D. P., & Pals, J. L. (2006). A new big five: Fundamental principles for an integrative science of personality. *American Psychologist, 61*, 204–217.

McWilliams, N. (2005). Preserving our humanity as therapists. *Psychotherapy: Theory, Research, Practice, Training, 42*(2), 139–151.

Nabokov, V. (1967). *Speak, memory*. New York: Penguin Books.

Nietzsche, F. (1954). *Thus spake Zarathustra*. (Trans. Thomas Common). New York: Modern Library.

Norcross, J. C. (Ed.). (2002). *Psychotherapy relationships that work: Therapist contributions and responsiveness to patients*. New York: Oxford University Press.

Safran, J. D., & Muran, J. C. (1996). The resolution of ruptures in the therapeutic relationship. *Journal of Consulting and Clinical Psychology, 64*, 447–458.

Sartre, J. P (1956). *Being and nothingness*. New York: Philosophical Library.

Schneider, K. (2007). *Existential–integrative psychotherapy: Guideposts to the core of practice*. New York: Routledge.

Schneider, K. J., & Krug, O. T. (2010). *Existential-humanistic therapy: Theories of psychotherapy*. Washington, DC: American Psychological Association.

Schulenberg, S. E., Hutzell, R. R., Nassif, C.,. Rogina, J. M. (2008). Logotherapy for clinical practice. *Psychotherapy: Theory, Research, Practice, Training, 45*, 4, 447–463.

Spinoza, B. de (1954). *L'éthique* (Trans. Roger Caillois). Paris: Gallimard/Folio Essais.

Taylor, M. J., & Nanney, J. T. (2011). An existential gaze at multiracial self-concept: Implications for psychotherapy. *Journal of Humanistic Psychology, 51*, 195-215.

Tolstoy, L. (1981). *The death of Ivan Ilych*. New York: Bantam Books.

Wampold, B. E. (2001). *The great psychotherapy debate*. Mahwah, NJ: Erlbaum.

Wheelis, A. (1973). *How people change*. New York: Harper & Row.

Wheelis, A. (1999). *The listener: A psychoanalyst examines his life*. New York: W.W. Norton.

Wong, P. T. P. (2010). Meaning therapy: An integrative and positive existential psychotherapy. *Journal of Contemporary Psychotherapy, 40*, 85–93.

Yalom, I. D. (1980). *Existential psychotherapy*. New York: Basic Books.

Yalom, I. D. (1989). *Love's executioner and other tales of psychotherapy*. New York: Basic Books.

Yalom, I. D. (1992). *When Nietzsche wept*. New York: Basic Books/Harper.

Yalom, I. D. (1996). *Lying on the couch*. New York: Harper.

Yalom, I. D. (1999). *Momma and the meaning of life*. New York: Basic Books.

Yalom, I. D. (2002). *The gift of therapy*. New York: HarperCollins.

Yalom, I. D. (2005). *The Schopenhauer cure*. New York: HarperCollins.

Yalom, I. D. (2008). *Staring at the sun: Overcoming the terror of death*. San Francisco: Jossey-Bass.

Yalom, I. D. (2012). *The Spinoza problem*. New York: Basic Books.

Yalom, I. D., & Lecscz, M. (2005). *The theory and practice of group psychotherapy* (5th ed.). New York: Basic Books.

Yalom, I. D., & Elkins, G. (1974). *Everyday gets a little closer*. New York: Basic Books.

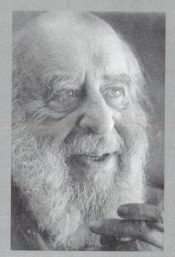

Fritz Perls (1893–1970)
Courtesy of the Gestalt Journal Press

9 | GESTALT THERAPY

Gary Yontef and Lynne Jacobs

OVERVIEW

Gestalt therapy was founded by Frederick ("Fritz") Perls and collaborators Laura Perls and Paul Goodman. They synthesized various cultural and intellectual trends of the 1940s and 1950s into a new gestalt, one that provided a sophisticated clinical and theoretical alternative to the two other main theories of their day: behaviorism and classical psychoanalysis.

Gestalt therapy began as a revision of psychoanalysis (Perls, 1942/1992) and quickly developed as a wholly independent, integrated system (Perls, Hefferline, & Goodman, 1951/1994). Because Gestalt therapy is an experiential and humanistic approach, it works with patients' awareness and awareness skills rather than using the classic psychoanalytic reliance on the analyst's interpretation of the unconscious. Also, in Gestalt therapy, the therapist is actively and personally engaged with the patient rather than fostering transference by remaining in the analytic role of neutrality. Gestalt therapy replaced the mechanistic, simplistic, Newtonian system of classical psychoanalysis with a process-based postmodern relational field theory.

Gestalt therapists use active methods that develop not only patients' awareness but also their repertoires of awareness and behavioral tools. Active methods and active personal engagement of Gestalt therapy are used to increase the awareness, freedom, and self-direction of patients rather than to direct them toward preset goals as in behavior therapy and encounter groups.

The Gestalt therapy system is truly integrative and includes affective, sensory, cognitive, interpersonal, and behavioral components (Joyce & Sills, 2009). In Gestalt therapy, therapists and patients are encouraged to be creative in doing the awareness work. There are no prescribed or proscribed techniques in Gestalt therapy.

Basic Concepts

Holism and Field Theory

Most humanistic theories of personality are holistic. Holism asserts that humans are inherently self-regulating, that they are growth oriented, and that persons and their symptoms cannot be understood apart from their environment. Holism and field theory are interrelated in Gestalt theory. Field theory is a way of understanding how one's context influences one's experiencing. Described elegantly by Einstein's theory of relativity, it is a theory about the nature of reality and our relationship to reality. It represents one of the first attempts to articulate a contextualist view of reality. Field theory, born in science, was an early contributor to the current postmodern sensibility that influences nearly all psychological theories today. Schools of thought that emphasize contextually emergent processes build on the work of Einstein and other field theorists. The combination of field theory, holism, and Gestalt psychology forms the bedrock for the Gestalt theory of personality.

Fields have certain properties that lead to a specific contextual theory. As with all contextual theories, a field is understood to be composed of mutually interdependent elements. But there are other properties as well. For one thing, variables that contribute to shaping a person's behavior and experience are said to be present in one's current field, and therefore people cannot be understood without understanding the field, or context, in which they live. A patient's life story cannot tell you what actually happened in his or her past, but it can tell you how the patient experiences his or her history in the here and now. That rendition of history is shaped to some degree by the patient's current field conditions.

What happened three years ago is not a part of the current field and therefore cannot affect one's experience. What *does* shape one's experience is how one holds a memory of the event and the fact that an event three years ago has altered how one may organize one's perception in the field. Another property of the field is that the organization of one's experience occurs in the here and now and is ongoing and subject to change based on field conditions. Also, no one can transcend embeddedness in a field; therefore, all attributions about the nature of reality are *relative* to the subject's position in the field. Field theory renounces the belief that anyone, including a therapist or scientist, can have an objective perspective on reality.

The *Paradoxical Theory of Change* is the heart of the Gestalt therapy approach (Beisser, 1970). The paradox is that the more one tries to become who one is not, the more one stays the same. The more one tries to force oneself into a mold that does not fit, the more one is fragmented rather than whole. Knowing and accepting the truth of one's feelings, beliefs, situation, and behavior builds wholeness and supports growth.

Organismic self-regulation requires knowing and owning—that is, identifying with—what one senses, feels emotionally, observes, needs or wants, and believes. Growth starts with conscious awareness of what is occurring in one's current existence, including how one is affected and how one affects others. One moves toward wholeness by identifying with ongoing experience, being in contact with what is actually happening, identifying and trusting what one genuinely feels and wants, and being honest with self and others about what one is actually able and willing to do—or not willing to do.

When one knows, senses, and feels one's self here and now, including the possibilities for change, one can be fully present, accepting or changing what is not satisfying. Living in the past, worrying about the future, or clinging to illusions about what one should be or could have been diminishes emotional and conscious awareness and the immediacy of experience that is the key to organismic living and growth.

Gestalt therapy aims for self-knowledge, acceptance, and growth by immersion in current existence, aligning contact, awareness, and experimentation with what is actually happening at the moment. It focuses on the here and now, not on what should be, could be, or was. From this present-centered focus, one can become clear about the needs, wishes, goals, and values of self and the situation.

The concepts emphasized in Gestalt therapy are contact, conscious awareness, and experimentation.

- *Contact* means being in touch with what is emerging here and now, moment to moment.

- *Conscious awareness* is a focusing of attention on what one is in touch with in situations requiring such attention. Awareness, or focused attention, is needed in situations that require higher contact ability, situations involving complexity or conflict, and situations in which habitual modes of thinking and acting are not working and in which one does not learn from experience. For example, in a situation that produces numbness, one can focus on the experience of numbness and cognitive clarity can emerge.

- *Experimentation* is the act of trying something new in order to increase understanding. The experiment may result in enhanced emotions or in the realization of something that had been kept from awareness. Experimentation, trying something new, is an alternative to the purely verbal methods of psychoanalysis and the behavior control techniques of behavior therapy.

Trying something new, without commitment to either the status quo or the adoption of a new pattern, can facilitate organismic growth. For example, patients often repeat stories of unhappy events without giving any evidence of having achieved increased clarity or relief. In this situation, a Gestalt therapist might suggest that the patient express affect directly to the person involved (either in person or through role playing). The patient often experiences relief or closure and the emergence of other feelings such as sadness or appreciation.

Contact, awareness, and experimentation have technical meanings, but these terms are also used in a colloquial way. The Gestalt therapist improves his or her practice by knowing the technical definitions. However, for the sake of this introductory chapter, we will try to use the colloquial form of these terms. Gestalt therapy starts with the therapist making contact with the patient by getting in touch with what the patient and therapist are experiencing and doing. The therapist helps the patient focus on and clarify what he or she is in contact with and deepens the exploration by helping focus the patient's awareness.

Awareness Process

Gestalt therapy focuses on the awareness process—in other words, on the continuum of one's flow of awareness. People have patterned processes of awareness that become foci for the work of therapy. The act of focusing enables the patient to become clear about what he or she thinks, feels, and decides in the current moment—and about how he or she does it. This includes a focus on what does not come to awareness. Careful attention to the sequence of the patient's continuum of awareness and observation of nonverbal behavior can help a patient recognize interruptions of contact and become aware of what has been kept out of awareness. For example, whenever Jill starts to look sad, she does not report feeling sad but moves immediately into anger. The anger cannot end as long as it functions to block Jill's sadness and vulnerability. In this situation, Jill can not only gain awareness of her sadness but also gain in skill at self-monitoring by being made aware of her tendency to block her sadness. That second order of awareness (how she interrupts awareness of her sadness) is referred to as *awareness of one's awareness process.*

Awareness of awareness can empower by helping patients gain greater access to themselves and clarify processes that had been confusing, improving the accuracy of perception and unblocking previously blocked emotional energy (Joyce & Sills, 2009). Jill had felt stymied by her lover's defensive reaction to her anger. When she realized that she actually felt hurt and sad, and not just angry, she could express her vulnerability, hurt, and sadness. Her lover was much more receptive to this than he was to her anger. In further work, Jill realized that blocking her sadness resulted from being shamed by her family when she had expressed hurt feelings as a child.

Gestalt therapists focus on patients' awareness and contact processes with respect, compassion, and commitment to the validity of the patients' experiential reality. Therapists model the process by disclosing their awareness and experience and being open to learning from the patient's perspective. Therapists are present in as mutual a way as possible in the therapeutic relationship and take responsibility for their own behavior and feelings. In this way, the therapist not only can be active and make suggestions but also can fully accept the patient in a manner consistent with the paradoxical theory of change.

Other Systems

Classical Freudian Psychoanalysis and Gestalt Therapy

At the heart of Freudian psychoanalysis was a belief in the centrality of basic biological drives and the establishment of relatively permanent structures created by the inevitable conflict between these basic drives and social demands—both legitimate demands and those stemming from parental and societal neurosis. All human development, behavior, thinking, and feeling were believed to be determined by these unconscious biological and social conflicts.

Patients' statements of their feelings, thoughts, beliefs, and wishes were not considered reliable because they were assumed to disguise deeper motivations stemming from the unconscious. The unconscious was a structure to which the patient did not have direct access, at least before completing analysis. However, the unconscious manifested itself in the transference neurosis; through the analyst's interpretation of the transference, "truth" was discovered and understood.

Psychoanalysis proceeded by a simple paradigm. Through free association (talking without censoring or focusing), the patient provided data for psychoanalytic treatment. These data were interpreted by the analyst according to the particular version of drive theory that he or she espoused. The analyst provided no details about his or her own life or person. He or she was supposed to be completely objective, eschewing all emotional reactions. The analyst had two fundamental rules: the *rule of abstinence* (gratifying no patient wish) and the *rule of neutrality* (having no preferences in the patient's conflict). Any deviation by the analyst was considered countertransference. Any attempt by the patient to know something about the analyst was interpreted as resistance, and any ideas about the analyst were considered a projection from the unconscious of the patient.

Although interpretation of the transference helped bring the focus back to the here and now, unfortunately, the potential of the here-and-now relationship is not realized in classical psychoanalysis because the focus is drawn away from the actual contemporaneous relationship, and the patients' feelings are interpreted as the result of unconscious drives and unresolved conflicts. Discussion in psychoanalysis was usually focused on the past and not on what is actually happening between analyst and patient *in the moment.*

This simple summary of psychoanalysis is not completely accurate because Adler, Rank, Jung, Reich, Horney, Fromm, Sullivan, and other analysts deviated from core Freudian assumptions in many ways and provided the soil from which the Gestalt therapy system arose. In these derivative systems, as in Gestalt therapy, the pessimistic Freudian view of a patient driven by unconscious forces was replaced by a belief in the potential for human growth and by appreciation for the power of relationships and conscious awareness. These approaches did not limit the data to free association; instead, they valued an explicitly compassionate attitude by the therapist and allowed a wider range of interventions. However, these approaches were still fettered by remaining in the psychoanalytic tradition. Gestalt therapy took a more radical position.

Behavior modification provided a simple alternative: Observe the behavior, disregard the subjective reports of the patient, and control problematic behavior by using either classical or operant conditioning to manipulate stimulus–response relationships. In the behavioral approaches, the emphasis was on what could be measured, counted, and "scientifically" proved.

The behavioral approach was the inverse of the intrapsychic approach of Freudian psychoanalysis. Here-and-now behavior was observed and taken as important data in its own right, but the patient's subjective, conscious experience was not considered reliable data.

A third choice was provided by Gestalt therapy. In Gestalt therapy, the patient's awareness is not assumed to be merely a cover for some other, deeper motivation. Unlike psychoanalysis, Gestalt therapy uses any and all available data. Like behavior modification, Gestalt therapy carefully observes behavior, including observation of the body, and it focuses on the here and now and uses active methods. The patient's self-report is considered real data. And, in a departure from both behavior modification and psychoanalysis, the therapist and the patient co-direct the work of therapy.

Client-Centered Therapy, Rational Emotive Behavior Therapy, and Gestalt Therapy

Gestalt therapy and client-centered therapy share common roots and philosophy. Both believe in the potential for human growth, and both believe that growth results from a relationship in which the therapist is experienced as warm and authentic (congruent). Both client-centered and Gestalt therapy are phenomenological therapies that work with the subjective awareness of the patient. However, Gestalt therapy has a more active phenomenological approach. The Gestalt therapy phenomenology is an experimental phenomenology. The patient's subjective experience is made clearer by using awareness experiments. These experiments are often similar to behavioral techniques, but they are designed to clarify the patient's awareness rather than to control her or his behavior.

Another difference is that the Gestalt therapist is more inclined to think in terms of an encounter in which the subjectivity of both patient and therapist is valued. The Gestalt therapist is much more likely than a person-centered therapist to tell the patient about his or her own feelings or experience.

Gestalt therapy provides an alternative to both the confrontational approach of rational emotive behavior therapy (REBT) and the nondirective approach of Carl Rogers. A person-centered therapist completely trusts the patient's subjective report, whereas a practitioner of REBT confronts the patient, often quite actively, about his or her irrational or dysfunctional ways of thinking. Gestalt therapy uses focused awareness experiments and personal disclosure to help patients enlarge their awareness. (During the 1960s and 1970s, Fritz Perls popularized a very confrontive model for dealing with avoidance, but this model is not representative of Gestalt therapy as it is practiced today.)

Gestalt therapy has become more like the person-centered approach in two important ways. First, Gestalt therapists have become more supportive, compassionate, kind, and oriented to the patient's experience. In addition, it has become clear that the therapist does not have an "objective" truth that is more accurate than the truth that the patient experiences.

Newer Models of Psychoanalysis and Relational Gestalt Therapy

There have been parallel developments in Gestalt therapy and psychoanalysis. The concept of the relationship in Gestalt therapy is modeled on Martin Buber's I–Thou relationship (Hycner & Jacobs, 1995; Yontef, 1993). In its emerging focus on the relationship, Gestalt therapy has moved away from classical psychoanalysis and drive theory, away from confrontation as a desired therapeutic tool, and away from the belief that the therapist is healthy and the patient is sick (Staemmler, 2011). Gestalt therapy has embraced such notions as intersubjectivity, mutual, reciprocal emotional influence, and the search for shared meanings as part and parcel of explorations of awareness (Wheeler, 2000).

Psychoanalysis has undergone a similar paradigm shift, and the two systems have somewhat converged. This is possible in part because contemporary psychoanalytic theories (especially relational and intersubjective theories) have rejected the limitations of classical Freudian psychoanalysis. The new theories eschew reductionism and determinism and reject the tendency to minimize the patient's own perspective. This movement brings psychoanalysis and Gestalt therapy closer in theory and practice (Orange, 2011). Gestalt therapy was formed in reaction to the same aspects of psychoanalysis that contemporary psychoanalysis is now rejecting.

Basic tenets now shared by contemporary psychoanalysis and Gestalt therapy include the following:

- an emphasis on the whole person and sense of self;
- an emphasis on process thinking;
- an emphasis on subjectivity and affect;
- an appreciation of the impact of life events (such as childhood sexual abuse) on personality development;
- a belief that people are motivated toward growth and development rather than regression;
- a belief that infants are born with a basic motivation and capacity for personal interaction, attachment, and satisfaction;
- a belief that there is no "self" without an "other"; and
- a belief that the structure and contents of the mind are shaped by interactions with others rather than by instinctual urges.

It is meaningless to speak of a person in isolation from the relationships that shape and define his or her life.

Cognitive Behavior Therapy, REBT, and Gestalt Therapy

The assumption that Gestalt therapy does not engage with patients' thinking processes is inaccurate. Gestalt therapy has always paid attention to what the patient is thinking.

Gestalt therapists, like their cognitive therapy colleagues, stress the role of "futurizing" in creating anxiety and, like REBT therapists, discuss the creation of guilt by moralistic thinking and thoughts of unreasonable conditions of worth ("shoulds"). Many of the thoughts that would be labeled irrational in REBT or cognitive behavior therapy have also traditionally been an important focus for Gestalt therapy.

There is one major difference between contemporary Gestalt therapy and REBT or cognitive behavior therapy. In modern Gestalt therapy, the therapist does not pretend to know the truth about what is irrational. The Gestalt therapist observes the process, directs the patient to observe his or her thoughts, and explores alternate ways of thinking in a manner that values and respects what the patient experiences and comes to believe.

HISTORY

Precursors

Gestalt therapy was less a font of substantial original "discoveries" than a groundbreaking integrative system for understanding personality and therapy that developed out of a seedbed of rich and varied sources. Fritz and Laura Perls, and the later American collaborators with whom they wrote, taught, and practiced from the 1940s through the 1960s (Isadore From, Paul Goodman, and others), swam in the turbulent waters of the 20th-century revolutions in science, philosophy, religion, psychology, art, literature, and politics. There was tremendous cross-fertilization between intellectuals in all disciplines during this period.

Frankfurt-am-Main of the 1920s, where Fritz Perls got his MD and Laura Perls her DSc, was a center of intellectual ferment in psychology. They were directly or indirectly exposed to leading Gestalt psychologists, existential and phenomenological philosophers, liberal theologians, and psychoanalytic thinkers.

Fritz Perls was intimately acquainted with psychoanalysis and in fact was a training analyst. However, he chafed under the dogmatism of classical psychoanalysis. For Perls, the revolutionary basic idea that Freud brought to Western culture—the existence of motivations that lay outside of conscious awareness—had to be woven into other streams of thought, particularly holism, Gestalt psychology, field theory, phenomenology, and existentialism.

These intellectual disciplines, each in its own way, were attempting to create a new vision of what it means to be human. Their vision came to be called a *humanistic* vision, and Gestalt therapy introduced that vision into the world of psychotherapy. Freudian analysts asserted the essential truth that human life is biologically determined, conflicted, and in need of constraint; the existentialists asserted the primacy of existence over essence, the belief that people choose the direction of their lives, and the argument that human life is not biologically determined. Within psychoanalysis, Perls was influenced by the more renegade analysts, especially Otto Rank and Wilhelm Reich. Both Rank and Reich emphasized conscious experience, the body as carrier of emotional wisdom and conflicts, and the active process of engagement between the therapist and the patient in the here and now. Reich introduced the important notion of *character armor:* repetitive patterns of experience, behavior, and body posture that keep the individual in fixed, socially determined roles. Reich also thought that how a patient spoke or moved was more important than what the patient said.

Rank emphasized the creative powers and uniqueness of the individual and argued that the client was his or her own best therapist. Like Fritz Perls, Rank stressed the importance of the experience of the here-and-now therapeutic relationship.

Providing a major source of inspiration to Fritz and Laura Perls were European continental philosophers who were breaking away from Cartesian dualism, arguing that the split between subject and object, self and world, was an illusion. These included the existentialists, the phenomenologists, and philosophers such as Ludwig Wittgenstein.

The new approach was influenced by field theory, the Gestalt psychologists, the holism of Jan Smuts, and Zen thought and practice. This thinking was blended by Fritz Perls with the Gestalt psychology of figure-and-ground perception and with the strongly Gestalt-influenced work of psychologists Kurt Goldstein and Kurt Lewin.

In his first book, *Ego, Hunger, and Aggression* (1942/1992), Perls described people as embedded in a person–environment field; this field was developed by the emergence into consciousness of those needs that organized perception. Perls also wrote about a "creative indifference" that enables a person to differentiate according to what is really needed in a particular situation. With the differentiation emerges the experience of contrast and awareness of the polarities that shape our experience of ourselves as separate. Perls thought of this as a Western equivalent to the Eastern practice of Zen.

Fritz and Laura left Germany during the Nazi era and later fled Nazi-occupied Holland. They went to South Africa, where they started a psychoanalytic training center. During this same period, Jan Smuts, South African prime minister in the 1940s, coined the term *holism* and wrote about it. In time, Fritz and Laura Perls left South Africa because of the beginning of the apartheid policies that Jan Smuts helped to initiate.

The fundamental precept of *holism* is that the organism is a self-regulating entity. For Fritz Perls, Gestalt psychology, organismic theory, field theory, and holism formed a happy union. Gestalt psychology provided Perls with the organizing principles for Gestalt therapy, as well as with a cognitive scheme that would integrate the varied influences in his life.

The word *Gestalt* has no literal English translation. It refers to a perceptual whole or configuration of experience. People do not perceive in bits and pieces, which are then added up to form an organized perception; instead, they perceive in patterned wholes. Patterns reflect an interrelationship among elements such that the whole cannot be gleaned by a study of component parts but only by a study of the relationship of parts to each other and to the whole. The leading figures in the development of Gestalt psychology were Max Wertheimer, Kurt Koffka, and Wolfgang Kohler.

Kurt Lewin extended this work by applying Gestalt principles to areas other than simple perceptual psychology and by explicating the theoretical implications of Gestalt psychology. He is especially well known for his explication of the field theory philosophy of Gestalt psychology, although this concept did not originate with him. Lewin (1938) discussed the principles by which field theory differed from Newtonian and positivistic thinking. In field theory, the world is studied as a systematic web of relationships, continuous in time, and not as discrete or dichotomous particles. In this view, everything is in the process of becoming, and nothing is static. Reality in this field view is configured by the relationship between the observer and the observed. "Reality," then, is a function of perspective, not a true positivist fact. There may be multiple realities of equal legitimacy. Such a view of the nature of reality opens Gestalt theory to a variety of formerly disenfranchised voices, such as those of women, gays, and non-Europeans.

Lewin carried on the work of the Gestalt psychologists by hypothesizing and researching the idea that a Gestalt is formed by the interaction between environmental possibilities and organismic needs. Needs organize perception and action. Perception is organized by the state of the person-in-relation and the environmental surround. A Gestalt therapy theory of organismic functioning was based on the Gestalt psychology principles of perception and holism. The theory of organismic self-regulation became a cornerstone of the Gestalt therapy theory of personality.

The philosophical tenets of phenomenology and existentialism were popular during the Perlses' years in Germany and in the United States. Gestalt therapy was influenced profoundly by the work of the dialogic existential thinkers, especially Martin Buber, with whom Laura Perls studied directly. Buber's belief in the inextricable existential fact that a self is always a self-with-other was a natural fit with Gestalt thinking, and his theory of the I–Thou relation became, through the teachings of Laura Perls, the basis for the patient–therapist relationship in Gestalt therapy.

Beginnings

Although Fritz Perls's earliest publication was *Ego, Hunger, and Aggression* (1942/1992), the first comprehensive integration of Gestalt therapy system is found in *Gestalt Therapy* (Perls et al., 1951/1994). This seminal publication represented the synthesis, integration, and new Gestalt formed by the authors' exposure to the intellectual zeitgeist already described. A New York Institute of Gestalt Therapy was soon formed, and the early seminar participants became teachers who spread the word to other cities by running regular training workshops, especially in New York, Cleveland, Miami, and Los Angeles. Intensive study groups formed in each of these cities. Learning was supplemented by the regular workshops of the original study group members, and eventually all of these cities developed their own Gestalt training institutes. The Gestalt Institute of Cleveland has made a special effort to bring in trainees from varied backgrounds and to develop a highly diverse faculty.

Gestalt therapy pioneered many ideas that have influenced humanistic psychotherapy. For instance, Gestalt therapy has a highly developed methodology for attending to experience phenomenologically and for attending to how the therapist and patient experience each other in the therapeutic relationship. *Phenomenology* assumes the reality is formed in the relationship between the observed and the observer. In short, reality is interpreted.

The dialogic relationship in Gestalt therapy derived three important principles from Martin Buber's thought (Hycner & Jacobs, 1995). First, in a dialogic therapeutic relationship, the therapist practices inclusion, which is similar to empathic engagement. In this, the therapist puts him- or herself into the experience of the patient, imagines the existence of the other, feels it as if it were a sensation within his or her own body, and simultaneously maintains a sense of self. Inclusion is a developed form of contact rather than a merger with the experience of the patient. Through imagining the patient's experience in this way, the dialogic therapist confirms the existence and potential of the patient. Second, the therapist discloses him- or herself as a person who is authentic and congruent and someone who is striving to be transparent and self-disclosing. Third, the therapist in dialogic therapy is committed to the dialogue, surrenders to what happens between the participants, and thus does not control the outcome. In such a relationship, the therapist is changed as well as the patient.

Underlying most existential thought is the existential phenomenological method. Gestalt therapy's phenomenology is a blend of the existential phenomenology of Edmund Husserl and his descendants and the phenomenology of Gestalt psychology.

Phenomenological understanding is achieved by taking initial perceptions and separating what is actually experienced at the moment from what was expected or merely logically derived. The phenomenological method increases the clarity of awareness by descriptively studying the awareness process. To do this, phenomenologists put aside assumptions, especially assumptions about what constitutes valid data. All data are considered valid initially, although they are likely to be refined by continuing phenomenological exploration. This is quite consistent with the Gestalt therapy view that the patient's awareness is valid and should be explored rather than explained away in terms of unconscious motivation.

Although other theories have not fully incorporated the I–Thou relation or systematic phenomenological focusing, they have been influenced by the excitement and vitality of direct contact between therapist and patient; the emphasis on direct experience; the use of experimentation; emphasis on the here and now, emotional process, and awareness; trust in organismic self-regulation; emphasis on choice; and attention to the patients' context as well as their experiential world.

Current Status

Gestalt institutes, literature, and journals have proliferated worldwide in the past 60 years. There is at least one Gestalt therapy training center in every major city in the United States, and there are many Gestalt therapy training institutes in most countries in Europe, North and South America, Australia, and Asia. Gestalt therapists practice all over the world.

Various countries and regions have begun to form umbrella organizations that sponsor professional meetings, set standards, and support research and public education. The Association for the Advancement of Gestalt Therapy is an international membership organization. This organization is not limited to professionals. The association was formed with the intention of governing itself through adherence to Gestalt therapy principles enacted at an organizational level. Regional conferences are also sponsored by the European Association for Gestalt Therapy and the Australian and New Zealand association, GANZ.

Gestalt therapy is known for a rich oral tradition, and, historically, Gestalt writings have not reflected the full depth of its theory and practice. Gestalt therapy has tended to attract therapists inclined to an experiential approach. The Gestalt therapy approach is almost impossible to teach without a strong experiential component.

Since the publication of a seminal book by the Polsters (1973), the gap between the oral and written traditions of Gestalt therapy has closed. There is now an extensive Gestalt therapy literature, and a growing number of books address various aspects of Gestalt therapy theory and practice. There are now four English-language Gestalt journals: the *International Gestalt Journal* (formerly *The Gestalt Journal*), the *British Gestalt Journal,* the *Gestalt Review,* and the *Gestalt Journal of Australia and New Zealand*. The Gestalt Journal Press also lists a comprehensive bibliography of Gestalt books, articles, videotapes, and audiotapes. This listing can be accessed through the Internet at www.gestalt.org. Another Internet site, Gestalt! (www.g-gej.org), the journal of the Association for the Advancement of Gestalt Therapy, provides resources for articles and research and is also an online journal. Gestalt therapy literature has also flourished around the world. There is at least one journal in most languages in Europe, North and South America, and Australia. In addition to the books written in English, translated, and widely read in other countries, there have been important original theoretical works published in French, German, Italian, Portuguese, Danish, Korean, and Spanish.

The past decade has witnessed a major shift in Gestalt therapy's understanding of personality and therapy. There has been a growing, albeit sometimes controversial, change in understanding the relational conditions for growth, both in general and (especially) in the therapeutic relationship. There is an increased appreciation for interdependence, a better understanding of the shaming effect of the cultural value placed on self-sufficiency, and greater realization of how shame is created in childhood and triggered in interpersonal relationships (Fairfield & O'Shea, 2008; Lee & Wheeler, 1996; Yontef, 1993). As Gestalt therapists have come to understand shame and its triggers more thoroughly, they have become less confrontive and more accepting and supportive than in earlier years (Jacobs, 1996).

PERSONALITY

Theory of Personality

Gestalt therapy theory has a highly developed, somewhat complicated theory of personality. The notions of healthy functioning and neurotic functioning are actually quite simple and clear, but they are built on a paradigm shift, not always easy to grasp, from linear cause-and-effect thinking to a process, field theory worldview.

Gestalt therapy is a radical ecological theory that maintains there is no meaningful way to consider any living organism apart from its interactions with its environment—that is, apart from the organism–environment field of which it is a part (Perls et al., 1951/1994). Psychologically, there is no meaningful way to consider a person apart from interpersonal relations just as there is no meaningful way to perceive the environment except through someone's perspective. According to Gestalt therapy field theory, it is impossible for perception to be totally "objective."

The "field" that human beings inhabit is replete with other human beings. In Gestalt theory, there is no self separate from one's organism and environmental field; more specifically, self does not exist without other. Self implies self-in-relation (Philippson, 2001). Contact is an integral aspect of all experience—in fact, experience does not exist without contact—but it is the contact between humans that dominates the formation and functions of our personalities.

The field is differentiated by *boundaries*. The contact boundary has dual functions: It not only connects people with each other but also maintains separation. Without emotionally connecting with others, one starves; without emotional separation, one does not maintain a separate, autonomous identity. Connecting meets biological, social, and psychological needs; separation creates and maintains autonomy and protects against harmful intrusion or overload.

Needs are met, and people grow through contact with and withdrawal from others. By separating and connecting, a person establishes boundary and identity. Effective self-regulation includes contact in which one is aware of what is newly emerging that may be either nourishing or harmful. One identifies with that which is nourishing and rejects that which is harmful. This kind of differentiated contact leads to growth (Polster & Polster, 1973). The crucial processes regulating this discrimination are awareness and contact.

The most important processes for psychological growth are interactions in which two persons each acknowledge the experience of the other with awareness and respect for the needs, feelings, beliefs, and customs of the other. This form of dialogic contact is essential in therapy.

Organismic Self-Regulation

Gestalt therapy theory holds that people are inherently self-regulating, context sensitive, and motivated to solve problems. Needs and desires are organized hierarchically so that in health the most urgent need takes precedence and claims attention until this need is met. When this need is met, the next need or interest becomes the center of attention.

Gestalt (Figure–and–Ground) Formation

A corollary to the concept of organismic self-regulation is called *Gestalt formation*. Gestalt psychology has taught us that we perceive in unified wholes and also that we perceive through the phenomenon of contrast. A figure of interest forms in contrast to a relatively dull background. For instance, the words on this page are a visual figure to the reader, whereas other aspects of the room are visually less clear and vivid until this reference to them leads the reader to allow the words on the page to slip into the background, at which time the figure of a table, chair, book, or soda emerges. One can only perceive one clear figure at a time, although figures and grounds may shift very rapidly.

Consciousness and Unconsciousness

A most important consequence of adapting Gestalt psychology to a theory of personality functioning is that ideas about consciousness and unconsciousness are radically different from those of Freud. Freud believed the unconscious was filled with impersonal, biologically based urges that constantly pressed for release. Competent functioning depended on the successful use of repression and sublimation to keep the contents of the unconscious hidden; these urges could be experienced only in symbolic form.

Gestalt therapy's "unconscious" is quite different. In Gestalt therapy theory, the concepts of awareness and unawareness replace the unconscious. Gestalt therapists use the concepts of awareness–unawareness to reflect the belief in the fluidity between what is momentarily in awareness and what is momentarily outside of awareness. When something vital, powerful, and relevant is not allowed to emerge into foreground, one is unaware. What is background is outside of awareness for the moment, but it could instantly become the figure in awareness. This is in keeping with the Gestalt psychology understanding of perception, which is the formation of a figure against a background.

In neurotic patients, some aspect of the phenomenal field is purposely and regularly relegated to the background. This concept is roughly similar to the Freudian dynamic unconscious. However, Gestalt therapists do not believe in a "primary process" unconscious that needs to be translated by the therapist before it can be comprehensible to the patient.

Gestalt therapists maintain that what is being relegated to permanent background status reflects the patient's current conflicts as well as the patient's perspective on current field conditions. When a patient perceives the conditions of the therapy relationship to be safe enough, more and more aspects of previously sequestered subjective states can be brought into awareness through the therapeutic dialogue.

Health

The Gestalt therapy notion of health is actually quite simple. In healthy organismic self-regulation, one is aware of shifting need states; that is, what is of most importance becomes the figure of one's awareness. Being whole, then, is simply identifying with one's ongoing, moment-by-moment experiencing and allowing this identification to organize one's behavior.

Healthy organismic awareness includes awareness of the human and nonhuman environment and is not unreflective or inconsiderate of the needs of others. For example, compassion, love, and care for the environment are all part of organismic functioning.

Healthy functioning requires being in contact with what is actually occurring in the person–environment field. Contact is the quality of being in touch with one's experience in relation to the field. By being aware of what is emerging and by allowing action to be organized by what is emerging, people interact in the world and learn from the experience. By trying something new, one learns what works and what does not work in various situations. When a figure is not allowed to emerge, when it is somehow interrupted or misdirected, there is a disturbance in awareness and contact.

Tendency Toward Growth

Gestalt therapists believe that people are inclined toward growth and will develop as fully as conditions allow. Gestalt therapy is holistic and asserts that people are inherently self-regulating and growth oriented and that people and their behavior, including symptoms, cannot be understood apart from their environment and what needs organize specific behaviors.

Gestalt therapy is interested in the existential themes of existence—connection and separation, life and death, choice and responsibility, authenticity and freedom. Gestalt therapy's theory of awareness is a bedrock phenomenological orientation toward experience derived from an existential and humanistic ethos. Gestalt therapy attempts to understand human beings by the study of experience. Meaning is understood in terms of what is experienced and how it is experienced.

Life Is Relational

Gestalt therapy regards awareness and human relations as inseparable. Awareness starts developing at birth through a matrix of relations; that process continues throughout life. Relationships are regulated by how people experience them. From birth to death, people define themselves by how they experience themselves in relation to others. This derives from how people are regarded by others and how they think and behave toward others. In Gestalt therapy theory, derived from Martin Buber, there is no "I," no sense of self, other than self in relation to others. There is only the "I" of the "I–Thou" or the "I" of the "I–[I]t." As Buber said, "All real living is meeting" (1923/1970, p. 11).

Living is a progression of needs, met and unmet. One achieves homeostatic balance and moves on to whatever need emerges next. In health, the boundary is permeable enough to allow exchange with that which promotes health (connecting) and firm enough to preserve autonomy and exclude that which is unhealthful (separation). This requires the identification of those needs that are most pressing at a particular time and in a particular environment.

Variety of Concepts

Disturbances at the Boundary

Under optimal conditions, there is ongoing movement between connecting and withdrawal. When the experience of coming together is blocked repetitively, one is left in a state of *isolation,* which is a boundary disturbance. It is a disturbance because it is fixed, does not respond to a whole range of needs, and fails to allow close contact to emerge. By the same token, if the need to withdraw is blocked, there is a corresponding boundary disturbance known as *confluence.* Confluence is the loss of the experience of separate identity.

In optimal functioning, when something is taken in—whether it is an idea, food, or love—there is contact and awareness. The person makes discriminations about what to take in and what meaning to attach to that which is taken in. When things (ideas, identity, beliefs, and so on) are taken in without awareness, the boundary disturbance of *introjection* results. Introjects are not fully integrated into organismic functioning.

For one to integrate and be whole, what is taken in must be assimilated. *Assimilation* is the process of experiencing what is to be taken in, deconstructing it, keeping what is useful, and discarding what is not. For example, the process of assimilation allows the listener to select and keep only what is useful from a lecture she or he attends.

When a phenomenon that occurs in one's self is falsely attributed to another person in an effort to avoid awareness of one's own experience, the boundary disturbance of *projection* occurs. When an impulse or desire is turned into a one-person event instead of a two-person event (an example is caressing oneself when one wants another person to do the caressing), there is the boundary disturbance of *retroflection*. In each process, some part of the person is disowned and not allowed to become figural or to organize and energize action.

Creative Adjustment

When all the pieces are put together, people function according to an overarching principle called *creative adjustment*. "All contact is creative adjustment of the organism and the environment" (F. Perls et al.,1994, p. 6). All organisms live in an environment to which they must adjust. Nevertheless, people also need to shape the environment so that it conforms to human needs and values.

The concept of creative adjustment follows from the notion that people are growth oriented and will try to solve their problems in living in the best way possible. This means solving the problem in a way that makes the fullest use of their own resources and those of the environment. Because awareness can be concentrated on only one figure at a time, those processes that are not the object of creative awareness operate in a habitual mode of adjustment until it is their turn to come into full awareness.

The term *creative adjustment* reflects a creative balance between changing the environment and adjusting to current conditions. Because people live only in relation, they must balance adjusting to the demands of the situation (such as societal demands and the needs of others) and creating something new according to their own, individual interests. This is a continual, mutual, reciprocal negotiation between one's self and one's environment.

The process whereby a need becomes figural, is acted on, and then recedes as a new figure emerges is called a *Gestalt formation cycle*. Every Gestalt formation cycle requires creative adjustment. Both sides of the polarity are necessary for the resolution of a state of need. If one is hungry, one must eat new food taken from the environment. Food that has already been eaten will not solve the problem. New actions must occur, and the environment must be contacted and adapted to meet the individual's needs.

On the other hand, one cannot be so balanced on the side of creating new experience that one does not draw on prior learning and experience, established wisdom, and societal mores. For example, one must use yesterday's learning to be able to recognize aspects of the environment that might be used as a source of food, while at the same time being creative in experimenting with new food possibilities.

Maturity

Good health has the characteristics of a good Gestalt. A *good Gestalt* consists of a perceptual field organized with clarity and good form. A well-formed figure clearly stands out against a broader and less distinct background. The relation between that which stands out (figure) and the context (ground) is meaning. In a good Gestalt, meaning is clear.

Health and maturity result from creative adjustment that occurs in a context of environmental possibility. Both health and maturity require a person whose Gestalt formation process is freely functioning and one whose contact and awareness processes are relatively free of excessive anxiety, inhibition, or habitual selective attention.

In health, the figure changes as needed; that is, it shifts to another focus when a need is met or superseded by a more urgent need. It does not change so rapidly as to prevent satisfaction (as in hysteria) or so slowly that new figures have no room to assume dominance (as in compulsivity). When the figure and ground are dichotomized, one is left with a figure out of context or a context without focus (as in impulsivity) (F. Perls et al., 1951/1994).

The healthy person is in creative adjustment with the environment. The person adjusts to the needs of the environment and adjusts the environment to his or her own needs. Adjustment alone is conformity and breeds stagnation. On the other hand, unbridled creativity in the service of the isolated individual would result in pathological narcissism.

Disrupted Personality Functioning

Mental illness is simply the inability to form clear figures of interest and identify with one's moment-by-moment experience and/or to respond to what one becomes aware of. People whose contact and awareness processes are disrupted often have been shaped by environments that were chronically impoverished or intrusive. Impoverished or intrusive environments diminish one's capacity for creative adjustment.

However, even neurotic self-regulation is considered a creative adjustment. Gestalt therapists assume that neurotic regulation is the result of a creative adjustment that was made in a difficult situation in the past and then not readjusted as field conditions changed. For example, one patient's father died when she was eight years old. The patient was terribly bereft, frightened, and alone. Her grief-stricken mother, the only adult in her life, was unavailable to help her assimilate her painful and frightening reactions to her father's death. The patient escaped her unbearable situation by busying herself to the point of distraction. That was a creative adjustment to her needs in a field with limited resources. But as an adult, she continues to use the same means of adjustment, even though the field conditions have changed. This patient's initial creative adjustment became hardened into a repetitive character pattern. This often happens because the original solution worked well enough in an emergency, and current experiences that mimic the original emergency trigger one's emergency adaptation.

Patients frequently cannot trust their own self-regulation because repeated use of a solution from an earlier time erodes their ability to respond with awareness to the current self-in-field problem. Organismic self-regulation is replaced by "shoulds"—that is, by attempts to control and manage one's experience rather than accepting one's experience. Part of the task of therapy is to create, in the therapy situation, a new "emergency"—but a "safe emergency," one that not only includes some elements reminiscent of the old situation (such as rising emotional intensity), but also contains health-facilitating elements that can be used (for instance, the therapist's affirming and calming presence). The new situation, if safe enough, can promote a new, more flexible and responsive creative adjustment.

Polarities

Experience forms as a Gestalt, a figure against a ground. Figure and ground stand in a polar relation to each other. In healthy functioning, figures and grounds shift according to changing needs and field conditions. What was previously an aspect of the ground can emerge almost instantly as the next figure.

Life is dominated by polarities: life–death, strength-vulnerability, connection–separation, and so on and on. When one's creative adjustments are flowing and responsive to current field conditions, the interaction and continually recalibrating balance of these polarities make up the rich tapestry of existence.

In neurotic regulation, some aspects of one's ground must be kept out of awareness (for instance, the patient's unbearable loneliness), and polarities lose their fluidity and become hardened into dichotomies. In neurotic regulation, a patient may readily identify with his or her strength but may instead ignore or disavow the experience of vulnerability. Such selective awareness results in a life filled with insoluble conflicts and plagued by crises or dulled by passivity.

Resistance

The ideas of holism and organismic self-regulation have turned the theory of resistance on its head. Its original meaning in psychoanalysis referred to a reluctance to face a painful truth about one's self. However, the theory of self-regulation posits that all phenomena, even resistance can be shown to serve an organismic purpose when taken in context.

In Gestalt theory, resistance is an awkward but crucially important expression of the organism's integrity. Resistance is the process of opposing the formation of a figure (a thought, feeling, impulse, or need) or the imposition of the therapist's figure (or agenda) that threatens to emerge in a context that is judged to be dangerous. For instance, someone may choke back tears, believing the tears would be more for the therapist than for the patient or that crying would expose him or her to ridicule. Or someone who has been ridiculed in the past for showing any vulnerability may assume that the current environmental surround is harsh and unforgiving. The inhibited experience is resisted—usually without awareness. For example, a patient may have pushed all experience of vulnerability out of awareness; however, the experience of vulnerability still lives in the background, quietly shaping and shadowing the figure formation process. Instead of a fluid polar relationship, the patient develops a hardened dichotomy between strength and vulnerability and inevitably experiences anxiety whenever he or she feels vulnerable. The result may be a man who takes risks demonstrating great physical courage but who is terrified by the thought of committing himself to a woman he loves. As the conflict is explored in therapy, he becomes aware that he is terribly frightened of his vulnerable feelings and resists allowing those feelings to be activated and noticed. The resistance protects him by ensuring that his habitual mode of self-regulation remains intact. When the original creative adjustment occurred, the identification with his strength and the banishment of his vulnerability were adaptive. Gestalt theory posits that he has "forgotten" that he made such an adjustment and so remains unaware that he even *has* any vulnerability that might be impeding his ability to make decisions in support of his current figure of interest, the commitment.

Even when the patient becomes vaguely aware, he may not be sure that the current context is sufficiently different that he can dare to change his dichotomized adjustment. Repetitive experiments within the relative safety of the therapeutic relationship may enable him to contact his vulnerable side enough to reenliven the polarity of strength–vulnerability such that he can resume a more moment-by-moment creative adjustment process.

Emotions are central to healthy functioning because they orient one to one's relationship to the current field, and they help establish the relative urgency of an emergent figure. Emotional process is integral to the Gestalt formation process and functions as a "signal" in a healthy individual. For instance, on suddenly experiencing shame, the healthy person takes it as a sign that perhaps he or she should not persist in whatever he or she is doing. Unfortunately, the person whose self-regulation has been disrupted cannot experience shame as a signal but instead tends to be overwhelmed by it.

Contact and Support

"*Contact* is possible only to the extent that *support* for it is available. . . . *Support* is everything that facilitates the ongoing assimilation and integration of experience for a person, relationship or society" (L. Perls, 1992). Adequate support is a function of the total field. It requires both self-support and environmental support. One must support oneself by breathing, but the environment must provide the air. In health, one is not out of touch with the current set of self and environmental needs and does not live in the past (unfinished business) or future (catastrophizing). It is only in the present that individuals can support themselves and protect themselves.

Anxiety

Gestalt therapy is concerned with the process of anxiety rather than the content of anxiety (what one is anxious about). Fritz Perls first defined anxiety as excitement minus support (Perls, 1942/1992; Perls et al., 1951/1994). Anxiety can be created cognitively or through unsupported breathing habits. The cognitive creation of anxiety results from "futurizing" and failing to remain centered in the present. Negative predictions, misinterpretations, and irrational beliefs can all trigger anxiety. When people futurize, they focus their awareness on something that is not yet present. For example, someone about to give a speech may be preoccupied with the potentially negative reaction of the audience. Fears about future failure can have a very negative effect on current performance. Stage fright is a classic example in which physical arousal is mislabeled and misattribution triggers a panic attack.

Anxiety can also be created by unsupported breathing. With arousal there is an organismic need for oxygen. "A healthy, self-regulating individual will automatically breathe more deeply to meet the increased need for oxygen which accompanies mobilization and contact" (Clarkson & Mackewn, 1993, p. 81). When people breathe fully, tolerate increased mobilization of energy, are present centered and cognitively flexible, and put energy into action, they experience excitement rather than anxiety. Breath support requires full inhalation and exhalation, as well as breathing at a rate that is neither too fast nor too slow. When one breathes rapidly without sufficient exhaling, fresh, oxygenated blood cannot reach the alveoli because the old air with its load of carbon dioxide is not fully expelled. Then the person has the familiar sensations of anxiety: increased pulse rate, inability to get enough air, and hyperventilation (Acierno, Hersen, & Van Hasselt, 1993; Perls, 1942/1992; Perls et al., 1951/1994).

The Gestalt therapy method, with its focus on both body orientation and characterological issues, is ideal for the treatment of anxiety. Patients learn to master anxiety cognitively and physically through cognitive and body-oriented awareness work (Yontef, 1993).

Impasse

An impasse is experienced when a person's customary supports are not available and new supports have not yet been mobilized. The experience is existentially one of terror. The person cannot go back and does not know whether he or she can survive going forward. People in the impasse are paralyzed as forward and backward energy fight each other. This experience is often expressed in metaphorical terms: void, hollow, blackness, going off a cliff, drowning, or being sucked into a whirlpool.

The patient who stays with the experience of the impasse may experience authentic existence—that is, existence with minimal illusion, good self-support, vitality, creativity, and good contact with the human and nonhuman environment. In this mode, Gestalt formation is clear and lively, and maximum effort is put into what is important. When support is not mobilized to work through the impasse, the person continues to repeat old and maladaptive behaviors.

Development

Gestalt therapy has not, until recently, had a well-developed theory of childhood development, but current psychoanalytic research and theory support a perspective that Gestalt therapists have held for quite a while. This theory maintains that infants are born with the capacity for self-regulation, that the development and refinement of self-regulatory skills are contingent on mutual regulation between caretaker and infant, that the contact between caretaker and infant must be attuned to the child's emotional states for self-regulation to develop best, and that children seek relatedness through emotionally attuned mutual regulation (Stern, 1985). Gestalt therapist Frank (Frank & La Barre, 2011) has used the research of Stern and others to formulate a comprehensive Gestalt theory of development based on embodiment and relatedness. McConville and Wheeler (2003) have used field theory and relatedness in articulating their theories of child and adolescent development.

PSYCHOTHERAPY

Theory of Psychotherapy

People grow and change all through life. Gestalt therapists believe growth is inevitable as long as one is engaged in contact. Ordinarily, people develop increasing emotional, perceptual, cognitive, motoric, and organismic self-regulatory competence. Sometimes, however, the process of development becomes impaired or derailed. To the extent that people learn from mistakes and grow, psychotherapy is not necessary. Psychotherapy is indicated when people routinely fail to learn from experience. People need psychotherapy when their self-regulatory abilities do not lead them beyond the maladaptive repetitive patterns that were developed originally as creative adjustments in difficult circumstances but that now make them or those around them unhappy. Psychotherapy is also indicated with patients who do not deal adequately with crises, feel ill equipped to deal with others in their lives, or need guidance for personal or spiritual growth.

Gestalt therapy concentrates on helping patients become aware of how they avoid learning from experience, how their self-regulatory processes may be closed ended rather than open ended, and how inhibitions in the area of contact limit access to the experience necessary to broaden awareness. Of course, awareness is developed through interactions with other people. From the earliest moment of a person's life, both functional and dysfunctional patterns emerge from a matrix of relationships.

Psychotherapy is primarily a relationship between a patient and a therapist, a relationship in which the patient has another chance to learn, to unlearn, and to learn how to keep learning. The patient and the therapist make explicit the patterns of thought and behavior that are manifest in the psychotherapy situation. Gestalt therapists hold that the patterns that emerge in therapy recapitulate the patterns that are manifest in the patient's life.

Goal of Therapy

The only goal of Gestalt therapy is awareness. This includes achieving greater awareness in particular areas and also improving the ability to bring automatic habits into awareness as needed. In the former sense, awareness refers to content; in the latter sense, it refers to process, specifically the kind of self-reflective awareness that is called *awareness of awareness*. Awareness of awareness is the patient's ability to use his or her skills with awareness to rectify disturbances in his or her awareness process. Both awareness as content and awareness as process broaden and deepen as the therapy proceeds. Awareness requires self-knowledge, knowledge of the environment, responsibility for choices, self-acceptance, and the ability to contact.

Beginning patients are chiefly concerned with the solution of problems, often thinking that the therapist will "fix" them the way a physician often cures a disease. However, Gestalt therapy does not focus on curing disease, nor is it restricted to talking about problems. Gestalt therapy uses an active relationship and active methods to help patients gain the self-support necessary to solve problems. Gestalt therapists provide support through the therapeutic relationship and show patients how they block their awareness and functioning. As therapy goes on, the patient and the therapist turn more attention to general personality issues. By the end of successful Gestalt therapy, the patient directs much of the work and is able to integrate problem solving, characterological themes, relationship issues with the therapist, and the regulation of his or her own awareness.

How Is the Therapy Done?

Gestalt therapy is an exploration rather than a direct attempt to change behavior. Therapist and patient work together to increase understanding. The goal is growth and autonomy through an increase in consciousness. The method is one of direct engagement, whether that engagement is the meeting between therapist and patient or engagement with problematic aspects of the patient's contacting and awareness process. The model of engagement comes directly from the Gestalt concept of contact. Contact is the means whereby living and growth occur, so lived experience nearly always takes precedence over explanation. Rather than maintaining an impersonal professional distance and making interpretations, the Gestalt therapist relates to the patient with an alive, excited, warm, and direct presence.

In this open, engaged relationship, patients not only get honest feedback but also, in the authentic contact, can see, hear, and be told how they are experienced by the therapist, can learn how they affect the therapist, and (if interested) can learn something about the therapist. They have the healing experience of being listened to by someone who profoundly cares about their perspectives, feelings, and thoughts.

What and How, Here and Now

Gestalt therapy holds a dual focus: a constant and careful emphasis on *what* the patient does and *how* it is done and also a similar focus on the interactions between therapist and patient. What does the patient do to support him- or herself in the therapy hour in relation to the therapist and in the rest of his or her life?

Direct experience is the primary tool of Gestalt therapy, and the focus is always on the here and now. The present is a transition between past and future. Not being primarily present centered reflects a time disturbance—but so does not being able to contact the relevant past or not plan for the future. Frequently, patients lose their contact with the present and live in the past. In some cases, patients live in the present as though they had no past, with the unfortunate consequence that they cannot learn from the past. The most common time disturbance is living in anticipation of what could happen in the future as though the future were now.

Now starts with the present awareness of the patient. In a Gestalt therapy session, what happens first is not childhood but what is experienced *now*. Awareness takes place *now*. Prior events may be the object of present awareness, but the awareness process is *now*.

Now I can contact the world around me, or *now* I can contact memories or expectations. "Now" refers to *this moment*. When patients refer to their lives outside of the therapy hour, or even earlier in the hour, the content is not considered *now*, but the action of speaking *is* now. We orient more to the now in Gestalt therapy than in any other form of psychotherapy. This "what and how; here and now" method frequently is used to work on characterological and developmental themes. Exploration of past experience is anchored in the present (for example, determining what in the present field triggers this particular old memory). Whenever possible, methods are used that bring the old experience directly into present experience rather than just recounting the past.

There is an emerging awareness in Gestalt therapy that the best therapy requires a binocular viewpoint: Gestalt therapy requires technical work on the patient's awareness process, but at the same time it involves a personal relationship in which careful attention is paid to nuances of what is happening in the contact between therapist and patient.

Awareness

One pillar of Gestalt therapy is developing awareness of the awareness process. Does the awareness deepen and develop fully—or is it truncated? Is any particular figure of awareness allowed to recede from the mind to make room for other awarenesses—or does one figure repeatedly capture the mind and shut out the development of other awareness?

Ideally, processes that need to be in awareness come into awareness when and as needed in the ongoing flow of living. When transactions get complex, more conscious self-regulation is needed. If this develops and a person behaves mindfully, the person is likely to learn from experience.

The concept of awareness exists along a continuum. For example, Gestalt therapy distinguishes between merely *knowing* about something and *owning* what one is doing. Merely knowing about something marks the transition between that something's being totally out of awareness and its being in focal awareness. When people report being aware of something and yet claim they are totally helpless to make desired changes, they are usually referring to a situation in which they *know about* something but do not fully feel it, do not know the details of how it works, do not fully know that they are making choices, and do not genuinely integrate it and make it their own. In addition, they frequently have difficulty imagining alternatives or believing that the alternatives can be achieved or know how to support experimenting with alternatives.

Being fully aware means turning one's attention to the processes that are most important for the person and environment; this is a natural occurrence in healthy self-regulating. One must know what is going on and how it is happening. What do I need and what am I doing? What are my choices? What is needed by others? Who is doing what? Who needs what? For full awareness, this more detailed descriptive awareness must be allowed to affect the patient—and he or she has to be able to own it and respond in a relevant way.

Contact

Contact, the relationship between patient and therapist, is another pillar of Gestalt therapy. The relationship is contact over time. What happens in the relationship is crucial. This is more than what the therapist says to the patient, and it is more than the techniques that are used. Of most importance is the *nonverbal subtext* (posture, tone of voice, syntax, and interest level) that communicates tremendous amounts of information to the patient about how the therapist regards the patient, what is important, and how therapy works.

In a good therapy relationship, the therapist pays close attention to what the patient is doing moment to moment and to what is happening between the therapist and the patient. The therapist not only pays close attention to what the patient experiences but also deeply believes that the patient's subjective experience is just as real and valid as the therapist's "reality."

The therapist is in a powerful position in relation to the patient. If the therapist regards the patient with honesty, affection, compassion, kindness, and respect, then an atmosphere can be created in which it is relatively safe for the patient to become more deeply aware of what has been kept from awareness. This enables the patient to experience and express thoughts and emotions that she or he has not habitually felt safe to share. The therapist is in a position to guide the awareness work by entering into the patient's experience deeply and completely. Martin Buber refers to "inclusion" as feeling the experience of the other much as one would feel something within one's own body while simultaneously being aware of one's own self.

There is some tension between the humane urge of the therapist to relieve the patient's pain and the indispensable need of the patient for someone who willingly enters into and understands his or her subjective pain. The therapist's empathic experience of the patient's pain brings the patient into the realm of human contact. However, trying to get the patient to feel better is often experienced by a patient as evidence that the patient is acceptable only to the extent that he or she feels good. The therapist may not intend to convey this message, but this reaction is often triggered when the therapist does not abide by the paradoxical theory of change.

Experiment

In client-centered therapy, the phenomenological work by the therapist is limited to reflecting what the patient subjectively experiences. In psychoanalytic work, the therapist is limited to interpretations or reflections. These interventions are both part of the Gestalt therapy repertoire, but Gestalt therapy has an additional experimental phenomenological method. Put simply, the patient and therapist can experiment with different ways of thought and action to achieve genuine understanding rather than mere changes in behavior. As in any research, the experiment is designed to get more data. In Gestalt therapy, the data are the phenomenological experience of the patient.

The greatest risk with experiments is that vulnerable patients may believe that change has been mandated. This danger is magnified if a therapist's self-awareness becomes clouded or if she or he strays from a commitment to the paradoxical theory of change. It is vitally important in Gestalt therapy that the therapist remain clear that the mode of change is the patient's knowledge and acceptance of self, knowing and supporting what emerges in contemporaneous experience. If the therapist makes it clear that the experiments are experiments in awareness and not criticism of what is observed, the risk of adding to the patient's self-rejection is minimized.

In Gestalt therapy experiments arise out of the interactions between therapist and patient and function to help the relationship develop. (See for example, Swanson, 2009).

Self-Disclosure

One powerful and distinguishing aspect of Gestalt therapy is that therapists are both permitted and encouraged to disclose their personal experience, in the moment as well as in their lives. Unlike classical psychoanalysis, in Gestalt therapy data are provided by both the patient and the therapist, and both the patient and the therapist take part in directing therapy through a process of mutual phenomenological exploration.

This kind of therapeutic relationship requires that therapists be at peace with the differences between themselves and their patients. In addition, therapists most truly believe that the patient's sense of subjective reality is as valid as their own. With an appreciation of the relativity of one's subjectivity, it becomes possible for therapists to disclose their reactions to patients without *requiring* that patients change. These conversations, entered into with care and sensitivity, are generally quite interesting and evocative, and they often enhance the patient's sense of efficacy and worthiness.

Dialogue is the basis of the Gestalt therapy relationship. In dialogue, the therapist practices inclusion, empathic engagement, and personal presence (for example, self-disclosure). The therapist imagines the reality of the patient's experience and, in so doing, confirms the existence and potential of the patient. However, this is not enough to make the interaction a real dialogue.

Real dialogue between therapist and patient must also include the therapist surrendering to the interaction and to what emerges from that interaction. The therapist must be open to being changed by the interaction. This sometimes requires the therapist to acknowledge having been wrong, hurtful, arrogant, or mistaken. This kind of acknowledgment puts therapist and patient on a horizontal plane. This sort of open disclosure requires personal therapy for the therapist to reduce defensiveness and the need to pridefully maintain his or her personal self-image.

Process of Psychotherapy

People form their sense of self and their style of awareness and behavior in childhood. These become habitual and often are not refined or revised by new experiences. As a person moves out of the family and into the world, new situations are encountered and the old ways of thinking, feeling, and acting are no longer needed or adaptive in new situations. But the old ways sometimes persist because they are not in awareness and hence are not subject to conscious review.

In Gestalt therapy, the patient encounters someone who takes his or her experience seriously, and through this different, respectful relationship, a new sense of self is formed. By combining the Gestalt therapy relationship with phenomenological focusing techniques, the patient becomes aware of processes that previously could not be changed because they were out of awareness. Gestalt therapists believe the contact between therapist and patient sets the stage for development of the capacity to be in contact with one's shifting figures of interest on a moment-by-moment basis.

Gestalt therapy probably has a greater range of styles and modalities than any other system. Therapy can be short term or long term. Specific modalities include individual, couple, family, group, and large systems. Styles vary in degree and type of structure; quantity and quality of techniques used; frequency of sessions; confrontation versus compassionate relating; focus on body, cognition, affect, or interpersonal contact; knowledge of and work with psychodynamic themes; emphasis on dialogue and presence; use of techniques; and so forth.

All styles of Gestalt therapy share a common emphasis on direct experience and experimenting, use of direct contact and personal presence, and a focus on the what and how, here and now. The therapy varies according to context and the personalities of both therapist and patient.

Gestalt therapy starts with the first contact between therapist and patient. The therapist inquires about the desires or needs of the patient and describes how he or she practices therapy. From the beginning, the focus is on what is happening now and what is needed now. The therapist begins immediately to help clarify the patient's awareness of self and environment. In this case, the potential relationship with the therapist is part of the environment.

The therapist and prospective Gestalt therapy patient work together to become clear about what the patient needs and whether this particular therapist is suitable. If there seems to be a match between the two, then the therapy proceeds with getting acquainted. The patient and therapist begin to relate to and understand each other, and the process of sharpening awareness begins. In the beginning, it is often not clear whether the therapy will be short- or long-term or even whether the match between patient and therapist will prove to be satisfactory on further examination.

Therapy typically begins with attention to the immediate feelings of the patient, the current needs of the patient, and some sense of the patient's life circumstances and history. A long social history is rarely taken, although there is nothing in Gestalt theory to prevent it. Usually, history is gathered in the process of therapy as it becomes relevant to current therapy work and at a pace comfortable for the patient.

Some patients start with their life story, others with a contemporaneous focus. The therapist helps patients become aware of what is emerging and what they are feeling and needing as they tell their stories. This is done by reflective statements of the therapist's understanding of what the patient is saying and feeling and by suggestions about how to focus awareness (or questions that accomplish that same goal).

For example, a patient might start telling a story of recent events but not say how he was affected by the events. The therapist might ask either what the patient felt when the reported event happened or what the patient is feeling in telling the story. The therapist also might go back over the story, focusing on recognizing and verbalizing the feelings associated with various stages in the story.

The therapist also makes an assessment of the strengths and weaknesses of patients, including personality style. The therapist looks for specific ways in which the patient's self-support is either precarious or robust. Gestalt therapy can be adapted and practiced with virtually any patient for whom psychotherapy is indicated. However, the practice must be adapted to the particular needs of each person. The competent Gestalt therapist, like any other kind of therapist, must have the training and ability to make this determination. A good therapist knows the limits of his or her experience and training and practices within these limits.

Treatment usually starts with either individual or couples therapy—or both. Group therapy is sometimes added to the treatment plan, and the group may become the sole modality for treatment. Fritz Perls claimed that patients could be treated by Gestalt group therapy alone. This belief was never accepted by most Gestalt therapists and is thoroughly rejected today. Gestalt group therapy complements individual and couples work but does not replace it.

Gestalt therapists work with people of all ages, although specialized training is required for work with young children. Gestalt therapy with children is done individually, as part of Gestalt family therapy, and occasionally in groups (Lampert, 2003; Oaklander, 1969/1988).

Mechanisms of Psychotherapy

All techniques in Gestalt therapy are considered experiments, and patients are repeatedly told to "Try this and see what you experience." There are many "Gestalt therapy techniques," but the techniques themselves are of little importance. Any technique consistent with Gestalt therapy principles can and will be used. In fact, Gestalt therapy explicitly encourages therapists to be creative in their interventions.

Focusing

The most common techniques are the simple interventions of focusing. Focusing ranges from simple inclusion or empathy to exercises arising largely from the therapist's experience while being with the patient. Everything in Gestalt therapy is secondary to the actual and direct experience of the participants. The therapist helps clarify what is important by helping the patient focus his or her awareness.

The prototypical experiment is some form of the question "What are you aware of, or experiencing, right here and now?" Awareness occurs continuously, moment to moment, and the Gestalt therapist pays particular attention to the *awareness continuum,* the flow or sequence of awareness from one moment to another.

The Gestalt therapist also draws attention to key moments in therapy. Of course, this requires that the therapist have the sensitivity and experience to recognize these moments when they occur. Some patients feel abandoned if the therapist is quiet for long periods; others feel it is intrusive when the therapist is active. Therefore, the therapist must weigh the possible disruption of the patient's awareness continuum if he or she offers guiding observations or suggestions against the facilitative benefit that can be derived from focusing. This balance is struck via the ongoing communication between the therapist and patient and is not solely directed by the therapist.

One key moment occurs when a patient interrupts ongoing awareness before it is completed. The Gestalt therapist recognizes signs of this interruption, including the nonverbal indications, by paying close attention to shifts in tension states, muscle tone, or excitement levels. The therapist's interpretation of the moment is not presumed to be relevant or useful unless the patient can confirm it. One patient may tell a story about events with someone in his life and at a key moment grit his teeth, hold his breath, and not exhale. This may turn out to be either an interruption of awareness or an expression of anger. On another occasion, a therapist might notice that an angry look is beginning to change to a look of sadness—but a sadness that is not reported. The patient might change to another subject or begin to intellectualize. In this case, the sadness may be interrupted either at the level of self-awareness or at the level of expression of the affect.

When the patient reports a feeling, another technique is to "stay with it." This encourages the patient to continue with the feeling being reported and builds the patient's capacity to deepen and work through a feeling. The following vignette illustrates this technique (P = patient; T = therapist).

P: [Looks sad.]
T: What are you aware of?
P: I'm sad.
T: Stay with it.
P: [Tears well up. The patient tightens up, looks away, and becomes thoughtful.]
T: I see you are tightening. What are you aware of?
P: I don't want to stay with the sadness.
T: Stay with the not wanting to. Put words to the not wanting to. [This intervention is likely to bring awareness of the patient's resistance to vulnerability. The patient might respond "I won't cry here—it doesn't feel safe," or "I am ashamed," or "I am angry and don't want to admit I'm sad."]

There is an emerging awareness in Gestalt therapy that the moments in which patients change subjects often reflect something happening in the interaction between therapist and patient. Something the therapist says or his or her nonverbal behavior may trigger insecurity or shame in the patient. Most often this is not in the patient's awareness until attention is focused on it by the therapist and explored by dialogue (Jacobs, 1996).

Enactment

The patient is asked to experiment with putting feelings or thoughts into action. This technique might be as simple as encouraging the patient to "say it to the person" (if the person involved is present), or it might be enacted using role playing, psychodrama, or Gestalt therapy's well-known empty-chair technique.

Sometimes enactment is combined with the technique of asking the patient to exaggerate. This is not done to achieve catharsis but is actually a form of experiment that sometimes results in increased awareness of the feeling.

Creative expression is another form of enactment. For some patients, creative expression can help clarify feelings in a way that talking alone cannot. The techniques of expression include journal writing, poetry, art, and movement. Creative expression is especially important in work with children (Oaklander, 1969/1988).

Mental Experiments, Guided Fantasy, and Imagery

Sometimes visualizing an experience here and now increases awareness more effectively than enacting it, as is illustrated in the following brief vignette (P = patient; T = therapist).

P: I was with my girlfriend last night. I don't know how it happened but I was impotent. [Patient gives more details and history.]

T: Close your eyes. Imagine it is last night and you are with your girlfriend. Say out loud what you experience at each moment.

P: I am sitting on the couch. My friend sits next to me and I get excited. Then I go soft.

T: Let's go through that again in slow motion, and in more detail. Be sensitive to every thought or sense impression.

P: I am sitting on the couch. She comes over and sits next to me. She touches my neck. It feels so warm and soft. I get excited—you know, hard. She strokes my arm and I love it. [Pause. Looks startled.] Then I thought, I had such a tense day, maybe I won't be able to get it up.

One can use imagery to explore and express an emotion that does not lend itself to simple linear verbalization. For example, a patient might imagine being alone on a desert, being eaten alive by insects, being sucked in by a whirlpool, and so forth. There are infinite possible images that can be drawn from dreams, waking fantasy, and the creative use of fantasy. The Gestalt therapist might suggest that the patient imagine the experience happening right now rather than simply discussing it. "Imagine you are actually in that desert, right now. What do you experience?" This is often followed by some version of "Stay with it."

An image may arise spontaneously in the patient's awareness as a here-and-now experience, or it may be consciously created by the patient or therapist (or both). The patient might suddenly report, "Just now I feel cold, like I'm alone in outer space." This might indicate something about what is happening between the therapist and the patient at that moment; perhaps the patient is experiencing the therapist as not being emotionally present.

Imagery techniques can also be used to expand the patient's self-supportive techniques. For example, in working with patients who have strong shame issues, at times it is helpful for them to imagine a metaphorical good mother, one who is fully present and loving and accepts and loves the patient just as he or she is (Yontef, 1993).

Meditative techniques, many of which are borrowed from Asian psychotherapies, can also be very helpful experiments.

Body Awareness

Awareness of body activity is an important aspect of Gestalt therapy, and there are specific Gestalt therapy methodologies for working with body awareness (Frank, 2001; Kepner, 1987). The Gestalt therapist is especially interested in patterns of breathing. For example, when a person is breathing in a manner that does not support centering and feeling, he or she will often experience anxiety. Usually the breathing of the anxious patient involves rapid inhalation and a failure to fully exhale. One can work with experiments in breathing in the context of an ordinary therapy session. One can also practice a thoroughly body-oriented Gestalt therapy (Frank, 2001; Kepner, 1987).

Loosening and Integrating Techniques

Some patients are so rigid in their thinking—a characteristic derived from either cultural or psychological factors—that they do not even consider alternative possibilities. Loosening techniques such as fantasy, imagination, or mentally experimenting with the opposite of what is believed can help break down this rigidity so that alternatives can at least be considered. Integrating techniques bring together processes that the patient either just doesn't bring together or actively keeps apart (splitting). Asking the patient to join the positive and negative poles of a polarity can be very integrating ("I love him and I abhor his flippant attitude"). Putting words to sensations and finding the sensations that accompany words ("See if you can locate it in your body") are other important integrating techniques.

APPLICATIONS

Who Can We Help?

Because Gestalt therapy is a process theory, it can be used effectively with any patient population the therapist understands and feels comfortable with. Yontef, for instance, has written about its application with borderline and narcissistic patients (1993). If the therapist can relate to the patient and understands the basic principles of Gestalt therapy and how to adjust these principles to fit the unique needs of each new patient, the Gestalt therapy principles of *awareness* (direct experience), *contact* (relationship), and *experimenting* (phenomenological focusing and experimentation) can be applied. Gestalt therapy does not advocate a cookbook of prescribed techniques for specialized groups of individuals. Therapists who wish to work with patients who are culturally different from themselves find support by attending to the field conditions that influence their understanding of the patient's life and culture (for example, see Jacobs, 2000). The Gestalt therapy attitude of dialogue and the phenomenological assumption of multiple valid realities support the therapist in working with a patient from another culture, enabling patient and therapist to mutually understand the differences in background, assumptions, and so forth.

Both Gestalt therapy philosophy and Gestalt therapy methodology dictate that *general principles must always be adapted for each particular clinical situation*. The manner of relating and the choice and execution of techniques must be tailored to each new patient's needs, not to diagnostic categories *en bloc*. Therapy will be ineffective or harmful if the patient is made to conform to the system rather than having the system adjust to the patient.

It has long been accepted that Gestalt therapy in the confrontive and theatrical style of a 1960s Fritz Perls workshop is much more limited in application than the Gestalt therapy described in this chapter. Common sense, professional background, flexibility, and creativity are especially important in diagnosis and treatment planning. Methods, emphases, precautions, limitations, commitments, and auxiliary support (such as medication, day treatment, and nutritional guidance) must be modified with different patients in accordance with their personality organization (for example, the presence of psychosis, sociopathy, or a personality disorder).

The competent practice of Gestalt therapy requires a strong general clinical background and training in more than Gestalt therapy. In addition to training in the theory and practice of Gestalt therapy, Gestalt therapists need to have a firm grounding in personality theory, psychopathology and diagnosis, theories and applications of other systems of psychotherapy, knowledge of psychodynamics, comprehensive personal therapy, and advanced clinical training, supervision, and experience.

This background is especially important in Gestalt therapy because therapists and patients are encouraged to be creative and experiment with new behavior in and outside of the session. The individual clinician has a great deal of discretion in Gestalt therapy. Modifications are made by the individual therapist and patient according to therapeutic style, personalities of therapist and patient, and diagnostic considerations. A good knowledge of research, other systems, and the principles of personality organization are needed to guide and limit the spontaneous creativity of the therapist. The Gestalt therapist is expected to be creative, but he or she cannot abdicate responsibility for professional discrimination, judgment, and proper caution.

Gestalt therapy has been applied in almost every setting imaginable. Applications have varied from intensive individual therapy multiple times per week to crisis intervention. Gestalt therapists have also worked with organizations, schools, and groups; they have worked with patients with psychoses, patients suffering from psychosomatic disorders, and patients with posttraumatic stress disorders. Many of the details about how to modify Gestalt techniques in order to work effectively with these populations have been disseminated in the oral tradition—that is, through supervision, consultation, and training. Written material too abundant to cite has also become available.

Treatment

Patients often present similar issues but need different treatment because of differences in their personality organization and in what unfolds in the therapeutic relationship. In the following two examples, both patients were raised by emotionally abandoning parents.

Tom was a 45-year-old man proud of his intelligence, self-sufficiency, and independence. He was not aware that he had unmet dependency needs and resentment. This man's belief in his self-sufficiency and denial of dependency required that his therapist proceed with respect and sensitivity. The belief in self-sufficiency met a need, was in part constructive, and was the foundation for the patient's self-esteem. The therapist was able to respond to the patient's underlying need without threatening the patient's pride (P = patient; T = therapist).

P: [With pride.] When I was a little kid my mom was so busy I just had to learn to rely on myself.
T: I appreciate your strength, but when I think of you as such a self-reliant kid, I want to stroke you and give you some parenting.
P: [Tearing a little.] No one ever did that for me.
T: You seem sad.
P: I'm remembering when I was a kid . . .

Tom evoked a sympathetic response in the therapist that was expressed directly to the patient. His denial of needing anything from others was not directly challenged. Exploration led to awareness of a shame reaction to unavailable parents and a compensatory self-reliance.

Bob was a 45-year-old man who felt shame and isolated himself in reaction to any interaction that was not totally positive. He was consistently reluctant to support himself, conforming to and relying totally on others. Previous empathic or sympathetic responses only served to reinforce the patient's belief in his own inadequacy.

P: [Whiny voice.] I don't know what to do today.
T: [Looks and does not talk. Previous interventions of providing more direction had resulted in the patient following any slight lead by the therapist into talk that was not felt by the patient.]

P: I could talk about my week. [Looks questioningly at therapist.]

T: I feel pulled on by you right now. I imagine you want me to direct you.

P: Yes, what's wrong with that?

T: Nothing. I prefer not to direct you right now.

P: Why not?

T: You can direct yourself. I believe you are directing us now away from your inner self. I don't want to cooperate with that. [Silence.]

P: I feel lost.

T: [Looks alert and available but does not talk.]

P: You are not going to direct me, are you?

T: No.

P: Well, let's work on my believing I can't take care of myself. [The patient had real feelings about this issue, and he initiated a fruitful piece of work that led to awareness of abandonment anxiety and feelings of shame in response to unavailable parents.]

Groups

Group treatment is frequently part of an overall Gestalt therapy treatment program. There are three general models for doing Gestalt group therapy (Frew, 1988; Yontef, 1990). In the first model, participants work one-on-one with the therapist while the other participants remain relatively quiet and work vicariously. The work is then followed by feedback and interaction with other participants, with an emphasis on how people are affected by the work. In the second model, participants talk with each other with emphasis on direct here-and-now communication between the group members. This model is similar to Yalom's model for existential group therapy. A third model mixes these two activities in the same group (Yontef, 1990). The group and therapist creatively regulate movement and balance between interaction and the one-on-one focus.

All the techniques discussed in this chapter can be used in groups. In addition, there are possibilities for experimental focusing that are designed for groups. Gestalt therapy groups usually start with some procedure for bringing participants into the here and now and contacting each other. This is often called *rounds* or *check-in*.

A simple and obvious example of Gestalt group work occurs when the therapist has each group member look at the other members of the group and express what he or she is experiencing in the here and now. Some Gestalt therapists also use structured experiments, such as experiments in which participants express a particular emotion ("I resent you for . . . ," "I appreciate you for . . . "). The style of other Gestalt therapists is fluid and organized by what emerges in the group.

Couples and Families

Couples therapy and family therapy are similar to group therapy in that there is a combination of work with each person in the session and work with interaction among the group members. Gestalt therapists vary in where they prefer to strike this balance (see Lee, 2008; Yontef, 2012). There is also variation in how structured the intervention style of the therapist is and in how much the therapist follows, observes, and focuses the spontaneous functioning of the couple or family.

Partners often start couples therapy by complaining and blaming each other. The work at this point involves calling attention to this dynamic and to alternative modes of interaction. The Gestalt therapist also explores what is behind the blaming. Frequently, one party experiences the other as shaming him or her and blames the other, without awareness of the defensive function of the blaming.

Circular causality is a frequent pattern in unhappy couples. In circular causality, A causes B and B causes A. Regardless of how an interaction starts, A triggers a response in B to which A then reacts negatively without being aware of his or her role in triggering the negative response. B likewise triggers a negative response by A without being aware of his or her role in triggering the negative response. Circular causality is illustrated in the following example.

A wife expresses frustration with her husband for coming home late from work every night and not being emotionally available when he comes home. The husband feels unappreciated and attacked; at an unaware level, he also feels ashamed of being criticized. The husband responds with anger, blaming the wife for not being affectionate. The wife accuses the husband of being defensive, aggressive, insensitive, and emotionally unavailable. The husband responds in kind. Each response in this circle makes it worse. In the worst cases, this circular causality can lead to total disruption in the relationship and may trigger drinking, violence, or sexual acting out.

Underneath the wife's frustration is the fact that she misses her husband, is lonely, worries about him working so hard, really wants to be with him, and assumes that he does not want to be home with her because she is no longer attractive. However, these fears are not expressed clearly. The husband might want to be home with his wife and might resent having to work so hard but might also feel a need to unwind from the stress of work before being emotionally available. The caring and interest of each spouse for the other often get lost in the circular defensive–offensive battle.

Blaming statements often trigger shame, and shame triggers defense. In this kind of toxic atmosphere, no one listens. There is no true contact and no repair or healing. Expressing actual experience rather than judgments and allowing oneself to really hear the experience of the spouse are first steps toward healing. Of course, this requires that both of the partners know or learn how to recognize their actual experience.

Sometimes structured experiments are helpful. In one experiment, the couple is asked to face each other, pulling their chairs toward each other until they are close enough to touch knees and then instructed to look at each other and express what they are aware of at each moment. Other experiments include completing sentences such as "I resent you for . . . " or "I appreciate you for . . . " or "I spite you by . . . " or "I feel bad about myself when you . . . . "

It is critical in couples therapy for the therapist to model the style of listening he or she thinks will enhance each spouse's ability to verbalize his or her experience and to encourage each partner to listen as well as to speak. The various experiments help to convey to patients that verbal statements are not something written in stone but are part of an ongoing dialogue. The restoration of dialogue is a sign that therapy is progressing.

As described in the earlier section on psychotherapy, patients may move into various treatment modalities throughout treatment. They may have individual therapy, group therapy, or couples therapy, and they may occasionally participate in workshops. It is not unusual for patients to make occasional use of adjunctive workshops while engaged in ongoing individual therapy.

Gestalt therapists tend to see patients on a weekly basis. As more attention comes to be focused on the therapist–patient relationship, patients are eager to come more often, so some Gestalt therapists see people more often than once a week. Many Gestalt therapists also run groups, and there are therapists who teach and conduct workshops for the general public. Others primarily teach and train therapists. The shape of one's practice is limited only by one's interests and by the exigencies of the work environment.

Evidence

Can Gestalt Therapy Be Evidence Based?

There is no straightforward simple approach to the discussion of "evidence" when it comes to Gestalt therapy, and the subject of research is controversial in the Gestalt therapy community. There are some who are skeptical about whether even the most sophisticated research paradigms can adequately support a dialogical endeavor that revolves primarily around one's values and personal meanings. (The authors of this chapter are more allied with this perspective.) This is not to deny the value of scientific findings as *one* useful perspective. Scientific research on broader themes pertaining to human behavior: trauma, attachment, development, cognition, emotional process, and neuropsychology have been sources of information and validation for Gestalt therapists, as long as such research is integrated in a nonreductionistic manner into the overall structure of Gestalt therapy theory and practice (see, for example, Staemmler, 2011). However, we become concerned when nomothetic data are privileged over the individual values, capacities, preferences, and experiences of the particular patient–therapist pair.

Meanwhile, efforts are underway to develop and refine research methods that are sensitive to personal meanings. For example, at a 2013 Gestalt therapy research conference, there was one major presentation on critical realism and how it fits with both Gestalt therapy and the endeavors of research and another on the phenomenological philosophies of Merleau-Ponty and Heidegger, relating them to the process of doing research. Likewise, there are many who are quite enthusiastic about Gestalt research around the world, as exemplified by attendance at a 2013 Gestalt therapy research conference; the French, Czech, and Spanish translations of Gestalt therapy research; Koreans and Portuguese translations in progress; MA programs in Mexico that are instituting research; and a Chilean institute that is going to require all its trainees to conduct single-case, timed-series studies as part of their competencies.

We shall discuss first our concerns and then describe research interests and findings that excite many Gestalt therapists. In the world of psychotherapy, research increasingly takes the shape of a search for "best practices." In the United States, research on "evidence-based practice" and "empirically supported treatments" are partly a capitulation to the demands of insurance companies and managed care providers that have evolved as therapists struggle to establish parity with physical medicine (Reed, Kihlstrom, & Messer, 2006). The search for measurably efficacious manualized treatment approaches is a direct response to pressure from insurers and managed care providers (Reed et al., 2006; Wachtel, 2010).

Those who question this approach to psychotherapy research are often the researchers themselves (Reed et al., 2006; Wachtel, 2010; Zeldow, 2009)! Messer (2005) uses two case studies to demonstrate something that psychotherapy researchers themselves have discovered: The manualized approaches of evidence-based practices are of little use in the face of "co-morbidity," and yet co-morbidity is ubiquitous in clinical settings (Westen, Novotny, & Thompson-Brenner, 2004). As noted by Messer,

> Diagnoses cannot capture the unique qualities and concerns that patients bring to the clinician, nor the specifics of the context in which their problems emerged in the past and are taking place in the present. . . . The strength of EST's [empirically supported treatments] . . . is their application to patients in general. The clinician, although needing to attend to such empirical findings, must go beyond them to take cognizance of patients' unique qualities, circumstances and wishes. (2005, p. 32)

In a delightful article that explored the relationship between research and clinical practice, Wolfe (2012), engaged in a "two-chair dialogue" between his "practitioner head" and his "researcher head." In doing so, he clearly captures the problems of turning the complex art of therapy—with its reliance on experience, tact, and creativity in the immediacy of moment-to-moment conversation—into a scientific practice. Ironically, he noted that the two-chair dialogue he used has its origins in Gestalt therapy and has been shown through research to support patients to expand awareness, illuminate emotional process, and resolve emotional conflicts.

Wolfe (2012) points to the limitations of a positivist epistemology, noting that randomized controlled trials, which are considered "strong evidence" by researchers, decontextualize the patient, and bear no resemblance to the clinical situation.

Hoffman (2008) poses similar arguments from a postmodern perspective:

First, postmodernism questions the ability of empirical research to be objective. Different types of research are more appropriate for evaluating different approaches to therapy. The measurement must be consistent with the theory; otherwise epistemological problems threaten the validity of the research.

Second, while all psychotherapies share the goal to decrease symptoms, at least to some degree, and to increase the quality of life, they disagree on what this looks like. In other words, not all psychotherapies seek the same ends. This makes it very difficult to consider which approach to therapy is best for which client.

A third concern relates to client values. If different therapies have different values and lead to slightly different ends, then which approach to therapy is best for a client is, in part, a values decision. In other words, both values and effectiveness need to be considered when making choices about which approach to psychotherapy is best.

The field of psychotherapy has often looked foolish by engaging in petty debates over which approach to therapy is best. Postmodernism responds by stating this is not even the right question! It is not possible to determine which therapy is superior because it depends upon too many client and therapist factors. Furthermore, when therapists are making the determination of which approach is best, they are taking responsibility away from their clients and imposing their values system upon them. Instead, therapists should work with client to help them decide which therapy approach best fits the client's goals and values. (p. 2)

The most productive research, rather than trying to identify one therapy as better than another, searches out what Wolfe (2012) describes as "empirically supported principles of change" (pg. 105) and seeks to identify core processes that apply to all forms of psychotherapy (e.g., the relationship between therapist and client).

Evidence Does Exist

Although relationship research validates the dialogic relationship that Gestalt therapy encourages, each psychotherapy relationship is necessarily unique and unrepeatable. Obviously, this creates difficulties for standard approaches to research. Nonetheless, some researchers and therapists who value the science (as well as the art) of therapy have tried to link existential values and research. These investigators seek ways to provide experimental support for the difficult work of making clinical decisions that help patients to have a fuller life (Brownell, in press). Among these are Gestalt therapists who are pioneering research approaches that aim to bridge the gap between traditional psychotherapy research and our complex, awareness-oriented holistic dialogic process Brownell, 2008). They are developing research models that are sensitive to the complexities of clinical work and that can obtain evidence, especially of the medium- and long-term effects of clinical practice. This has led to a substantial increase in new studies

(Strümpfel, 2006). Activity promoting research is also described on Gestalt therapy list-serves and in journals and books (e.g., Finlay & Evans, 2009). Of special note is the work of Brownell (2008), who helped plan and prepare a major conference in 2013, The Challenge of Establishing a Research Tradition for Gestalt Therapy, which was co-hosted by the Gestalt International Study Center and the Association for the Advancement of Gestalt Therapy, An International Community.

Strümpfel (2006) reviewed data from 74 published research studies on therapeutic process and outcome reanalyzed in 10 meta-analyses and added his own calculations. Many of the studies that Strümpfel analyzed reported more positive findings for the humanistic therapies than for the behavioral and the psychodynamic approaches.

Although Strümpfel's research makes Gestalt therapy look good, research that pits one therapeutic approach against another is suspect for two reasons, both first illuminated by Lester Luborsky and since reaffirmed numerous times (Luborsky et al., 2003). First, there is the finding that the particular therapeutic orientation of the practitioner is relatively insignificant compared with the experience, skill, and personhood of the practitioner. Second, researchers tend to find significant positive effects for the orientation that most closely matches their own allegiances.

Common Factors

Common factors research also transcends any one particular therapy. Research on the therapeutic relationship and its predictive power is well established. This research inevitably finds relational conditions such as acceptance, warmth, and genuineness on the part of the therapist are important predictors of successful therapy. These conditions are core components of Gestalt therapy's dialogic relationship (Jacobs, 2009; Staemmler, 2011; Yontef, 2002).

Likewise, meta-analytic studies of evidence-based practices, summarized by Norcross and Wampold (2011), document that (1) the relationship makes a substantial and consistent contribution to outcome independent of the specific type of treatment, (2) the therapeutic relationship accounts for why clients improve (or fail to improve) at least as much as the particular treatment method, (3) efforts to advance evidence-based practices without including the relationship are incomplete and potentially misleading, and (4) the relationship acts in concert with treatment methods, patient characteristics, and practitioner qualities in determining effectiveness.

It is interesting that recent research on infant–parent interaction has added a new wrinkle to research on relational factors. Lyons-Ruth, a psychoanalytic developmental researcher and clinician, studied communication patterns and attachment in infants and children and found that "collaborative communication" best supported the development of what Gestalt therapy would define as resilient organismic self-regulation. She suggests that treatment should focus less on reflective understanding and more on "expanding areas of collaborative communication in the interactions between patient and therapist" (2006, p. 612). This conclusion and the research of the humanistic therapists lines up nicely with the dialogical attitude that is so vital in Gestalt therapy.

Studies in neurology and infant development, elaborated and summarized thoroughly in Staemmler (2011), support the Gestalt therapy viewpoint on the importance of the here and now and the inseparability of emotion and thought (Damasio, 1999; Stern, 2004). In addition, Gestalt therapy's inclusion of work with the body in the methodology of psychotherapy gives it an added power that ideally would be included in the evaluation of psychotherapy efficacy, but body work is almost never evaluated in psychotherapy research (Strümpfel, 2006).

Leslie Greenberg and his colleagues have conducted a large series of studies over the last 20 years in which process and outcome studies are brought together with appreciation for context and of the interaction between technique and relationship factors (e.g., Greenberg, Rice & Elliott, 1993). Gestalt therapy is primarily a therapy of contact and relationship. It is also an experiential method and an experimental method, and it is supported by the research that Greenberg and his colleagues have pursued.

To conclude this section, we suggest a word of caution about using research evidence when endeavoring to understand and evaluate therapeutic efficacy, whether by comparing different approaches or by assessing the value of therapy as a healing enterprise. Any treatment dyad and treatment process has vastly more complex meanings than can possibly be measured. Added to the mix is the fact that each therapist is unique and can practice well only by working within a framework matched to his or her personality. Therefore, even if research suggests most generally that, say, Gestalt therapy is very well suited to support a patient's strivings for enduring relationships, if the therapist is not attracted to working with close attention to moment-by-moment emotional experience, then he or she would probably need to work in another framework to be at all helpful to his or her patients. In fact, it is possible that therapists' comfort within their orientations may prove to be a more significant factor for positive outcomes than their specific orientations. Our current research results are limited as always by the questions we ask and by the research tools available to us.

Psychotherapy in a Multicultural World

The founders of Gestalt therapy were all cultural and political outsiders. Some were Jews, and some of them were immigrants—including Fritz and Laura Perls—who had fled persecution in Europe. Some were gay. All were interested in developing a process-oriented theory that could provide support and encouragement for people to explore their own life paths, even if those life paths did not fit neatly within extant cultural values. Thus, instead of establishing content goals for successful therapy (e.g., achievement of genital sexuality), they established a process goal: awareness.

Gestalt therapists throughout the world have been involved with and written about their involvement in multicultural and intercultural projects, be they the provision of mental-health services or community organizational consulting (Bar-Yoseph, 2005). Heiberg (2005) interviewed non-European immigrants and residents of Norway about their experiences and found that shame and a shaming process constantly infused their interactions with members of Norway's dominant culture. Almost all of his respondents had been in therapy with white therapists, and the Gestalt patients spoke most enthusiastically of the chance to explore their experience—especially their shame—on their own terms rather than being analyzed and interpreted. Gaffney (2008) wrote about the subtle and gross difficulties of providing supervision in the divided society of Northern Ireland. Bar-Yoseph (2005) edited a collection of articles by Gestalt therapists engaged in various multicultural endeavors. Articles by American therapists are included.

A common thread in almost all of the literature is that efficacious multicultural interaction requires that the therapist recognize the implications of his or her social, cultural, and political *situatedness*. There are two reasons for this. First, such awareness helps the therapist relativize his or her own cultural norms to help navigate the inevitable strong emotional reactions that emerge when coming into intimate contact with profoundly different and sometimes disturbing worldviews. Knowing one's own situatedness and relativizing it supports wanting to know about the cultural and personal situation of the other. Second, awareness of the difference between the relative insider status of being a professional and the often marginalized status of the cultural outsider is crucial for opening up meaningful dialogue with one's client. Billies (2005), Jacobs (2005), and

McConville (2005) elaborate this point in exploring what it means to be a white therapist in racially divided America.

All of the authors referred to field theory as a strong support for phenomenological, experiential explorations with their clients. They also emphasized that attention to the contacting and awareness processes and how these processes are shaped by field conditions enhanced the capacity of the therapist and the client to make creative adjustments in their work together.

Another strongly emphasized dimension of Gestalt therapy is the dialogical attitude, a humble attitude that includes a willingness to be affected and changed by the client. In dialogue, the therapist learns from the patient about the patient's culture. This attitude enables the therapist to learn more about his or her own biases, and it also fosters contacting that is often experienced by the client as empowering.

CASE EXAMPLE

Background

Miriam often spoke in a flat voice, seemingly disconnected from her feelings and even from any sense of the meaningfulness of her sentences. She had survived terrifying and degrading childhood abuse, and now, some 35 years after leaving home, she had the haunted, pinched look of someone who expected the abuse to begin again at any moment. She could not even say that she wanted therapy for herself because she claimed not to want or need people in her life. She thought that being in therapy could help her to develop her skills as a consultant more fully. Miriam was quite wary of therapy, but she had attended a lecture given by the therapist and had felt a slight glimmer of hope that this particular therapist might actually be able to understand her.

Miriam's experiential world was characterized by extreme isolation. She was ashamed of her isolation, but it made her feel safe. When she moved about in the world of people, she felt terrified, often enraged, and deeply ashamed. She was unrelentingly self-critical. She believed she was a toxic presence, unwillingly destructive of others. She was unable to acknowledge wants or needs of her own because such an acknowledgment made her vulnerable and (in her words) a "target" for humiliation and annihilation. Finally, she was plagued by a sense of unreality. She never knew whether what she thought or perceived was "real" or imagined. She knew nothing of what she felt, believed that she had no feelings, and did not even know what a feeling was. At times, these convictions were so strong that she fantasized she was an alien.

Miriam's fundamental conflicts revolved around the polarity of isolation versus confluence. Although she was at most times too ashamed of her desires to even recognize them, when her wish to be connected to others became figural, she was overcome with dread. She recognized that she wanted to just "melt" into the other person, and she could not bear even a hint of distance, for the distance signaled rejection, which she believed would be unbearable to her. She was rigidly entrenched in her isolated world. A consequence of her rigidity was that she was unable to flow back and forth in a rhythm of contact and withdrawal. The only way she could regulate the states of tension and anxiety that emerged as she dared to move toward contact with the therapist and others was to suddenly shrink back in shame, retreat into isolation, or become dissociated, which happened quite often. Then she would feel stuck, too ashamed and defeated to dare to venture forward again. She was unable to balance and calibrate the experience of desiring contact while at the same time being afraid of contact.

The following sequence occurred about four years into therapy. Miriam was much better at this point in being able to identify with and express feeling, but navigating a contact boundary with another person was still daunting. She had begun this session with a deep sense of pleasure because she finally felt a sense of continuity with the therapist, and she reported that for the first time in her life she was also connected to some memories. The air of celebration gave way to desperation and panic later as therapist and patient struggled together with her wishes and fears for a closer connection to the therapist.

In a conversation that had been repeated at various times, Miriam's desperation grew as she wanted the therapist to "just reach past" her fear, to touch the tiny, disheveled, and lonely "cave girl" who hid inside. Miriam felt abandoned by the therapist's "patience" (Miriam's word).

P: You're so damn patient!
T: . . . and this is a bad thing? [Said tentatively.]
P: Right now it is.
T: Because you need . . .
P: [Pause.] Something that indicates *something*. [Sounding frightened and exasperated, and confused.]
T: What does my patience indicate to you right now?
P: That I am just going to be left scrambling forever!
T: It sounds like I am watching from too far away—rather than going through this with you—does that sound right?
P: Sounds right . . .
T: So you need something from me that indicates we will get through this together, that I won't just let you drown. [Said softly and seriously.]

A few minutes later, the exploration of her need for contact and her fear had continued, with Miriam even admitting to a wish to be touched physically, which was a big admission for her to make. Once again, Miriam started to panic. She was panicked with fear of what may happen now that she has exposed her wish to be touched. She feared the vulnerability of allowing the touch, and she was also panicky about being rejected or cruelly abandoned. The therapist had been emphasizing that Miriam's wish for contact is but one side of the conflict, and that the other side, her fear, needed to be respected as well. The patient was experiencing the therapist's caution as an abandonment, whereas the therapist was concerned that "just reaching past" the patient's fear would reenact a boundary violation and would trigger greater dissociation.

T: . . . so, we need to honor *both* your fear and your wish. [Miriam looks frightened, on the verge of dissociating.] . . . now you are moving into a panic—speak to me . . .
P: [Agonized whisper.] It's too much.
T: [Softly.] Yeah, too much . . . what's that . . . "it's too much"?
P: Somehow if you touch me I will disappear. And I don't want to—I want to—I want to use touch to *connect,* not to disappear!
T: Right, OK, so the fear side of you is saying that the risk in touching is that you'll disappear. Now we have to take that fear into account. And I have a suggestion—that I will move and we sit so that our fingertips can be just an inch or so from each other—and see how that feels to you. Do you want to try? [Therapist moves as patient nods assent. Miriam is still contorted with fear and desperation.] Okay, now, I am going to touch one of your fingers—keep breathing—how is that?
P: [Crying] How touch-phobic I am! I shift between "it feels nice" and "it feels horrid!"

T: That is why we have to take this slowly. . . . Do you understand that . . . if we didn't take it slowly you would have to disappear—the horror would make you have to disappear [all spoken slowly and carefully and quietly] . . . do you understand that . . . so it's worth going slowly . . . your fingers feel to me . . . full of feeling?

P: Yes . . . as if all my life is in my fingers . . . not disappeared here, warm . . .

The patient attended a weeklong workshop the next week, after which she reported, with a sense of awe, that she had stayed "in her body" for the whole week, even when being touched. After this session, the patient reported that she felt a greater sense of continuity, and as we continued to build on it (even the notion of being able to "build" is new and exciting), she felt less brittle, more open, more "in touch."

As more time has passed, and we continued to work together several times per week, long-standing concerns about feeling alien and about being severely dissociated and fragmented began to be resolved. The patient felt increasingly human, able to engage more freely in intimate participation with others.

SUMMARY

Gestalt therapy is a system of psychotherapy that is philosophically and historically linked to Gestalt psychology, field theory, existentialism, and phenomenology. Fritz Perls and his wife, Laura Perls, and their collaborator, Paul Goodman, initially developed and described the basic principles of Gestalt therapy.

Gestalt therapists focus on contact, conscious awareness, and experimentation. There is a consistent emphasis on the present moment and on the validity and reality of the patient's phenomenological awareness. Most of the change that occurs in Gestalt therapy results from an I–Thou dialogue between therapist and patient, and Gestalt therapists are encouraged to be self-disclosing and candid, about both their personal history and their feelings in therapy.

The techniques of Gestalt therapy include focusing exercises, enactment, creative expression, mental experiments, guided fantasy, imagery, and body awareness. However, these techniques themselves are relatively insignificant and are only the tools traditionally employed by Gestalt therapists. Any mechanism consistent with the theory of Gestalt therapy can and will be used in therapy.

Therapeutic practice is in turmoil in a time when the limitations associated with managed care have encroached on clinical practice. At a time of humanistic growth in theorizing, clinical practice seems to be narrowing, with more focus on particular symptoms and an emphasis on people as products who can be fixed by following the instructions in a procedure manual.

The wonderful array of Gestalt-originated techniques for which Gestalt therapy is famous can be easily misused for just such a purpose. We caution the reader not to confuse the use of technique for symptom removal, however imaginative, with Gestalt therapy. The fundamental precepts of Gestalt therapy, including the paradoxical theory of change, are thoroughly geared toward the development of human freedom, not human conformity; in that sense, Gestalt therapy rejects the view of persons implied in the managed care ethos. Gestalt practice, when true to its principles, is a protest against the reductionism of mere symptom removal and adjustment; it is a protest for a client's right to develop fully enough to be able to make conscious and informed choices that shape her or his life.

Because Gestalt therapy is so flexible, creative, and direct, it is very adaptable to both short- and long-term therapies. The direct contact, focus, and experimentation can sometimes result in important insight. This adaptability is an asset in dealing with managed care and related issues of funding mental-health treatment.

In the 1960s, Fritz Perls prophesied that Gestalt therapy would come into its own during the decade ahead and become a significant force in psychotherapy during the 1970s. His prophecy has been more than fulfilled.

In 1952, perhaps a dozen people were actively involved in the Gestalt therapy movement. Today there are hundreds of training institutes here and abroad and thousands of well-trained Gestalt therapists practicing worldwide. Unfortunately, there are also large numbers of poorly trained therapists who call themselves Gestalt therapists after attending a few workshops but who do not have adequate academic preparation. It behooves students and patients who are interested in exposure to Gestalt therapy to inquire in depth about the training and experience of anyone who claims to be a Gestalt therapist or who claims to use Gestalt therapy techniques.

Gestalt therapy has pioneered many useful and creative innovations in psychotherapy theory and practice that have been incorporated into the general psychotherapy field. Now Gestalt therapy is moving to further elaborate and refine these innovations. The principles of existential dialogue, the use of direct phenomenological experience for both patient and therapist, the trust of organismic self-regulation, the emphasis on experimentation and awareness, the paradoxical theory of change, and close attention to the contact between the therapist and the patient all form a model of good psychotherapy that will continue to be used by Gestalt therapists and others.

 Counseling CourseMate Website:
See this text's Counseling CourseMate website at www.cengagebrain.com for learning tools such as chapter quizzing, videos, glossary flashcards, and more.

ANNOTATED BIBLIOGRAPHY

Jacobs, L., & Hycner, R. (Eds.) (2009). *Relational approaches in Gestalt therapy.* New York: Gestalt Press.
This edited volume includes uniformly interesting, thoughtful articles that acquaint the reader with topics of current interest in Gestalt therapy.

Mann, D. (2010). *Gestalt therapy: 100 key points and techniques.* New York: Routledge.
This book is part of a series that introduces readers to the main points of various theoretical approaches. This volume is written in a wise, personable style that exemplifies the humanity of Gestalt therapy at the same time that it teaches. It is an excellent introduction to Gestalt therapy.

Polster, E., & Polster, M. (1999). *From the radical center: The heart of Gestalt therapy. Selected writings of Erving and Miriam Polster.* A. Roberts (Ed.). Cambridge, MA: GIC Press.
This is an enjoyable book with illustrative vignettes for people who want to get a sense of what Gestalt therapy is like. The book is written at the level of clinical theory and covers the basics of Gestalt therapy: process, here and now, contact, awareness, and experiments. The writing is so lively that the reader is bound to come away with a feel for the Gestalt therapy experience as practiced by some of its finest senior practitioners.

Staemmler, F.-M. (2011). *Empathy in psychotherapy: How therapists and clients understand each other.* New York: Springer Publishing.

This award-winning book is scholarly and thoroughly researched. The author documents that Gestalt therapy has an empathic orientation, and the knowledge and insights in this book will help anyone who wants to increase his or her understanding of, and skill with, empathic engagement.

Wheeler, G. (2000). *Beyond individualism: Toward a new understanding of self, relationship and experience.* Hillsdale, NJ: Gestalt Press/Analytic Press.
The author manages to walk the reader, in a simple, lucid, and evocative manner, through the paradigm shift that Gestalt therapy brings to the field of psychotherapy. He offers illustrative experiments along the way. The reader cannot help but have his or her experience of living changed by this book. This book, coupled with the clinical flavor of the Polsters' book *Gestalt Therapy Integrated*, provides a well-rounded beginning for the interested clinician.

Yontef, G. (1993). *Awareness, dialogue and process: Essays on Gestalt therapy.* Highland, NY: Gestalt Journal Press.
A compendium of articles written over a span of 25 years. Some of the articles are for those who are new to Gestalt therapy, but most are for the advanced reader. The essays are sophisticated probes into some of the thornier theoretical and clinical problems that any theory must address. The book comprehensively traces the evolution of Gestalt theory and practice and provides a theoretical scaffolding for its future.

CASE READINGS

Feder, B., & Ronall, R. (1997). *A living legacy of Fritz and Laura Perls: Contemporary case studies*. New York: Feder Publishing.

> This edited collection provides a look at how different clinicians work from a Gestalt perspective. The variety of styles encourages the reader to find his or her own.

Hycner, R., & Jacobs, L. (1995). Simone: Existential mistrust and trust. *The healing relationship in Gestalt therapy: A dialogic, self-psychology approach* (pp. 85–90). Highland, NY: Gestalt Journal Press.

Hycner, R., & Jacobs, L. (1995). Transference meets dialogue. *The healing relationship in Gestalt therapy: A dialogic, self-psychology approach* (pp. 171–195). Highland, NY: Gestalt Journal Press.

> The first case is an example drawn from a workshop conducted in Israel; the second is an interesting case report by a psychoanalytically oriented Gestalt therapist, including verbatim transcripts of three sessions. The second case is analyzed in a panel discussion by two Gestalt therapists and two psychoanalysts in Alexander, Brickman, Jacobs, Trop, and Yontef (1992), Transference meets dialogue. *Gestalt Journal, 15,* 61–108.

Lampert, R. (2003). *A child's eye view: Gestalt therapy with children, adolescents and their families*. Highland, NY: Gestalt Journal Press.

> Case material is provided throughout this book.

Perls, F. S. (1992). Jane's three dreams. In *Gestalt therapy verbatim* (pp. 284–310). Highland, NY: Gestalt Journal Press.

> Three dreams are presented verbatim. The third dream work is a continuation of unfinished work from the second dream. Portions of this case are also found in D. Wedding & R. J. Corsini (Eds.). (2005). *Case studies in psychotherapy*. Belmont, CA: Brooks/Cole.

Perls, L. P. (1968). Two instances of Gestalt therapy. In P. D. Purlsglove (Ed.), *Recognition in Gestalt therapy* (pp. 42–68). New York: Funk & Wagnalls. (Originally published in 1956)

> Laura Perls presents the case of Claudia, a 25-year-old woman of color who comes from a lower-middle-class West Indian background, and the case of Walter, a 47-year-old Central European Jewish refugee.

Staemmler, F. (Ed). (2003). The IGJ Transcript Project. *International Gestalt Journal, 26*(1), 9–58.

> In this intriguing project, British Gestalt therapist Sally Denham-Vaughan provides a brief summary of her work with a patient and then an extended transcript of a session. Four therapists from Europe and the United States offer their commentaries on the session, and then Denham-Vaughan replies. The result is not only a good example of a Gestalt therapy process but also a lively discussion of some points of interest and controversy in Gestalt therapy. [Reprinted in D. Wedding & R. J. Corsini. (2013). *Case studies in psychotherapy* (7th ed.). Belmont, CA: Brooks/Cole.]

Swanson, C. (2009). The scarf that binds: A clinical case navigating between the individualist paradigm and the "between" of a relational Gestalt approach. In L. Jacobs & R. Hycner (Eds.) *Relational approaches in Gestalt therapy* (pp. 171–186). New York: Gestalt Press.

> A delightful tale of the therapeutic process of disruption and repair with a good example of how experimentation emerges from the therapeutic dialogue.

REFERENCES

Acierno, R., Hersen, M., & Van Hasselt, V. (1993). Interventions for panic disorder: A critical review of the literature. *Clinical Psychology Review, 13,* 561–578.

Bar-Yoseph, T. (Ed.). (2005). *Making a difference: The bridging of cultural diversity*. New Orleans: Gestalt Institute Press.

Beisser, A. (1970). The paradoxical theory of change. In J. Fagan & I. Shepherd (Eds.), *Gestalt therapy now* (pp. 77–80). Palo Alto: Science & Behavior Books.

Billies, M. (2005). Therapist confluence with social systems of oppression and privilege. *International Gestalt Journal, 28*(1), 71–92.

Brownell, P. (2008). Practice-based evidence. In P. Brownell (Ed.) *Handbook for theory, research, and practice in Gestalt therapy* (pp. 90-103). Newcastle, UK: Cambridge Scholars.

Brownell, P. (in press). Assimilating/integrative: The case of Gestalt therapy. In T. Plante (Ed.), *Abnormal psychology through the ages*. Santa Barbara, CA: Praeger/ABC-CLIO.

Buber, M. (1923/1970). *I and thou* (Trans. W. Kaufmann). New York: Scribner's.

Clarkson, P., & Mackewn, J. (1993). *Fritz Perls*. London: Sage.

Damasio, A. (1999). *The feeling of what happens: Body and emotion in the making of consciousness*. New York: Harvest Books.

Fairfield, M., & O'Shea, L. (2008). Getting beyond individualism. *British Gestalt Journal, 17*(2), 24–38.

Finlay, L., & Evans, K. (2009). *Relational-centered research for psychotherapists: Exploring meanings and experience*. New York: Wiley-Blackwell.

Frank, R. (2001). *Body of awareness: A somatic and developmental approach to psychotherapy*. Hillsdale, NJ: GIC/Analytic Press.

Frank, R., & La Barre, F. (2011). *The first year and the rest of your life: Movement, development, and psychotherapeutic change*: New York: Routledge.

Frew, J. (1988). The practice of Gestalt therapy in groups. *Gestalt Journal, 11,* 1, 77–96.

Gaffney, S. (2008). Gestalt group supervision in a divided society: Theory, practice, perspective and reflections. *British Gestalt Journal, 17*(1), 27–39.

Greenberg, L., Rice, L., & Elliott, R. (1993). *Facilitating emotional change: The moment-by-moment process*. New York: Guilford Press.

Heiberg, T. (2005). Shame and creative adjustment in a multicultural society. *British Gestalt Journal, 14*(2), 188–127.

Hycner, R., & Jacobs, L. (1995). *The healing relationship in Gestalt therapy: A dialogic, self-psychology approach*. Highland, NY: Gestalt Journal Press.

Jacobs, L. (1996). Shame in the therapeutic dialogue. In R. Lee & G. Wheeler (Eds.), *The voice of shame* (pp. 297–314). San Francisco: Jossey-Bass.

Jacobs, L. (2000). Respectful dialogues. [Interview]. *British Gestalt Journal, 9*(2), 105–116.

Jacobs, L. (2005). For whites only. In T. Bar-Yoseph (Ed.), *Making a difference: The bridging of cultural diversity* (pp. 225–244). New Orleans: Gestalt Institute Press.

Jacobs, L. (2009).Relationality: Foundational assumptions. In D. Ullman & G. Wheeler (Eds.), *Cocreating the field: Intention and practice in the age of complexity*. New York: Gestalt Press/Routledge.

Jacobs, L., & Hycner, R. (Eds.). (2009). *Relational approaches in Gestalt therapy*. New York: Gestalt Press.

Joyce, P., & Sills, C. (2009). *Skills in Gestalt counseling & psychotherapy* (2nd ed.). London: Sage.

Kepner, J. (1987). *Body process: A Gestalt approach to working with the body in psychotherapy*. New York: Gestalt Institute of Cleveland Press.

Lampert, R. (2003). *A child's eye view: Gestalt therapy with children, adolescents, and their families*. Highland, NY: Gestalt Journal Press.

Lee, R., & Wheeler, G. (Eds.). (1996). *The voice of shame: Silence and connection in psychotherapy*. San Francisco: Jossey-Bass.

Lee, R. G. (2008). *The secret language of intimacy*. New York: Routledge.

Lewin, K. (1938). The conflict between Aristotelian and Galilean modes of thought in contemporary psychology. In K. Lewin, *A dynamic theory of personality* (pp. 1–42). London: Routledge & Kegan Paul.

Luborsky, L., Rosenthal, R., Diguer, L., Andrusyna, T., Levitt, J., Seligman, D., Berman, J., & Krause, E. (2003). Are some psychotherapies much more effective than others? *Journal of Applied Psychoanalytic Studies, 5*(4), 455–460.

Lyons-Ruth, K. (2006). The interface between attachment and intersubjectivity: Perspective from the longitudinal study of disorganized attachment. *Psychoanalytic Inquiry, 26*, 595–616.

McConville, M. (2005). The gift. In T. Bar-Yoseph (Ed.), *Making a difference: The bridging of cultural diversity* (pp. 173–182). New Orleans: Gestalt Institute Press.

McConville, M., & Wheeler, G. (2003). *Heart of development* (Vols. 1 & 2). Hillsdale, NJ: Gestalt Press/Analytic Press.

Messer, S. (2005). Patient values and preferences. Evidence-based practices in mental health: Debate and dialogue on the fundamental questions. In J. Norcross, L. Beutler & R. Levant, *Evidence-based practices in mental health* (pp. 31–40). Washington, DC: American Psychological Association.

Norcross, J., & Wampold, B. (2011). Evidence-based therapy relationships: Research conclusions and clinical practices. *Psychotherapy, 48*(1), 98–102.

Oaklander, V. (1988). *Windows to our children: A Gestalt therapy approach to children and adolescents*. New York: Gestalt Journal Press. (Original work published 1969)

Orange, D. (2011). *The suffering stranger*. New York: Routledge.

Perls, F. (1992). *Ego, hunger, and aggression*. New York: Gestalt Journal Press. (Original work published 1942)

Perls, F., Hefferline, R., & Goodman, P. (1994). *Gestalt therapy: Excitement & growth in the human personality*. New York: Gestalt Journal Press. (Original work published 1951)

Perls, L. (1992). *Living at the boundary*. New York: Gestalt Therapy Press.

Philippson, P. (2001). *Self in relation*. New York: Gestalt Journal Press.

Polster, E., & Polster, M. (1973). *Gestalt therapy integrated*. New York: Brunner/Mazel.

Polster, E., & Polster, M. (1999). *From the radical center: The heart of Gestalt therapy. Selected writings of Erving and Miriam Polster*. A. Roberts (Ed.). Cambridge, MA: GIC Press.

Reed, G. M., Kihlstrom, J. F., & Messer, S. B. (2006). *What qualifies as evidence of effective practice*. Washington, DC: American Psychological Association.

Staemmler, F. (Ed) (2003). The IGJ Transcript Project. *International Gestalt Journal, 26*(1), 9–58.

Staemmler, F.-M. (2011). *Empathy in psychotherapy: How therapists and clients understand each other*. New York: Spring Publishing.

Stern, D. (1985). *The interpersonal world of the infant*. New York: Basic Books.

Stern, D. N. (2004). *The present moment in psychotherapy and everyday life*. New York: London.

Swanson, C. (2009). The scarf that binds: A clinical case navigating between the individualist paradigm and the "between" of a relational Gestalt approach. In L. Jacobs & R. Hycner (Eds.), *Relational approaches in Gestalt therapy* (pp. 171–186). Cambridge, MA: Gestalt Press.

Wachtel, P. L. (2010). Beyond "ESTs": Problematic assumptions in the pursuit of evidence-based practice. *Psychoanalytic Psychology, 27*(3), 251–272.

Westen, D., Novotny, C., & Thompson-Brenner, H. (2004). The empirical status of empirically supported psychotherapies: Assumptions, findings, and reporting in controlled clinical trials. *Psychological Bulletin, 130*(4), 631–663.

Wheeler, G. (2000). *Beyond individualism: Toward a new understanding of self, relationship and experience*. Hillsdale, NJ: GIC/Analytic Press.

Wolfe, B. E. (2012). Healing the research–practice split: Let's start with me. *Psychotherapy, 49*(2), 101–108.

Yontef, G. (1990). Gestalt therapy in groups. In I. Kutash & A. Wolf (Eds.), *Group psychotherapist's handbook* (pp. 191–210). New York: Columbia University Press.

Yontef, G. (1993). *Awareness, dialogue and process: Essays on Gestalt therapy*. Highland, NY: Gestalt Journal Press.

Yontef, G. (2002). The relational attitude in Gestalt therapy theory and practice. *International Gestalt Journal, 25*(1), 15–36.

Yontef, G. (2012). The four relationships of Gestalt therapy couples work. In T. Bar-Joseph (Ed.), *Gestalt therapy: Advances in theory & practice* (pp. 123–135). London: Routledge.

Zeldow, P. B. (2009). In defense of clinical judgment, credentialed clinicians, and reflective practice. *Psychotherapy: Theory, Research, Practice, Training, 46*(1), 1.

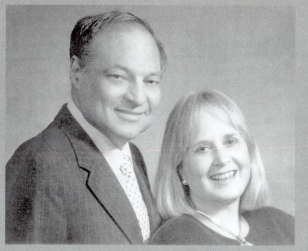

Gerald Klerman (1929–1992) and Myrna Weissman
Courtesy of Dr. Myrna Weissman

10 | INTERPERSONAL PSYCHOTHERAPY

Helen Verdeli and Myrna M. Weissman

OVERVIEW

Basic Concepts

Interpersonal psychotherapy (IPT) is a time-limited, symptom-focused therapy that was originally developed by Gerald Klerman and Myrna Weissman in the 1970s to treat unipolar, nonpsychotic depression in adults (Klerman, Weissman, Rounsaville, & Chevron, 1984; Weissman, Markowitz, & Klerman, 2000, 2007). The fundamental principle of IPT is that depression occurs in an interpersonal context. Regardless of the *causes* of depression, the *triggers* of depressive episodes involve disruptions of significant attachments and social roles. Four interpersonal problem areas have been defined as depressogenic triggers and become the focus of IPT: grief, interpersonal disputes, role transitions, and interpersonal deficits. While recognizing the genetic, personality, and early childhood factors that contribute to depression, the IPT therapist focuses on the recovery from the current depressive episode by (1) clarifying the relationship between the onset of patient's current depressive symptoms and interpersonal problems and (2) building interpersonal skills to resolve or manage more effectively these interpersonal problems.

The foundation of IPT as an operationalized and manual-based approach has facilitated extensive testing against other psychotherapeutic and pharmacological interventions (Weissman et al., 2007). In the last 30 years, randomized controlled clinical trials (RCTs) have established IPT as a major evidence-based psychotherapy for:

- several mood disorders (e.g., major depression, bipolar disorder, postpartum depression);
- other conditions (e.g., bulimia, binge-eating disorder, posttraumatic stress disorder, or PTSD);
- certain populations (adolescents, adults);
- certain settings (hospital clinics—inpatient and outpatient, school-based clinics, primary care, prisons);
- certain modalities (individual, group, conjoint, via telephone);
- various stages of disorder (prevention, acute treatment, maintenance); and
- different cultural contexts (Western countries, sub Saharan Africa, Asia, and Latin America).

Each adaptation adheres to the fundamental elements of the original treatment manual for depression while emphasizing, adding, and modifying techniques to address the unique needs of the patient population served. The description of the theoretical and empirical basis and principles of IPT can be found in the original manual (Klerman et al., 1984). More recent data on efficacy can be found in Weissman and colleagues' comprehensive guide (2000), and a simplified clinical manual has been published by Weissman and her coauthors (2007).

Theory of Depression or Psychopathology

In IPT, depression is conceptualized as having three components:

1. symptom formation,
2. social functioning, and
3. personality factors.

Historically, IPT has focused on the first two components. Although IPT recognizes the contribution of personality factors in the etiology and maintenance of mental disorders, because of its short-term nature, it has not focused on entrenched aspects of personality that typically take longer to change. Instead, IPT has addressed current symptoms and interpersonal problems that can be improved. Social functioning, symptom formation, and personality factors are all linked, and improvements in interpersonal relations help assuage problems in the other areas of functioning (Weissman et al., 2000). In recent years, however, Markowitz and colleagues have adapted and tested IPT to address the more chronic mood disturbances in borderline personality disorder by extending the duration of treatment while preserving its fundamental strategies and techniques (Markowitz, Skodol, & Bleiberg, 2006).

Phases of Treatment

IPT has a "phasic" structure in that it is conducted in three distinct phases: initial, middle, and termination. The specific content of each phase is described later in "Process of Psychotherapy." In that sense, IPT is different from a modular approach to treatment, which characterizes cognitive behavior therapy or dialectical behavior therapy where, for example, cognitive or mindfulness strategies can be conducted before and also after behavioral ones.

Medical Model

Following a medical model of conceptualizing depression, the patient is diagnosed and prescribed the "sick role" in the very beginning of the treatment. The therapist educates the patient about depression, emphasizing that it is a treatable medical problem similar to other illness such as pneumonia, receptive to treatment, and not the patient's fault or failure (Klerman et al., 1984). Giving patients' symptoms a name, allowing them to take on the sick role, and instilling hope about recovery is in itself a powerful therapeutic strategy that (1) demystifies the patients' symptoms by grouping them as part of a known syndrome, (2) excuses patients from blame for the illness and what it makes them do or renders them incapable of doing, (3) separates patients' disorder from their personality and identifies it as a treatable condition, and (4) gives patients permission to experiment with implementation of new interpersonal strategies.

Interpersonal Problem Areas

IPT identifies four classes of interpersonal problem that may trigger depression: grief, interpersonal disputes, role transitions, and interpersonal deficits. Identifying and addressing these problem areas becomes the central axis of the IPT clinical focus. Right at the outset of the treatment, the therapist and patient review current relationship problems that could be associated with the onset and maintenance of depression symptoms. Together they select and focus on the interpersonal problem area associated with the current episode.

The four interpersonal problem areas of IPT are:

1. *grief* (actual death of a significant other or pet),
2. *interpersonal disputes* (overt or covert disagreements with family members, friends and peers, neighbors, etc.),
3. *role transitions* (difficulty making transitions between stages in life or changes in life circumstances such as divorce, moving to a new home, promotion, birth of a child, illness in the family, transition to college, etc.), and
4. *interpersonal deficits* (social isolation or significant communication problems that lead to difficulty in starting or maintaining relationships).

Although many patients present with a variety of problems, to organize therapy and maintain focus, one or at most two areas should be identified as initial targets for therapy. It is not necessary to address all the interpersonal problems occurring in a patient's life to reduce depressive symptoms and alleviate the current episode. Developing a sense of mastery in one interpersonal context may transfer to other areas of a patient's life.

Transcultural adaptations of IPT have shown that the interpersonal problem areas are found across cultures and are universal elements of the human condition. For some disorders (e.g., depression, bulimia nervosa), they are seen as triggers for an episode; in others (e.g., PTSD), they are seen as consequences of the illness that contribute to its maintenance. More generally, the interpersonal context is a paradigm that people universally recognize, unlike intrapsychic or cognitive behavioral perspectives that are much more informed by our Western and anglophonic cultural background, values, and assumptions. Likewise, in parts of the world where there may be a stigma against psychological problems and their treatment, the focus in IPT on resolving interpersonal and often group conflict may be more acceptable and less threatening than other approaches.

Time-Limited Duration

The length of treatment is also established in the initial phase and typically ranges between 12 and 16 consecutive weekly sessions. This structure presents a clear, positive expectation of rapid relief from symptoms and improvement in interpersonal functioning and generates mobilization and optimism. It helps establish patient–therapist rapport by promoting confidence in the patient's ability to change. By focusing on the here and now, it also protects against potential risks of long-term treatment such as patient dependency on the therapist, regression, and the reinforcement of avoidance behaviors (Weissman et al., 2000).

Testability

IPT was originally developed as part of a clinical drug trial to be directly comparable to the other treatment arms. This influenced the character and structure of the therapy in two fundamental ways: (1) It is manualized to ensure consistency of treatment delivery and, from a research perspective, to limit threats to internal reliability and validity (although there is considerable flexibility in the therapeutic techniques used, particularly in the middle phase of treatment); (2) regular assessment of the patients' depressive symptoms and functioning is built into the structure of the therapy. These elements are not simply by-products of the context in which the therapy was developed but may also have important therapeutic effects; for example, tracking patients' illness during treatment (using the Hamilton Rating Scale for Depression (HAM-D) or some other established measure) gives them and their therapists a clear and objective sense of changes in their clinical picture and so can be used to promote a sense of movement in therapy.

Evidence-Based

The development of IPT was also informed heavily by the scientific ethos of Klerman and colleagues and their conviction that all approaches should be tested empirically and that the strongest source of evidence for a treatment's efficacy derives from RCTs (Klerman et al., 1984). The testability of IPT has facilitated its comparison with other forms of psychotherapeutic and psychopharmacological intervention in a long series of clinical trials. The results of these studies have greatly influenced the evolution of IPT: its adaptation for a range of disorders in different populations, its modification for use in a variety of treatment modalities, and its employment in many different cultures around the world.

Other Systems

Klerman and Weissman's goal in developing IPT was to make explicit and operational a systematic psychotherapeutic approach to depression based on theory, clinical observation, and empirical evidence. Given the genesis of IPT, it is not surprising that its procedures and techniques have much in common with those used in other schools of psychotherapy: Clarification of mood states and linking them to interpersonal events, communication analysis and decision making, interpersonal skill building, and homework are hardly exclusive to IPT. Likewise, IPT shares many common goals with other schools of psychotherapy: helping patients gain a sense of mastery of current social roles, combating social isolation, restoring a sense of group belonging, and assisting patients in finding new meaning in their lives (Klerman et al., 1984).

The focus on reduction of depressive symptoms and interpersonal issues in the here and now distinguishes IPT from more traditional psychoanalytic and dynamic psychotherapies. Whereas psychodynamic psychotherapy focuses heavily on early childhood experiences as determinants of unconscious mental processes and intrapsyhic conflict.

IPT does not attempt to explore the patient's behavior as a manifestation of internal conflict but rather in terms of current interpersonal relations. Although the influence of early childhood experiences is recognized as significant, it is not emphasized in IPT. Instead, therapy focuses on patients' current disputes, frustrations, anxieties, and wishes as defined in the interpersonal context. Whereas psychodynamic therapies emphasize unconscious thoughts, IPT works largely at the conscious and preconscious levels. Psychodynamic therapies intervene at the level of personality organization, whereas IPT seeks to improve symptom formation and social adjustment. Psychodynamic therapies are concerned with internalized object relations, whereas IPT looks at interpersonal relations. A psychodynamic therapist listens for a patient's intrapsychic wishes, whereas the IPT therapist listens for the patient's role expectations and interpersonal disputes (Klerman et al., 1984).

These differences between IPT and psychodynamic approaches are not necessarily the result of fundamental theoretical differences. In exploring current interpersonal problems with the patient, an IPT therapist may recognize intrapsychic defense mechanisms such as projection, denial, isolation, undoing, or repression but does so without making internal conflict a focus of treatment. Nor do the techniques used in the two forms of therapy necessarily differ greatly: Many dynamically trained and psychoanalytically oriented psychotherapists report that they already routinely use many of the concepts and techniques of IPT in their practice.

The interpersonal focus of IPT is quite different from that of another time-limited treatment, cognitive-behavioral therapy (CBT). Aaron Beck's work in defining and describing the procedures of cognitive therapy (CT), from which CBT developed, provided a model for the development of IPT by Klerman and Weissman. In common with CBT, IPT focuses on the here and now, is structured, shares techniques, and addresses patients' limited sense of options available to them. Unlike CBT, IPT neither attempts to uncover distorted thoughts systematically through homework nor attempts to help the patient develop alternative thought patterns through prescribed practice. Instead, the IPT therapist draws attention to patients' exploration and modification of maladaptive communication patterns that trigger and maintain their depressive symptoms. Unlike CBT, negative cognitions and behaviors such as guilt, lack of assertiveness, and negative bias are focused only through the examination of their impact on the person's relationships and social roles.

Like rational emotive behavior therapy (REBT), IPT views the therapist's role as active and directive. Unlike REBT, IPT does not focus on uncovering irrational thoughts and beliefs through direct confrontation but uses as a point of departure the functional impact of discordant interpersonal and role expectations between the patient and the other parties involved in the interpersonal problem.

Finally, several principles of Rogerian psychotherapy—such as the importance of creating a genuine, accepting, validating, and safe therapeutic environment to promote desire for exploration and growth in the patient—are shared by IPT. However, unlike the Rogerian tradition, IPT therapists believe that making the patient feel safe is a necessary but not sufficient condition for good therapy. Patients need to develop a thorough understanding of how they affect and are affected by their interpersonal problems and then learn and practice concrete skills to manage these problems more effectively.

HISTORY

Precursors

The formative work by Klerman, Weissman, and colleagues was informed by contemporary theories and empirical findings from three different areas.

Interpersonal Context of Depression.   The creators of IPT believed that depression was essentially a biological illness but that the onset and recurrence of symptoms were triggered by stress, particularly the loss or threat of an important interpersonal attachment. This idea has its theoretical origins in Adolph Meyer's psychobiological framework of mental illnesses (Meyer, 1957) and the work of Harry Stack Sullivan (Sullivan, 1955).

Meyer was perhaps the most influential figure in American psychiatry during the first decades of the 20th century. Strongly influenced by evolution theory, his concept of psychobiology modified the Darwinian principle of biological adaptation to include the adaptation of the organism to its social environment. Within this model, Meyer viewed mental illness as the result of an individual's *maladaptive* attempt to adjust to the changing environment. Although he considered patients' response to environmental stress and change in adulthood to be determined by early experiences in the family and other important social groups, Meyer put great emphasis on patients' current experience, social relations, and relationship to their environments. He noted that a variety of common life events could be important etiological factors in the development of a disorder and created the "life chart" to track the relationship between life history, illness (physical and psychiatric), and stressful events (Meyer, 1957).

Although the interpersonal approach has its basis in Meyer's ideas, it was Sullivan who developed and fully articulated the interpersonal paradigm. Sullivan went so far as to describe psychiatry as the field of interpersonal relations and defined the discipline as the study of people and the processes between them rather than focusing exclusively on the brain, the individual, or society. Along with his associates, he developed a comprehensive theory of the relationship between psychiatric disorders and interpersonal relations, rooted for the developing child in the family and for the adult in life's many interactions. He maintained that one can only understand and address mental illness by making sense of the person's interpersonal matrix (Sullivan, 1955).

Attachment Theory.   If the work of Meyer and then Sullivan established the interpersonal approach to psychiatric practice formalized in IPT, it is John Bowlby's *attachment theory* that provides the theoretical basis for the interpersonal context of depression and the mechanisms underpinning the therapy. Bowlby proposed that humans have an innate tendency to make strong *affectional bonds* (attachments) and that separation or threat of separation of these bonds causes emotional distress, sadness, and in some cases more severe depression. The underlying premise is that there is a universal human need to develop lasting affectional bonds with primary caregivers. These attachments make it possible for the individual to develop the ability to construct and maintain mental representations of the self and others—namely, "internal working models" that organize cognition, affect, and behavior (Bowlby, 1980).

Loss or threat of disruption to these affectional bonds causes emotional distress, sadness, and anxiety. In her famous "Strange Situation" study, Ainsworth (1978, with Blehar, Waters, & Wall) was able to identify three major *attachment styles*: secure attachment, ambivalent–insecure attachment, and avoidant–insecure attachment. A fourth attachment style known as disorganized–insecure attachment was added later (Main & Solomon, 1986). Anxious–ambivalent, avoidant, and disorganized styles are insecure attachment patterns and are considered to be secondary behavioral strategies in response to an insensitive or unavailable caregiver. Although somewhat adaptive, they are considered to be pathogenic because they signify important self-deficits (Peluso, Peluso, White, & Kern, 2004).

Based on these observations, Bowlby proposed that psychotherapy should help patients examine current interpersonal relationships and consider how these relationships developed from experiences with attachment figures earlier in life. In addition, therapeutic strategies should seek to correct the distortions produced by faulty earlier attachments and teach patients how to develop more adaptive and salutary interpersonal relationships. This in turn makes patients less vulnerable to the threats to attachment that might trigger future mental-health problems. Contemporary theories and studies of attachment have continued to inform IPT; this research is reviewed later in "Theory of Personality."

Life Events.   IPT has also been influenced heavily by the psychosocial and life events literature of depression. Since IPT was first developed, the use of systematic life events interviews within long-term epidemiological studies has begun to clarify the role of life events in the complex matrix of factors that contribute to the development of psychiatric disorders. Eugene Paykel has been an important figure in the development of this research. In an influential 1978 study, he used the measure of *relative risk*—the ratio of the disease rate among those exposed to a putative causal factor versus the disease rate among people not exposed—to examine the impact of stressful life events on depression. He found the relative risk of developing depression after the most stressful category of events to be a striking 6:1 (Paykel, 1978). Since then, evidence corroborating the role of life stress in the genesis of depression has accumulated from large-scale epidemiological and genetic studies (see "Theory of Personality").

Beginnings

IPT was not originally developed with the intention of creating a new psychotherapy for depression. The motivation was to formulize a psychotherapy for a clinical trial testing the efficacy of antidepressant medication as a maintenance treatment for unipolar depression. Tricyclic antidepressants had shown promise in reducing the acute symptoms of depression, but there were no data on the efficacy of medication in maintaining long-term symptom reduction for depression. Klerman and Weissman felt that as far as possible, clinical trials should mimic clinical practice (Klerman et al., 1984). As the majority of patients at that time received both medication and therapy, they felt a therapy arm should be included, if only to create a milieu effect. Thus an eight-month-long clinical trial was designed for subjects who had shown symptom reduction while on antidepressant medication during their acute phase of depression. Patients were randomly assigned to conditions in which they received amitriptyline, placebo, or no medication with or without weekly psychotherapy sessions.

Before conducting the study, the team first needed to define the psychotherapy it would use and the techniques it would incorporate. Psychotherapists could then be trained in this standardized approach and the quality and consistency of the treatment could be tested. A cornerstone of the new therapy was its *time-specific* nature, focus on current problems, and the use of a manual to standardize the procedure. The psychotherapy, initially called *high contact*, differed markedly from the open-ended structure of psychodynamic psychotherapy, the predominant treatment method of the time. Another novel feature of the treatment, again reflecting the psychopharmacologic trial of which it was a part, was the use of *standardized assessments* to diagnose patients and follow their clinical course.

The development of the psychotherapy was governed by several guiding principles (Weissman, 2006):

1. It was important to test and establish the efficacy of all treatments, including psychotherapy, in RCTs. (There had been no positive randomized trials of psychotherapy.)

2. Outcomes should be measured across a broad range of standardized measures, including assessments of social functioning and quality of life.

3. Treatment results needed to be replicated before widespread dissemination.

The preliminary step in creating the therapy involved determining its dose, frequency, and diagnostic process. The latter evolved into the first phase of IPT and involved what have become many of IPT's most important and distinctive features: conducting an *interpersonal inventory* of important people currently in the patient's life; giving the patient the *sick role*; linking symptoms to *interpersonal situations*; and selecting *problem areas* associated with the onset of the current depressive episode. The four problem areas were chosen to cover the range of problems that lead to disrupted attachment and trigger depression and arose from Klerman and Paykel's ongoing work developing measures to assess the role of life events in depression onset and relapse. The high contact treatment manual was developed and revised by reviewing cases and developing scripts based on real practice. In this way, the treatment sequence and procedures were formalized so that therapists could be trained to deliver the therapy in a consistent manner.

The one-year follow-up results from the maintenance study found that medication prevented relapse and the psychotherapy improved social functioning (Klerman, Dimascio, Weissman, Prusoff, & Paykel, 1974). The positive findings for the therapy sparked the team to elaborate the principles of the therapy. It was first termed *interpersonal psychotherapy* at this time. An acute treatment trial involving IPT alone and in combination with medication was also positive, with the combination of IPT and medication proving the most efficacious intervention. This was followed by the National Institute of Mental Health's Multisite Collaborative Study testing IPT, cognitive therapy, and drugs as treatments for depression (Elkin et al., 1989). In 1984, the efficacy of IPT was documented by another team, and Klerman, Weissman, and colleagues (1984) published the first IPT manual, *Interpersonal Psychotherapy of Depression*. Since that time, numerous studies and adaptations of IPT for different patient populations have been conducted across a variety of settings and in many different countries.

Current Status

Since it was first developed in the 1970s, clinical and research interest in IPT has grown steadily. IPT has been adapted, tested, and shown to be efficacious as a treatment for a variety of mood and other disorders. Adaptations for mood disorders include IPT as a maintenance treatment of depression; IPT for pregnancy, miscarriage, and postpartum depression; IPT for depression in adolescents and children; IPT for depression in older adults, IPT for depression in medical patients; IPT for dysthymic disorder; and IPT for bipolar disorder. IPT has also been adapted for eating disorders, substance abuse, anxiety disorders, borderline personality disorder, and PTSD. The evidence for the efficacy of IPT is strongest for mood disorders (where the most trials have taken place), varies for other adaptations, and remains untested for some of the newest ones.

Although it was developed as an individual psychotherapy, IPT has also been adapted and tested across a variety of treatment modalities: in group, conjoint couple, and telephone formats. These adaptations have been made based on for both practical reasons (to address barriers to care such as limited funding, poor transportation, and time constraints) and a clinical rationale (e.g., to foster a sense of constructive collaboration between patients and destigmatize their problems). Positive evidence has been found for each adaptation, with group therapy in particular supported by several RCTs for a variety of disorders, cultures, and patient populations (e.g., Bolton et al., 2003; Wilfley et al., 1993). An abbreviated form of IPT called *interpersonal counseling* (IPC) has also been developed and tested (Weissman & Klerman, 1986) to address the practical restraints of treating patients in certain settings (e.g., patients with depression as a secondary diagnosis being treated for a medical problem in a general hospital setting). A new adaptation that includes evaluation, support, and triage (IPT-EST), developed by Weissman and Verdeli (2012), provides a three-session intervention based on the first phase of the standard IPT (diagnosis, identification of the interpersonal problem area, and management of depression). IPT-EST is designed to be followed by an assessment of the need for ongoing treatment. It is currently being tested domestically and internationally.

IPT not only has been tested and used for a range of disorders in several different modalities, but also it is increasingly being used across a variety of cultures, both within and outside the United States. There have been IPT training programs in Australia, Austria, Brazil, the Czech Republic, Ethiopia, Finland, France, Germany, Greece, Haiti, Hungary, Iceland, India, Italy, Ireland, Japan, Kenya, the Netherlands, New Zealand, Norway, Portugal, Romania, South Korea, Spain, Sweden, Switzerland, Thailand, Turkey, Uganda, and the United Kingdom. In many of these countries, clinical trials have established the efficacy of important new adaptations such as trials of group IPT (IPT-G) with depressed adults in rural southwest Uganda and depressed adolescents in camps for internally displaced persons (IDPs) in northern Uganda. In the United States, IPT has shown efficacy in clinical trials with black and Hispanic (mainly Puerto Rican and Dominican) minorities. IPT manuals have been translated into French, Spanish, Italian, German, Japanese, Portuguese, and Danish.

Ease of training was a priority in the development of IPT, and learning the psychotherapy should be straightforward for anyone with a basic knowledge of clinical psychiatric diagnosis and prior training in standard psychotherapeutic techniques: how to show empathy and warmth, formulate a problem, develop a therapeutic alliance, maintain professional boundaries, and so forth (Weissman, 2006). Within its prescribed, goal-oriented, and three-phased structure, IPT nevertheless affords the therapist considerable autonomy and flexibility to employ a variety of therapeutic techniques common to other forms of therapy.

Despite its widespread dissemination and proven efficacy, few professional training programs for mental health workers—psychiatrists, psychologists, social workers, or psychiatric nurses—teach IPT as part of a program in evidence-based psychotherapy. Among those that do, typically only a didactic course is offered without the very important training component of hands-on clinical supervision (Weissman et al., 2006).

For students and professionals who are interested in being trained, many of the professional organizational meetings (e.g., the American Psychiatric Association's annual meetings) offer continuing education courses in IPT. These short half- or full-day courses are primarily didactic. The two- to four-day workshops offered by academic centers around the world are much more intensive and include practical, hands-on training. Clinicians interested in becoming trained in IPT should obtain supervision with an experienced IPT therapist. Three supervised IPT cases following didactic training usually suffice for experienced psychotherapists to learn to perform IPT competently (Weissman, 2006). Guidelines for becoming an IPT therapist or trainer can be found at www.interpersonalpsychotherapy.org, the Web site of the International Society for Interpersonal Psychotherapy. Every other year, the organization holds an international meeting at which IPT researchers, students, and clinicians come together to discuss developments in the field and take part in workshops. For clinicians wanting a glimpse of IPT procedures with scripts, the 2007 manual is recommended (Weissman et al., 2007).

PERSONALITY

Theory of Personality

A theory of personality is not relevant to IPT. Within the theoretical framework of IPT, pathology is considered to have three component processes: symptom function, social and interpersonal relations, and personality and character problems. IPT research and practice have historically focused on the first two. IPT investigators were reluctant to focus on personality traits and disorders for a number of reasons. One is the difficulty in reliably diagnosing personality pathology while in a depressive episode: for example, research by Fava and colleagues (2002) has shown that although axis II diagnoses are common among acutely depressed patients, they drop significantly following successful antidepressant treatment. Therefore, IPT does not make definitive axis II diagnostic assessment during the acute phase of the depression. Another reason is that a significant number of patients do not want or cannot be in long-term psychotherapy. Even if a personality disorder emerges, brief treatment focuses on acute symptom relief and not on personality restructuring, which has not been shown empirically to be possible to change in a short time. However, there is some evidence that the skills learned in IPT may have an effect on behavior, which is a reflection of personality. IPT aims for specific, measurable changes in how the person feels, relates, and communicates. As Markowitz and colleagues noted:

> [A]lthough IPT makes no claims to change personality, imparting interpersonal skills such as self-assertion, confrontation, and effective expression of anger is almost as good as effecting personality change. These skills frequently open up new possibilities for interpersonal functioning that patients may never have dared imagine and that can feel enormously empowering. (Markowitz et al., 2006, p. 442)

The terrain of personality traits as determinants and outcomes of the impact of IPT has changed over the last 10 years. One body of evidence comes from attachment research; another comes from work by Markowitz and colleagues on IPT for borderline personality disorder (2006).

Personality Variables and Environment: Contemporary Research on Attachment

As previously discussed in "Precursors," Bowlby's attachment theory and its evolution provide an important theoretical basis for IPT. The attachment framework offers a set of organizing principles for the understanding of the various aspects of normal and pathological interpersonal relations and the consequent psychological fitness across the life cycle.

Attachment patterns remain pertinent throughout the human life span. Based on Ainsworth's infant–caretaker attachment paradigm, contemporary research has identified similar attachment patterns in adults. According to Bartholomew's four-category model (Bartholomew & Horowitz, 1991), adult attachment is conceptualized as combinations of the internal working models of the self and others. The internal working model of the self constitutes the dimension of *anxiety* and refers to whether the individual has the inner resources for security and self-soothing vis-à-vis an important relationship, whereas the internal working model of others yields the dimension of *avoidance*—that is, whether security is maintained through proximity or, alternatively, self-reliance and emotional distance (Bartholomew & Horowitz, 1991). The combination of these two dimensions results in *four possible attachment styles*: (1) secure anxiety, (2) dismissing, (3) preoccupied, and (4) fearful.

Secure individuals (those with low scores on measures of *anxiety* and *avoidance attachment*) are relatively more protected against psychological distress in general (Hammen et al., 1995) and depression in particular (Mickelson, Kessler, & Shaver, 1997). In contrast, insecurely attached individuals tend to have lower self-esteem (Collins & Read, 1990), poorer affect-regulation strategies (Brennan & Shaver, 1995), and marked problems with emotional support (Simpson, Rholes, & Nelligan, 1992), and they tend to have a higher number of depressive symptoms (Murphy & Bates, 1997). Moreover, there is evidence that the fearful attachment pattern is correlated with depression. In a maintenance study of 162 female participants with major depression who received IPT, Cyranowski and colleagues (2002) identified 43% as fearfully attached compared to only 22% who were securely attached.

There is evidence that attachment style is associated with treatment response in IPT. Cyranowski and colleagues (2002) found a temporal effect of attachment style on depression remission: Although the proportion of subjects who remitted did not differ by attachment profile, among the patients who did remit, those with secure attachment had significantly more rapid remission compared to subjects with fearful–avoidant attachment. The finding indicates that IPT's brief course may not allow enough time for fearful–avoidant patients to develop a trusting relationship with the therapist.

At the same time, evidence is emerging that IPT can help improve patients' attachment styles as opposed simply to resolving the interpersonal crises to which insecure attachment may predispose them. Ravitz (2009) has hypothesized that IPT may ameliorate the anxious and avoidant behaviors of insecurely attached depressed patients. In a study of IPT with depressed adults, subjects whose symptoms fully remitted also showed significant decreases in measures of attachment avoidance and anxiety (Ravitz, 2009). Although these results need to be corroborated in future trials, they present an intriguing possibility: IPT may intervene at the level of attachment style as well as influence the current interpersonal environment and in this way reduce vulnerability to future psychopathology.

IPT and Treatment of Borderline Personality Disorder (BPD)

Although IPT explicitly addresses only axis I disorders, Markowitz and colleagues (2006) note that there is a strong rationale for treating BPD with IPT. First, BPD is frequently co-morbid with mood disorders. Second, BPD is largely about maladaptive social interactions. Markowitz's team at Columbia University is currently investigating the effectiveness of IPT in an open trial of an 8-month (34 sessions) adaptation for BPD patients. According to the investigators, BPD is a "mood-inflected chronic illness" interspersed with explosive outbursts of anger, despair, and impulsivity. Because of the chronicity of the disorder, patients find it particularly difficult to link their mood symptoms with current life events and erroneously regard those symptoms as part of their personality.

Markowitz has outlined the therapeutic elements in IPT for BPD: IPT provides the patient *success experiences*, whereby patients learn new skills to deal effectively with their life crises. Overcoming the crisis is experienced as an interpersonal victory and results in significant improvement of their self-image and a sense of competence and control. The medical model of IPT allows patients to conceptualize BPD as a chronic yet treatable illness. Also, IPT aims at solving patients' problems in the relationships *outside the office*, which is thought to minimize the possibility of therapeutic rupture (in a clinical population in which rupture poses serious threat to therapeutic relationship). Finally, although IPT does not implement "direct" changes in personality, the patient is given tools to deal with those triggers of mood dysregulation characteristic of BPD (intense episodes of depression and anger) that result in *correction of interpersonal dysfunction*. The latter heralds new possibilities for interpersonal functioning that deeply alter the way patients see the world and themselves (Markowitz et al., 2006).

Variety of Concepts

The development and practice of IPT have been informed by several fields of research that variously place emphasis on the impact of life events, biology, social interaction, and personality in the development of psychopathology. Together they suggest that the etiology of psychiatric disorders is complex and multidetermined, with the various genetic, personality, and environmental factors interacting with one another.

Methodological advances over the years, in particular the use of systematic life-event interviews within long-term epidemiological studies, have helped to clarify the role of life events in the complex matrix of factors that coincide in the development of psychiatric disorders. As the isolation of genes related to specific psychiatric disorders becomes a reality, important new advances are being made in our understanding of gene X environment interactions in the development of pathology.

In a landmark study, Caspi and colleagues (2003) examined how genetic differences in the 5-HTT (serotonin transporter) gene moderated the influence of stressful life events on depression. They found that people with one or two copies of the short allele were more likely to become depressed in response to stressful life events than people with a double long allele. In other words, the study showed a *gene X environment interaction* in which the 5-HTT genotype moderated the depressogenic influence of adverse life events. These findings show that psychiatric disorders are genetically complex illnesses in which, like diabetes or hypertension, a genetic predisposition may interact with the environment to produce pathology; the *phenotype* (clinical picture) results from the interaction of the *genotype* and the environment (Weissman et al., 2007). These genetic findings highlight the importance of addressing the pathology of genetically susceptible individuals with treatment that emphasizes current life events.

Although the replication of the Caspi findings has been called into question, these questions have to do more with the design of the replications than with the original findings of Caspi and colleagues. Their important findings based on observational epidemiology are being supported by numerous controlled human and animal studies. This work showing the relationship between genes and environmental stress for depression is in its early phase. Most relevant to psychotherapy is the work of Champagne and colleagues (2003) showing that attachment stress in mice can be reversed by maternal licking and grooming.

There is strong evidence for a relationship between type of life event and the genesis of depression. Kendler, Prescott, Myers, and Neale (2003) have found that humiliating events are more strongly associated with depression onset compared to other types of life events. Moreover, personality characteristics influence the impact of life events on the onset of depression (Shahar, Blatt, Zuroff, & Pilkonis, 2003).

Although genetic and personality variables that place people at risk for disorders such as depression cannot readily be altered, people's reactions and responses to their social environment can be. IPT aims to improve patients' depression by improving interpersonal relations, thus reducing life stress and increasing social support. These improvements in the people's social world are hypothesized to moderate the effects of the genetic, personality, and environmental factors that place the individual at risk for depression.

PSYCHOTHERAPY

Theory of Psychotherapy

IPT aims to improve symptoms and interpersonal functioning by improving the way distressed individuals relate to others. As emphasized previously, this interpersonal focus is the hallmark of IPT. IPT has not invented new techniques. However, although many of the techniques it uses are common to other time-limited therapies, IPT specifically applies them to interpersonal issues. Much more than collecting a set of techniques, the developers of IPT codified *strategies* organized around active management of depression and the four problem areas into a cohesive therapeutic system.

The language of affect is used more in IPT than in other time-limited therapies such as CBT or REBT. Commenting on how the affect is communicated (verbally and nonverbally) is the bread and butter of IPT: "Your eyes seem so sad as you are talking about her"; "You say you are mad at him, but I noticed you are smiling"; "How did you let your boss know that you were not happy about his decision?"

IPT is also different from simple interpersonal skills training: Although IPT therapists often work with patients on assertiveness, they put the skills within the much bigger context of patients' expectations of other people. This helps patients mourn what was lost or never given and encourages change and mobilization. The goal is to break patients' social isolation, helplessness, and hopelessness by assisting them in generating new options and enabling them to access sources of interpersonal support.

IPT does not maintain that all relationships need to be maintained at all costs. Some ties are destructive for patients by not fostering growth and closeness. In other relationships, one of the parties has moved on and does not wish to continue. Helping patients have a balanced view of the strengths and weaknesses of the relationship and a thorough understanding of their own and the other person's desires would determine the outcome of what is frequently asked by the IPT therapist: "Do you think you would like to try one more time?"

A big challenge in IPT, especially for new therapists, is the difficulty in staying focused on problem areas defined as targets for treatment. Dealing with patients' daily crises without putting them into a larger context of a problem area can diffuse and derail the treatment. What often happens is that a general "antidepressant" method of approaching interpersonal situations is learned systematically through work in one problem area. The learning that was generated is frequently transferred to other interpersonal issues that emerge along the way. There are times, of course, when 16 sessions have not been enough and the person, although better, is still not well. In those cases, therapists renew the contract with the patient, setting as new goals the specific interpersonal aims the patient wants to work on in the next set of sessions.

The Therapeutic Relationship

IPT therapists are active, ask questions, and make comments, especially in the first sessions (see "Process of Psychotherapy" next). Although therapists are directive, they are not prescriptive; in other words, they try to let patients generate options, ideas, and resources, as opposed to providing them themselves. They do not work through forms (like the dysfunctional thought records or mood-monitoring forms used in CBT). They do not interpret dreams or other material that communicates unconscious desires, and they do not encourage regression (like analytic treatment).

Process of Psychotherapy

The usual course of IPT for acute depression is 16 sessions for adults or 12 for adolescents divided into three phases: initial, middle, and termination. For a detailed account of clinical practice, see Weissman and colleagues (2007). Here we will briefly illustrate the clinical work through a case vignette with segments from the three phases. The patient, Paul, is a 22-year-old college student who presented to his university's student health services with symptoms of depression. Note that prior to initiation of IPT, the therapist had already conducted a thorough clinical interview, evaluated suicidality, and assessed the need for medication (in case of melancholic depression, severe neurovegetative symptoms, etc.).

Initial Phase (First 3–4 Sessions)

During the initial phase, therapists administer depression rating scales or symptoms checklists (e.g., the Hamilton Rating Scale for Depression, the Beck Depression Inventory). In addition, therapists evaluate patients' idiosyncratic symptoms of depression. For example, when depressed, some patients become particularly jealous or anxious; some drink or smoke more, whereas others stop smoking and drinking; some may develop somatic symptoms, such as nausea, headaches, and the like. Following an in-depth clinical interview to determine patients' diagnosis and psychosocial functioning, the initial phase is conducted over three to four sessions.

In this phase, therapists aim to (1) educate patients about depression and give them hope that it is a treatable condition, (2) help patients manage the consequences of depression and create space in their lives to heal from the episode, (3) understand how depression affects and is affected by patients' important social ties and roles, and (4) agree with patients to focus during the rest of the treatment on one or two interpersonal problem areas that are associated with the current depressive episode. Therapists complete the following tasks (Weissman et al., 2007):

- confirm diagnosis of depression and give syndrome a name;

- give patients hope;

- assign the "sick role"—that is, explain to patients they are suffering from a depression that does not let them function at an optimal level, that they may temporarily need to lower expectations for what they are able to accomplish but that they need to do the therapeutic work to get out of the current episode; and

- help patients rationalize and manage the impact of depression on their lives (e.g., lower expectations, suspend major decisions until depression remission)

The following is a dialogue between Paul and his therapist from the initial phase:

Therapist: Paul, you described today a number of difficulties you've had in the last 2 months . . . trouble concentrating, which led to a low grade in your stats test and your difficulty in finishing your sociology assignment . . . you also have trouble falling asleep, and you've been waking up at 5:30 every day . . . you told me that you have been feeling sad and empty and that your friends noticed it . . . you get tired easily and need to go to bed . . . and since you don't feel like eating, you've also lost 11 pounds in the last 7 weeks. These are symptoms of depression. Depression is . . .

Paul: I'm screwing everything up (on the verge of tears) . . . I should have . . . I'm just failing in everything . . . now I *am* depressed (covers face with hands).

Therapist: It's not your fault that you have depression. It's not your failure, Paul. Depression is common and the good news is that we have a number of great treatments for it. You will get better. Right now it's important for you to take care of yourself and make sure that the circumstances around you allow you to get better.

Paul: But I don't have the time for that. I'm failing at school, I'm in trouble big time . . . (is tearful and panicked).

Therapist: If you had any other illness right now, say if you had pneumonia . . . have you ever had pneumonia, or a really bad flu? (Paul nods in agreement.) Would you expect yourself to do well in your classes, "business as usual"?

Paul: Well, that's different, that's a real illness.

Therapist: Depression is also a real illness. It has symptoms, exactly the types of things you mentioned before: sadness, sleep and appetite problems, low energy and motivation, difficulty concentrating and making decisions . . . This is typical depression. The good news is that we have some very effective ways to treat it. Right now, to get your everyday work done you may need a little extra help from family and friends. For the time being, you may not even be able to do all of the things that you need and want to do. As we make progress in the treatment, you'll start improving, but it's going to take a little time.

Paul: I hope so, this can't go on. I feel terrible that I may fail my stats class . . . maybe I don't have what it takes to be in the program any more, it's crushing me, I may have to just drop out . . .

Therapist: Paul, this is not the right time to make decisions about leaving the program. Depression colors everything in your world and you may not see any options available to you. Why don't we discuss the program some more after you recover from your depression? If you still feel the same, it might be something to consider.

Paul: Ok, I guess . . . (seems somewhat less overwhelmed). But what am I going to do about the stats?

Therapist: Well, given that you are in the midst of a depressive episode, it makes sense that you are struggling a lot with stats. It requires good concentration, maybe more than other classes. What are your options right now for that class?

Paul: It's too late to drop it.

Therapist: I see.

Paul: Maybe I can get an incomplete, I don't know.

Therapist: You came up with a really good idea there. How can you find out what you need to do to get an incomplete?

They then discussed ways in which Paul might go about talking to the professor about getting an incomplete grade because of his depression. Paul said that he wanted to talk to his professor about getting some extra time to complete the outstanding assignments before considering asking for an incomplete. When the therapist asked him about people who could help him through the stats course, Paul thought of asking the class teaching assistant go over some recent difficult material with him. At the end of this part of the discussion, Paul seemed somewhat relieved, "lighter," and less anxious.

The therapist then proceeded to explore the interpersonal context of Paul's depression. She did so through the following strategies: (1) by finding out what was happening in Paul's life around the onset of his symptoms, and (2) by conducting the interpersonal inventory, a detailed exploration of Paul's significant current interpersonal relationships, to understand which contributed to his depression and which were important resources.

Therapist: Paul, you said that you started noticing the first depression symptoms at the beginning of the spring semester.

Paul: Yeah, when I came back after I visited home for the holidays.

Therapist: Did anything happen then, during or after the visit?

Here the therapist wanted to explore what problem area had triggered Paul's depression. She asked questions such as, "Did anyone important to you die around that time? Or maybe a pet? Did you have a fight with or feel distant from a person who was close to you? Have you felt very lonely or isolated? Were there any big changes in your life around then?"

Paul: No big changes, not yet. I have got some big decisions to make about the future, though. I'm not sure what to do after I graduate. . . . I have no idea right now. . . . I told my parents that during the visit. They asked me, and I told them the truth, I have no idea. I don't know what to do next, I'm not even sure what I want to do.

The therapist started gathering information about an impending role transition that seemed to be preoccupying Paul. She also wanted to explore the possibility of a dispute (overt or covert) with his parents because Paul referred emphatically and repeatedly to that interaction.

Therapist: How did they react?

Paul: They didn't say much. . . .

Therapist: Do you know how they felt about it?

Paul: I don't know, I don't think they lost sleep over it. We did the usual family stuff. I don't know what happened, it wasn't different from other times, kind of boring. . . .

Therapist: Did you expect it to be boring?

Paul: Well, I guess every time I get ready to go home, I have the stupid idea that this time it's going to be different, but nothing ever is.

Therapist: You were disappointed, Paul. You were hoping that this time things would be better, but they were not. (Paul nods) I wonder what you wish was better.

Paul: Well, I know they love me and everything, but . . . I don't know, my sister Sarah was there and . . . Sarah and I are close, she just got engaged and Bill was there as well . . . I guess they didn't have much time for me, so many things to celebrate about Sarah, I guess. She just got accepted into law school, Dad has this ridiculous expression when he looks at her, like she'll continue his practice or something . . . she won't, she's moving to California, where Bill is from, and they're going to school together there. Don't get me wrong, I am really close to Sarah and all, but I don't know, these visits are too much . . .

Therapist: It sounds like this one was especially rough. . . .

The therapist had started to form an idea about Paul's problems linked to his depression (a role transition and a covert dispute with his father, who seemed to show preference for his successful sister) but felt she needed to get more information. She proceeded to conduct the interpersonal inventory. The therapist elicited examples of interactions and communications to identify strengths and weaknesses in Paul's interpersonal communication patterns.

Therapist: To get a more complete understanding of your life circumstances right now, I think it'd be useful to talk about the important people in your life. Who would you like to start with?

What do you like about ____?
What don't you like about ____?
Have you ever told ____ how you feel?
What stops you? What do you think would happen?
Are there any times that you and ____ enjoy hanging out? What do you guys do?
Are there things that you would like to change in that relationship? What are they?
How would you feel about _____ if those things changed?
Are there things in that relationship that you would like to keep the same? What are they?

Following the inventory, the therapist suspected that Paul's current episode was triggered by two sets of problems: One was his current difficulty in figuring out what to do after he graduated. Paul did not think he would like to pursue graduate studies in sociology (his major). He described being interested in becoming an emergency medical technician (EMT); he had taken and enjoyed an introductory course. However, he was not sure how to investigate this option further. During the inventory, Paul described a strained relationship with his father, a successful attorney, who had always been proud of Paul's older sister's strong personality and academic excellence and who, by contrast, was dismissive and frequently sarcastic toward Paul. Paul reported reacting to his father's comments by leaving the room or "pretending I don't hear him . . . he is full of it . . . I don't care." Paul described being close to his mother and sister, although the latter's success has been hard on him at times ("It's not her fault, but she always gets it right. . . . I'm not jealous or anything , that's juvenile, but it's too much, man . . ."). Paul had a few friends, was on "the quiet side," but talked to a couple of friends daily and was particularly close to a female friend, Lisa. He said that he was not dating much this year.

At this point, the therapist shared her understanding of Paul's problems, explained the treatment course, and made a treatment contract, also known as the *interpersonal formulation*.

Therapist: From all the information we gathered these three weeks, Paul, it seems to me that your depression began shortly after the Christmas vacation. It seems to me like a couple of things were going on for you around that time. Firstly, you started worrying a bit about what you're going to do after you graduate this May, you're not sure what you want to do next. Secondly, the situation isn't helped by the pressure from your father . . . it sounds like he has very high expectations, and can make you feel pretty bad. I think that your anxieties about what to do next, after you finish school, have been made worse by your father's attitude, and that together these two things triggered your depression . . . all the problems you started experiencing about the time you came back to school: your trouble in some of your classes, your difficulty sleeping, the concentration problems, your loss of appetite. Does this sound right to you?

Paul: Sure, I guess.

Therapist: We'll be talking about these important changes that triggered your depression, and we'll try to find ways to help you feel confident to negotiate these problems . . . finishing up with school and thinking about what you want to do next, and how to manage your interactions with your father. I want to remind you that we will be meeting every week for the next 13 weeks. It's important that you come on time and that you reschedule if you need to miss an appointment. Does all that make sense?

Middle Phase

During this phase of treatment, the majority of the interpersonal work takes place: assisting patients in clarifying how they are affected by and affect their interpersonal environments and building antidepressant relational skills to handle interpersonal difficulties better. In Paul's case, the therapist helped clarify his role transition and made him aware of how his father's derogatory remarks affected his depression. Although Paul's difficulties with his father had started a long time previously, the therapist focused on how the dispute manifested itself in the here and now.

The following is an excerpt from session 8:

Therapist: Hi Paul, how have you been since we saw each other last week?

Paul: Kind of mixed.

Therapist: How have your depression symptoms been?

Paul: I don't feel like doing much, I'm sleeping a bit better but still have trouble concentrating

Therapist: How's your appetite? [The therapist asks about whatever depression symptoms the patient has not mentioned.]

Paul: Same.

Therapist: How would you rate your depression on our 1–10 scale (10 being the worst depression you ever felt)?

Paul: I guess a 6.

Therapist: Was it 6 all week?

Paul: No, after I left here on Wednesday it was, I'd say 4, maybe even 3 for a couple of days. Then it kind of went downhill.

Therapist: So you felt really well for a short time. That's wonderful. What happened during those days?

Paul: Lisa called on Wednesday evening, I went over and we watched a couple of movies, Josh and Annie were there too, it was good. Also, I guess what we talked about last time was helpful, how I don't like theoretical stuff and prefer more hands-on work, how happy I felt when I did my EMT work . . . I felt useful, and I was really good at it, Mr. Harris told me so in front of everybody . . . I pulled some info from the Web and made an appointment with the career counselor to see if she can help me find out some more.

Therapist: How did you feel about doing that?

Paul: I felt good, kind of proud, relieved, I guess. I was thinking that things may get better. I also went to speak to the stats professor again. She thinks it makes more sense now to go for the incomplete than trying to finish. She's right, I guess.

Therapist: These were very important steps, Paul. You did a number of things we discussed: you took action and got information to help you decide about your career; you talked with your professor about your stats course; you had a good time with your friends. And look how well you felt after all that. Then things became tough again. When did you start noticing it?

Paul: I'd say on Saturday, I woke up and . . . well, I didn't really feel like getting up.

Therapist: Hmm, that's quite a change. Did something happen on Friday?

Paul: Well, nothing much, I stayed home and watched TV, my parents called, nothing dramatic.

Therapist: Well, as we discussed, subtle things can at times deeply affect people's mood . . . what happened during the call?

Paul: Well, nothing. My mom was telling me about Sarah's new apartment, the furniture they plan to buy and stuff. My father was also on the line, on the other phone. I was yawning, I was tired, they were going on and on about how her in-laws' plan to get them tickets for a trip to Morocco. On and on and on . . . I am failing my stats, I don't know what to do in my life, and I have to hear about Sarah's vacation . . . My dad asked me why I was yawning, and I told him I was tired and wanted to go to bed.

Therapist: What did he say?

Paul: He said, "You're always tired, not quite sure why."

Therapist: How did you feel when he said that?

Paul: I just said, "Oh! Come on, Dad . . . I'm tired, going to bed." Mom said goodnight, he kind of said "alright . . ." or something like that, and we hung up. I went to bed and fell asleep, but woke up at 5 again. I couldn't go back to sleep, so I watched some TV. I was really tired all day, so I cancelled my plans to go out with Annie and Josh.

Therapist: Paul, as you are talking about the event, are you clearer about what affected your mood?

Paul: I guess that discussion with my dad, it didn't sound that bad, but now that I'm talking about it . . .

Therapist: What are you feeling right now?

Paul: I'm pissed . . . he always puts me down, I don't need this shit right now . . .

Therapist: You're right, you sure don't.

Paul: I have so much crap on my plate right now, the least he could do is to leave me alone, just leave me alone . . . (Paul looks tearful but animated).

Therapist: You seem sad and rightfully angry right now, but you don't seem lost. You do have a lot on your plate: you're trying to finish school and decide what your next professional step is, and you are doing this while you're struggling with depression. Have you ever tried to let your father know the effect his remarks have on you?

Paul: I bet he knows.

Therapist: He may know, but I would like now to focus on whether you have tried to make him understand how his comments affect you.

Paul: Not really, we don't get along; I try to stay away from him.

Therapist: From what you said before though, this seems to work only sometimes. Take last week as an example. You were doing a number of things that were making you feel better: you saw your friends, you *were* better, and then after that discussion you felt depressed again, but thankfully not as much as before. As we said in the beginning, you need to make some space for you to heal from your depression and make the changes that will help you move on. Remember what we said about how important it is to have options, not to let yourself be cornered. What are your options right now about contact with your father?

Paul: I can't just stop talking to him, when Mom calls, he says he wants to talk to me, Mom always lets him talk to me. They do the same with Sarah . . . family tradition, I guess.

Therapist: You've said that you feel well after you talk to your mother. Is there any way you can ask her to talk to you without your father present?

Paul: Knowing her, no. She'll be kind of hurt and ask me why, and insist . . . My Mom likes to pretend that everything is fine . . . she won't do that.

Therapist: I wonder if you could have a direct discussion with your father.

Paul: And what would I say?

Therapist: Good question. What would you like to get across?

Paul: (smiles) You asshole, you are ruining my life . . .

Therapist: (laughs) There you go . . .

Paul: (laughing) OK, OK . . . Maybe, I don't know, I could tell him that I'm depressed right now, and listening to him saying things like that isn't really helpful.

Therapist: You know, that was a very clear message. How about we role play that . . .

Termination Phase (Last 2 Sessions)

During the initial phase of IPT, the duration of treatment is determined. In IPT, every two to three meetings, therapists explicitly make patients aware of the number of remaining sessions. Having a "deadline" facilitates mobilization and a sense of momentum and keeps patients active. During termination, therapists:

1. evaluate patients' depressive symptoms with them to determine if they are full or partial responders;

2. address patients' sadness or anxiety about ending treatment (differentiating this from depression);

3. increase patients' competence and independence in continuing therapeutic gains;

4. review what skills were useful; and

5. reduce guilt if IPT has not been successful (e.g., "the treatment failed you, you did not fail the treatment, and we have other options available to you").

One of the therapeutic options after termination is maintenance IPT. The maintenance model consists of monthly therapy sessions for a year after termination of the acute treatment. Therapists emphasize the interpersonal skills learned and practiced during acute treatment while addressing any new interpersonal stressors that could potentially trigger further depressive episodes.

The following is an excerpt from Paul's penultimate therapy session.

Therapist: Paul, you have made some significant gains in the last four months. First of all, your depression symptoms have improved: you're sleeping better, you're eating better, you're feeling more motivated and energetic, and your concentration has improved. All these improvements have helped you pass all your courses this semester. You also negotiated the problem with your stats professor by arranging to receive an incomplete. On top of all that, you've found the time to think about you want to do next, once you graduate. You've looked into a career as an EMT and signed up to take another course to help decide if it's the right job for you. Also, you've done really well in finding a way to communicate effectively with your father. Now that he understands that you've been depressed, he's interfering less. In addition, you've identified people in your life who you can look to for support and encouragement moving forward. I'd like to hear what you think about what I've just said.

Paul: Yeah, I'm happy about the semester. I didn't think I'd make it. But I'm feeling better than I did. But even though Dad has gotten off my back, I don't think he really gets it. He still wants me to be a success, which in his mind doesn't include becoming an EMT.

Therapist: That's one of the things that remain for you to keep working on going forward from here. But what you've done during the last few months has been enough to improve your mood. The work you'll do in the future should help keep you from getting depressed again. We're almost finished for today. Next week is our last session, and I'd like to hear about your feelings about termination, to look at what situations might arise in your future that you think might trigger another depression, and to look at what skills you've developed during our work that you might use to manage those situations.

During the final session, therapists complete the tasks of termination that were not addressed in the penultimate session.

Mechanisms of Psychotherapy

IPT aims to reduce the helplessness and hopelessness inherent in depression. Its therapeutic power involves:

demystifying depression (it is an illness and can be treated; it does not happen out of the blue but is triggered by interpersonal problems),

generating options for interpersonal communication and action,

increasing mastery,

realizing the antidepressant effect of healthy expression of anger,

clarifying expectations from individuals and roles, and

reducing social isolation.

At the beginning of each session, therapists assess patients' depressive symptoms, noting any changes that occurred over the course of the week and linking symptom changes to interpersonal interactions and events. Following the review of symptoms, together they address the tasks specific to each IPT phase. The strategies in Table 10.1 are associated with each problem area used in the middle phase.

APPLICATIONS

Who Can We Help?

IPT was originally developed for the treatment of unipolar, nonpsychotic depression. However, since its development, the treatment has been adapted to other depressed populations with good results. In all these adaptations, the founding principles of IPT remain the same, with therapy focusing on the interpersonal context. A growing body of literature suggests that no single treatment is appropriate for all patients with the same disorder. Indeed, outcome research has recently begun to focus not on what works in general but on what works for whom and under what circumstances. Thus, through randomized controlled trials, researchers have been trying to identify those characteristics that influence clinical outcome differently, depending on the treatment modality. These characteristics are commonly cited in clinical and epidemiological research as *moderators* or *effect modifiers*.

A moderator suggests for whom or under what conditions a treatment works (Baron & Kenny, 1986). It is a pretreatment or baseline characteristic that is independent of received treatment and has an interactive effect with treatment modalities on therapeutic

TABLE 10.1 Goals and Strategies for Addressing Problems in the Middle Phase

Goals	Strategies
Grief—death of people (or animals) important to the patient	
• Facilitate mourning of the deceased loved one. • Reengage with the world by breaking social isolation and refocusing on relationships and interests.	• Start with the sequence of events before, during, and after the death. • Help the patient reconstruct the relationship with the deceased and view it in a balanced way. • Assist the patient in facing the future without the loved one, developing new skills, and deepening social support.
Interpersonal Disputes—overt or covert disagreements with a significant other	
• Identify the stage of the dispute (see part b of this table). • Identify and modify mismatched expectations or maladaptive communication between the two parties. • Assist the patient in actively resolving the dispute.	• Explore interactions between the parties to identify discordant expectations that led to the dispute. • Explore patient's wishes about the relationship. • Modify maladaptive communication patterns. • Support the patient in trying out new communication skills to resolve the dispute (and as a result either improve a relationship or end a destructive one).
Role Transitions—positive or negative life changes	
• Mourn the loss of the old role. • Develop new skills and social support to handle the new role.	• Elicit feelings about loss of the old role. • Identify positive and negative aspects of the old role. • Identify positive and negative aspects of the new role. • Assist patient in reducing social isolation and finding resources and skills to handle the new role better.
Interpersonal Deficits—difficulty in starting or sustaining relationships	
• Reduce social isolation by improving social skills.	• Review past and current relationships to identify recurrent patterns. • Rehearse new social skills for the formation of new relationships and the deepening of existing relationships.
Stages of Disputes	
Renegotiation	The two parties are still communicating, and both want to resolve the dispute but have been unsuccessful so far.
Impasse	The parties have failed in resolving the dispute and have stopped trying. They still want to be together but are "stuck." The therapist helps to move the impasse into either a renegotiation or a dissolution.
Dissolution	One or both parties want to end the relationship. The therapist explores whether the person wants to try one more time. If this fails, the therapist helps the patient in moving away from the relationship.

outcome. Identifying moderators of treatment is central for both researchers and clinicians: Moderators clarify the best choice for exclusion or inclusion criteria and stratification to maximize power in subsequent RCTs, and they help clinicians identify the most appropriate treatment for a patient (Kraemer, Frank, & Kupfer, 2006). Although the literature in the area of moderators of response to IPT is in its infancy, some moderating characteristics have been identified.

Evidence for *baseline depressive severity* as a moderator of treatment outcome is equivocal. Findings from some studies (e.g., Elkin et al., 1989) suggest that the benefits of IPT (particularly in combination with medication) compared to other psychotherapeutic interventions such as CBT may only emerge in relation to more depressed individuals, with patients with less severe baseline depression faring equally well across different treatments. However, this association has not been found consistently across all trials.

Somatic anxiety (anxiety of a more physiological nature) appears to reduce response to IPT. Feske and colleagues (1998) found that patients whose depression did not remit following IPT experienced significantly higher levels of somatic anxiety and were more likely to meet lifetime criteria for panic disorder compared to those who did remit. Whereas depression with co-morbid anxiety disorder is generally responsive to IPT, when that anxiety is more somatic in nature (as in the case of panic disorder), pharmacotherapy may be required as well.

Social functioning has been shown to moderate the relationship between treatment condition and depression outcome, with patients with low baseline social dysfunction responding significantly better to IPT (Sotsky et al., 1991). This led Sotsky and colleagues to hypothesize that for IPT to be effective, a minimum baseline level of social functioning may be required.

Attachment avoidance also seems to moderate treatment outcome in depression, with findings from McBride and colleagues (2006) suggesting that patients with high attachment avoidance do better in CBT than IPT. They proposed that avoidant individuals' tendency to deny the importance of close relationships and to value cognition over emotion as a defense against attachment insecurity may mean they respond better to CBT, which focuses on cognitions and behaviors, than to IPT, which focuses on interpersonal relationships (McBride, Atkinson, Quilty, & Bagby, 2006).

Treatment

IPT works in depression by providing understanding of the symptoms and their origin within the current context, changing the context and making the symptoms understandable and manageable, identifying the problem, and providing ways of resolving it to generate mastery. In the preceding sections, we outlined the strategies through which the interpersonal goals are realized. We will now present the IPT techniques used to carry out those strategies.

1. *Linking mood to the interpersonal event.*

   Example: "Patient: I am sad." "Therapist: What happened?" or "Patient: I had a terrible fight with my boyfriend" "Therapist: how did it make you feel?"

   This is a very important technique because it provides the interpersonal context in patients' communications and behavior. By understanding that context, patients start realizing which interpersonal interactions contribute to their depression and also which contribute to their recovery.

2. *Conducting communication analysis (analyzing frame-by-frame an interpersonal situation to understand where communication strayed).*

   Example: "Justin, you told me how the argument with your boss worsened your mood for the rest of the week. It is important to understand what happened during that argument. How did it start? What did you say? How did he respond? How did you feel when he said that? What did you say in turn? What did you wish you had said?"

The aim of communication analysis is to help patients understand the interpersonal message they wish to convey and clarify what stood in the way of conveying that message or whether the message conveyed was not what they wanted or needed to get across.

Many times, the therapist uses the metaphor of the camera ("I would like to get a sense of what happened with the detail of a video camera"). Communication analysis helps patients increase their awareness and responsibility for the interpersonal message they need to send.

3. *Generating options (e.g., conducting decision analysis).* In contrast with analytic work, in IPT therapists always ask patients, "What do you plan to do about his?" Teaching patients to generate options counters the hopelessness and helplessness of depression. Therapists help patients come up with alternative ways of dealing with the situation at hand and support them in thinking how to choose one or a combination of them.

4. *Role playing.* After a specific option is chosen, therapists and patients play it out (like a dress rehearsal for action). They may take turns playing the roles of the different parties involved. Therapists give feedback on how patients' communications came across; they also instruct patients about interpersonal skills needed to carry out the communication effectively. For example, the need to find an appropriate time for an important discussion when both parties will be receptive; the importance of focusing on the current issue as opposed to talking about similar issues from the past; characterizing the action but not the person; and being direct in what one is asking for.

5. *Assigning homework (to implement the options that came out of the session guided by the role play).* Homework in IPT is less prescriptive than in CBT. Patients are instructed to try to implement a certain interpersonal interaction before the next session, when they review how the interaction went.

Evidence

The rules of evidence should apply equally to studies of psychotherapy and studies of medication. We believe that a controlled clinical trial with randomization of treatment (RCT) is the highest level of evidence. *Efficacy testing* typically tests the treatment within a relatively homogenous group, under optimal clinical circumstances, and with the therapy performed by highly trained experts. In contrast, *effectiveness studies* include a broad range of participants and are typically conducted in real-life settings by community clinicians; they are the next step in the psychotherapy development sequence (Weissman et al., 2007).

This section offers an overview of the evidence for the various adaptations of IPT. For a more complete discussion of the studies that have contributed evidence for the efficacy of IPT, please refer to Weissman et al. (2007).

IPT for Mood Disorders

In the trial of maintenance antidepressant medication for which it was developed, IPT was shown to improve social functioning. This positive clinical trial, the first for any form of psychotherapy, was followed by a series of studies that established IPT as a leading evidence-based treatment for acute adult unipolar depression. These showed the efficacy of IPT as both in a monotherapy and in combination with medication (e.g., Elkin et al., 1989).

Since then, IPT has been adapted to several depressed populations. In their adaptation of IPT for *depressed adolescents* (IPT-A), Mufson and colleagues (1999) tailored the therapy through several important modifications: (1) reduction of treatment from 16 to 12 sessions, because adolescents generally do not want to be in treatment for a long time; (2) telephone contact, especially during the initial phase, to increase active participation in the treatment; and (3) engaging in a collaborative relationship with the parents and school. The efficacy of IPT-A has been validated through several RCTs (e.g., Mufson, Dorta, & Wickramaratne, 2004). In addition, Young and colleagues have used group IPT focused on interpersonal skills training as a preventive intervention for adolescents at risk for depression (Young, Mufson, & Davies, 2006). At the opposite end of the age spectrum, IPT has also shown efficacy as a treatment for *geriatric depression* across several studies (see Hinrichsen & Clougherty, 2006).

IPT has been successfully adapted and tested for *pregnancy* and *postpartum depression*, based on the following rationale: (1) Given the potentially damaging effects of medication on fetus development, psychotherapeutic alternatives for pregnant, depressed women may be especially important; (2) IPT lends itself to the issues most frequently encountered in pregnancy and childbirth: major role transition, disputes, and grief (e.g., from miscarriage).

IPT has also been used for *medical patients*, who often suffer from depression comorbid with their primary diagnosis. Serious medical illness frequently results in social and interpersonal distress: role transitions because of the incapacitating effects of the illness, interpersonal disputes with family and medical staff, and in some cases grief in anticipation of one's impending death. IPT has shown efficacy in treating depression in primary care patients, to include patients with medical syndromes such as human immunodeficiency virus (HIV), cancer, and coronary disease.

Although it is widely acknowledged that *bipolar disorder* has a major biological component and that treatment requires pharmacotherapy, some aspects of the clinical picture suggest that psychotherapy—and IPT in particular—may make a useful adjunct to medication. The depressive, manic, and psychotic symptoms of the disorder are often extremely disruptive to interpersonal relationships. IPT treats the depressive phase of the illness much like unipolar depression: focusing on interpersonal disputes, role transitions associated with depressive episodes, and—in a variation on the grief problem area—patients' "grief for the lost healthy self." However, because IPT is not equipped to deal with the manic aspect of the illness, in their adaptation Frank and colleagues integrated a behavioral component, social rhythm therapy (SRT), aimed at helping patients avoid the disruptions to their daily routine that can trigger manic episodes. Interpersonal and social rhythm therapy (IPSRT) aims not to treat mania once it has arisen, but to prevent its recurrence by regularizing daily social activities and improving interpersonal relationships. In combination with medication, IPSRT has shown efficacy in increasing the length of time between episodes (see Frank, 2005).

Adapting IPT for *dysthymia* has necessitated some important theoretical modifications. The IPT model, which identifies and targets an interpersonal problem as a trigger of the current depressive episode, makes less sense for a disorder characterized by chronically impaired mood and psychosocial functioning. Thus, IPT for dysthymia (IPT-D) has developed the concept of an iatrogenic role transition: Here the doctor makes treatment itself a role transition through which patients start to understand maladaptive interpersonal patterns, explore new options, and realize that dysthymia is a treatable disorder (Markowitz, 1998). The efficacy of IPT as an adjunct to medication has been established as both individual therapy and group therapy for dysthymia.

IPT for Nonmood Disorders

IPT for *bulimia nervosa* (IPT-BN) focuses on the interpersonal problems that may trigger binge episodes. One significant modification from IPT for depression is the lack of focus on the primary symptoms of the illness. In IPT-BN, the therapist tries to steer discussion away from eating topics and toward their interpersonal context and to explore with the patient the affective and interpersonal problems that may be triggering and maintaining eating symptomatology. In clinical trials that compared IPT-BN to CBT for bulimia nervosa (e.g., Fairburn, Jones, Peveler, Hope, & O'Connor, 1993), IPT patients took longer to attain symptom reduction but caught up over the course of treatment and showed significant and lasting improvement. These findings support IPT-BN's putative mediating mechanism: Rather than addressing eating problems head-on (like CBT), IPT helps patients improve the interpersonal problems driving their illness, which then leads to reduction in disordered eating. IPT has also shown efficacy in trials for *binge eating disorder*. IPT has also been tested as a treatment for *anorexia nervosa*, but failed to demonstrate efficacy.

In the case of PTSD, which by definition occurs in response to a traumatic event, it is less appropriate to conceptualize an interpersonal trigger of pathology. Instead, IPT for PTSD focuses on the management of interpersonal relationships that may become difficult as a result of the disorder: Many patients with PTSD become mistrustful, have difficulty expressing their emotions, and retreat from their social environment. Unlike most treatments, IPT for PTSD does not use exposure as a means of confronting past trauma. However, as patients improve, often they voluntarily expose themselves to reminders of past traumas. An RCT of IPT for PTSD with low-income women showed that the treatment was effective for PTSD and co-morbid depression (Krupnick et al., 2008). Adaptations of IPT for *social phobia* and *panic disorder* have also shown promise in open trials, but CBT remains the treatment of choice for these conditions.

Some of the central characteristics of IPT, such as its short time frame and attention to the reduction of acute symptoms, reflect its development as a treatment for axis I disorders. The adaptation of IPT for *borderline personality disorder* by Markowitz and colleagues (2006) therefore represents a new departure for the treatment and remains under testing. For further discussion of IPT for BPD, see the preceding "Theory of Personality" section.

The use of IPT to treat *substance abuse* is based on a double rationale: Patients may abuse drugs or alcohol to compensate for poor interpersonal relationships, or substance abuse may damage existing relationships and in turn intensify the disorder in a vicious cycle. The goal of IPT with this population is to help patients resolve current interpersonal problems and interpersonal deficits and in doing so counter the need for further substance use. In initial trials, IPT has failed to demonstrate efficacy for substance abuse. However, IPT has shown effectiveness in reducing depression in people with co-morbid substance use disorders, such as in Johnson and Zlotnick's (2012) trial of IPT with incarcerated women.

Other Applications

The adaptation of IPT to a group format has a number of potential benefits. In clinical terms, *group IPT* (IPT-G) can help validate the sick role by showing patients that other people suffer from the same illness, reducing patients' social isolation, allowing them to practice interpersonal skills within therapy, and providing gratification for patients who feel they are helping one another. On a practical level, the group format allows therapists to see a larger number of patients, making it a potentially cost-effective alternative to individual treatment. One potential drawback of IPT-G, especially if different members of a group present with different problem areas, is diminished focus on each individual's particular interpersonal difficulty. Wilfley and colleagues (1993) successfully developed IPT-G as an adaptation for nonpurging bulimic women. To counteract some of the potential problems of the group format, their treatment included two individual sessions before starting the group format (during which the interpersonal inventory was conducted and the case formulation presented), the issuing of homework specific to each patient's case throughout therapy, and the assigning of the interpersonal deficits problem area to all group members. Subsequent studies have provided additional support for the efficacy of IPT-G, including an adaptation of IPT-G for depressed adults in Uganda, which is discussed in detail in the following section.

Interpersonal counseling is a form of IPT with fewer, shorter sessions. IPC was developed by for use with medical patients with co-morbid depression (Weissman & Klerman, 1986) and is currently being tested as a treatment for use in primary care settings.

Conjoint (couples) IPT has been used to treat couples in which one or both spouses are depressed. Before the conjoint phase of treatment, therapists conduct individual sessions with each spouse during which they make their diagnosis, complete the interpersonal inventory, and propose a case formulation. Interpersonal disputes and role transitions have emerged as common problem areas with this population. A pilot study by Foley and colleagues (1989) found that although conjoint IPT and individual IPT resulted in similar reduction in depressive symptoms, subjects from the conjoint IPT arm reported greater improvements in marital satisfaction.

Telephone IPT has been tested successfully in several small pilot studies and open trials for populations to include homebound cancer patients with co-morbid depression who were too ill to come to sessions, depressed patients in partial remission, and patients with subsyndromal depression following miscarriage (Weissman et al., 2007). Following an initial in-person session to determine the patient's diagnosis and level of suicidality, all sessions take place over the phone. However, in other respects the approach is the same as that used in standard IPT.

Psychotherapy in a Multicultural World

IPT has been successfully practiced with patients in many countries and cultures throughout the globe. Often with minimal modifications, IPT has been used effectively with minority populations in the United States and in more than 30 countries on 6 continents. Moreover, even when adapting IPT for use in sub-Saharan Africa, researchers and clinicians have been struck by the similarity in the issues faced by people in rural Uganda and urban areas of the United States despite the considerable cultural and socioeconomic differences between the two societies.

Several features illustrated in the work in sub-Saharan Africa were prerequisites to make IPT *feasible, acceptable, ecologically valid, effective*, and *sustainable* (Verdeli, 2008):

understand the mental-health issues and needs of the community;

validate assessment scales (not just translate and back-translate) to capture local mental-health syndromes;

intervene when the community recognizes the need for assistance and consents to the intervention plans;

choose and adapt the therapy for ecological validity by engaging in ongoing dialogue with the trainees and key informants;

develop a practical and feasible intervention by choosing as mental-health providers educated local laypeople;

develop collaborations among domestic and international academic centers, nongovernment organizations (NGOs), and local communities to test and, if found effective, disseminate the treatment; and have a strong commitment from the international experts to gradually make themselves redundant by withdrawing and letting the local experts take over.

An Example of IPT Adaptation: Group IPT in Southwest Uganda

The adaptation of IPT for use in southwest Uganda serves as a model for the psychotherapy adaptation process. Bolton and colleagues tested the efficacy of IPT to treat adults suffering from depression in the Masaka and Rakai districts of southwestern Uganda, with the long-term goal of making IPT sustainable following the end of the project (Bolton et al., 2003).

Qualitative Research to Inform the Adaptation.   Epidemiological studies conducted over the last 25 years have indicated an elevated level of depression in Uganda, with prevalence rates as high as 21% (Bolton et al., 2003). Local people cited the HIV epidemic in Uganda, a country with one of the highest rates of HIV infection in the world, as the cause of this depression. In 2000, an ethnographic study was conducted and two local syndromes were found to be particularly prevalent: *y'okwetchawa* (self-loathing) and *okwekubagiza* (self-pity). The symptoms experienced within these syndromes overlapped considerably with the *Diagnostic and Statistical Manual* (DSM-IV) criteria for depression (e.g., sadness, poor sleep and appetite, low energy, and feelings of worthlessness). However, these local syndromes also included several additional symptoms not recognized with the DSM criteria, such as not responding when greeted and not appreciating assistance when it was provided. The lack of physicians and high cost of medication prohibited the use of antidepressants. Psychotherapy was seen as a viable alternative provided that (1) laypeople with no previous experience as therapists could be trained to deliver the intervention (because of the scarcity of mental-health professionals), (2) the therapy could be conducted in groups to increase coverage and reduce cost, and (3) its effectiveness could be established.

IPT seemed like a potentially good fit for this population for three principal reasons: the established efficacy of IPT for depression, its compatibility with the importance local Ugandan culture gives to interpersonal relations, and the match between the IPT problem areas and the types of issues the population surveyed seemed to be experiencing (Verdeli et al., 2003). Grief in the local communities was typically associated with the death of a family member or a close friend, often because of AIDS or other illnesses. Some sources of interpersonal dispute were disagreements with neighbors about property boundaries, political fights, and wives protesting an HIV-infected husband's demands to have sex without using condoms. Role transitions included becoming sick with AIDS and other illnesses, getting married and moving into the husband's home, and dealing with a husband's decision to marry a second wife. Local workers deemed interpersonal deficits less relevant to the local culture, and as a result this problem area was dropped from the treatment (Verdeli et al., 2003).

Task Shifting.   A group of workers from World Vision, the organization sponsoring the project, were selected as group leaders. Despite the fact that the majority had no background in mental-health work, a two-week training with IPT experts followed by supervision by telephone during the trial itself proved an effective means of instruction. This approach is consistent with the World Health Organization's *task-shifting model:* the delegation of tasks to less-specialized local health workers in order to make the most efficient use possible of available resources and thereby improve health care coverage (WHO, 2007).

Adaptations Made for the Local Context.   The language used during therapy was informed by the Ugandan cultural context. For example, grief was referred to as "death of a loved one," role disputes were termed "disagreements," and transitions were referred to as "life changes" (Clougherty, Verdeli, & Weissman, 2003). In addition, the strategies employed were adapted to local cultural norms. For instance, in the local context, direct confrontation could be interpreted as inappropriate and disrespectful, so indirect forms of communication had to be used. One effective strategy was for women to cook bad meals, which indicated to their husbands that something was amiss. In another cultural modification, group members understandably had difficulty drawing positives from many of the devastating life changes that had brought about role transitions in Uganda—the AIDS epidemic, tyrannical regimes, and civil war. This problem area was therefore adapted such that therapists worked with group members to identify aspects of life that were under their control and worked on identifying options and building skills that would improve their sense of mastery in these areas (Verdeli et al., 2003).

Results of the Clinical Trial in Southwest Uganda.   An RCT found modified IPT-G for depression to be significantly more effective than the control condition (Bolton et al., 2003). The treatment was very well received by the local community, with excellent attendance and a dropout rate of only 7.8%. Moreover, the groups continued to meet on their own following the official termination.

IPT in Northern Uganda

Effectiveness.   One of the deadliest humanitarian emergencies in the world is the 22-year-old civil war in northern Uganda. More than 20,000 children have been abducted and forced to serve and fight for the Lord's Resistance Army rebel movement. In 2005, the Columbia IPT team participated in the adaptation of group IPT for adolescents living in internally displaced persons camps in northern Uganda. Ethnographic studies showed elevated levels of both depression and anxiety in this population (Bolton et al., 2007). Two additional treatment conditions to those used in the adult study in southwest Uganda were included: creative play (CP), which is what NGOs routinely administer in these settings, and wait-list. CP was included to control for nonspecific group effects and to discern whether any improvements observed resulted from specific elements in IPT over and above generic inclusion in a group. The results of the RCT showed significant improvement of depression in the IPT group compared to the other two conditions (Bolton et al., 2007). Since the study, IDP camp officials have been working with World Vision employees to promote the use of IPT-G among the locally depressed youth, and once again the group leaders have been working extraordinarily hard to cope with the high demand for the treatment.

Sustainability.   Since the initial Ugandan study in 2003, the IPT-G project has been expanded to form new groups and provide services in other provinces. To date, more than 2,500 people in southwest Uganda have been treated as well as adolescents in eight IDP camps in northern Uganda. This stands in contrast to many international projects implemented in developing countries that have dissolved after the initial study (Verdeli, 2008).

Dissemination.   To facilitate the continued development of the IPT work in Africa, a training of trainers was held in Nairobi in 2007. Twelve of the most experienced trainers from the Ugandan projects spent two weeks working on including quality assurance and delineation of training standards for trainers and supervisors, clarification of theoretical and technical issues, and teaching of training skills.

Since the RCT testing of IPT in Uganda, other adaptations have been evaluated in many different cultural contexts domestically and internationally. For example, IPT has been tested with distressed primary care patients in Goa, India, as part of a stepped-care approach. There was strong evidence for the intervention in clients attending public but not private facilities (Patel et al., 2010). IPT has also been adapted for use with Spanish-speaking patients with major depressive disorder in the United States. Blanco and colleagues (Markowitz et al., 2009) identified several cultural issues that emerged from therapy with Hispanic patients: (1) the centrality of the family (*familismo*); (2) conflicts because of migration and acculturation, because migration is a major role transition; (3) gender issues (*machismo*) aimed at constructing a more desirable and also culturally acceptable gender-based sense of self; and (4) the need for culturally acceptable confrontational approaches.

CASE EXAMPLE

This summary refers to the case of Paul, whose treatment was used to illustrate aspects of IPT in the "Process of Psychotherapy" section. As noted, 22-year-old Paul presented to his university's student health services complaining of a number of symptoms he had been experiencing over the past couple of months: feeling sad and empty, difficulty concentrating, poor sleep, loss of appetite, and fatigue.

Paul's clinical interview confirmed a diagnosis of major depression, and his score of 18 on the Hamilton Rating Scale for Depression (HAM-D) confirmed that he was suffering from a severe depressive episode. Based on his low scores on measures of suicidality and neurovegetative symptoms, the therapist decided not to recommend medication at this time.

While taking a psychiatric history, the IPT therapist learned that Paul was the second of two children. His father was a partner in a big law firm; his mother had stayed at home to raise Paul and his sister, Sarah. Paul had been an anxious child, and although he had always had two or three close friends, he struggled to meet new people. He had always been close to Sarah, who was very protective of her younger brother. On the one hand, his relationship with his sister gave him a sense of security, but on the other it occasionally left him feeling deficient. Whereas Paul was shy, an average student, and lacked confidence, by contrast Sarah was outgoing and academically gifted. Paul felt close to his mother but had a difficult relationship with his father, who seemed to identify much more with his sister. He was quick to praise Sarah and celebrate her academic excellence, but he was often dismissive and sarcastic toward Paul, whose lack of direction seemed to puzzle and frustrate him.

Paul had always gotten by at college with mediocre grades, despite having suspected attention deficit hyperactivity disorder (ADHD), although a formal assessment was inconclusive. He was not passionate about any particular subject area and had chosen to major in sociology because it "seemed easy and kind of general." However, now that he was in the spring semester of his final year, this choice of major had left Paul unsure what he wanted after he graduated in the summer. He felt like he might do better with a career that was concrete and action oriented: "less academic and, you know, more practical."

Paul's depressive episode started after the winter break. He was finding it hard to concentrate and struggling with his courses; in particular, his anxiety that he might fail stats had led Paul think that maybe he should "just drop out." Being given the "sick role" at this point in treatment seemed to reduce somewhat Paul's anxiety and persuade him to hold off making drastic decisions about his college and professional future. It also helped him start considering practical solutions to his most pressing current problems, in particular how to handle his failing grade in his stats class.

Having conducted the interpersonal inventory, the IPT therapist hypothesized that Paul's depressive episode had been triggered by his uncertainty about what to do after college (a role transition) and exacerbated by the pressure and high expectations resulting from his tense relationship with his father (an interpersonal dispute). The fact that his sister had recently gotten engaged and been accepted into law school had left Paul feeling even more inadequate and lost. This interpersonal formulation made sense to Paul, and he and the therapist agreed to focus their work together in therapy on his upcoming postcollege role transition and his interpersonal dispute with his father.

In the middle phase of treatment, the therapist worked with Paul to help him clarify his role transition by separating his feelings and views from other people's, coming up with options about his next career step, and identifying individuals who could help him in this transition by providing information or support. The therapist also helped Paul become more aware of how his father's derogatory remarks affected his depression and assisted Paul in learning to set limits with him.

Over the next few weeks, Paul's depressive symptoms began to improve, and increasingly he took an active role in therapy. Paul explained his situation to his stats professor and, based on her advice, decided to take an incomplete grade for the course. He also made an effort to spend more time with his friend Lisa, and in doing so became friends with her roommates. These accomplishments gave Paul a sense of interpersonal mastery and a new sense of confidence. Paul also became more proactive about planning what to do after college. Reflecting on how much he had enjoyed taking an introductory EMT course, he did some Internet research and talked with a career counselor about next steps in exploring this as a potential career. Paul also worked hard at setting limits in his interactions with his father. Although he felt they "weren't any closer," he became better at establishing limits and over the course of therapy their phone conversations began to affect Paul's mood less.

Having declined steadily, four sessions before treatment termination, Paul's HAM-D depression score briefly increased by several points. Reflecting that this was quite normal for a patient nearing the end of treatment, the therapist assuaged Paul's anxiety about ending therapy, reminding him of the considerable progress he had made over the previous few months. In the final phase of treatment, Paul and his therapist took stock of the progress he had made: the improvements in his depression, his increased interpersonal mastery, and the progress he had made in his postcollege role transition and interpersonal dispute with his father. This discussion became a springboard to discuss Paul's ongoing progress after therapy, the problems that might trigger a future depressive episode, and the resources available to Paul to deal with them. Paul reflected that he felt proud of his gains during therapy and pleased about his decision to take a second EMT course after graduating. He was realistic about his relationship with his father, noting that although he was now giving him more space, when it came to his career plans, his father still did not really "get it." He felt good about his relationship with his mother, who had been very supportive of his treatment and encouraging with regard to his plans for the future. Now that Paul felt more secure in himself and his future, he was also able to enjoy his sister's success more. When, in the last session, Paul and the therapist discussed treatment termination, Paul reflected that although things "weren't perfect," he felt he would "do all right."

Before the termination of treatment, the therapist made sure to keep the door open by letting Paul know that if ever he needed more help he could recontact her. Eighteen months later, Paul did call. He reported that in general things were going well. He had not had any more depressive episodes, had become a full-time EMT, and was enjoying the work. He had made a few new friends, and although mostly he was focusing on his career, had been dating casually. However, although he was getting on well with his mother and sister, his relationship with his father remained distant. Paul still felt that in his father's eyes he was "just an EMT" and resented feeling "like I somehow disappointed him, or something." Recently, Paul's father had suffered a heart attack, which had left Paul feeling anxious and as though he should try to "patch things up between us." The therapist congratulated Paul on the gains he had made and reminded him of the importance of separating his own feelings and views from those of others. She helped him accept that his current relationship with his father might be "as good as it gets" and gave him an opportunity to mourn the fact that he might not ever get to be as close to his father as he would have liked. This realization, while sad for Paul, made him feel "less bad, less . . . responsible for how things are between Dad and me" and appeared to reduce his anxiety about their relationship.

SUMMARY

Initially designed to represent the psychotherapy arm of a psychopharmacological trial, in IPT Gerald Klerman, Myrna Weissman, and their colleagues sought to create a therapy that brought together a variety of best psychotherapeutic practices and strategies within a cohesive, systematic structure. What they developed was a logical framework within which therapists from different theoretical approaches and backgrounds could place and use their clinical expertise in a coherent and testable fashion. These characteristics also turned out to be the greatest strength of the approach. IPT is neither doctrinaire nor prescriptive; it allows therapists considerable flexibility to incorporate a broad variety of therapeutic tools within a short-term framework that provides shape to therapy and facilitates patient movement and symptom reduction.

This structure has not only made IPT accessible to clinicians from a variety of professional and cultural backgrounds but also allowed for ready adaptation of the treatment to a range of disorders and settings. This flexibility and usability within a uniform, overarching structure has allowed IPT to evolve through continuous testing and adaptation.

The interpersonal context of psychopathology on which IPT focuses and the problem areas of grief, interpersonal deficits, role transitions, and interpersonal deficits that it identifies as triggers of mental illness appear to hold constant across cultures. Research has established IPT as a feasible and efficacious treatment for a variety of disorders spanning political, economic, and cultural contexts. Currently, it is being used to treat patient populations ranging from depressed American adolescents to sub-Saharan trauma survivors.

Weissman has suggested that psychotherapy in the Western world is in crisis. Rendered prohibitively expensive by the exigencies of insurance companies and the pressures of managed care, psychotherapy is being replaced by pharmacotherapy even where there is evidence to support its use as either in monotherapy or in combination with medication. Paradoxically, psychotherapy is beginning to flourish in resource-poor parts of the world, where it is frequently much more cost-effective than pharmacological approaches. As the first psychotherapeutic treatment to show efficacy in places such as Africa, IPT is at the forefront of this movement.

Counseling CourseMate Website:

See this text's Counseling CourseMate website at www.cengagebrain.com for learning tools such as chapter quizzing, videos, glossary flashcards, and more.

ANNOTATED BIBLIOGRAPHY

Klerman, G. L., Weissman, M. M., Rounsaville, B. J., & Chevron, E. S. (1984). *Interpersonal psychotherapy of depression.* New York: Basic Books.
This book was the first IPT manual (published by Klerman, Weissman, and colleagues) to show efficacy for IPT beyond their research group. The nature and prevalence of depression are discussed, the theoretical basis for IPT is described, and detailed treatment strategies are provided for the four IPT problems areas.

Weissman, M. M., Markowitz, J. C., & Klerman, G. L. (2000). *Comprehensive guide to interpersonal psychotherapy.* New York: Basic Books.
This second IPT manual builds on the first by providing an updated description of IPT for depression, discussing the adaptations of IPT for mood and nonmood disorders, and presenting the efficacy research to support these approaches. Case examples and clinical scripts are included.

Weissman, M. M., Markowitz, J. C., & Klerman, G. L. (2007). *Clinician's quick guide to interpersonal psychotherapy.* New York: Oxford University Press.

Designed for busy clinicians, this condensed manual describes how to conduct IPT for depression and provides adaptations of the approach for a variety of disorders (e.g., mood and nonmood), populations (e.g., older adults, medical patients), and settings (e.g., developing countries). This text provides clinicians with the outline and course of IPT treatment in a concise and practical format.

Mufson, L., Pollack Dorta, K. P., Moreau, D., & Weissman, M. M. (2004). *Interpersonal psychotherapy for depressed adolescents* (2nd ed.). New York: Guildford Press.

This text (IPT-A) presents readers with developmental adaptations for this age group, including the various presentations of depression in teens and the need for parental involvement in treatment. IPT-A is illustrated through case examples.

Frank, E. (2005). *Treating bipolar disorder: A clinician's guide to interpersonal and social rhythm therapy.* New York: Guildford Press.

In this manual, Frank describes the framework and process of IPSRT, an evidence-based treatment for bipolar disorder that incorporates the principles and practice of IPT as part of a broader therapy. This book provides practical guidelines for employing this intervention, outlines efficacy data, and provides clinical vignettes.

Hinrichsen, G. A., & Clougherty, K. F. (2006). *Interpersonal psychotherapy for depressed older adults.* Washington: American Psychological Association.

This manual describes the adaptation of IPT for depressed older adults, addresses issues specific to this population, and discusses the empirical and theoretical basis of the approach.

Web Resources

www.interpersonalpsychotherapy.org

The Web site of the International Society for Interpersonal Psychotherapy provides students, clinicians, and researchers with information about meetings, training, and developments in IPT research and practice.

CASE READINGS

Crowe, M., & Luty, S. (2005). The process of change in interpersonal psychotherapy (IPT) for depression: A case study for the new IPT therapist. *Psychiatry, 68* (1), 43–54. [Reprinted in D. Wedding & R. J. Corsini (2013). *Case studies in psychotherapy.* Belmont, CA: Brooks/Cole.]

This case provides detailed examples of how IPT was used to treat a 42-year-old divorced woman with a major depressive disorder.

Markowitz, J. C., & Weissman, M. M. (Eds.). (2012). *Casebook of interpersonal psychotherapy.* New York: Oxford University Press.

This book provides case material to illustrate the use of IPT for patients with a variety of conditions and across a range of modalities and contexts.

Mufson, L., Verdeli, H., Clougherty, K. F., & Shoum, K. (2009). How to use interpersonal psychotherapy for adolescents (IPT-A). In J. M. Rey & B. Birmaher (Eds.), *Treating child and adolescent depression.* Baltimore: Lippincott Williams & Wilkins.

The chapter provides a session-by-session description of Bill, a depressed adolescent who received IPT-A.

Weissman, M. M., Markowitz, J. C., & Klerman, G. L. (2000). *Comprehensive guide to interpersonal psychotherapy.* New York: Basic Books.

The case of Ellen, a 27-year-old depressed suicidal woman, is described in detail in this book. The case provides a meaningful introduction to key features of IPT.

Weissman, M. M., Markowitz, J. C., & Klerman, G. L. (2007). *Clinician's quick guide to interpersonal psychotherapy.* Oxford: Oxford University Press.

This book includes a number of case examples illustrating the adaptation of IPT to a variety of disorders.

REFERENCES

Ainsworth, M., Blehar, M., Waters, E., & Wall, S. (1978). *Patterns of attachment.* Hillsdale, NJ: Erlbaum.

Baron, R. M., & Kenny, D. A. (1986). The moderator–mediator variable distinction in social psychological research: conceptual, strategic, and statistical considerations. *Journal of Personality and Social Psychology, 51,* 1173–1182.

Bartholomew, K., & Horowitz, L. M. (1991). Attachment styles among young adults: A test of a four-category model. *Journal of Personality and Social Psychology, 61*(2), 226–244.

Bolton, P., Bass, J., Betancourt, T., Speelman, L., Onyango, G., Clougherty, K. F., et al. (2007). Interventions for depression symptoms among adolescent survivors of war and displacement in northern Uganda: A randomized controlled trial. *Journal of the American Medical Association, 298,* 519–527.

Bolton, P., Bass, J., Neugebauer, R., Clougherty, K., Verdeli, H., Ndogoni, L., et al. (2003). Results of a clinical trial of a group intervention for depression in rural Uganda. *Journal of the American Medical Association, 289,* 3117–3124.

Bowlby, J. (1980). *Loss: Sadness and depression.* New York: Basic Books.

Brennan, K. A., & Shaver, P. R. (1995). Dimensions of adult attachment, affect regulation, and romantic relationship functioning. *Personality and Social Psychology Bulletin*, *21*, 267–283.

Caspi, A., Sugden, K., Moffitt, T. E., Taylor, A., Craig, I. W., Harrington, H., et al. (2003). Influence of life stress on depression: Moderation by a polymorphism in the 5-HTT gene. *Science, 301*, 386–389.

Champagne, F. A., Francis, D. D., Mar, A., & Meaney, M. (2003). Variations in maternal care in the rat as a mediating influence for the effects of environment on development. *Physiology and Behavior, 79*, 359–371.

Clougherty, K. F., Verdeli, H., & Weissman, M. M. (2003). *Interpersonal psychotherapy adapted for a group in Uganda (IPT-G-U).* Unpublished manual available through M. M. Weissman, PhD, 1051 Riverside Drive, Unit 24, New York 10032 (mmw3@columbia. edu).

Collins, N. L., & Read, S. J. (1990). Adult attachment, working models, and relationship quality in dating couples. *Journal of Personality and Social Psychology*, *58*, 644–663.

Cyranowski, J. M., Shear, M. K., Rucci, P., Fagiolini, A., Frank, E., Grochocinski, V. J., et al. (2002). Adult separation anxiety: Psychometric properties of a new structured clinical interview. *Journal of Psychiatric Research*, *36*, 77–86.

Elkin, I., Shea, T. M., Watkins, J. T., Imber, S., Sotsky, S. M., Collins, J. F., et al. (1989). National Institute of Mental Health Treatment of Depression Collaborative Research Program: General effectiveness of treatments. *Archives of General Psychiatry, 46*, 971– 982.

Fairburn, C. G., Jones, R., Peveler, R. C., Hope, R. A., & O'Connor, M. (1993). Psychotherapy and bulimia nervosa. Longer-term effects of interpersonal psychotherapy, behavioral therapy, and cognitive behavior therapy. *Archives of General Psychiatry, 50*(6), 419–428.

Fava, M., Farabaugh, A. H., Sickinger, A. H., Wright, E., Alpert, J. E., Sonawalla, S., et al. (2002). Personality disorders and depression. *Psychological Medicine*, 32(6):1049–1057.

Feske, U., Frank, E., Kupfer, D. J., Shear, M. K., & Weaver, E. (1998). Anxiety as a predictor of response to interpersonal psychotherapy for recurrent major depression: An exploratory analysis. *Depression and Anxiety, 8*, 135–141.

Foley, S. H., Rounsaville, B. J., Weissman, M. M., Sholomskas, D., & Chevron, E. (1989). Individual versus conjoint interpersonal psychotherapy for depressed patients with marital disputes. *International Journal of Family Psychiatry, 10*, 29–42.

Frank, E. (2005). *Treating bipolar disorder: A clinician's guide to interpersonal and social rhythm therapy.* New York: Guildford Press.

Frank, E., Kupfer, D. J., & Thase, M. E. (2005). Two-year outcomes for interpersonal and social rhythm therapy in individuals with bipolar I disorder. *Archives of General Psychiatry, 62*, 996–1004.

Hammen, C., Burge, D., Daley, S., Davila, J., Paley, B., & Rudolph, K. D. (1995). Interpersonal attachment cognitions and prediction of symptomatic responses to interpersonal stress. *Journal of Abnormal Psychology*, *104*, 436–443.

Hinrichsen, G. A., & Clougherty, K. F. (2006). *Interpersonal psychotherapy for depressed older adults.* Washington, DC: American Psychological Association.

Johnson, J. E., & Zlotnick, C. (2012). Pilot study of treatment for major depression among women prisoners with substance use disorder. *Journal of Psychiatric Research*. E-publication ahead of print.

Kendler, K. S., Prescott, C. A., Myers, J., & Neale, M. C. (2003). The structure of genetic and environmental risk factors for common psychiatric and substance use disorders in men and women. *Archives of General Psychiatry*, *60*, 929–937.

Klerman, G. L., Dimascio, A., Weissman, M. M., Prusoff, B., & Paykel, E. S. (1974). Treatment of depression by drugs and psychotherapy. *American Journal of Psychiatry, 131* (2): 186–191.

Klerman, G. L., Weissman, M. M., Rounsaville, B. J., & Chevron, E. (1984). *Interpersonal psychotherapy for depression.* New York: Basic Books.

Kraemer, H. C., Frank, E., & Kupfer, D. J. (2006). Moderators of treatment outcomes: Clinical, research, and policy importance. *JAMA, 296*(10), 1286–1289.

Krupnick, J. L., Green, B. L., Stockton, P., Miranda, J., Krause, E., & Mete, M. (2008). Group interpersonal psychotherapy for low-income women with posttraumatic stress disorder. *Psychotherapy Research: Journal of the Society for Psychotherapy Research, 18*(5), 497–507.

Main, M., & Solomon, J. (1986). Discovery of an insecure–disorganized/disoriented attachment pattern: Procedures, findings, and implications for the classification of behavior. In T. B. Brazelton & M. Yogman (Eds.), *Affective development in infancy* (pp. 95–124). Norwood, NJ: Ablex.

Markowitz, J. C. (1998). *Interpersonal psychotherapy for dysthymic disorder.* Washington, DC: American Psychiatric Press.

Markowitz, J. C., Patel, S. R., Balan, I. C., Bell, M. A., Blanco, C., Brave Heart, M. Y. H., Buttacavoli Sosa, S., & Lewis-Fernandez, R. (2009). Toward an adaptation of Interpersonal Psychotherapy for Hispanic patients with DSM-IV Major Depressive Disorder. *Journal of Clinical Psychiatry*, *70*(2), 214–222.

Markowitz, J. C., Skodol, A. E., & Bleiberg, K. (2006). Interpersonal psychotherapy for borderline personality disorder: Possible mechanisms of change. *Journal of Clinical Psychology*, *62*(4), 431–444.

Markowitz, J. C., & Weissman, M. M. (Eds.). (2012). *Casebook of interpersonal psychotherapy.* New York: Oxford University Press.

McBride, C., Atkinson, L., Quilty, L. C., & Bagby, R. M. (2006). Attachment as a moderator of treatment outcome to major depression: A randomized control trial of interpersonal psychotherapy vs. cognitive behavior therapy. *Journal of Consulting and Clinical Psychology, 74*, 1041–1054.

Meyer, A. (1957). *Psychobiology: A science of man.* Springfield, IL: Charles C. Thomas.

Mickelson, K. D., Kessler, R. C., & Shaver, P. R. (1997). Adult attachment in a nationally representative sample. *Journal of Personality and Social Psychology*, *73*, 1092–1106.

Mufson, L., Dorta, K. P., & Wickramaratne, P. (2004). A randomized effectiveness trial of interpersonal psychotherapy for depressed adolescents. *Archives of General Psychiatry, 61*, 577–584.

Mufson, L., Pollack Dorta, K., Moreau, D., & Weissman, M. M. (2004). *Interpersonal psychotherapy for depressed adolescents* (2nd ed.). New York: Guilford Publications.

Mufson, L., Verdeli, H., Clougherty, K. F., & Shoum, K. (2009). How to use interpersonal psychotherapy for adolescents (IPT-A). In J. M. Rey & B. Birmaher (Eds.), *Treating child and adolescent depression.* Baltimore: Lippincott Williams & Wilkins.

Mufson, L., Weissman, M. M., Moreau, D., & Garfinkel, R. (1999). Efficacy of interpersonal psychotherapy for depressed adolescents. *Archives of General Psychiatry, 56,* 573–579.

Murphy, B., & Bates, G. W. (1997). Adult attachment style and vulnerability to depression. *Personality & Individual Differences, 22,* 835–844.

Patel, V., Weiss, H. A., Chowdhary, N., Naik, S., Pednekar, S., Chatterjee, S., et al. (2010). Effectiveness of an intervention led by lay health counsellors for depressive and anxiety disorders in primary care in Goa, India (MANAS): A cluster randomised controlled trial. *Lancet, 376*(9758), 2086–2095.

Paykel, E. S. (1978). Contributions of life-events to causation of psychiatric illness. *Psychological Medicine, 8*(2), 245–253.

Peluso, P. R., Peluso, J. P., White, J. F., & Kern, R. M. (2004). A comparison of attachment theory and individual psychology: A review of the literature. *Journal of Counseling and Development, 82,* 139–145.

Ravitz, P. (2009). *Changes in self-reported attachment and interpersonal problems in depressed patients treated with IPT.* Paper presented at the Third International Conference on Interpersonal Psychotherapy: Global Update, New York.

Shahar, G., Blatt, S. J., Zuroff, D. C., & Pilkonis, P. A. (2003). Role of perfectionism and personality disorder features in response to brief treatment for depression. *Journal of Consulting and Clinical Psychology, 71*(3), 629–633.

Simpson, J. A., Rholes, W. S., & Nelligan, J. S. (1992). Support seeking and support giving within couples in an anxiety-provoking situation: The role of attachment styles. *Journal of Personality and Social Psychology, 62,* 434–446.

Sotsky, S. M., Glass, D. R., Shea, M. T., Pilkonis, P. A., Collins, J. F., Elkin, I., et al. (1991). Patient predictors of response to psychotherapy and pharmacotherapy: Findings in the NIMH Treatment of Depression Collaborative Research Program. *American Journal of Psychiatry, 148,* 997–1008.

Sullivan, H. S. (1955). *The interpersonal theory of psychiatry.* London: Tavistock Publications.

Verdeli, H. (2008). Toward building feasible, efficacious and sustainable treatments for depression. *Depression and Anxiety, 25*(11), 899–902.

Verdeli, H., Clougherty, K., Bolton, P., Speelman, L., Ndogoni, L., Bass, J., et al. (2003). Adapting group interpersonal psychotherapy for a developing country: Experience in rural Uganda. *World Psychiatry, 2,* 114–120.

Weissman, M. M. (2006). A brief history of interpersonal psychotherapy. *Psychiatric Annals, 36*(8), 553–557.

Weissman, M. M., & Klerman, G. L. (1986). Interpersonal Counseling (IPC) for stress and distress in primary care settings. Unpublished manual available through M. M. Weissman, PhD, 1051 Riverside Drive, Unit 24, New York 10032 (mmw3@columbia. edu).

Weissman, M. M., Markowitz, J. C., & Klerman, G. L. (2000). *Comprehensive guide to interpersonal psychotherapy.* New York: Basic Books.

Weissman, M. M., Markowitz, J. C., & Klerman, G. L. (2007). *Clinician's quick guide to interpersonal psychotherapy.* New York: Oxford University Press.

Weissman, M. M., Verdeli, H., Gameroff, M. J., Bledsoe, S. E., Betts, K., Mufson, L., et al. (2006). National Survey of Psychotherapy Training in Psychiatry, Psychology, and Social Work. *Archives of General Psychiatry, 63,* 925–934.

Weissman, M., & Verdeli, H. (2012). Interpersonal psychotherapy: evaluation, support, triage. *Clinical Psychology & Psychotherapy, 19*(2). E publication ahead of print.

Wilfley, D. E., Agras, W. S., Telch, C. F., Rossiter, E. M., Schneider, J. A., Cole, A. G., et al. (1993). Group cognitive-behavioral therapy and group interpersonal psychotherapy for the nonpurging bulimic individual: A controlled comparison. *Journal of Consulting and Clinical Psychology, 61*(2), 296–305.

World Health Organization (WHO). (2007). Treat train retain. Task shifting: Global recommendations and guidelines. Retrieved 20 June, 2009, from www.who.int/healthsystems/task_shifting/en/

Young, J. F., Mufson, L., & Davies, M. (2006). Efficacy of interpersonal psychotherapy-adolescent skills training: An indicated preventive intervention for depression. *Journal of Child Psychology and Psychiatry, 47*(12), 1254–1262.

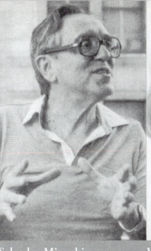

Salvador Minuchin
Courtesy of Dr. Salvador Minuchin,
The Minuchin Center

Virginia Satir
(1916–1988)
© Cengage Learning

Michael White
(1948–2008)
Courtesy of Michael White

11 | FAMILY THERAPY

Irene Goldenberg, Herbert Goldenberg, and Erica Goldenberg Pelavin

Family therapy is both a theory and a treatment method. It offers a way to view clinical problems within the context of the family's transactional patterns. Family therapy also represents a form of intervention in which members of a family are assisted in identifying and changing problematic, maladaptive, repetitive relationship patterns, as well as self-defeating or self-limiting belief systems.

Unlike individually focused therapies, in family therapy the *identified patient* (the family member considered to be the problem in the family) is viewed as manifesting troubled or troubling behavior maintained by problematic transactions within the family or perhaps between the family and the outside community. Helping families to change leads to improved functioning of individuals as well as families. In recent years, therapeutic efforts have been directed at broadening the context for understanding family functioning, adopting an ecological focus that takes the individual, the family, and the surrounding cultural community into account (Robbins, Mayorga, & Szapocznik, 2003).

OVERVIEW

Basic Concepts

When a single attitude, philosophy, point of view, procedure, or methodology dominates scientific thinking (and thus assumes the character of a *paradigm*), solutions to problems are sought within the perspectives of that school of thought. If serious problems arise that do not appear to be explained by the prevailing paradigm, however, efforts are made to expand or replace the existing system. Once the old belief system changes, perspectives shift and previous events may take on entirely new meanings. The resulting transition to a new paradigm, according to Kuhn (1970), was a scientific revolution.

In the field of psychotherapy, such a dramatic shift in perspective occurred in the mid-1950s as some clinicians, dissatisfied with slow progress when working with individual patients or frustrated when change in their patients was often undermined by other family members, began to look at the family as the locus of pathology. Breaking away from the traditional concern and investigation of individual personality characteristics and behavior patterns, they adopted a new perspective—a family frame of reference—that provided a new way of conceptualizing human problems, especially the development of symptoms and their alleviation. As is the case with all paradigm shifts, this new viewpoint called for a new set of premises about the nature of psychopathology and stimulated a series of family-focused methods for collecting data and understanding individual functioning.

When the unit of analysis is the individual, clinical theories inevitably look to internal events, psychic organization, and the patient's intrapsychic problems to explain that person's problems. Based on a heritage dating back to Freud, such efforts turn to the reconstruction of the past to seek out root causes of current difficulties, producing hypotheses or explanations for *why* something happened to this person. With the conceptual leap to a family framework, attention is directed to the family context in which individual behavior occurs, to behavioral sequences between individuals, and to *what* is now taking place and *how* each participant influences and is influenced by other family members.

This view of *reciprocal causality* provides an opportunity to observe repetitive ways in which family members interact and to use such data to initiate therapeutic interventions. Family therapists therefore direct their attention to the dysfunctional or impaired family unit rather than to a symptomatic person, who is only one part of that family system and, by his or her behavior, is seen as expressing the family's dysfunction.

The Family as a System

By adopting a relationship frame of reference, family therapists pay attention to both the family's *structure* (how it arranges, organizes, and maintains itself at a particular cross section of time) and its *processes* (the way it evolves, adapts, or changes over time). These therapists view the family as an ongoing, living system, a complex, durable, causal network of related parts that together constitute an entity larger than the simple sum of its individual members. That system, in turn, is part of a larger social context—the outside community.

Several key concepts are central to understanding how systems operate. *Organization* and *wholeness* are especially important. Systems are composed of units that stand in some consistent relationship to one another, and thus we can infer that they are organized around those relationships. In a similar way, units or elements, once combined, produce an entity—a whole—that is greater than the sum of its parts. A change in one part causes a change in the other parts and thus in the entire system. If this is indeed the case, argue systems theorists, then adequate understanding of a system requires study of the whole rather than separate examination of each part. No element within the system can ever be understood in isolation because elements never function separately. The implications for understanding family functioning are clear: A family is a system in which members organize into a group, forming a whole that transcends the sum of its individual parts.

The original interest in viewing a family as a system stems in part from the work of Gregory Bateson, an anthropologist who led an early study in which he and his colleagues hypothesized that schizophrenia might be the result of pathological family interaction

(Bateson, Jackson, Haley, & Weakland, 1956). Although not a family therapist himself, Bateson (1972) deserves special credit for first seeing how a family might operate as a *cybernetic system*. Current views of the origins of schizophrenia emphasize genetic predispositions exacerbated by environmental stresses, but Bateson's team should be recognized for first focusing attention on the flow of information and the back-and-forth communication patterns that exist within families. Rather than studying the content of what transpires, family therapists were directed to attend to family processes, the interactive patterns among family members that define a family's functioning as a unit.

A Cybernetic Epistemology

Several significant shifts in clinical outlook occur with the adoption of a cybernetic epistemology. For example, the locus of pathology changes from the identified patient to the social context, and the interaction between individuals rather than the troubled person is analyzed. Instead of assuming that one individual causes another's behavior ("You started it. I just reacted to what you did"), family therapists believe both participants are caught up in a circular interaction, a chain reaction that feeds back on itself, because each family member has defined the situation differently. Each argues that the other person is the cause; both are correct, but it is pointless to search for a starting point in any conflict between people because a complex, repetitive interaction is occurring, not a simple, linear, cause-and-effect situation with a clear beginning and end.

The simple, nonreciprocal view that one event leads to another in stimulus–response fashion represents *linear causality*. Family therapists prefer to think in terms of *circular causality:* Reciprocal actions occur within a relationship network by means of a network of interacting loops. From this perspective, any cause is seen as an effect of a previous cause and becomes in turn the cause of a later event. Thus, the attitudes and behavior of system members, as in a family, are tied to one another in powerful, durable, reciprocal ways and in a never-ending cycle.

The term *cybernetics*, which is based on a Greek word for "steersman," was coined by mathematician Norbert Wiener (1948) to describe regulatory systems that operate by means of *feedback loops*. The most familiar example of such a mechanism is the thermostat in a home heating system; set to a desired temperature, the furnace will turn on when the heat drops below that setting, and it will shut off when the desired temperature is reached. The system is balanced around a set point and relies on information fed back into it about the temperature of the room. Thus, it maintains a dynamic equilibrium and undertakes operations to restore that equilibrium whenever the balance is upset or threatened.

So, too, with a family. When a crisis or other disruption occurs, family members try to maintain or regain a stable environment—*family homeostasis*—by activating family-learned mechanisms to decrease the stress and restore internal balance.

Family members rely on the exchange of information—a word, a look, a gesture, or a glance—that acts as a feedback mechanism, signaling that disequilibrium has been created and that some corrective steps are needed to help the relationship return to its previous balanced state. In effect, information about a system's output is fed back into its input to alter, correct, or govern the system's functioning. *Negative feedback* has an attenuating effect, restoring equilibrium, whereas *positive feedback* leads to further change by accelerating the deviation. In negative feedback, a couple may exchange information during a quarrel that says, in effect, "It is time to pull back or we will regret it later." In positive feedback, the escalation may reach dangerous, runaway proportions; the quarreling couple may escalate an argument to the point that neither one cares about the consequences. In some situations, however, positive feedback, although temporarily destabilizing, may be beneficial if it does not get out of control and if it helps the couple reassess a dysfunctional transactional pattern, reexamine their methods of engagement, and change the system's rules. In other words, a system need not revert to its previous level but may instead, as a result of positive feedback, change and function more smoothly at a higher homeostatic level (Goldenberg & Goldenberg, 2013).

Subsystems, Boundaries, and Larger Systems

Following largely from the work of Minuchin, Nichols, and Lee (2006), family therapists view families as comprising several coexisting subsystems in which members group together to carry out certain family functions or processes. Subsystems are organized components within the overall system, and they may be determined by generation, sex, or family function. Each family member is likely to belong to several subsystems at the same time. A wife may also be a mother, daughter, younger sister, and so on, thus entering into different complementary relationships with other members at various times and playing different roles in each. In certain dysfunctional situations, family members may split into separate long-term coalitions: males opposed to females, parents against children, father and daughter in conflict with mother and son.

Although family members may engage in temporary alliances, three key subsystems will always endure: the spousal, parental, and sibling subsystems (Minuchin, Rosman, & Baker, 1978). The first is especially important to the family: Any dysfunction in the spousal subsystem is bound to reverberate throughout the family, resulting in the scapegoating of children or co-opting them into alliances with one parent against the other. Effective spousal subsystems provide security and teach children about commitment by presenting a positive model of marital interaction. When effective, the parental subsystem provides child care, nurturance, guidance, limit setting, and discipline; problems here frequently take the form of intergenerational conflicts with adolescents, often reflecting underlying family disharmony and instability. Sibling subsystems help members learn to negotiate, cooperate, compete, and eventually attach to others.

Boundaries are invisible lines that separate a system, a subsystem, or an individual from outside surroundings. In effect, they protect the system's integrity, distinguishing between those considered insiders and those viewed as outsiders. Boundaries within a family vary from being rigid (overly restrictive, permitting little contact among the members of different groups) to being diffuse (overly blurred so that roles are interchangeable and members are overinvolved in each other's lives). Thus, the clarity of the boundary between subsystems and its permeability are more important than the subsystem's membership. Excessively rigid boundaries characterize *disengaged families* in which members feel isolated from one another, and diffuse boundaries identify *enmeshed families* in which members are intertwined in one another's lives.

Boundaries between the family and the outside world need to be sufficiently clear to allow information to flow to and from the environment. In systems terms, the more flexible the boundaries, the better the information flow. The family is open to new experiences, able to alter and discard unworkable or obsolete interactive patterns, and operates as an *open system*. When boundaries are not easily crossed, the family is insular, not open to what is happening around it, suspicious of the outside world, and said to be operating as a *closed system*. In reality, no family system is either completely open or completely closed; rather, all exist along a continuum.

Cybernetics Revisited and the Postmodern Challenge

The early, radical assumptions proposed by systems theory (circular causality, feedback loops, boundaries, subsystems) were groundbreaking in their relationship-focused and holistic character but were limited because they were confined to outside observers attempting to describe what was occurring within a system (Becvar, 2003). A later refinement, sometimes called *second-order cybernetics*, acknowledged the effect of the observer (the family therapist) on his or her observations; by helping define the problem, the observer influences goals and outcomes. Each family member's perceptions of the presenting problem began to be acknowledged as important and valid because how each member constructs reality influences and is influenced by a larger social context. Postmodern views, popular today, are especially rejecting of the systems metaphor as based on mechanistic models. Postmodernists argue that our notion of reality is inevitably subjective; there are no universal truths out there ready to be described by "objective observers" (Gergen, 1999).

All family systems thus are influenced by one or more of society's larger systems—the courts, the health-care system, schools, welfare, probation, and most currently the psychological challenges inherent in the cybersystem. This frontier presents new challenges to therapists who must be aware of and understand the complications of virtual relationships and boundaries. Untangling the web of relationships, both perceived and real, can be difficult for the practitioner and presents both legal and ethical issues (Pelavin & Moskowitz-Sweet, 2009).

Although such contact with the larger system may be time limited and generally free of long-term conflict, numerous families become entangled with such systems, and this entanglement sometimes impedes the development of family members. Family therapists today pay close attention to such interactions, looking beyond the dysfunctional family itself and integrating the recommendations of the various agencies in order to provide a broad, coordinated set of interventions to achieve maximum effectiveness.

Gender Awareness and Culture Sensitivity

Challenged by postmodern inquiries into the diversity of perspectives for viewing life, as well as by the feminist movement, family therapists have begun to look beyond observable interactive patterns within a family, and today they examine how gender, culture, and ethnicity shape the perspectives and behavior patterns of family members. Indoctrinated early into gender-role behavior in a family, men and women have different socialization experiences and as a result develop distinct behavioral expectations, are granted disparate opportunities, and have differing life experiences. Work and family roles and responsibilities have changed dramatically in the last 30 years, requiring new male–female interactions and family adaptations (Barnett & Hyde, 2001).

Gender, cultural background, ethnicity membership, sexual preference, and social class are interactive; one cannot be considered without the others. As Kliman (1999) notes, the experience of being male or female shapes and is shaped by being poor, middle class, or wealthy—or being African American, Chinese, or Armenian. Contemporary views of family therapy emphasize taking a *gender-sensitive outlook* in working with families, being careful not to reinforce (as therapists sometimes did in the past) stereotyped sexist, patriarchal attitudes or class differences. Today, family therapists pay more attention to differences in power, status, and position within families and in society in general.

Similarly, family therapists today believe a comprehensive picture of family functioning at the minimum requires an understanding of the cultural context (race, ethnic-group membership, social class, religion, sexual orientation) and the form of family organization (stepfamily, single-parent family, gay couples, etc.) of the family seeking help. Adopting a broad, multicultural framework leads to a pluralistic outlook, one that recognizes that attitudes and behavior patterns are often deeply rooted in the family's cultural background. That pluralistic viewpoint also enables therapists to better understand the unique problems inherent in the multitude of families today that do not fit the historical model of the intact family (Sue & Sue, 2007).

Developing a *culturally sensitive therapy* (Prochaska & Norcross, 1999) necessitates moving beyond the white, middle-class outlook from which many therapists operate (prizing self-sufficiency, independence, and individual development) and recognizing that such values are not necessarily embraced by all ethnic groups. For example, many clients from traditional Asian backgrounds are socialized to subordinate their individual needs to those of their families or of society in general. In developing a multicultural framework, the family therapist must recognize that acculturation is an ongoing process that occurs over generations and that ethnic values continue to influence a client family's child-rearing practices, intergenerational relationships, family boundaries, and so forth.

A culturally competent family therapist remains alert to the fact that how he or she accesses or counsels a family is influenced not only by professional knowledge but also by his or her own "cultural filters"—values, attitudes, customs, religious beliefs and practices, and (especially) beliefs regarding what constitutes normal behavior (Madsen, 2007). To ignore such built-in standards is to run the risk of misdiagnosing or mislabeling as abnormal an unfamiliar family pattern that might be perfectly appropriate to that family's cultural heritage (McGoldrick & Hardy, 2008). Similarly, the culturally sensitive therapist must be careful not to overlook or minimize deviant behavior by simply attributing it to cultural differences. According to Falicov (2000), the family therapy encounter is really an engagement between a therapist's and a family's cultural and personal constructions about family life. This includes the role of spirituality on the part of both the clinician and the client, tapping spiritual resources for coping, healing, and resiliency (Walsh, 2009). If religious or previously established family rituals do not satisfy the system's needs, then creating collaborative rituals can be healing to the family (Imber-Black, Roberts, & Alva Whiting, 2003).

Therapeutic intervention with a wide variety of families requires the therapist to help family members understand any restrictions imposed on them as a result of such factors as gender, race, religion, social class, or sexual orientation. Cultural narratives (White, 2007) specifying the customary or preferred ways of being in a society are sometimes toxic (racism, sexism, ageism, class bias) and thus inhibiting and subjugating to the individual, family, and group. Here the therapist must provide help in addressing the limitations imposed by the majority culture if the family is to overcome societal restrictions.

Other Systems

Differences between family therapy and other therapeutic approaches are less clear-cut than in the past as systems ideas have permeated other forms of psychotherapy. Although therapists may focus on the individual patient, many have begun to view that person's problems within a broader context, of which the family is inevitably a part, and have adapted family systems methods to individual psychotherapy (Wachtel & Wachtel, 1986). For example, *object relations theory* has emphasized the search for satisfactory "objects" (persons) in our lives, beginning in infancy. Practitioners of psychoanalytically based object relations family therapy, such as Scharff and Scharff (2006), help family members uncover how each has internalized objects from the past, usually as a result of an unresolved relationship with one's parents, and how these imprints from the past—called *introjects*—continue to impose themselves on current relationships, particularly with one's spouse or children. Object relations family therapists search for unconscious relationship seeking from the past as the primary determinant of adult personality formation, whereas most family therapists deal with current interpersonal issues to improve overall family functioning.

Conceptually, Adlerian psychotherapy is compatible with family therapy formulations. Being far less reliant on biological or instinctual constructs than psychoanalysis is, Adlerian theory emphasizes the social context of behavior, the embeddedness of the individual in his or her interpersonal relationships, and the importance of current circumstances and future goals rather than unresolved issues from childhood. Both Adlerian psychotherapy and family therapy take a holistic view of the person and emphasize intent and conscious choices. Adler's efforts to establish a child-guidance movement, as well as his concern with improving parenting practices, reflect his interest beyond the individual to family functioning. However, the individual focus of his therapeutic efforts fails to change the dysfunctional family relationships that underlie individual problems.

The person-centered approach developed by Carl Rogers is concerned with the client's here-and-now issues, is growth oriented, and is applicable to helping families move in the direction of self-actualization. Its humanistic outlook was particularly appealing to experiential family therapists such as Virginia Satir (1972) and Carl Whitaker (Whitaker & Bumberry, 1988), who believed families were stunted in their growth and would find solutions if provided with a growth-facilitating therapeutic experience. Experiential family therapists are usually more directive than Rogerians and, in some cases, act as teachers to help families open up their communication processes (for instance, using methods developed by Virginia Satir).

Existential psychotherapies are phenomenological in nature, emphasizing awareness and the here and now of the client's existence. Considered by most family therapists to be too concerned with the organized wholeness of the single person, this viewpoint nevertheless has found a home among some family therapists, such as Walter Kempler (1991), who argued that people define themselves and their relationships with one another through their current choices and decisions and what they choose to become in the future rather than through their reflections on the past.

Behavior therapists traditionally take a more linear view of causality regarding family interactions than do most systems theory advocates. A child's tantrums, for example, are viewed by behaviorists as maintained and reinforced by parental responses. Systems theorists view the tantrum as an interaction, including an exchange of feedback information, occurring within a family system.

Most behaviorists now acknowledge that cognitive factors (attitudes, thoughts, beliefs, expectations) influence behavior, and cognitive-behavior therapy has become a part of mainstream psychotherapy (Dattilio & Epstein, 2005). However, rational emotive behavior therapy's view that problems stem from maladaptive thought processes seems too individually focused for most family therapists (Ellis & Dryden, 2007).

Evidence-based treatments identify specific groups and the cultural adaptations that are necessary (Cardona et al., 2012).

HISTORY

Precursors

Freud, Adler, and Sullivan

Family therapy can trace its ancestry to efforts begun early in the last century, led largely by Sigmund Freud, to discover intervention procedures for uncovering and mitigating symptomatic behavior in neurotic individuals. However, although Freud acknowledged in theory the often-powerful impact of individual fantasy and family conflict and alliances (e.g., the oedipal conflict) on the development of such symptoms, he steered clear of involving the family in treatment, choosing instead to help the symptomatic person resolve personal or intrapsychic conflicts.

Adler went further than Freud in emphasizing the family context for neurotic behavior, stressing the importance of the family constellation (e.g., birth order, sibling rivalry) on individual personality formation. He drew attention to the central role of the family in the formative years, contending that family interactive patterns are the key to understanding a person's current relationships both within and outside the family.

Harry Stack Sullivan, beginning in the 1920s, adopted an interpersonal relations view in working with hospitalized schizophrenics. Sullivan (1953) argued that people were the product of their "relatively enduring patterns of recurrent interpersonal situations." Even though he did not work directly with families, Sullivan speculated on the role that family played in the transitional period of adolescence, thought to be the typical time for the onset of schizophrenia. Sullivan's influence on Don Jackson and Murray Bowen, two pioneers in family therapy who trained under Sullivan, as well as on his colleague Frieda Fromm-Reichmann, is apparent both in their adoption of Sullivan's early notion of redundant family interactive patterns and in their active therapeutic interventions with families.

General Systems Theory

Beginning in the 1940s, Ludwig von Bertalanffy (1968) and others began to develop a comprehensive theoretical model embracing all living systems. General systems theory challenged the traditional reductionistic view in science that complex phenomena could be understood by carefully breaking them down into a series of less complex cause-and-effect reactions and then analyzing in linear fashion how A causes B, B causes C, and so forth. Instead, this new theory argued for a systems focus in which the interrelations between parts assume far greater significance: A may cause B, but B affects A, which in turn affects B, and so on in a circular causality. General systems theory ideas can be seen in such family systems concepts as circular causality and the belief that symptoms in one family member signal family dysfunction rather than individual psychopathology.

Group Therapy

John Bell (1961) developed a therapeutic approach called *family group therapy*, applying some of the social psychological theories of small-group behavior to the natural group that is the family. Adopting group therapy's holistic outlook, family therapists involve entire families in the therapeutic process, believing that kinship groups provide more real situations and provide a greater opportunity for powerful and longer-lasting system changes as a result of family-level interventions.

Beginnings

Research on Schizophrenia

Several researchers, working independently, began in the 1950s to zero in on schizophrenia as an area where family influences might be related to the development of psychotic symptoms. Taking a linear viewpoint at first and seeking causes of the schizophrenic condition in early family child-rearing practices, the researchers ultimately branched out into a broader systems point of view. Early efforts by the following are particularly noteworthy: Bateson's group in Palo Alto, Theodore Lidz's project at Yale, and the efforts at the National Institute of Mental Health (NIMH) of Murray Bowen and Lyman Wynne. The idea of seeing family members together for therapeutic purposes came later as a result of research discoveries and subsequent theorizing.

A landmark paper by Bateson and colleagues (1956) speculated that *double-bind* communication patterns within a family may account for the onset of schizophrenia in one of its members. Double-bind situations exist when an individual, usually a child, habitually receives simultaneous contradictory messages from the same important person, typically a parent, and concurrently is forbidden comment on the contradiction. The overall message might be, "I'm interested in what you are telling me," but the nonverbal message might signal, "Go away, you are bothering me, I don't care about you."

Compelled to respond, but doomed to failure whatever the response, the child becomes confused and ultimately withdraws after repeated exposure to such incongruent messages, unable to understand the true meaning of his or others' communications. Schizophrenia was thus reformulated as an interpersonal phenomenon and as a prototype of the consequences of failure in a family's communication system.

Lidz and his colleagues (Lidz, Cornelison, Fleck, & Terry, 1957) hypothesized that schizophrenics did not receive the necessary nurturance as children and thus failed to achieve autonomy as adults. According to this premise, one or both parents' own arrested development was responsible, especially because the parents were likely to have a conflict-ridden marriage, providing poor role models for children. These researchers distinguished two patterns of chronic marital discord that were common in schizophrenic families. In one, labeled *marital skew,* extreme domination by one emotionally disturbed partner is accepted by the other, who implies to the children that the situation is normal. In the *marital schism* scenario, parents undermine their spouses, threats of divorce are common, and each parent vies for the loyalty and affection of the children.

Bowen was especially interested in the symbiotic mother–child bonds that he hypothesized might lead to schizophrenia. Hospitalizing entire families on the research wards for months at a time in order to observe ongoing family interactions, Bowen (1960) broadened his outlook, observing emotional intensity throughout these families. As a result, he moved from his previous psychoanalytic viewpoint to one that emphasized reciprocal functioning in what he labeled the *family emotional system.*

Lyman Wynne, who succeeded Bowen at NIMH, turned his attention to the blurred, ambiguous, confused communication patterns he and his associates found in families with schizophrenic members (Wynne, Ryckoff, Day, & Hirsch, 1958). Wynne coined the term *pseudomutuality* to describe a false sense of family closeness in which the family gives the appearance of taking part in a mutual, open, and understanding relationship without really doing so. The members of these families have poorly developed personal identities and doubt their ability to accurately derive meaning from personal experiences outside the family, preferring to remain within the safe and familiar family system with its enclosed boundaries.

Psychodynamics of Family Life

Trained in psychoanalytic work with children, Nathan Ackerman nevertheless saw the value of treating entire families as a unit in assessing and treating dysfunctional families. In his landmark book *The Psychodynamics of Family Life,* which is often considered the first text to define the new field, Ackerman (1958) argued for family sessions aimed at untangling interlocking pathologies, thus endorsing the systems view that problems of any one family member cannot be understood apart from those of all other members.

By working therapeutically with nonschizophrenic families, Ackerman demonstrated the applicability of family therapy to less disturbed patients. By 1962, he in New York and Don Jackson on the West Coast founded the first journal in the field, *Family Process,* with Jay Haley as editor. This periodical enabled researchers and practitioners to exchange ideas and identify with the growing field of family therapy.

Delinquent Families

One project combining theory and practice was led by Salvador Minuchin (Minuchin, Montalvo, Guerney, Rosman, & Schumer, 1967) at the Wiltwyck School for Boys in upper New York state, a residential setting for delinquent youngsters from urban slums.

Recognizing the limitations of traditional methods for reaching these boys, who were generally from poor, underorganized, fatherless homes, Minuchin developed several brief, action-oriented therapeutic procedures aimed at helping reorganize unstable family structures.

Current Status

A current trend in family therapy is toward eclecticism and integration of therapeutic approaches (Lebow, 1997) because no single technique fits all clients or situations. Multisystemic evidence-based approaches that are research-based are being used to treat a variety of behavioral and emotional problems in adolescents and entire families as therapists select and borrow from one another's theories to address a current therapeutic problem.

Two promising family approaches aimed at treating delinquency or other behavior problems in adolescents as well as at reducing recidivism are functional family therapy (Sexton & Alexander, 2002) and multisystemic therapy (known as *evidence-based therapies*) (Henggeler, Schoenwald, Borduin, Rowland, & Cunningham, 2009). Both have garnered considerable research support, and both offer systems-based, cost-effective programs that community providers can adopt in working with at-risk adolescents and their families.

As conceptualized by Goldenberg and Goldenberg (2013), eight theoretical viewpoints and corresponding approaches to family therapy can be identified.

Object Relations Family Therapy

The psychodynamic view is currently best expressed by object relations family therapists (Hughes, 2007; Scharff & Scharff, 2006), who contend that the need for a satisfying relationship with some "object" (i.e., another person) is the fundamental motive of life. From the object relations perspective, we bring *introjects*—memories of loss or unfulfillment from childhood—into current dealings with others, seeking satisfaction but sometimes "contaminating" family relations in the process. Thus, they argue, people unconsciously relate to one another in the present largely on the basis of expectations formed during childhood. Individual intrapsychic issues and family interpersonal difficulties are examined in a therapeutic setting. Helping family members gain insight into how they internalized objects from the past and how these objects continue to intrude on current relationships is the central therapeutic effort, along with providing understanding and instigating change. Treatment is aimed at helping members become aware of those unresolved objects from their families of origin and at increasing their understanding of the interlocking pathologies that have blocked both individual development and fulfillment from family relationships. Virginia Satir anticipated in her treatment methods today's mind–body approaches.

Experiential Family Therapy

Experiential family therapists such as Satir and Whitaker believe that troubled families need a *growth experience* derived from an intimate interpersonal experience with an involved therapist. By being real or authentic themselves, and often self-disclosing, experiential therapists contend that they can help family members learn to be more honest, more expressive of their feelings and needs, and better able to use their potential for self-awareness to achieve personal and interpersonal growth.

For Virginia Satir, building self-esteem and learning to communicate adequately and openly were essential therapeutic goals. Calling his approach *symbolic–experiential family therapy,* Carl Whitaker gave voice to his own impulses and fantasies and de-pathologized human experiences as he helped family members probe their own covert world of symbolic meanings, freeing them to activate their innate growth processes. Currently, experiential family therapy is best represented by *emotion-focused couple therapy* (Furrow, Johnson, & Bradley, 2011), an experiential approach grounded in attachment theory and based on humanistic and systemic foundations that attempts to change a couple's negative interactions while helping them cement their emotional connection to each other.

Transgenerational Family Therapy

Murray Bowen argued that family members are tied in thinking, feeling, and behavior to the family system and thus individual problems arise and are maintained by relationship connections with fellow members. Those persons with the strongest affective connections (or *fusion*) with the family are most vulnerable to personal emotional reactions to family stress. The degree to which an individualized, separate sense of self independent from the family (or *differentiation of self*) occurs is correlated with the ability to resist being overwhelmed by emotional reactivity in the family; the greater the differentiation, the less likely the individual will experience personal dysfunction.

Bowen (1978) believed that the child most vulnerable to dysfunction is the one most easily drawn into family conflict. He maintained that the most attached child will have the lowest level of differentiation, will be the least mature, and thus have the hardest time separating from the family and is likely to select a marital partner who is also poorly differentiated in his or her family. The least differentiated of their offspring will marry someone equally undifferentiated, and so forth. In this formulation, problems are passed along to succeeding generations by a multigenerational transmission process. Bowen maintained that schizophrenia could result after several generations of increased fusion and vulnerability.

Another transgenerational family therapist, Ivan Boszormenyi-Nagy (1987), emphasizes the ethical dimension (trust, loyalty, entitlements, and indebtedness) in family relationships, extending over generations. He focuses on the relational ethics within a family aimed at preserving fairness and ensuring fulfillment of each member's subjective sense of claims, rights, and obligations in relation to one another. To *contextual therapists* such as Boszormenyi-Nagy, the patterns of relating within a family that are passed down from generation to generation are the keys to understanding both individual and family functioning.

Structural Family Therapy

Minuchin's (1974) structural view focuses on how families are organized and on what rules govern members' transactions. He pays particular attention to family rules, roles, alignments, and coalitions, as well as to the boundaries and subsystems that make up the overall family system. Symptoms are viewed as conflict defusers, diverting attention from more basic family conflicts. Therapeutically, structuralists challenge rigid, repetitive transactions within a family, helping to "unfreeze" them to allow family reorganization (Minuchin et al., 2006).

Strategic Family Therapy

The strategic family approach involves the designing of novel strategies by the therapist to eliminate undesired behavior. Strategists such as Jay Haley (1996) are not particularly interested in providing insight to family members; they are more likely to assign tasks to get families to change those aspects of the system that maintain the problematic behavior. Sometimes indirect tasks in the form of *paradoxical interventions* are used to force clients to abandon symptoms. Therapists at the Mental Research Institute in Palo Alto believe families develop unworkable "solutions" to problems that become problems themselves. Consequently, these therapists have evolved a set of brief therapy procedures using various forms of paradox aimed at changing undesired family interactive patterns (Watzlawick, Weakland, & Fisch, 1974).

In Milan, Italy, Mara Selvini-Palazzoli and her colleagues (Selvini-Palazzoli, Boscolo, Cecchin, & Prata, 1978) developed *systemic family therapy,* a variation of strategic family therapy that has had its greatest success with psychotic and anorectic patients. Selvini-Palazzoli (1986) believed behavioral symptoms in families represent "dirty games" in which parents and symptomatic children engage in power struggles, the children using their symptoms to try to defeat one parent for the sake of the other. Boscolo and Cecchin (Boscolo, Cecchin, Hoffman, & Penn, 1987) in particular have refined several interviewing techniques such as *circular questioning* to help family members examine their family belief system in the process of helping to empower them to exercise their prerogative of making new choices for their lives. Boscolo and Cecchin offer a systemic epistemology based on second-order cybernetics in which the therapist, rather than attempting to describe the family system as an outside observer, is viewed as part of what is being observed and treated. Like other participants, the therapist is seen as someone with a particular perspective but not a truly objective view of the family or what is best for it. Their approach enhanced the development of the postmodern-influenced social construction therapies.

Cognitive–Behavior Family Therapy

The behavioral perspective—the idea that maladaptive or problematic behavior can be extinguished as the contingencies of reinforcement for that behavior are altered—has been expanded in recent years by including a cognitive viewpoint (Beck & Weishaar, 2007; Berg, Dolan, & Trepper, 2008; Ellis & Dryden, 2007). Working with couples or offering training in parenting skills, cognitive restructuring is designed to help clients overcome dysfunctional beliefs, attitudes, or expectations and to replace their self-defeating thoughts and perceptions with more positive self-statements about themselves and their future. Beyond changing current distorted beliefs, clients are taught how to better evaluate all beliefs. Cognitively based couples therapy is directed at restructuring distorted beliefs (called *schemas*) learned early in life (from the family of origin, mass media, or the family's ethnic and socioeconomic subculture). These negative schemas affect automatic thoughts and emotional responses to others and call for cognitive restructuring to modify or alter faulty perceptions (Wills, 2009).

Social Constructionist Family Therapy

Influenced primarily by postmodern thinking, social constructionists are at the forefront of challenging systems thinking, especially the simple cybernetic model presented by the early family therapists. They contend that each of our perceptions is not an exact duplication of the world but a point of view seen through the limiting lens of our assumptions about people. The view of reality each of us constructs is mediated through language and is socially determined through our relationships with others and with the culture's shared set of assumptions. Valuing diversity, these therapists maintain that ethnicity, cultural considerations, gender issues, sexual orientation, and so forth must be addressed in determining a family's functioning level.

Family therapy from a social constructionist outlook requires collaboration between therapist and family members without preconceived notions of what constitutes a functional family or how a particular family should change. Instead, therapist and family members together examine the belief systems that form the basis for the meaning they give to events, and then they jointly construct new options that change past accounts of their lives and allow them to consider new alternatives that offer greater promise. Leading proponents of this view included Steve de Shazer (1991), Berg (Berg et al., 2008) (solution-focused therapy) and Harlene Anderson (1997) (collaborative language systems approach).

Narrative Therapy

Narrative therapists such as Michael White (1995) argued that our sense of reality is organized and maintained through the stories by which we circulate knowledge about ourselves and the outside world. Families that present negative, dead-end stories about themselves typically feel overwhelmed, inadequate, defeated, and without future choices. Their self-narratives concede being beaten and fail to provide options that would allow change. The dominant cultural narratives also make them feel they cannot live up to what is expected of them. Therapeutic help comes in the form of learning to reduce the power of problem-saturated stories and reclaiming their lives by substituting previously subjugated stories in which they were successful. The therapist's role is not to help clients replace one story with another but to help them view life as multistoried, with numerous options and possibilities.

Narrative therapists are concerned not with how family patterns produced the problem but with how the problem affected the family. The therapist's task, according to narrative therapists, is to help liberate families from such feelings of hopelessness by collaborating with them in exploring alternative stories, making new assumptions about themselves, and opening them up to new possibilities by reauthoring their stories. *Externalization* (viewing the problem as outside themselves rather than as an internal part of their identity) helps them notice alternative choices and paves the way for alternative stories.

White is especially interested in helping clients reexamine the oppressive stories that formed the basis for how they have lived their lives and in working with them to construct new alternatives, whereas de Shazer helps clients view their problems differently, engaging them in dialogue directed at finding new and empowering solutions.

PERSONALITY

Family therapists as a group do not subscribe to a single, unified theory of personality, although all view individual development as embedded in the context of family life. Expanding on Sullivan's (1953) emphasis on the role of interpersonal relationships in personality development, family therapists believe that behavior is the product of one's relationships with others. Symptomatic conduct in any individual family member is a response to that person's current situation, although it may have its roots in past experiences within the family.

Theory of Personality

Clinicians who adopt a family systems outlook have varying theoretical bases. Individual personality is not overlooked but is instead recast as a unit of a larger system, the family, which in turn is seen as part of a larger societal system. Nevertheless, family therapists remain aware that no matter how much individual behavior is related to and dependent on the behavior of others in the family system, individual family members remain flesh-and-blood persons with unique experiences, private hopes, ambitions, outlooks, expectations, and potentials (Nichols, 1987). Most family therapists try to remain focused on family interaction without losing sight of the singularity of the individual. The ultimate goal is to benefit all those who make up the family.

How a therapist views personality development depends largely on her or his initial theoretical framework. In keeping with their psychoanalytic roots, object relations theorists (Hughes, 2007) believe that people's fundamental need is for attachments—that is, they seek closeness and emotional bonding to others based on how needy or insecure they are as adults as a result of early infant experiences. These therapists investigate individual "object-loss" growing up, believing that if one's relational needs are unmet by parents or other caregivers, then the child will internalize both the characteristics of the lost object and the accompanying anger and resentment over the loss. The resulting unresolved unconscious conflict develops into frustration and self-defeating habits in the adult, who continues, unconsciously and unsuccessfully, to choose intimate partners to repair early deprivation.

Behaviorally oriented family therapists believe that all behavior, normal and abnormal, is learned as a result of a process involving the acquisition of knowledge, information, experiences, and habits. Classical conditioning, operant conditioning, and modeling concepts are used to explain how personality is learned. Following the early lead of B. F. Skinner, some strict behaviorists question whether an inner personality exists, maintaining that what we refer to as "personality" is nothing more than the sum of the environmental experiences in one's life. Rejecting explanations that imply the development of internal traits, they search instead for relationships between observable behavior and observable variations in the person's environment. In their view, situations determine behavior.

Those behavior therapists who adopt a more cognitive orientation believe that people do develop personality traits and that their behavior is based at least in part on those traits and does not arise simply in response to situations. These family therapists contend that certain types of cognitions are learned, become ingrained as traits, and mediate a person's behavior. Perceptions of events, attitudes, beliefs, expectations of outcomes, and attributions are examples of such cognitions. Especially when negative or rigid, these cognitions can contribute to negative behavior exchanges within a family. Intervention is an attempt to change maladaptive cognitions.

Many family therapists view personality from a *family life cycle* perspective (Carter & McGoldrick, 2005). This developmental outlook notes that certain predictable marker events or phases (marriage, birth of first child, children leaving home, and so on) occur in all families, regardless of structure, composition or cultural background, compelling each family to deal in some manner with these events. Because there is an ever-changing family context in which individual members grow up, there are many chances for maladaptive responses. Situational family crises (such as the death of a parent during childhood or the birth of a handicapped child) and certain key transition points are periods of special vulnerability.

Both continuity and change characterize family systems as they progress through the life cycle. Ordinarily, such changes are gradual, and the family is able to reorganize as a system and adapt successfully. Certain discontinuous changes, however, may be disruptive, transforming a family system so that it will never return to its previous way of functioning. Divorce, becoming part of a stepfamily, serious financial reverses, and chronic illness in a family member are examples of sudden, disruptive changes that cause upheaval and disequilibrium in the family system. Symptoms in family members are especially likely to appear during these critical periods of change as the family struggles to reorganize while negotiating the transition. Family therapists may seize the crisis period as an opportunity to help families develop higher levels of functioning by helping them galvanize their inherent potential for resiliency to better cope with upheaval or loss (Walsh, 2003).

Variety of Concepts

Family Rules

A family is a rule-governed system in which the interactions of its members follow organized, established patterns. Growing up in a family, members all learn what is expected or permitted in family transactions. Parents, children, relatives, males, females, and older and younger siblings all have prescribed rules for the boundaries of permissible behavior—rules that may not be verbalized but are understood by all. Such rules regulate and help stabilize the family system.

Family therapists are especially interested in persistent, repetitive behavioral sequences that characterize much of everyday family life because of what these patterns reveal about the family's typical interactive patterns. The term *redundancy principle* is used to describe a family's usually restricted range of options for dealing with one another. Attending to a family's rules represents an interactive way of understanding behavior rather than attributing that individual behavior to some inferred inner set of motives. Don Jackson (1965), an early observer of family behavioral patterns, believed that family dysfunction resulted from a family's lack of rules for accommodating to changing conditions.

Family Narratives and Assumptions

All families develop paradigms about the world (enduring assumptions that are shared by family members). Some families view the world as friendly, trustworthy, orderly, predictable, and masterable and thus are likely to view themselves as competent; they can encourage members to share their views, even when disagreement is likely to ensue. Others perceive the world as mostly menacing, unstable, and thus unpredictable and potentially dangerous. This latter group is likely to insist on agreement from all family members on most if not all issues in an effort to present a united front against any intrusion or threat. The narrative the family develops about itself, derived largely from its history and passed from one generation to the next, has a powerful impact on its daily functioning.

Families inevitably create narratives or stories about themselves, linking certain family experiences together in a certain sequence to justify how and why they live as they do. Certain dominant stories (how they were orphaned at an early age, how they lived with alcoholic parents, how their parents' divorce frightened them about commitment to a relationship, how their grandmother's love and devotion made them feel loved and cared for, and so on) explain their current actions and attitudes. Narrative therapists such as White (2007) contend that our sense of reality is organized and maintained through the stories by which we circulate knowledge about ourselves and our view of the world we live in. Beyond personal experiences, the meanings and understandings that families attribute to events and situations they encounter are embedded in their social, cultural, and historical experiences (Anderson & Gehart, 2006).

Pseudomutuality and Pseudohostility

One result of Wynne's NIMH studies of families with schizophrenic members (Wynne et al., 1958) was his observation of their recurrent fragmented and irrational style of communication. He discovered an unreal quality about how they expressed both positive and negative emotion to one another, a process he labeled *pseudomutuality*. Wynne reported that members in these families were absorbed with fitting together at the expense of developing their separate identities. Rather than encourage a balance between separateness and togetherness, as occurs in well-functioning families, members in Wynne's group seemed concerned with the latter only, apparently dreading expressions of individuality as a threat to the family as a whole. By presenting a facade of togetherness, they learned to maintain a homeostatic balance but at the expense of not allowing either disagreements or expressions of affection. The tactic kept them from dealing with any underlying conflict; at the same time, the surface togetherness prevented them from experiencing deeper intimacy with one another.

Wynne's research also identified *pseudohostility,* a similar collusion in which apparent quarreling or bickering between family members is in reality merely a superficial tactic for avoiding deeper and more genuine feelings. Members may appear alienated from one another, and their antagonism may even appear intense, but the turmoil is merely a way of maintaining a connection without becoming either deeply affectionate or deeply hostile to one another. Like pseudomutuality, it represents a distorted way of communicating and fosters irrational thinking about relationships.

Mystification

Another masking effort to obscure the real nature of family conflict and thus maintain the status quo is called *mystification.* First described by R. D. Laing (1965) in analyzing the family's role in a child's development of psychopathology, the concept refers to parental efforts to distort a child's experience by denying what the child believes is occurring. Instead of telling the child, "It's your bedtime," or explaining that they are tired and want to be left alone, parents say, "You must be tired. Go to bed." In effect, they have distorted what the child is experiencing ("I'm not tired"), especially if they add that they know better than the child what he or she is feeling.

Mystification, then, occurs when families deal with conflict by befuddling, obscuring, or masking whatever is going on between members. This device does not deter conflict but rather clouds the meaning of conflict and is called into play when a family member threatens the status quo, perhaps by expressing feelings. A husband who says, in response to his wife's query about why he appears angry, "I'm not angry. Where do you dream up these things?" when he actually is angry is attempting to mystify her. His apparent intent to avoid conflict and return matters to their previous balance only leads to greater conflict within her. If she believes him, then she feels she must be "crazy" to imagine his anger; if she trusts her own senses, then she must deal with a deteriorating marital relationship. Mystification contradicts one person's perceptions and, in extreme or repeated cases, leads that person to question his or her grip on reality.

Scapegoating

Within some families, a particular individual is held responsible for whatever goes wrong with the family. *Scapegoating* directed at a particular child often has the effect of redirecting parental conflict, making it unnecessary for the family to look at the impaired father–mother relationship, something that would be far more threatening to the family. By conveniently picking out a scapegoat who becomes the identified patient, other family members can avoid dealing with one another or probing more deeply into what is really taking place.

Scapegoated family members are themselves often active participants in the family scapegoating process. They not only assume the role assigned to them but also may become so entrenched in that role that they are unable to act otherwise. Particularly in dysfunctional families, individuals may be repeatedly labeled as the "bad child"—incorrigible, destructive, unmanageable, troublesome—and they proceed to act accordingly. Scapegoated children are inducted into specific family roles that over time become fixed and serve as the basis for chronic behavioral disturbance. Because the family retains a vested interest in maintaining the scapegoated person in that role, blaming all their problems on one member, changes in family interactive patterns must occur before scapegoating will cease. Otherwise, the scapegoated person, usually symptomatic, will continue to carry the pathology for the family.

PSYCHOTHERAPY

Theory of Psychotherapy

There is no single theory of psychotherapy for family therapists, although all would probably agree with the following basic premises:

1. People are products of their social connections, and attempts to help them must take family relationships into account.

2. Symptomatic or problematic behavior in an individual arises from a context of relationships, and interventions to help that person are most effective when those faulty interactive patterns are altered.

3. Individual symptoms are maintained externally in current family system transactions.

4. Conjoint sessions, in which the family is the therapeutic unit and the focus is on family interaction, are more effective in producing change than attempts to uncover intrapsychic problems in individuals via individual sessions.

5. Assessing family subsystems and the permeability of boundaries within the family and between the family and the outside world offers important clues regarding family organization and susceptibility to change.

6. Traditional psychiatric diagnostic labels based on individual psychopathology fail to provide an understanding of family dysfunctions and tend to pathologize individuals.

7. The goals of family therapy are to change maladaptive or dysfunctional family interactive patterns or help clients construct alternative views about themselves that offer new options and possibilities for the future.

Systems thinking most often provides the underpinnings for therapeutic interventions with the family. By viewing causality in circular rather than linear terms, it keeps the focus on family transactional patterns, especially redundant maladaptive patterns that help maintain symptomatic behavior. When family interrelationships are emphasized over individual needs and drives, explanations shift from a *monadic* model (based on the characteristics of a single person) to a *dyadic* model (based on a two-person interaction) or a *triadic* model (based on interactions among three or more persons).

In a monadic outlook, a husband fails to pay attention to his wife because he is a cold and uncaring person. Adopting a dyadic mode, people are viewed in terms of their interlocking relationships and their impact on one another. Here the therapist looks beyond the separate individuals who make up the couple, focusing instead on how these two individuals organize their lives together and, more specifically, on how each helps define the other. From a dyadic viewpoint, a husband's indifference arouses his wife's emotional pursuit, and she demands attention. Her insistence arouses the fear of intimacy that led to his withdrawal to begin with, and he retreats further. She becomes more insistent and he less available as their conflict escalates. A family therapist helping such a couple will direct attention to their interactive effect, thus making the dyad (and not each participant) the unit of treatment. Seeing the couple conjointly rather than separately underscores the therapist's view that the problem arises from both partners and that both are responsible for finding solutions.

In a triadic model, the family therapist assumes that the presenting problems result from the dyad's inability to resolve the conflict, which causes other family members to be drawn into it. A preteenage son who frustrates his father by refusing to do his homework and thus is performing badly at school may be doing so in alliance with his mother against his father, indirectly expressing her resentment at her husband's authoritarian behavior. The couple's original dyadic conflict has become a triadic one in which multiple interactions occur. Merely to develop a behavioral plan or contract for the boy to receive money or special television or videogame privileges in return for completing school assignments would miss the complex family interaction involved. Family therapists would look at the overall impact of the symptomatic behavior in context; the youngster may or may not be included in the entire treatment, which certainly would deal with the unspoken and unresolved husband–wife conflicts and the recruitment of their child to express or act out their tensions.

In the example just presented, the child's symptom (the school problem) maintains the family homeostasis but obscures the underlying and unexpressed set of family conflicts. Symptoms often function in maintaining family homeostasis; in this case, attention to the school problem keeps the parents from quarreling with each other and upsetting the family balance. If the school problem did not at some level sustain the family organization, then it would not be maintained. Thus, the systems-oriented therapist might ask: (1) Is the family member expressing, through symptoms, feelings that the other members are denying or not permitting themselves to experience? (2) What would happen to other family members if the identified patient were to become symptom free? (Wachtel, 2007). Symptoms thus serve a protective purpose or are stabilizing devices used in families. As a consequence, although they may not do so consciously, families may be invested in the maintenance of the symptom for homeostatic purposes.

Even though the idea that symptoms may serve a purpose in helping maintain family stability has been a mainstay of family therapy theory, critics argue that it suggests that families need a "sick" member and are willing to sacrifice that person for the sake of family well-being. *Narrative therapists* such as White (2007) reject the notion that a child's problems necessarily reflect more serious underlying family conflict. In White's view, families may be oppressed rather than protected by the symptomatic behavior. White's efforts are directed at getting all family members to unite in wresting control of their lives from the oppressive set of symptoms.

Family therapists usually are active participants with families and concentrate on current family functioning. They attempt to help members achieve lasting changes in the functioning of the family system, not merely superficial changes that will allow the system to return to its former tenuous balance. Watzlawick, Weakland, and Fisch (1974) distinguish between *first-order changes* (changes within the system that do not alter the organization of the system itself) and *second-order changes* (fundamental changes in a system's organization and function). The former term refers to specific differences that take place within the system, and the latter involves rule changes in the system—in effect, changing the system itself.

For example, the following is a first-order change. The Ryan parents were concerned with the repeated school absences of their son Billy; in an attempt to correct his behavior, they told him that any time they learned he was truant from school, he would be grounded the following Saturday.

The following is a second-order change. The Ryan parents were concerned with the repeated school absences of their son Billy. After consulting with a family therapist for several sessions, they realized that by struggling with Billy, they only encouraged his rebelliousness and thus were involved in sustaining the truant behavior. They also came to recognize that Billy's relationship with the school was truly his own and that they should back off from intruding. Attempting to change the rules and pull themselves out of the struggle, they told Billy that from now on, whether or not he went to school was between him and the school and that henceforth he would be responsible for his education.

As in these examples, a problematic family on their own may try first-order changes by attempting to impose what appear to be logical solutions to their problems. Assuming the problem to be monadic—the result of Billy's rebelliousness—they are employing negative feedback, attempting to do the opposite of what has been occurring. The family actually may make some changes in behavior for a brief period, but they are still governed by the same rules, the cease-fire is not likely to hold, and Billy will probably return to his school absences sooner or later.

Second-order changes, based on positive feedback, call for a change in the way the family organizes itself. Here the rules of the game must change, viewpoints must be altered, and old situations must be seen in a new light, providing a revised context in which new behavior patterns may emerge. Most people try to solve everyday problems by attempting first-order changes and repeating the same solutions in a self-perpetuating cycle, which only makes things worse. Especially with seriously troubled families, fundamental second-order changes in the system are necessary so that the family members can give different meanings to old feelings and old experiences.

Process of Psychotherapy

The Initial Contact

Family therapy begins when the client asks for help. One family member or a coalition of members begins the process by seeking help outside the family, thus acknowledging that a problem exists and that the family has been unsuccessful in its attempts to resolve the problem by themselves. While the caller is assessing whether the right person has been contacted, the therapist is forming tentative hypotheses about the family. How self-aware is the caller? What sort of impression is he or she trying to make? What other members are involved? Are they all willing to attend the initial session?

Initial contact, whether in person or by telephone, provides an opportunity for a mini-evaluation and also represents the therapist's first opportunity to enter into the family system. If the therapist is careful not to get maneuvered into taking sides, be engulfed by family anxiety, or become excessively sympathetic or angry with any member on the basis of what the caller is reporting, then he or she can establish the rules of the game for further family sessions.

The Initial Session

The family therapist usually encourages as many family members as possible to attend the first session. Entering the room, members are encouraged to sit where they wish; their chosen seating arrangement (such as mother and child close together, father sitting apart) offers the therapist an early clue about possible family alliances and coalitions. Welcoming all members separately as equally important participants, the therapist becomes aware that some members may need extra support and encouragement to participate.

Each person's view of the problem must be heard, as well as the first-order solutions the family has attempted. Observing family interactive patterns, particularly repetitive behavioral sequences that occur around a problem, the therapist tentatively begins to redefine the identified patient's symptoms as a family problem in which each member has a stake. Together, therapist and family explore whether they wish to continue working together and who will attend; if they choose to discontinue, outside referrals to other therapists are in order. If they agree to stay, treatment goals are defined.

Engaging the Family

Beginning with the initial session, the therapist tries to build a working alliance with the family, accommodating to their transactional style as well as assimilating their language patterns and manner of affective expression. The therapist tries to create an atmosphere in which each member feels supported and able to voice previously unexpressed or unexplored problems. By "joining" them, the therapist is letting them know they are understood and cared about and that in such a safe climate they can begin to confront divisive family issues.

Assessing Family Functioning

Like all forms of psychotherapy, family therapy involves some form of assessment, formal or informal, as the clinician attempts, early in the course of therapy, to learn more about the family in order to make more informed treatment decisions. (1) Is treatment for the entire family needed? (2) Who are the appropriate family members with whom to work? (3) What underlying interactive patterns fuel the family disturbance and lead to symptoms in one or more of its members? (4) What specific interventions will most effectively help this family? In later sessions, the therapist continues to revise hypotheses, basing subsequent interventions on assessments of the success of previous attempts to alter dysfunctional repetitive family patterns.

Cognitive-behavior family therapists are apt to make a careful, systematic behavioral analysis of the family's maladaptive behavioral patterns, often using questionnaires, pinpointing precisely which behaviors need to be altered and which events typically precede and follow that behavioral sequence. What exactly does the family mean by their child's "temper tantrums"? How often do these occur, under what circumstances, how long do they last, what specific reactions does each family member have, and what antecedent and subsequent events are associated with the outburst? The therapist tries to gauge the extent of the problem, the environmental cues that trigger the behavior, and the behaviors of various family members that maintain the problem. The assessment, continuously updated, helps the therapist plan interventions to reduce undesired or problematic behaviors.

Experiential family therapists spend less time on a formal family history. They work more in the here and now, helping families examine current interactive patterns with little regard for historical antecedents. Assessment is an informal, ongoing process indistinguishable from the therapeutic process itself. Such therapists attempt to provide families with an experience, using themselves as models to explore their own feelings and give voice to their own impulses. Carl Whitaker, an experiential therapist, insists on controlling the structure of the therapy at the start of treatment, making certain that the family is not successful in imposing its own definition of the upcoming therapeutic relationship and how it should proceed. Later, he believes, the family members must be encouraged to take responsibility for changing the nature of their relationships.

Many family therapists agree with Salvador Minuchin (1974) that they get a better sense of how families function by interacting with them over a period of time than from any formal assessment process. Therapists observe how subsystems carry out family tasks, how alliances and coalitions operate within the family, how flexible family rules are in the face of changing conditions, and how permeable the boundaries are within the family and between the family and the outside world. These observations help family therapists modify and discard hypotheses and adjust intervention strategies on the basis of refined appraisals of family functioning.

History Taking

Consistent with their theoretical leanings, object relations family therapists such as Scharff and Scharff (2006) contend that an examination of family history is essential to understanding current family functioning. Because they believe people carry attachments of their parental introjects (memories from childhood) into their current relationships, these therapists are especially interested in such matters as how and why marital partners chose each other. That choice is seen as seeking to rediscover, through the other person, the lost aspects of primary object attachments that had split off earlier in life. Similarly, contextual family therapists (Boszormenyi-Nagy, 1987) examine with their patients those interconnections from the past that bind families together in an effort to help them discover new ways of making fresh inputs into stagnant relationships.

Bowen (1978) began with a set of evaluation interviews aimed at clarifying the history of the presenting problem, especially trying to understand how the symptoms affect family functioning. He tried to assess the family's pattern of emotional functioning as well as the intensity of the emotional process of the symptomatic person. What is this family's relationship system like? How well differentiated are the various members? What are the current sources of stress, and how adaptive is the family?

Because Bowen believed dysfunction may result from family fusion extending back over generations, he probed for signs of poor differentiation from families of origin. To aid in the process, Bowen constructed a family *genogram*, a schematic diagram in the form of a family tree, usually including at least three generations, to trace recurring family behavior patterns. Hypotheses developed from the genogram, such as fusion–differentiation issues or emotional cutoffs from family, are used to better understand the underlying emotional processes connecting generations. Careful not to become drawn into the family's emotional system, Bowen used this information to coach family members to modify their relationships and especially to differentiate themselves from their families of origin.

Satir (1972) attempted to get families to think about the relevant concepts that formed the basis of their developing relationships by compiling a family life chronology for each family member. More than simply gathering historical facts, this represented an effort to help people understand how family ideology, values, and commitments had emerged in the family and influenced current family functioning. Later, she used the therapeutic technique of family reconstruction, guiding family members back through stages of their lives in an attempt to discover and unlock dysfunctional patterns from the past.

Structural and strategic family therapists pay less attention to family or individual histories, preferring to focus on the current family organization, coalitions, hierarchies, and so on. They are concerned with developing ways to change ongoing dysfunctional family patterns, and they typically show less concern for how these patterns historically emerged.

Social constructionists pay particular attention to how the various family members view their world rather than attempting to act as outside observers evaluating client responses. From their perspective, any preconceived views by the therapist of what constitutes a functional family fail to attend to the diversity inherent in today's pluralistic society. The personal outlook of each family member is privileged, and all such outlooks are valued equally.

Facilitating Change

Family therapists use several therapeutic techniques to alter family functioning.

1. *Reframing.* This technique involves relabeling problematic behavior by viewing it
    in a new, more positive light that emphasizes its good intention. (To an adolescent
    angry because he believes his mother is invading his privacy: "Your mother is con-
    cerned about your welfare and hasn't yet found the best way to help." Labeling her
    as wishing to do well for her son rather than agreeing with her son's perception that
    she does not trust him alters the context in which he perceives her behavior, thus
    inviting new responses from him to her behavior.) Reframing changes the meaning
    attributed to a behavior without changing the "facts" of the behavior itself. Strate-
    gic family therapists are most likely to use this technique because it enables them to
    help clients change the basis for their perceptions or interpretation of events. This
    altered perspective leads to a change in the family system as the problematic behav-
    ior becomes understood from a new perspective. Reframing, then, is a method for
    bringing about second-order changes in the family system.

2. *Therapeutic double-binds.* Another technique favored by strategic and systemic fam-
    ily therapists is putting the family in a *therapeutic double-bind* by directing family
    members to continue to manifest their presenting symptoms: obsessive people are
    asked to think about their problem for a specific period of time each day; quar-
    reling husbands and wives are instructed to indulge in and even exaggerate their
    fighting. By instructing family members to enact symptomatic behavior, the thera-
    pist is demanding that the presentation of the symptom, which they have claimed is
    "involuntary" and thus out of their control, be done voluntarily. Such paradoxical
    interventions are designed to evoke one of two reactions, either of which is sought
    by the therapist. If the patient complies, continuing to be symptomatic, there is the
    admission that the symptomatology is under voluntary control, not involuntary as
    claimed, and thus can be stopped. On the other hand, if the directive to continue
    the symptom is resisted, the symptom will be given up.

3. *Enactment.* Most likely to be used by structural family therapists, *enactments* are
    role-playing efforts to bring the outside family conflict into the session so that fam-
    ily members can demonstrate how they deal with it and the therapist can start to
    devise an intervention procedure for modifying their interaction and creating struc-
    tural changes in the family. Encouraged by the therapist, the family members act
    out their dysfunctional transactions rather than talking about them. This gives the
    therapist an opportunity to observe the process directly instead of relying on family
    members' reports of what occurs at home. Also, because of the immediacy of this
    approach, the therapist can intervene on the spot and witness the results of such
    interventions as they occur.

    Helping "unfreeze" family members from repetitive family interactions that end
    in conflict, the therapist has a chance to guide them in modifying the interactions.
    By introducing alternative solutions calling for structural changes in the family, the
    therapist can help the family create options for new behavior sequences. Treating
    the family of an anorectic adolescent, Minuchin (Minuchin et al., 1978) might ar-
    range to meet the family for the first session and bring in lunch, thus deliberately
    provoking an enactment around eating. Observing their struggles over their daugh-
    ter's refusal to eat, Minuchin can demonstrate that the parental subsystem is not
    working effectively. If parents begin to cooperate with one another in encouraging
    their daughter to eat, they form a stronger union. At the same time, the daughter is
    relieved of the too-powerful and destructive position she has been maintaining. The
    enactment impels the family to look at the system they have created together and to
    change the dysfunctional behavior displayed in the session.

4. *Family sculpting*. Rather than putting their feelings or attitudes toward one another into words, which may be difficult or threatening, family members each take a turn at being a "director"—that is, placing each of the other members in a physical arrangement in space. The result is often revealing of how the director perceives his or her place in the family, as well as that person's perception of what is being done to whom, by whom, and in what manner. Individual perceptions of family boundaries, alliances, roles, and subsystems are typically revealed, even if the director cannot, or will not, verbalize such perceptions. The resulting graphic picture of individual views of family life provides active, nonverbal depictions for other members to grasp. Because of its nonintellectualized way of putting feelings into action, family sculpting is especially suited to the experiential approach of Satir.

5. *Circular questioning*. This technique is often used by systemic family therapists (Boscolo et al., 1987) to focus attention on family connections rather than individual symptomatology. Each question posed to the family by the therapist addresses differences in different members' perceptions about the same events or relationships. By asking several members the same question regarding their attitudes toward those situations, the therapist is able to probe more deeply without being confrontational or interrogating the participants in the relationship. In this nonconfrontational therapeutic situation, the family can examine the origin of the underlying conflict. Advocates of this technique believe questioning is a therapeutic process that allows the family to untangle family problems by changing the ways they view their shared difficulties.

6. *Cognitive restructuring*. This technique of cognitive-behavior therapists, based on the idea that problematic behavior stems from maladaptive thought processes, tries to modify a client's perceptions of events to bring about behavioral change. Thus, a partner may have unrealistic expectations about a relationship and catastrophize a commonplace disagreement ("I am worthless"). As Ellis & Dryden (2007) suggests, it is the interpretation that causes havoc, not the quarrel itself. Cognitive restructuring can significantly modify perceptions ("It's upsetting that we're arguing, but that doesn't mean I'm a failure or our marriage is doomed").

7. *Miracle question*. In this solution-focused technique (de Shazer, 1991), clients are asked to consider what would occur if a miracle took place and, upon awakening in the morning, they found the problem they brought to therapy solved. Each family member is encouraged to speculate on how things would be different, how each would change his or her behavior, and what each would notice in the others. In this way, goals are identified and potential solutions revealed.

8. *Externalization*. In an effort to liberate a family from its dominating, problem-saturated story, narrative therapists employ the technique of externalization to help families separate the symptomatic member's identity from the problem for which they sought help. The problem is recast as residing outside the family (rather than implying an internal family deficiency or individual pathological condition) and as having a restraining influence over the life of each member of the family. Instead of focusing on what's wrong with the family or with one of its members, all are called on to unite to deal with this external and unwelcome story with a will of its own that dominates their lives. Thus, rather than the family concluding that "Mother is depressed" and therefore creating problems for the family, the symptom is personified as a separate, external, burdensome entity ("Depression is trying to control Mother's life"). By viewing the problem as outside themselves, the family is better able to collaborate in altering their way of thinking and developing new options for dealing with the problem rather than merely being mired in it. This technique has been used in the narrative treatment of Michael White (Epston & White 1990).

Mechanisms of Psychotherapy

Family therapists generally take an active, problem-solving approach with families. Typically, they are more interested in dealing with current dysfunctional interactive issues within the family than in uncovering or helping resolve individual intrapsychic problems from the past. Past family transactional patterns may be explored, but this is done to hone in on ongoing behavioral sequences or limiting belief systems that need changing rather than to reconstruct the past.

Depending on their specific emphases, family therapists may try to help clients achieve one or more of the following changes.

1. *Structural change*. Having assessed the effectiveness of a family's organizational structure and its ongoing transactional patterns, family therapists may actively challenge rigid, repetitive patterns that handicap optimal functioning of family members. Minuchin, for example, assumes the family is experiencing sufficient stress to overload the system's adaptive mechanisms, a situation that may be temporary because of failure to modify family rules to cope successfully with the demands of transitions. Helping families modify unworkable patterns creates an opportunity to adopt new rules and achieve realignments, clearer boundaries, and more flexible family interactions. Through restructuring, the family is helped to get back on track so that it will function more harmoniously and maximize the growth potential of each member.

2. *Behavioral change*. All family therapists try to help clients achieve desired behavioral changes, although they may go about it in differing ways. Strategic therapists focus treatment on the family's presenting problems: what they came in to have changed. Careful not to allow families to manipulate or subdue the therapist and therefore control the treatment, strategic therapy is highly directive, and practitioners devise strategies for alleviating the presenting problem rather than exploring its roots or hidden meanings. Through directives such as paradoxical interventions, they try to force the symptom bearer to abandon old dysfunctional behavior. Similarly, *systemic therapists* (the Milan approach of Selvini-Palazzoli and her colleagues) may assign tasks or rituals for the family to carry out between sessions. These typically are offered in paradoxical form and call for the performance of a task that challenges an outdated or rigid family rule. Behavioral change follows from the emotional experience gained by the family through enactment of the directive.

3. *Experiential change*. Therapists such as Satir, Whitaker, and Kempler believe that families need to feel and experience what previously was locked up. Their efforts are directed at growth-producing transactions in which therapists act as models of open communication, willing to explore and disclose their own feelings. Satir was especially intent on helping families learn more effective ways of communicating with one another and on teaching them to express what they are experiencing. Kempler also tries to help family members learn to ask for what they want from one another, thus facilitating self-exploration, risk taking, and spontaneity. Whitaker champions family members giving voice to underlying impulses and symbols. Because he sees all behavior as human experience and not as pathological, clients are challenged to establish new and more honest relationships, simultaneously maintaining healthy separation and personal autonomy. Emotionally focused couples therapists, too, help clients recognize how they have hidden their primary emotions or real feelings (say, fear of rejection) and instead have displayed defensive or coercive secondary emotions (anger or blaming when afraid). Their therapeutic efforts are directed at accessing and reprocessing the emotions underlying the clients' negative interactional sequences.

4. *Cognitive change.* Psychodynamically oriented family therapists are interested in providing client families with insight and understanding. Boszormenyi-Nagy stresses intergenerational issues, particularly how relationship patterns are passed on from generation to generation, influencing current individual and family functioning. By gaining awareness of one's "family ledger," a multigenerational accounting system of who, psychologically speaking, owes what to whom, clients can examine and correct old unsettled or unredressed accounts. Framo (1992) also helped clients gain insight into introjects reprojected onto current family members to compensate for unsatisfactory early object relations. He had clients meet with members of their families of origin for several sessions to discover what issues from the past they may have projected onto current members and also to have a corrective experience with parents and siblings. Narrative therapists, such as White, open up conversations about clients' values, beliefs, and purposes so that they have an opportunity to consider a wide range of choices and attach new meanings to their experiences.

APPLICATIONS

Who Can We Help?

Individual Problems

Therapists who adopt a family frame of reference attend primarily to client relationships. Even if they work with single individuals, they look for the *context* of problematic behavior in planning and executing their clinical interventions. Thus, for example, they might see a college student, far away from family, for individual sessions but continue to view his or her problems within a larger context in which faulty relations with others have helped create the presenting troublesome behavior and still maintain it. Should the parents arrive for a visit, they might join their child for a counseling session or two to provide clues regarding relationship difficulties within the family system and assist in their amelioration.

Intergenerational Problems

Family therapists frequently deal with parent–child issues such as adolescents in conflict with their parents or with society in general. Minuchin's structural approach might be adopted to help families, particularly at transition points in the family life cycle, adapt to changes and modify outdated rules. Here they are likely to try to strengthen the parental subsystem, more clearly define generational boundaries, and help the family craft new and more flexible rules to account for changing conditions as adolescence is reached. To cite an increasingly common example, families in which the children are raised in this country by foreign-born parents often present intergenerational conflicts that reflect differing values and attitudes. Intervention at the family level is often required if changes in the family system are to be achieved.

Marital Problems

Troubled marriages are common today, and many of the problems involving symptomatic behavior in a family member can be traced to efforts by the family to deal with parents in conflict. In addition to personal problems of one or both spouses that contribute to their unhappiness, certain key interpersonal difficulties are frequently present: ineffective communication patterns; sexual incompatibilities; anxiety over making or maintaining a long-term commitment; conflicts over money, in-laws, or children; physical abuse; or conflicts over power and control. These issues, repeated without resolution over a period of time, escalate the marital dissatisfaction of one or both partners, placing the marriage in jeopardy. Couples who enter therapy conjointly, before one or both conclude that the costs of staying together outweigh the benefits, are better able to salvage their relationship than if either or both seek individual psychotherapy.

Treatment

The Family Therapy Perspective

Family therapy represents an outlook regarding the origin and maintenance of symptomatic or problematic behavior, as well as a form of clinical intervention directed at changing dysfunctional aspects of the family system. Adopting such an outlook, the therapist may see the entire family together or may see various dyads, triads, or subsystems, depending on what aspects of the overall problem are being confronted by the therapist. Methods of treatment may vary, depending largely on the nature of the presenting problem, the therapist's theoretical outlook, and her or his personal style.

However, family therapy involves more than seeing distressed families as a unit or group. Simply gathering members together and continuing to treat the individuals separately but in a group setting fails to make the paradigm shift called for in treating relationships. Nor is it enough to perceive individual psychopathology as the therapist's central concern while acknowledging the importance of the family context in which such psychopathology developed. Rather, family therapy calls for viewing the amelioration of individual intrapsychic conflicts as secondary to improving overall family functioning.

To work in a family systems mode, the therapist must give up the passive, neutral, nonjudgmental stance developed with so much care in conventional individual psychotherapy. To help change family functioning, the therapist must become involved in the family's interpersonal processes (without losing balance or independence), must be supportive and nurturing at some points and challenging and demanding at others, must attend to (but not overidentify with) family members of different ages, and must move swiftly in and out of emotional involvements without losing track of family interactions and transactional patterns (Goldenberg & Goldenberg, 2008).

The *social constructionist family therapies*, which are currently gaining in popularity, place particular emphasis on the egalitarian, collaborative nature of therapist–family relationships. Family members are encouraged to examine the "stories" about themselves that they have lived by as together the therapist–family system searches for new and empowering ways to view and resolve client problems.

Indications and Contraindications

Family therapy is a valuable option in a therapist's repertoire of interventions, not a panacea for all psychological disturbances. However, it is clearly the treatment of choice for certain problems within the family. Wynne (1965) suggests that family therapy is particularly applicable to resolving relationship difficulties (e.g., parent–children, husband–wife), especially those to which all family members contribute, collusively or openly, consciously or unconsciously. Many family therapists go beyond Wynne's position, arguing that all psychological problems of individuals and of groups, such as families, ultimately are tied to systems issues and thus amenable to intervention at the family level.

Under what circumstances is family therapy contraindicated? In some cases, it may be too late to reverse the forces of fragmentation or too difficult to establish or maintain a therapeutic working relationship with the family because key members are unavailable or refuse to attend. Sometimes one seriously emotionally disturbed member may so dominate the family with malignant and destructive motives, violent or abusive be-havior, or paranoid ideation that working with the entire family becomes impossible, although some members of the family may continue to benefit from the family therapy perspective.

Length of Treatment

Family therapy may be brief or extended, depending on the nature and complexities of the problem, family resistance to its amelioration, and the goals of treatment. Changes that most benefit the entire family may not in every case be in the best interest of each family member, and some members may cling to old and familiar ways of dealing with one another. In general, however, family therapy tends to be relatively short term com-pared to most individual therapy. In some cases, as few as 10 sessions may eliminate problematic behavior; others may require 20 sessions or more for symptoms to subside. Strategic therapy quickly focuses on what problems require attention, and then the ther-apist devises a plan of action to change the family's dysfunctional patterns in order to eliminate the presenting problem. Structural approaches tend to be brief as the therapist joins the family, learns of its transactional patterns, and initiates changes in its structure leading to changes in behavior and symptom reduction in the identified patient. The object relations approach, on the other hand, is consistent with its psychoanalytic foun-dations and tends to take longer and deal with material from earlier in clients' lives.

Settings and Practitioners

Outpatient offices, school counselor settings, and inpatient hospital wards all provide places where family therapy may be carried out. No longer out of the mainstream of psychotherapy, where it dwelt in its earlier years, family therapy has been accepted by nearly all psychotherapists. Marital or couples therapy, now considered a part of the family therapy movement, has grown at an astonishing rate since the 1970s, as recently reflected in the American Board of Professional Psychology change of name to Ameri-can Board of Couples and Family Psychology.

Psychiatrists, psychologists, social workers, marriage and family counselors, and pas-toral counselors practice family therapy, although their training and emphases may be different. Three basic kinds of training settings exist today: degree-granting programs in family therapy, freestanding family therapy institutes, and university-affiliated programs.

Stages of Treatment

Most family therapists want to see the entire family for the initial session because overall family transactional patterns are most apparent when all participants are together. (Very young children, although they are encouraged to attend the first session, are not always expected to attend subsequent meetings unless they are an integral part of the problem.) After establishing contact with each member present and assessing the suitability of fam-ily sessions for them, therapists who are interested in family history, such as Bowen, may begin to construct a family genogram. Others, such as Haley, may proceed to negotiate with the family about precisely what problem it wishes to eliminate. Minuchin's opening move is to "join the family" by adopting an egalitarian role within it, making suggestions rather than issuing orders. He accommodates to the family's style of communicating, analyzes problems, and prepares a treatment plan. Solution-focused therapists, such as de Shazer, discourage clients from the start from speculating on the origin of a particular problem, preferring instead to engage in collaborative "solution talk"—that is, discuss-ing solutions they want to construct together.

The middle phase of family therapy is usually directed at helping family members redefine the presenting problem or symptomatic behavior in the identified patient as a relationship problem to be viewed within the family context. Here the family becomes the "patient," and together its members begin to recognize that all have contributed to the problem and that all must participate in changing ingrained family patterns. If therapy is successful, then families, guided by the therapist, typically begin to make relationship changes.

In the final stage of family therapy, families learn more effective coping skills and better ways to ask for what the members want from one another. Although they are unlikely to leave problem free, they have learned problem-solving techniques for resolving relationship issues together. Termination is easier in family therapy than in individual therapy because the family has developed an internal support system and has not become overdependent on an outsider. The presenting complaint or symptom has usually disappeared, and it is time for disengagement.

Evidence

The early family therapy pioneers, eager to create new and exciting techniques for treating families, did so largely without benefit of research support. In the ensuing years, a kind of cultural war developed between researchers and practitioners. The former contended that clinicians too readily adopted trendy techniques without pausing to evaluate their effectiveness beyond anecdotal data, and the latter maintained that the research being published often seemed trivial and unrelated to their daily work with people with real problems. That schism is now being addressed by a set of research investigations that are better integrated with the delivery of clinical services by family therapists (Sprenkle & Piercy, 2012).

Partly as a response to pressure from managed care companies to provide validated treatment and partly as a result of increased funding for such research from government agencies such as the National Institute of Mental Health, meaningful studies are being undertaken to determine which family therapy procedures offer empirically proven evidence-based techniques for a variety of family-related problems. Some practitioners, accustomed to relying on their individual experiences rather than on research data, are starting to find themselves forced by third-party payers such as HMOs to justify their interventions by supplying evidence-based data, when available, to receive reimbursement for their services.

Evidence-based practice refers to an attempt by researchers to assess the strengths and limitations of the current research data on psychotherapy. It has been shown that the treatment method, the therapist, and the treatment relationship are major contributors to the success or failure of therapy. It is less clear from research what the contributions of the system are to the process. There remain many disorders, problems, constellations, and family dysfunctions for which data are sparse (Levant, 2005). Therapeutic research efforts typically are directed at *process research* (what actually occurs during a therapy session that leads to a desired outcome) and *outcome research* (what specific therapeutic approaches work best with which specific problems). The former—and more elusive—approach attempts to operationally describe what actually transpires during a successful session. Is it the therapeutic alliance between a caring, competent therapist and a trusting family that builds confidence and offers hope? Is it insight or greater understanding, or perhaps a shared therapeutic experience with a therapist and other family members, that leads to change? Is it the promotion of constructive dialogue encouraged by the therapist or the blocking of negative affect? Are there certain intervention techniques that work best at an early stage of family treatment and others that are more effective during later stages (Christensen, Russell, Miller, & Peterson, 1998; Heatherington, Friedlander, & Greenberg, 2005)?

Linking certain within-session processes with outcome results would lead to developing an empirically validated map to follow, but unfortunately this is not yet available for most models, with some exceptions. *Emotion-focused couple therapy* integrates research with attachment theory and spells out manualized procedures to be followed. *Functional family therapy* successfully combines systems and behavioral theories with carefully designed research backing. In general, evidence-supported studies thus far have been carried out primarily on behavioral and cognitive-behavioral approaches. These brief methods, with specific goals, are not necessarily the most effective, but they are easier to test using traditional research methodology than are other treatment methods.

Outcome research in family therapy must deal with the same problems that hinder such research in individual therapy, with the additional burden of gauging and measuring the various interactions taking place within a large and complex unit (the family) that is in a continuous state of change. Some family members may change more than others, different members may change in different ways, and the researcher must take into account intrapsychic, relationship, communication, and ordinary group variables in measuring therapeutic effectiveness. In addition, attention must be paid to types of families, ethnic and social backgrounds, level of family functioning, and the like. In recent years, qualitative research methods, discovery oriented and open to multiple perspectives, have become more popular. Unlike more traditional quantitative research methodology, qualitative analyses are apt to rely on narrative reports in which the researcher makes subjective judgments about the meaning of outcome data. Qualitative research (based on case studies, in-depth interviewing, and document analysis) is especially useful for exploratory purposes, whereas quantitative techniques are more likely to be used in evaluating or justifying a set of experimental hypotheses.

Published outcome research today is likely to take one of two forms: *efficacy studies* or *effectiveness studies* (Pinsof & Wynne, 1995). The former, which are more common, attempt to determine whether a particular treatment works under ideal conditions such as those in a university or medical center. Interview methodology is standardized, treatment manuals are followed, clients are randomly assigned to treatment or no-treatment groups, independent evaluators measure outcomes, and so on. Effectiveness studies seek to determine whether the therapy works under normal, real-life conditions such as in a clinic, social agency, or private practice setting. Most research to date is of the efficacy kind and is encouraging, but it is not always translatable into specific recommendations for therapy under more real-world, consultation room conditions. Overall results from surveys (Shadash, Ragsdale, Glaser, & Montgomery, 1995), based mainly on efficacy studies, indicate that clients receiving family therapy did significantly better than untreated control-group clients.

The current thrust of outcome research continues to explore the relative advantages (in terms of costs, length of treatment, and extent of change) of alternative treatment interventions for clients with different specific psychological or behavioral difficulties. Brief strategic family therapy, multisystemic therapy, and functional family therapy have all been used for conduct disorders and have been shown to be effective, especially with high-risk adolescents, acting-out problems, and parent management training. All of these treatment approaches are based on social-learning principles. Psychoeducational programs for marital discord have also proved effective, as have programs for reducing relapse and rehospitalization in schizophrenic patients.

The recent move to develop evidence-based family therapy represents a need for the accountability increasingly expected of professionals in medicine, education, and elsewhere. Within psychotherapy, there is increasing commitment to establishing an empirically validated basis for delivering services that work (Goodheart, Kazdin, & Sternberg, 2006; Nathan & Gorman, 2007). Clinical interventions backed up by research are intended to make the therapeutic effort more efficient, thereby improving the quality of health care and reducing health-care costs (Reed & Eisman, 2006), a goal practitioners and researchers share. However laudable, the effort is costly and time consuming, requiring a homogeneous client population, clients randomly assigned to treatment or no-treatment groups, carefully trained and monitored therapists who follow manuals indicating how to proceed, with multiple goals that need to be measured, follow-up studies over extended periods to see whether gains made during therapy are maintained, and so on.

Westen, Novotny, and Thompson-Brenner (2004) argue that researchers might do better by focusing on what works in real-world practice than by devoting their efforts to designing new treatments and manuals from the laboratory. Although everyone would agree that integration of the best available research and clinical expertise represents an ideal solution, the fact remains that practitioners and clinical researchers operate from different perspectives. (The former are client focused and dedicated to improving services; the latter are science focused and dedicated to understanding and testing clinical phenomena.) Experienced practitioners are likely to be integrationists, taking the best from different approaches on the basis of their experience with what works with whom. Now that students are trained in academia on manualized techniques, they are more likely to be able to follow manualized guidelines in treating their clients. Recent research has focused on the methodological strengths and limitations of quantitative research. However, research methodology has improved and family therapy research is now comparable to research on any of the other intervention strategies (Sprenkle & Piercy, 2012).

Psychotherapy in a Multicultural World

The 21st century sees an increasing number of challenges for therapists in dealing with the issues stimulated by a multicultural population. As our consulting rooms fill with immigrant populations and the number of mixed-heritage families increases exponentially, we must attend to basic principles in working with "the Other"—people different from ourselves in certain meaningful ways.

It is critical for therapists to understand the movements taking place in the general society and in specific cultural environments. The therapist must be aware of his or her personal strengths and, most important, any weaknesses, biases, or prejudices (Axelson, 1999).

Understanding when consultation is appropriate or when referral is necessary also is important. Tuning in to the client's internal–external frame of reference allows the therapist to see the world through the client's eyes. Because the family therapist has other members of the family in the room for corroboration, it is easier to differentiate idiosyncratic behavior from culturally determined thinking or action. It is a logical step for the therapist to move from the family to the family of origin to the multicultural family genogram to a global perspective in family therapy (Ng, 2003). That perspective should include information on ethnic, economic, religious, and political factors influencing family dynamics.

An important part of the development of the family therapy movement was the corrective action that occurred as a result of the women's movement in the 1980s (McGoldrick, Giordano, & Garcia-Preto, 2005) when the issue of "white male privilege" became a hot topic in family therapy circles. The awareness that gender bias determined the way people were seen and treated in the consulting room was a radical new idea and set the stage for future attention to issues beyond gender such as race, social class, immigration status, and religion and their influence on the therapy process. Multicultural expertise was recognized as necessary to understand a variety of areas such as boundary lines, communication rules, displays of emotions, gender expectations, rituals, immigrant and refugee status, and the way these variables affect therapy.

The theory of social construction in family therapy has provided an additional philosophical foundation for multicultural counseling. The narrative model of Michael White takes a stand against the imposition of dominant culture imperatives. White recognizes the misuse of power as a central construct in the presentation of dominant culture, giving voice to local alternative knowledges (Epston & White, 1990). Clients are the experts on their own experiences. Working with diverse ethnic and racial groups, including Australian aborigines, White used a reflecting team approach that included the participation of traditional and indigenous healers from the community. White believed that therapy does not exist in a vacuum; emerging stories of change must be shared with the client's larger cultural community to be meaningful. This somewhat obviates the problem of the personal feelings of the therapist, supplanting them with the reflections of the community. This process can be translated on an international level and can incorporate the voices of other groups within the client's community. It is central to White's philosophy that the therapist collaborates with clients to determine which audience can best witness their stories of change.

CASE EXAMPLE

Background

Although the appearance of troublesome symptoms in a family member is typically what brings the concerned family to seek help, it is becoming increasingly common for couples or entire families to recognize they are having relationship problems that need to be addressed at the family level. Sometimes, too, therapy is seen as a preventive measure. For example, adults with children from previous marriages who are planning to marry may become concerned enough about the potential problems involved in forming a stepfamily that they consult a family therapist before marriage.

Frank, 38, and Michelle, 36, who are to marry within a week, referred themselves because they worried about whether they were prepared or had prepared their children sufficiently for stepfamily life. The therapist saw them for two sessions, which were largely devoted to discussing common problems they had anticipated along with suggestions for their amelioration. Neither Frank's two children, Ann, 13, and Lance, 12, nor Michelle's daughter, Jessica, 16, attended these sessions.

Michelle and Frank had known each other since childhood, although she later moved to a large city and he settled in a small rural community. Their families had been friends in the past, and Frank and Michelle had visited and corresponded with each other over the years. When they were in their early 20s, before Frank went away to graduate school, a romance blossomed between Frank and Michelle and they agreed to meet again as soon as feasible. When her father died unexpectedly, Michelle wrote to Frank, and when he did not respond, she was hurt and angry. On the rebound, she married Alex, who turned out to be a drug user, verbally abusive to Michelle, and chronically unemployed. They divorced after two years, and Michelle, now a single mother, began working to support herself and her daughter, Jessica. Mother and daughter became unusually close in the 12 years before Michelle and Frank met again.

Frank also had been married. Several years after his two children were born, his wife developed cancer and lingered for five years before dying. The children, although looked after by neighbors, were alone much of the time, with Ann, Frank's older child, assuming the parenting role for her younger brother, Lance. When Frank met Michelle again, their interrupted romance was rekindled, and in a high state of emotional intensity they decided to marry.

Problem

Approximately three months after their marriage, Frank and Michelle contacted the therapist again, describing increasing tension between their children. Needing a safe place to be heard (apparently no one was talking to anyone else), the children—Ann and Lance (Frank's) and Jessica (Michelle's)—eagerly agreed to attend family sessions. What emerged was a set of individual problems compounded by the stresses inherent in becoming an "instant family."

Frank, never able to earn much money and burdened by debts accumulated during his wife's long illness, was frustrated and guilty over his feeling that he was not an adequate provider for his family. Michelle was jealous over Frank's frequent business trips, in large part because she felt unattractive (the reason for her not marrying for 12 years). She feared Frank would find someone else and abandon her again, as she felt he had done earlier, at the time of her father's death. Highly stressed, she withdrew from her daughter, Jessica, for the first time. Losing her closeness to her mother, Jessica remained detached from her stepsiblings and became resentful of any attention Michelle paid to Frank. In an attempt to regain a sense of closeness, she turned to a surrogate family—a gang—and became a "tagger" at school (a graffiti writer involved in pregang activities). Ann and Lance, who had not had the time or a place to grieve over the loss of their mother, found Michelle unwilling to take over mothering them. Ann became bossy, quarrelsome, and demanding; Lance, at age 12, began to wet his bed.

In addition to these individual problems, they were having the usual stepfamily problems: stepsibling rivalries, difficulties of stepparents assuming parental roles, and boundary ambiguities.

Treatment

From a systems viewpoint, the family therapist is able to work with the entire family or see different combinations of people as needed. Everyone need not attend every session. However, retaining a consistent conceptual framework of the system is essential.

The therapist had "joined" the couple in the two initial sessions, and they felt comfortable returning after they married and were in trouble. While constructing a genogram, the therapist was careful to establish contact with each of the children, focusing attention whenever she could on their evolving relationships. Recognizing that parent–child attachments preceded the marriage relationship, she tried to help them as a group develop loyalties to the new family. Boundary issues were especially important because they lived in a small house with little privacy, and the children often intruded on the parental dyad.

When seeing the couple together without the children present, the therapist tried to strengthen their parental subsystem by helping them learn how to support one another and share child-rearing tasks. (Each had continued to take primary responsibility for his or her own offspring in the early months of the marriage.) Jealousy issues were discussed, and the therapist suggested they needed a "honeymoon" period that they had never had. With the therapist's encouragement, the children stayed with relatives while their parents spent time alone with each other.

After they returned for counseling, Frank's concerns over not being a better provider were discussed. He and Michelle considered alternative strategies for increasing his income and helping more around the house. Michelle, still working, felt less exhausted and thus better able to give more of herself to the children. Frank and Lance agreed to participate in a self-help behavioral program aimed at eliminating bed-wetting, thus strengthening their closeness to one another. As Lance's problem subsided, the entire family felt relieved of the mess and smell associated with the bed-wetting.

The therapist decided to see Ann by herself for one session, giving her the feeling she was special. Allowed to be a young girl in therapy and temporarily relieved of her job as a parent to Lance, she became more agreeable and reached outside the family to make friends. She and Lance had one additional session (with their father), grieving over the loss of their mother. Michelle and Jessica needed two sessions together to work out their mother–daughter adolescent issues as well as Jessica's school problems.

Follow-Up

Approximately 12 sessions were held. At first the sessions took place weekly; they were later held biweekly and then took place at 3-month intervals. By the end of a year, the family had become better integrated and more functional. Frank had been promoted at work, and the family had rented a larger house, easing the problems brought about by space limitations. Lance's bed-wetting had stopped, and he and Ann felt closer to Michelle and Jessica. Ann, relieved of the burden of acting older than her years, enjoyed being an adolescent and became involved in school plays. Jessica still had some academic problems but had broken away from the gang and was preparing to go to a neighboring city to attend a junior college.

The family contacted the therapist five times over the next 3 years. Each time, they were able to identify the dyad or triad stuck in a dysfunctional sequence for which they needed help. And each time, a single session seemed to get them back on track.

SUMMARY

Family therapy, which originated in the 1950s, turned its attention away from individual intrapsychic problems and placed the locus of pathology on dysfunctional transactional patterns within a family. From this new perspective, families are viewed as systems with members operating within a relationship network and by means of feedback loops aimed at maintaining homeostasis. Growing out of research aimed at understanding communication patterns in the families of schizophrenics, family therapy later broadened its focus to include therapeutic interventions with a variety of family problems. These therapeutic endeavors are directed at changing repetitive maladaptive or problematic sequences within the system. Early cybernetic views of the family as a psychosocial system have been augmented by the postmodern view that rejects the notion of an objectively knowable world, arguing in favor of multiple views of reality.

Symptomatic or problematic behavior in a family member is viewed as signaling family disequilibrium. Symptoms arise from and are maintained by current, ongoing family transactions. Viewing causality in circular rather than linear terms, the family therapist focuses on repetitive behavioral sequences between members that are self-perpetuating and self-defeating. Family belief systems also are scrutinized as self-limiting.

Therapeutic intervention may take several forms, including approaches that assess the impact of the past on current family functioning (object relations, contextual), those largely concerned with individual family members' growth (experiential), those that focus on family structure and processes (structural) or transgenerational issues, those heavily influenced by cognitive-behavioral perspectives (strategic, behavioral), and those that emphasize dialogue in which clients examine the meaning and organization they bring to their life experiences (social constructionist and narrative therapies). All attend particularly to the context of people's lives in which dysfunction originates and can be ameliorated.

Interest in family systems theory and concomitant interventions will probably continue to grow in the coming years. The stress on families precipitated by the lack of models or strategies for dealing with divorce, remarriage, alternative lifestyles, or acculturation in immigrant families is likely to increase the demand for professional help at a family level.

Consumers and cost-containment managers will utilize family therapy even more often in the future because it is a relatively short-term procedure, solution oriented and dealing with real and immediate problems. Moreover, it feels accessible to families with relationship problems who don't wish to be perceived as pathological. Its preventive quality—helping people learn more effective communication and problem-solving skills to head off future crises—is attractive not only to families but also to practitioners of family medicine, pediatricians, and other primary care physicians to whom troubled people turn. As the field develops in both its research and clinical endeavors, it will better identify specific techniques for treating different types of families at significant points in their life cycles.

Counseling CourseMate Website:

See this text's Counseling CourseMate website at www.cengagebrain.com for learning tools such as chapter quizzing, videos, glossary flashcards, and more.

ANNOTATED BIBLIOGRAPHY

Goldenberg, H., & Goldenberg, I. (2008). *Family therapy: An overview* (7th ed.). Pacific Grove, CA: Brooks/Cole.
This text describes the major theories and the assessment and intervention techniques of family therapy. Systems theory and family life-cycle issues are outlined, a historical discussion of the field's development is included, and research, training, and ethical and professional issues are considered.

Goodheart, C. D., Kazdin, A. E., & Sternberg, R. J. (2006). *Evidence-based psychotherapy: Where practice and research meet*. Washington, DC: American Psychological Association.
This timely text outlines the current controversies surrounding the issue of developing an evidence-based body of knowledge to support psychotherapy approaches.

Haley, J., & Richeport-Haley, M. (2007). *Directive family therapy*. New York: Haworth.
This text provides practitioners with directive family techniques to identify client problems, formulate treatment plans, and then carry them out to achieve lasting therapeutic change. Using case examples, this text shows problem-solving directives in action.

McGoldrick, M., & Hardy, K. V. (Eds.). (2008). *Re-visioning family therapy: Race, culture, and gender in clinical practice* (2nd ed.). New York: Guilford Press.
These authors have brought together several dozen experts to provide detailed information about a wide variety of racial and ethnic groupings. Common family patterns are delineated for each group, and suggestions are offered for effective family interventions tied to the unique aspects of each set.

Sue, D. W., & Sue, D. (2007). *Counseling the culturally diverse: Theory and practice* (5th ed.). New York John Wiley.
Authors Derald Wing Sue and David Sue define and analyze the meaning of diversity and multiculturalism, covering racial and ethnic minority groups as well as multiracial individuals, women, gays and lesbians, the elderly, and those with disabilities. This book is up to date and includes new research and a discussion of future direction in the field.

Sexton, T. L., Weeks, G. R., & Robbins, M. S. (Eds.). (2003). *The science and practice of working with families and couples*. New York, Guilford Press.
This useful, up-to-date handbook is filled with discussions of the foundation and theories of family therapy and its application to special populations for whom family therapy is recommended. A large section is devoted to issues surrounding evidence-based couple and family intervention programs.

CASE READINGS

Family therapy trainers commonly make use of videotapes and DVDs of master therapists demonstrating their techniques with real families because these sources provide a richer sense of the emotional intensity of family sessions than is available from case readings alone. Tapes are available to rent or purchase from the Ackerman Institute in New York, the Philadelphia Child Guidance Center, the Georgetown University Family Center, the Family Institute of Washington, D.C., and many other training establishments.

The following three texts deal largely with descriptions and analyses of family therapy from the vantage point of leading practitioners.

Grove, D. R., & Haley, J. (1993). *Conversations on therapy: Popular problems and uncommon solutions*. New York: Norton.
Grove and Haley, apprentice and master therapist, respectively, offer a question-and-answer conversation regarding specific cases seen at the Family Therapy Institute of

Washington, D.C., and together they devise strategies for intervening effectively in problematic situations.

Napier, A. Y., & Whitaker, C. A. (1978). *The family crucible.* New York: Harper & Row.

This text gives a full account of cotherapy with one family, including both parents; a suicidal, runaway, teenage daughter; an adolescent son; and a six-year-old daughter.

Satir, V. M., & Baldwin, M. (1983). *Satir step by step: A guide to creative change in families.* Palo Alto, CA: Science and Behavior Books.

Using double columns, Satir presents a transcript of a session accompanied by an explanation for each intervention.

Two recent casebooks contain descriptions offered by family therapists with a variety of viewpoints. Both effectively convey what transpires as family therapists attempt to put theory into practice.

Dattilio, F. (Ed.). (1998). *Case studies in couple and family therapy: Systemic and cognitive perspectives.* New York: Guilford Press.

Leading figures from each school of family therapy briefly summarize their theoretical positions, followed by detailed case studies of actual sessions. The editor offers comments throughout in an attempt to integrate

cognitive-behavior therapy with a variety of current family therapy systems.

Golden, L. B. (2003). *Case studies in marriage and family therapy* (2nd ed.). Englewood Cliffs, NJ: Prentice Hall.

This text contains 19 case studies that highlight the major approaches taken to family therapy. Seasoned marriage and family therapists share real-life session data and explore their own decision making and personal experiences.

Other valuable works include the following:

Oxford, L. K., & Wiener, D. J. (2003). Rescripting family dramas using psychodramatic methods. In D. J. Wiener & L. K. Oxford (Eds.), *Action therapy with families and groups: Using creative arts improvisation in clinical practice* (pp. 45–74). Washington, DC: American Psychological Association. [Reprinted in D. Wedding & R. J. Corsini (Eds.). (2008). *Case Studies in Psychotherapy* (5th ed.). Belmont, CA: Brooks/Cole.]

This recent case illustrates how the techniques of psychodrama can be applied in a family therapy context.

Papp, P. (1982). The daughter who said no. In P. Papp, *The process of change* (pp. 67–120). New York: Guilford. [Reprinted in D. Wedding & R. J. Corsini (Eds.). (2013). *Case studies in psychotherapy* (7th ed.). Belmont, CA: Brooks/Cole.]

This classic case illustrates the way a master family therapist treats a young woman with anorexia nervosa.

REFERENCES

Ackerman, N. W. (1958). *The psychodynamics of family life.* New York: Basic Books.

Anderson, H. D. (1997). *Conversation, language, and possibilities: A postmodern approach to therapy.* New York: HarperCollins.

Anderson, H. D., & Gehart, D. R. (2006). *Collaborative therapy: Relationships and conversations that make a difference.* New York: Routledge.

Axelson, J. A. (1999). *Counseling and development in multicultural society* (3rd ed.). Pacific Grove, CA: Brooks/Cole.

Barnett, R. C., & Hyde, J. S. (2001). Women, men, work, family. *American Psychologist, 56,* 781–796.

Batcson, G. (1972). *Steps to an ecology of mind.* New York: Dutton.

Bateson, G., Jackson, D. D., Haley, J., & Weakland, J. (1956). Towards a theory of schizophrenia. *Behavioral Science, 1,* 251–264.

Beck, A. T., & Weishaar, M. (2007). Cognitive therapy. In R. J. Corsini & D. Wedding (Eds.), *Current psychotherapies* (8th ed., pp. 263–294). Belmont, CA: Brooks/Cole.

Becvar, D. S. (2003). Eras of epistemology: A survey of family therapy thinking and theorizing. In T. L. Sexton, G. R. Weeks, & M. S. Robbins (Eds.), *Handbook of family therapy: The science and practice of working with families and couples* (pp. 3–20). New York: Brunner-Routledge.

Bell, J. E. (1961). *Family group therapy.* Public Health Monograph No. 64. Washington, DC: U.S. Government Printing Office.

Berg, I. K., Dolan, Y., & Trepper, T. (Eds.). (2008). *More than miracles: The state of the art of solution-focused brief therapy.* New York: Haworth.

Bertalanffy, L. von. (1968). *General systems theory: Foundation, development, applications.* New York: Braziller.

Boscolo, L., Cecchin, G., Hoffman, L., & Penn, P. (1987). *Milan systemic family therapy: Conversations in theory and practice.* New York: Basic Books.

Boszormenyi-Nagy, I. (1987). *Foundations of contextual therapy: Collected papers of Ivan Boszormenyi-Nagy.* New York: Brunner/Mazel.

Bowen, M. (1960). A family concept of schizophrenia. In D. D. Jackson (Ed.), *The etiology of schizophrenia* (pp. 346–373). New York: Basic Books.

Bowen, M. (1978). *Family therapy in clinical practice.* New York: Jason Aronson.

Cardona, J. R. P., Domenech-Rodriguez, M., Forgatch, M., Sullivan, C., Bybee, D., Holtrop, K., Escobar-Chew, A. R., Tams, L., Dates, B., Bernal, G., (2012). Culturally adapting an evidence-based parenting intervention for Latino immigrants: The need to integrate fidelity and cultural relevance. *Family Process, 51,* 56–72.

Carter, B., & McGoldrick, M. (2005). *The expanded family life cycle: Individual, family, and social perspectives* (3rd ed.). Boston: Allyn & Bacon.

Christensen, L. L., Russell, C. S., Miller, R. B., & Peterson, C. M. (1998). The process of change in couple therapy: A qualitative investigation. *Journal of Marital and Family Therapy, 24,* 177–188.

Dattilio, F. M., & Epstein, N. B. (2005). Introduction to the special section: The role of cognitive-behavioral interventions in couple and family therapy. *Journal of Marital and Family Therapy, 31*, 7–13.

de Shazer, S. (1991). *Putting differences to work.* New York: Norton.

Ellis, A., & Dryden, W. (2007). *The practice of rational emotive behavior therapy* (2nd ed.). Thousand Oaks, CA: Sage.

Epston, D., & White, M. (1990). *Narrative means to therapeutic ends.* Adelaide, Australia: Dulwich Centre.

Falicov, C. J. (2000). *Latino families in therapy: A guide to multicultural practice.* New York: Guilford Press.

Framo, J. L. (1992). *Family-of-origin therapy: An intergenerational approach.* New York Brunner Mazel Inc.

Gergen, K. J. (1999). *An invitation to social construction.* Thousand Oaks, CA: Sage.

Goldenberg, H., & Goldenberg, I. (2008). *Family therapy: An overview* (7th ed.). Pacific Grove, CA: Brooks/Cole.

Goldenberg, I., & Goldenberg, H. (2013). *Family therapy: An Overview* (8th ed.). Pacific Grove, CA: Brooks/Cole.

Goodheart, C. D., Kazdin, A. E., & Sternberg, R. J. (2006). *Evidence-based psychotherapy: Where practice and research meet.* Washington, DC: American Psychological Association.

Haley, J. (1996). *Learning and teaching therapy.* New York: Guilford Press.

Heatherington, L., Friedlander, M. L., & Greenberg, L. (2005). Change process research in couple and family therapy: Methodological challenges and opportunities. *Journal of Family Psychology, 19*, 18–27.

Henggeler, S. W., Schoenwald, S. K., Borduin, C. M., Rowland, M. D., & Cunningham, P. B. (2009). *Multisystemic therapy for antisocial behavior in children and adolescents.* New York: Guillford Press.

Hughes, D. (2007). *Attachment-focused family therapy.* New York: Norton.

Imber-Black, E., Roberts, J., & Alva Whiting, R. (2003). *Rituals in families and family therapy* (Rev. ed.). New York: Norton.

Jackson, D. D. (1965). Family rules: Marital quid pro quo. *Archives of General Psychiatry, 12*, 589–594.

Furrow, J., Johnson, S., & Bradley, B. (2011). *Emotionally focused casebook: New directions in treating couples.* New York: Routledge, Taylor & Francis Group.

Kempler, W. (1991). *Experiential psychotherapy with families.* New York: Brunner/Mazel.

Kliman, J. (1999). Social class and the family life cycle. In B. Carter & M. McGoldridge, *The expanded family life cycle: Individual, family and social perspectives* (pp. 1–24). Boston: Allyn & Bacon.

Kuhn, T. (1970). *The structure of scientific revolutions.* Chicago: University of Chicago Press.

Laing, R. D. (1965). Mystification, confusion, and conflict. In I. Boszormenyi-Nagy & J. L. Framo (Eds.), *Intensive family therapy: Theoretical and practical aspects* (pp. 343–362). New York: Harper & Row.

Lebow, J. (1997). The integrative revolution in couple and family therapy. *Family Process, 36*, 1–17.

Levant, R. F. (2005, July). *Report of the 2005 Presidential Task Force on Evidence-Based Practice.* Washington, DC: American Psychological Association.

Lidz, T., Cornelison, A., Fleck, S., & Terry, D. (1957). The intrafamilial environment of schizophrenic patients: II. Marital schism and marital skew. *American Journal of Psychiatry, 114*, 241–248.

Madsen, C. W. (2007). *Collaborative therapy with multistressed families* (2nd ed.). New York: Guilford Press.

McGoldrick, M., Giordano, J., & Garcia-Preto, N. (Eds.). (2005). *Ethnicity and family therapy* (3rd ed.). New York: Guilford Press.

McGoldrick, M., & Hardy, K. V. (Eds.). (2008). *Re-visioning family therapy: Race, culture, and gender in clinical practice* (2nd ed.). New York: Guilford Press.

Minuchin, S. (1974). *Families and family therapy.* Cambridge, MA: Harvard University Press.

Minuchin, S., Montalvo, B., Guerney, B. G., Jr., Rosman, B. L., & Schumer, F. (1967). *Families of the slums: An exploration of their structure and treatment.* New York: Basic Books.

Minuchin, S., Nichols, M. P., & Lee, W. Y. (2006). *Assessing families and couples: From symptom to system.* Boston: Allyn & Bacon.

Minuchin, S., Rosman, B. L., & Baker, L. (1978). *Psychosomatic families: Anorexia nervosa in context.* Cambridge, MA: Harvard University Press.

Nathan, P. E., & Gorman, J. M. (2007). *A guide to treatment that works* (3rd ed.). London: Oxford University Press.

Nichols, M. P. (1987). *The self in the system: Expanding the limits of family therapy.* New York: Brunner/Mazel.

Ng, K. S. (2003). *Global perspectives in family therapy: Development, practice, trends.* New York: Brunner-Routledge.

Pelavin, E., & Moskowitz-Sweet, G. (2009). *From common sense to cybersense: A families guide to prevention and response.* Unpublished manuscript, Palo Alto.

Pinsof, W. M., & Wynne, L. C. (1995). The effectiveness and efficacy of marital and family therapy: Introduction to the special issue. *Journal of Marital and Family Therapy, 21*, 341–343.

Prochaska, J. O., & Norcross, J. C. (1999). *Systems of psychotherapy: A transtheoretical analysis* (4th ed.). Pacific Grove, CA: Brooks/Cole.

Reed, G. M., & Eisman, E. J. (2006). Uses and misuses of evidence: Managed care, treatment guidelines, and outcome measurements in professional practice. In C. D. Goodheart, A. E. Kazdin, & R. J. Sternberg (Eds.), *Evidence-based psychotherapy: Where practice and research meet* (pp. 13–36). Washington, DC: American Psychological Association.

Robbins, M. S., Mayorga, C. C., & Szapocznik, J. (2003). The ecosystemic "lens" to understanding family functioning. In T. L. Sexton, G. R. Weeks, & M. S. Robbins (Eds.), *Handbook of family therapy: The science and practice of working with families and couples* (pp. 23–40). New York: Brunner-Routledge.

Satir, V. (1972). *Peoplemaking*. Palo Alto, CA: Science and Behavior Books.

Scharff, J. S., & Scharff, D. E. (2006). *The primer of object relations* (2nd ed.). New York: Jason Aronson.

Selvini-Palazzoli, M. (1986). Towards a general model of psychotic games. *Journal of Marital and Family Therapy, 12,* 339–349.

Selvini-Palazzoli, M., Boscolo, L., Cecchin, G. F., & Prata, G. (1978). *Paradox and counterparadox: A new model in the therapy of the family schizophrenic transaction*. New York: Jason Aronson.

Sexton, T. L., & Alexander, J. F. (2002). Functional family therapy: An empirically supported, family-based intervention model for at-risk adolescents and their families. In T. Patterson (Ed). *Comprehensive handbook of psychotherapy: Vol. II. Cognitive, behavioral and functional approaches* (pp. 117–140). New York: John Wiley.

Shadash, W. R., Ragsdale, K., Glaser, R. R., & Montgomery, L. M. (1995). The efficacy and effectiveness of marital and family therapy: A perspective from meta-analysis. *Journal of Marital and Family Therapy, 21,* 345–360.

Sprenkle, D. H., & Piercy, F. P. (Eds.). (2012). *Research methods in family therapy* (2nd ed.). New York: Guilford Press.

Sue, D. W., & Sue, D. (2007). *Counseling the culturally diverse: Theory and practice* (5th ed.). New York John Wiley.

Sullivan, H. S. (1953). *The interpersonal theory of psychiatry*. New York: Norton.

Wachtel, P. L. (2007). *Relational theory and the practice of psychotherapy*. New York: Guillford Press.

Wachtel, E. E., & Wachtel, P. L. (1986). *Family dynamics in individual psychotherapy: A guide to clinical strategies*. New York: Guilford Press.

Walsh, F. (2003). Strengths forged through adversity. In F. Walsh (Ed.), *Normal family processes: Growing diversity and complexity* (3rd ed., pp. 356–377). New York: Guilford Press.

Walsh, F. (2009). *Spiritual resources in family therapy* (2nd ed.). New York: Guilford Press.

Watzlawick, P., Weakland, J. H., & Fisch, R. (1974). *Change: Principles of problem formation and problem resolution*. New York: Norton.

Westen, D., Novotny, C. M., & Thompson-Brenner, H. (2004). Empirical status of empirically supported psychotherapies: Assumptions, findings, and reporting in controlled clinical trials. *Psychological Bulletin, 130,* 631–663.

Whitaker, C. A., & Bumberry, W. M. (1988). *Dancing with a family: A symbolic–experiential approach*. New York: Brunner/Mazel.

White, M. (1995). *Re-authoring lives: Interviews and essays*. Adelaide, South Australia: Dulwich Centre Publications.

White, M. (2007). *Maps of narrative practice*. New York: Norton.

Wiener, N. (1948). Cybernetics. *Scientific American, 179*(5), 14–18.

Wills, F. (2009). *Beck's cognitive therapy: Distinctive features*. New York: Routledge.

Wynne, L. C. (1965). Some indications and contraindications for exploratory family therapy. In I. Boszormenyi-Nagy & J. L. Framo (Eds.), *Intensive family therapy: Theoretical and practical aspects* (pp. 289–322). New York: Harper & Row.

Wynne, L. C., Ryckoff, I. M., Day, J., & Hirsch, S. I. (1958). Pseudomutuality in the family relationships of schizophrenics. *Psychiatry, 21,* 205–220.

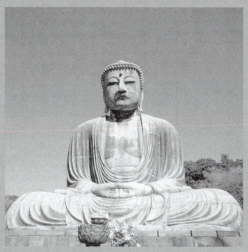

12 | CONTEMPLATIVE PSYCHOTHERAPIES

Roger Walsh

OVERVIEW

Something remarkable is happening. After centuries of separate development, two great disciplines—both designed to explore, heal, and enhance the human mind—are finally meeting. History is being made and psychology changed as contemplative and traditional Western therapies finally meet, mingle, challenge, and enrich each other. In just a few decades, contemplative therapies have gone from marginal practices to the most intensively researched psychotherapies. For thousands of years, millions of people have practiced contemplation, and now these practices are benefiting Western therapists, clients, and the public.

Basic Concepts

Varieties of Practices

Contemplative practices such as contemplation, meditation, and yoga are found worldwide. They occur in most cultures and are part of every major religion. They include the traditional practices of Taoist and Hindu yogas, Confucian quiet sitting, Buddhist meditations, Jewish Tzeruf, Islamic Sufi Zikr, and Christian contemplation. In their traditional settings, contemplative practices are usually part of a larger worldview and way of life. For example, they are usually framed and explained by a corresponding psychology and philosophy such as Buddhist psychology or yogic philosophy. They are also integrated with other practices intended to optimize well-being such as supportive exercises (e.g., yogic breathing) and lifestyles (e.g., diet, ethics, time in nature, and service to others). Originally practiced primarily for religious and spiritual goals, they are now widely used for their many psychological and psychosomatic benefits. The terms *meditation* and *contemplation* are both used in several ways but are treated here as synonymous.

There are many kinds of contemplative and meditative practices. The most researched are yogic transcendental meditation (TM) and Buddhist mindfulness, which is also known as *vipassana* (clear seeing) or insight meditation. TM is a mantra (inner sound) practice that begins by directing attention to a repetitive mantra, which then allows the mind to settle into a clear, peaceful state. Mindfulness meditation cultivates clear sensitive awareness by carefully investigating each experience, and this results in deep insight into the mind and oneself. Mindful movement practices include Indian yoga and Chinese tai chi and qigong. Dozens of other meditations await research.

Definitions

Despite many variations between practices, common themes are evident, and these commonalities suggest the following definitions.

The term *meditation* refers to a family of introspective self-regulation practices that train attention and perception in order to bring mental processes under greater voluntary control and to foster mental capacities, well-being, and maturation.

The term *yoga* refers to a family of multimodal practices with aims similar to those of meditation. However, yogas are more inclusive disciplines that, in addition to meditation, can encompass ethics, lifestyle, body postures, diet, breath control, study, and intellectual analysis. In the West, the best-known yogic practices are the body postures, but these are only one aspect of a far more comprehensive training that was the first integrative psychotherapy.

Central Assumptions

Contemplative psychologies are based on a "good-news, bad-news" understanding of the mind.

- The *bad news* is that our ordinary state of mind is considerably less controlled, developed, and functional than we usually recognize. The result is significant unnecessary suffering.

- The *good news* is that we can train and develop our minds, even far beyond conventional levels. The results include enhanced mental capacities, well-being, and maturity.

This good news and bad news can be expanded into five central assumptions underlying contemplative therapies:

1. Our usual state of mind is significantly uncontrolled, underdeveloped, and dysfunctional.

2. The full extent of this "normal" dysfunction goes unrecognized for two reasons:
   - First, we all share this dysfunction, so it seems "normal."
   - Second, this dysfunction is *self-masking*. Just as psychological defenses distort awareness and conceal themselves, so too our usual state of psychological dysfunction (which is partly constituted by defenses) distorts awareness and conceals itself.

3. Psychological suffering is largely a function of this mental dysfunction.

4. Contemplative practices can be used to train the mind and thereby reduce dysfunction, enhance well-being, and develop exceptional capacities such as heightened calm, concentration, insight, and joy.

5. These claims can be tested for oneself.

A Developmental Perspective

Developmental psychology helps us understand contemplative goals and compare them with other therapies. Developmental psychologists currently recognize three broad levels of development: prepersonal, personal, and transpersonal, which are also called *preconventional, conventional,* and *postconventional* (Wilber, 2000a). We are born into the prepersonal, preconventional stage in which we have no coherent sense of self or of social conventions. As we grow, we gradually acculturate and mature to the personal and conventional stage. Here we establish a more coherent sense of self and largely accept the conventional cultural assumptions about ourselves and the world. Until recently, this conventional stage was assumed to be the peak of our developmental potential.

Yet for centuries, philosophers and sages have lamented the limitations of conventional development and pointed to further possibilities. Their concern was that at the conventional stage our usual state of mind is limited, distorted, and unclear in ways we don't usually recognize. Plato famously compared our usual mental state to living in a darkened cave; Asian contemplative psychologies describe it as illusory and dreamlike; and some Western psychologists call it a *consensus trance* or a *shared hypnosis* (Tart, 1986).

Likewise, existentialists describe conventional ways of life as unnecessarily superficial, defensive, and inauthentic. Too often, they say, we accept cultural beliefs and values unquestioningly, follow fads and fashions unreflectively, and avoid facing the deeper questions about life and ourselves. The tragic result is a semiconscious submersion in "herd mentality" in which we fail to live fully or authentically (Yalom & Josselson, 2013). Unfortunately, much of contemporary culture—with its commercial superficiality and constant distraction—reinforces this herd mentality and collective semiconsciousness. According to Abraham Maslow (1968), a founder of humanistic and transpersonal psychology, the result is that the "normal adjustment of the average, common sense, well-adjusted [person] implies a continued successful rejection of much of the depths of human nature . . ." (p. 142).

This is not a new idea. In fact, Maslow was echoing the words of numerous contemplatives who for centuries have claimed that, as yoga puts it, "You are not fully grown up, there are levels left undeveloped because unattended" (Nisargadatta, 1973, p. 40). Likewise, for Jewish contemplatives:

> One's normal mode of thinking is referred to the "mentality of childhood" (*mochin de-katnuth*). More advanced modes of thought and states of consciousness, on the other hand, are referred to as the "mentality of adulthood" (*mochin de-gadluth*). One learns these methods of "adult thought" through meditation. (Kaplan, 1985, p. 8)

These diverse views—from East and West, from philosophy and religion, and now from psychology—all converge on a startling conclusion of enormous importance: *We are only half-grown and half-awake.* Development proceeds from preconventional to conventional but then usually grinds to a semiconscious halt. What we call *normality* may be a form of collective developmental arrest! As William James (1911/1924), America's most famous psychologist, put it, "Compared to what we ought to be, we are only half awake" (p. 237).

Fortunately, there is also good news: Further development is possible. The conventional stage can be a stepping stone rather than a stopping place. Such has long been the claim of contemplative psychologies, a claim now supported by developmental researchers who recognize postconventional stages of motivation, cognition, moral thinking, and the sense of self (Maslow, 1971; Wilber, 1999, 2000b).

With this developmental background, we can now compare psychotherapeutic systems in two ways. The first is according to the developmental levels they aim to foster. For example, most psychotherapies aim to foster healthy conventional development. Meditative therapies, on the other hand, though capable of facilitating conventional adjustment, traditionally aim for postconventional growth.

A related idea is that psychological systems address three major levels of concerns: pathological, existential, and transpersonal. As this book demonstrates, Western professionals have devised sophisticated techniques for alleviating pathologies and have begun to focus on the existential issues—such as meaning, isolation, and death—that all of us inevitably face (Yalom, 2002; Yalom & Josselson, 2013). However, only recently have Western psychologies begun to explore the transpersonal domains that interest contemplative disciplines.

Other Systems

Principles for Optimal Comparisons of Different Psychotherapies

Each psychotherapy is a rich and complex system, and brief comparisons necessarily do them an injustice. When making comparisons, it is wise to assume the following.

1. Each system offers a *valuable but only partial* contribution to understanding and treatment.
2. Claims for blanket supremacy of any one approach are suspect.
3. Effective therapies share a variety of methods and mechanisms.
4. Different therapies may be complementary rather than necessarily conflictual.
5. Therapists familiar with only one system are likely to fall into the procrustean trap of interpreting and treating all clients in the same way. As Abraham Maslow put it, if the only tool you have is a hammer, everything begins to look like a nail. If you know only one therapy, then all clients and conditions appear appropriate for it.
6. Good therapists are flexible and familiar with multiple methods. They assess which approach is likely to work best for each client at each stage and treat or refer clients appropriately.

These principles are demonstrated well by integrative, integral, and outcome informed therapies (Duncan, Miller, & Sparks, 2004; Norcross & Beutler, 2013; Wilber, 2000b).

Comparisons with Other Systems

The following comparisons highlight the contributions of contemplative approaches. However, this is in no way to deny the many contributions of the following therapies.

Psychoanalysis focuses above all on psychological conflict. It sees humans as necessarily locked and lost in a never-ending inner struggle and assumes that "mental life represents an unrelenting conflict between the conscious and unconscious parts of the mind" (Arlow, 1995, p. 20). Psychoanalysis has made enormous pioneering contributions to our understanding of the unconscious, defenses, the childhood roots of some pathologies, and a variety of therapeutic processes. In fact, it has made major advances over contemplative disciplines in the areas of childhood development, transference, and unconscious dynamics and defenses.

However, from a contemplative perspective, psychoanalysis has tragically underestimated our human nature and potentials. By focusing on conflict, problems, and pathology, it largely overlooks human strengths and possibilities and what Abraham Maslow (1971) famously called "the farther reaches of human nature." Consequently, psychoanalysis does not recognize possibilities of, for example, exceptional health and well-being or how to foster transpersonal maturation and exceptional capacities. In short, "Freudianism institutionalized the underestimation of human possibility" (Needleman, 1980, p. 60).

Both ancient contemplative claims and recent research call into question psychoanalytic assumptions about the universality of psychological conflict. Contemplative psychologies suggest that conflicts may largely resolve in the higher reaches of development, becoming far less powerful and problematic. Studies of advanced mindfulness meditation teachers showed "no evidence of sexual or aggressive drive conflicts" (Wilber, Engler, & Brown, 1986, p. 214).

Unfortunately, psychoanalysis often overestimates its own scope and supremacy. Consider, for example, two claims: "Psychoanalysis is the most extensive, inclusive and comprehensive system of psychology" (Arlow, 1995, p. 16) and "When it comes to unraveling the mysteries of the human mind, no body of knowledge approaches that of psychoanalytic theory" (Gabbard, 1995, p. 431). Comparisons with other schools offer little support for such grandiose claims. Overestimating the supremacy of one's own school seems directly related to one's ignorance of others.

In spite of their differences, meditation practices and psychoanalysis (together with other psychodynamic therapies) share certain goals and understandings. Both are based on the recognition that, as Freud (1917/1943, p. 252) put it, "man is not even master in his own house . . . his own mind." Likewise, the two systems agree on the value of deep introspection, and Freud acknowledged that meditative disciplines "may be able to grasp happenings in the depths of the ego and in the id which were otherwise inaccessible to it. . . . It may be admitted that the therapeutic efforts of psychoanalysis have chosen a similar line of approach" (Freud, 1933/1965, p. 71).

Analytical (Jungian) and contemplative psychologies agree on several major issues. These include the mind's innate drive toward growth, the beneficial effects of transpersonal experiences, and the multilayered nature of the unconscious, including levels below the Freudian.

Meditation traditions tend to agree with Jungian, humanistic, and person-centered Rogerian schools that, in addition to motives such as sex and aggression, the psyche possesses an innate drive toward growth and development. Although the concepts are not perfectly synonymous, there is overlap among Jung's drive for *individuation*, Abraham Maslow's *self-actualization* and *self-transcendence*, Carl Rogers's *formative tendency*, and the contemplative motive for self-transcendence and awakening. All would agree with Abraham Maslow's (1968, p. iv) poignant observation: "Without the transcendent and the transpersonal, we get sick, violent, and nihilistic, or else hopeless and apathetic. We need something 'bigger than we are' to be awed by and to commit ourselves to."

Both Jungian and contemplative perspectives, and now contemporary research, agree that transpersonal experiences can foster psychological healing and growth (Walsh & Vaughan, 1993). Transpersonal experiences are experiences in which the sense of identity or self expands beyond (trans) the individual or personal to encompass wider aspects of humankind and the world. Here one experiences oneself as intimately linked and identified with others, the world, and even the cosmos. As Jung (1973) put it, "the approach to the numinous is the real therapy and inasmuch as you attain to the numinous experience you are released from the curse of pathology" (p. 377).

Historically, most Western therapies recognized only the first two developmental stages, the prepersonal and personal, and this left them prey to a specific trap. Because transpersonal experiences went unrecognized, they were often confused with prepersonal ones and were therefore mistakenly diagnosed as regressive or pathological. The unfortunate result was "the pre/post fallacy" (Wilber, 1999). For example, Freud interpreted transpersonal experiences as indicative of infantile helplessness, Albert Ellis viewed them as examples of irrational thinking, and the classic text *The History of Psychiatry* referred to "The obvious similarities between schizophrenic regressions and the practices of Yoga and Zen" (Alexander & Selesnich, 1966, p. 372).

However, careful comparisons reveal major differences between prepersonal regression and transpersonal progression. As Ken Wilber (1999) points out, "pre and trans can be seriously equated only by those whose intellectual inquiry goes no further than superficial impressions" (p. 157). Nevertheless, the pre- and post- fallacy was widespread until recently and led to a tragic underestimation of contemplative therapies and human potentials.

Cognitive, rational emotive, and contemplative therapies share an appreciation of the enormous power of thoughts and beliefs. They agree that we are all prone to numerous erroneous thoughts that all too easily become unrecognized erroneous assumptions and beliefs, a process that acceptance and commitment therapy calls *fusion* with one's thoughts. These assumptions are mistaken for reality, and they then bias cognition, distort experience, and produce pathology. These mistaken beliefs are described as *basic mistakes* (Alfred Adler), *cognitive distortions* (cognitive therapy), *irrational beliefs* (Albert Ellis), and *delusion* (Asian therapies). Rumi, one of Sufism's greatest contemplatives—and now, eight centuries after his death, one of the world's most popular poets—wrote, "Your thinking . . . drives you in every direction under its bitter control" (Helminski, 2000, p. 19). Likewise, Jewish wisdom holds that "A person's entire destiny—for good or ill—depends on the thoughts in his heart" (Hoffman, 1985, p. 103) and therefore recommends the practice of "elevating strange thoughts." The great Indian leader Mahatma Gandhi, who was a devoted yogic practitioner, summarized it this way: "What you think you become" (Fischer, 1954, p. 146).

Of course, there are also significant differences between schools. On the one hand, cognitive therapy has made several advances over contemplative approaches such as recognizing specific cognitive profiles for each psychopathology.

On the other hand, meditators can identify and modify layers of thought below those accessible to cognitive and rational emotive therapies. Meditators are able to observe thoughts and their effects with remarkable precision (as will be described), to unearth deep and distorted beliefs and cognitive schemas, and to develop remarkable degrees of cognitive control. Advanced meditators may observe each thought that arises and then reduce harmful thoughts and cultivate beneficial ones, or they may simply allow harmful thoughts to self-correct as they tend to do when held clearly in awareness.

Cognitive therapies recognize the possibility of brief *thought stopping*. However, contemplatives can extend thought stopping for prolonged periods and then rest in the profound calm and clarity that result, a claim now supported by electroencephalogram (EEG) studies.

Reduction of the usually incessant torrent of thoughts calms and clarifies the mind. This fosters healing and growth, and it reveals hidden depths of the psyche, just as the depths of a lake become visible only when its surface waves are calmed. Taoism's great philosopher Chuang Tzu wrote, "if water derives lucidity from stillness, how much more the faculties of the mind?" (Giles, 1926/1969, p. 47).

Contemplative therapies can therefore do more than heal the erroneous thoughts and beliefs that underlie clinical psychopathologies. They can also help us recognize, transform, and disidentify from deeper thoughts that keep us trapped at conventional levels of development and unaware of our deeper identity and further potentials. So important are thoughts that the Buddha began his teaching with the words:

> We are what we think. All that we are arises with our thoughts. . . .
> It is good to control them, and to master them brings happiness. . . .
> The task is to quieten them, and by ruling them to find happiness. (Byrom, 1976, p. 3, 13)

Existential and contemplative therapies both center on *ultimate concerns*—those fundamental challenges of life that all of us inevitably face. These include the inescapable challenges of meaning and purpose, suffering and limitation, isolation and death. Both schools agree that these challenges leave us prey to a deep sense of anxiety (*angst*). Moreover, this anxiety is not just circumstantial but also existential because of the nature of our human existence.

Both schools also emphasize the many ways in which we live superficially and inauthentically, hiding from and deceiving ourselves about these ultimate concerns. Conventional culture often reflects and fosters this inauthenticity, creating what Nietzsche described as a *herd mentality* that functions as a collective defense. This herd mentality encourages *automation conformity*: superficial, unreflective, conventional lifestyles in which, according to Kierkegaard, we "tranquilize ourselves with trivia." Contemporary media offers innumerable examples of tranquilization with trivia.

Contemplative and existential psychologies offer overlapping but distinct solutions. They both urge us to recognize rather than deny our existential challenges and then to face them as fully and defenselessly as we can. Only in this way can we escape the conventional slumber of our herd mentality, go beyond unthinking conformity, and live more fully and authentically. However, for most existentialists, the best we can do is to adopt a heroic attitude, such as courage and authenticity, which involves unflinching openness to the harsh realities of life (Yalom, 2002).

Contemplative therapies agree completely that we need authenticity and courage. However, contemplative practices enable us to deal with life's existential challenges in two additional ways. The first is by cultivating mental qualities—such as courage, equanimity, and insight—that help in facing life's challenges. The second is by fostering maturation to transpersonal stages in which the separate *egoic* self that suffers isolation and meaningness is transcended in a larger transpersonal identity. This transpersonal self recognizes its inherent interconnection with others and with all life, and it finds inherent meaning and purpose in this larger identity and in the service of all.

Integrative, integral, and contemplative therapies all agree that the best way to promote healing and growth is by judiciously combining multiple approaches and techniques. *Contemplative therapies go further, and suggest that all of life—each experience, activity, and relationship—can become an opportunity for learning.* "The wise man learns from every phrase he hears, from every event he observes, and from every experience he shares" (Hoffman, 1985, p. 94). The aim is not just to foster healthy qualities such as calm and clarity during formal therapy sessions, but also to both foster and apply these healthy qualities in all activities for the benefit of everyone. The goal is to go into oneself so as to go out into the world more effectively and helpfully and to go out into the world so as to go into oneself more effectively and deeply.

What Makes Psychotherapy and Psychotherapists Effective? Supershrinks and Pseudoshrinks

One of the most consistent findings in psychotherapy research is that most of the benefits come from so-called nonspecific factors—such as the clients' and therapists' personal qualities and the quality of the relationship—rather than from the unique elements of a particular therapy. Moreover, therapists differ enormously in their effectiveness, with "supershrinks" far outperforming "pseudoshrinks." Unfortunately, most research still tries to demonstrate the superiority of one therapy over another in spite of decades of minimal success. Clearly, more effort should go into identifying characteristics of supershrinks and discovering how to emulate them. For example, obtaining feedback is crucial, and using rating scales to obtain immediate feedback from clients about each session *dramatically* improves therapy success rates (Duncan et al., 2004; Miller, Hubble, & Duncan, 2007).

So what qualities characterize contemplative supershrinks? Probably the beneficial qualities of effective psychotherapists identified by Carl Rogers—such as presence, accurate empathy, and a nonjudgmental attitude— and meditation foster all of these qualities. In addition, meditation promotes other helpful qualities in therapists such as psychological maturity, insight, and sensitivity (Irving, Dobkin, & Park, 2009).

Therapists of any persuasion and their clients can benefit from contemplative practices. Therapists can learn these practices and then continue to offer other kinds of therapies to clients while bringing contemplative qualities—such as greater calm, clarity, and empathy—to their work. As a result, they may feel better themselves and also have better therapeutic outcomes (Grepmair et al., 2007; Shapiro & Carlson, 2009).

HISTORY

Precursors

The human quest for healing and self-understanding extends back to the dawn of history. The earliest systematic seekers and therapists were ancient healers called *shamans*, whose remarkable 20,000-year-old paintings decorate cave walls. Shamans were the original general practitioners who functioned as physicians, therapists, and spiritual counselors. To fill these multiple roles, they drew on diagnostic and healing techniques that ranged from rituals to projective testing, herbal medications, individual counseling, and group therapy (Walsh, 2007). As such, they exemplify psychiatrist Jerome Frank's (1982) famous claim that all psychotherapy methods "are elaborations and variations of age-old procedures of psychological healing" (p. 49).

However, their distinctive practice was the induction and use of altered states of consciousness. Many thousands of years ago, they learned how to alter their consciousness through techniques such as fasting, drumming, dancing, and psychedelics. With the heightened sensitivity conferred by these altered states, they accessed intuitive knowledge to make diagnoses and recommend treatments. Today, shamanism still plays a vital role in many cultures, making it by far the most enduring of all current psychotherapies (Walsh, 2007).

Beginnings

Meditative and yogic practices emerged when practitioners learned to induce desired states of consciousness without external aids by focusing attention and refining awareness. Their origins are lost in the mists of history but can be traced back at least 3,000 years.

Beginning some 2,500 years ago, there was a dramatic stirring of human consciousness called the *Axial Age*. In diverse countries, remarkable individuals pioneered new techniques for training the mind and thereby developed the first systematic meditative, philosophical, and psychological disciplines. In Greece, the first systematic thinkers—and especially the remarkable trio of Socrates, Plato, and Aristotle—established rational inquiry and thereby laid the foundation for Western philosophy and psychology.

Similar breakthroughs occurred in the East. In India, sages developed yoga and the yoga-based philosophy and psychology that would undergird subsequent centuries of

Indian thought. Meanwhile, the Buddha devised new meditations and a corresponding psychology and philosophy. In China, Confucius, a veritable one-man university, and Lao Tzu, a semilegendary sage, laid the foundations of Confucianism and Taoism, respectively. Consequently, "All the traditions that were developed during the Axial Age pushed forward the frontiers of human consciousness and discovered a transcendent dimension in the core of their being" (Armstrong, 2006, p. xvii). The result was a dramatic leap in the understanding of the mind, human nature, and human potentials.

Subsequent Evolution

Each tradition evolved over time. For example, Confucius lived in a time of horrendous social turmoil and so focused on ethical and social reform. Only centuries later, when Confucianism incorporated elements of Taoism and Buddhism did the tradition come to include major meditative and yogic components.

In India, yoga developed into several schools that emphasized different but complementary approaches to mind training and self-transformation. Four main approaches—or *yogas*—emerged that focused respectively on transforming thoughts, emotions, attention, and motivation.

Buddhism eventually developed a sophisticated introspective psychology that analyzed the contents and processes of mind into some 50 elements of experience. Then it used these elements to describe psychological health and pathology and to guide mental training.

Early Western psychology was also introspective. However, whereas Western introspectionists failed to create a useful replicable map of experience, the Buddhists succeeded (perhaps because of their far more rigorous training in introspection), and their map has guided meditators for more than 2,000 years.

Common Discoveries and Practices

Whenever people search deeply into the great questions and mysteries of life, common themes emerge. Inevitably, seekers come to recognize the need for wise teachers, silent introspection, and the development of their own minds. Only in periods of quiet can we disentangle ourselves from the superficial busyness of our lives and then reflect on what is truly important—calm and clear our minds—and access our inner wisdom.

Contemplative practices and traditions therefore became part of each of the great religions. Christian contemplatives claimed, for example, "Good speech is silver, but silence is pure gold" (Savin, 1991, p. 127), and Judaism says, "I grew up among the sages. All my life I listened to their words. Yet I have found nothing better than silence" (Shapiro, 1993, p. 18). Likewise, Islamic contemplatives, who are known as *Sufis*, echoed the words of their founder, Muhammad: "Silent is wise; alas, there are not enough who keep silent. . . . Bring your heart to meditation" (Angha, 1995, pp. 68, 74). Similar themes also echo through Eastern traditions and through the lives of secular contemplatives.

Over time, it became increasingly obvious that mental training is essential for psychological health, wisdom, and maturity. Contemplative practices therefore evolved over the centuries, becoming increasingly refined, systematic, and diverse. Each tradition developed a family of practices aimed at cultivating specific mental capacities—for example, attentional capacities such as concentration and focus, cognitive skills such as insight and wisdom, and valued emotions such as love and compassion. And each tradition came to the life-changing recognition that within us are untapped potentials, sources of wisdom, and kinds of satisfaction far richer and more profound than we suspect.

"Know yourself" is the key maxim of the contemplative traditions, and it has been stated in numerous ways. The great contemplative Plotinus, who fathered neoplatonic philosophy, advised, "We must close our eyes and invoke a new manner of seeing . . . a wakefulness that is the birthright of us all, though few put it to use" (O'Brien, 1964, p. 42). Early female Christian contemplatives, who were known as the Christian Desert Mothers, quickly learned that "Self-awareness is not selfishness but self-connectedness. It is a deep and intense listening to our inner being, learning to be conscious and alert to what our inner world is trying to say to us" (Swan, 2001, p. 36).

In summary, contemplatives from diverse countries and cultures discovered what Western psychology is now rediscovering. The great contemplative philosopher Marcus Aurelius, who was also emperor of Rome, put it this way: "Dig within. Within is the wellspring of good; and it is always ready to bubble up, if you just dig" (Harvey, 1996, p. 135).

Current Status

For a long time, Western mental-health professionals knew little and misunderstood much about contemplative practices, but recently both popular and professional interest have exploded. Worldwide, these practices remain the most widespread and popular of all current psychotherapies, practiced by thousands of therapists and hundreds of millions of people around the world. Hundreds of research studies demonstrate psychological, spiritual, and somatic benefits, and combination therapies and psychologies that synthesize contemplative and standard Western approaches are proliferating.

Integration of Therapies

Attempts to forge integrations across different Western psychologies and therapies are of three major kinds: (1) the search for underlying common factors, (2) technical eclecticism (combining techniques), and (3) theoretical integration. Similarly, attempts are now being made to integrate contemplative and traditional therapies.

Contemplative technical eclecticism is proceeding rapidly and most often combines mindfulness with traditional therapeutic techniques. The original inspiration was Jon Kabat-Zinn's (2003) widely used mindfulness-based stress reduction (MBSR). MBSR is an eight-week group program that offers mindfulness meditation and yoga posture training, individual and group support, education, and daily practices. Tens of thousands of people have completed the program.

Mindfulness combination therapies are proliferating. Examples include mindfulness-based cognitive therapy (MBCT); mindfulness-based art, sleep, relationship, and eating therapies; and relapse prevention for drug abuse. Most such approaches have initial research support, and several—such as MBSR and MBCT—already meet the APA criteria for "well established and empirically supported" (Fjorback & Walach, 2012). Nonwestern psychotherapies that incorporate meditative elements include the Japanese Naikan and Morita therapies.

The success of these combination therapies raises several intriguing questions. An obvious one is, "What other combinations will prove efficacious?" A more provocative question, given the many successes so far, is "Would most mainstream therapies benefit from the addition of mindfulness training?" And, just as provocative, "Would most mainstream therapists benefit from mindfulness or some other kind of contemplative training?"

Theoretical Integrations

A growing movement now seeks to create integrative theories that synthesize contemplative and Western psychological perspectives. The best-known examples are transpersonal and integral psychologies. Transpersonal psychology was founded as the first explicitly integrative school of Western psychology, and as such it sought to honor and synthesize valid insights of all schools, including East and West, psychology and meditation, personal and transpersonal (Walsh & Vaughan, 1993).

The most comprehensive theoretical integration to date is the *integral psychology* of Ken Wilber. His approach traces psychological development, pathologies, and appropriate therapies from infancy to adulthood using primarily Western psychological resources, and then from personal to transpersonal using primarily contemplative resources (Wilber, 1999, 2000b; Wilber et al., 1986).

Integral psychotherapy is a multimodal approach that addresses multiple psychological and somatic dimensions, as well as prepersonal, personal, and transpersonal levels. Integral therapies recommend a judicious mix, tailored to the individual, of educational, psychotherapeutic, contemplative, social, and somatic approaches. Somatic approaches include exercise, mindful movement such as tai chi, yogic postures, and diet.

Diet has long been a central concern of yoga, which holds "As one's food, so is one's mind" (Feuerstein, 1996, p. 63). Considerable research support suggests that an optimal diet for both mental and physical health consists primarily of multicolored fruits and vegetables (a rainbow diet), some fish, and minimal excess calories.

Such diets enhance mental health across the lifespan. They improve cognitive and academic performance in children, ameliorate affective disorders in adults, and reduce cognitive decline and dementia in the elderly. In fact, "dietary factors are so important that the mental health of nations may be linked to them. . . . As such, dietary assessment and recommendations are appropriate and important elements of mental health care" (Walsh, 2011, pp. 581, 583). As the great Indian leader Gandhi—who was himself a yoga practitioner—put it, "Diet is a powerful factor not to be neglected" (Feuerstein, 1996, p. 66).

Learning Contemplative Practices

For those who want to learn contemplative practices, there are many popular books (see the Case Readings in this chapter). However, it is extremely helpful to have the guidance of a teacher–therapist. Good teachers have extensive personal practice, and they live and relate in ways consistent with their message, treating everyone with kindness and respect. Therapists who wish to teach these techniques or counsel people already using them, need considerable personal practice themselves under expert guidance. Ideally, this includes long-term daily practice as well as periods of retreat where, over several days or weeks, one engages in continuous practice that can dramatically accelerate learning and growth.

PERSONALITY

Just as there are many meditations, there are many contemplative psychologies. These not only vary significantly but also display recurrent themes. We can therefore outline a contemplative view of mind and human nature while remembering that specific systems may differ.

Theory of Personality

Contemplative practices stem from and lead to views of human nature, pathology, health, and potential that are in some ways very different from traditional Western assumptions. We can discuss these views under the following headings: consciousness, identity, motivation, development, and higher capacities.

Consciousness

All of us have experienced impaired states of consciousness (states of mind) such as illnesses, stress, sleep deprivation, and alcohol intoxication. These states are associated with suboptimal mental functions such as distorted perception, reduced concentration, impaired cognition, and negative emotions. When we recover, we return to our usual waking state of consciousness that we, and traditional Western psychology, assume to be optimal.

Contemplative psychologies disagree and make a provocative claim: Our usual waking state is not optimal, and more effective and functional states are available to us through contemplative training.

This claim raises two crucial questions. First, in what ways is our usual waking state suboptimal? Second, how could we be unaware of its limitations?

Contemplative psychologies answer by pointing us to our own experience. All of us recognize that we often daydream and become lost in thoughts and fantasies. Contemplative psychologies simply suggest that these thoughts and fantasies are significantly more pervasive, distorting, and confusing than we realize.

This claim, like other contemplative claims, can be tested for ourselves through meditation. Meditative observation quickly reveals that our minds are filled with a continual flux of unrecognized thoughts, images, and fantasies that distort and reduce awareness, resulting in unappreciated trance-like states. As in any hypnotic state, the trance and its constricted distorted awareness easily go unrecognized. The result is a clouding and distortion of daily experience that causes much of our mental suffering yet remains unrecognized until we subject our perceptual-cognitive processes to direct rigorous scrutiny as in meditation.

Thus the "normal" person is considered to be partly "asleep," "dreaming," or in a "consensus trance." When such a "dream" is especially painful or disruptive, it becomes recognized as pathology. However, because the vast majority of the population "dreams," the usual more subtle forms remain unrecognized. Contemplative therapies enable people to "awaken" from this waking dream, and this awakening is known by such names as *liberation*, *enlightenment*, and *salvation* and *satori*, *fana*, and *nirvana* (Walsh, 1999).

To some extent, these concepts simply extend Western psychology. Research reveals that we are far less aware of our own cognitive processes than we usually assume and that we suffer from multiple unrecognized cognitive-perceptual distortions. Contemplative psychologies suggest that meditative or yogic training can help us recognize and reduce these distortions, and studies of advanced meditators demonstrate enhanced perceptual speed, sensitivity, and accuracy (Murphy & Donovan, 1997).

The contemplative suggestion that there are many other functional waking states available to us echoes William James's famous claim:

> Our normal waking consciousness . . . is but one special type of consciousness, whilst all about it, parted from it by the filmiest of screens, there lie potential forms of consciousness entirely different. We may go through life without suspecting their existence; but apply the requisite stimulus, and at a touch they are there in all their completeness. . . . No account of the universe in its totality can be final which leaves those other forms of consciousness quite disregarded. (James, 1958, p. 298)

Contemplative psychologies agree completely. They describe a broad spectrum of states—many as yet unrecognized by mainstream Western psychology—and provide practices for attaining them.

Many of these states offer heightened capacities such as unwavering concentration, perceptual clarity, penetrating insight, and deep compassion. States of consciousness that possess the usual waking capacities plus additional ones are known as *higher states* (Tart, 1986). Contemplative practices cultivate these higher states in order to heal the mind, foster heightened capacities, and make these capacities available in daily life. These ideas have important implications for both individuals and cultures.

Anthropologists divide cultures into monophasic and polyphasic. *Monophasic* cultures such as the West, value and derive their view of reality almost entirely from the usual waking state of consciousness. *Polyphasic* cultures value, explore, and derive their view of reality from multiple states such as dreams, meditations, and yogas. The Western world is currently beginning a major historical and cultural shift from monophasic to polyphasic as contemplative practices make multiple beneficial states widely available.

Identity

Who am I? What am I? These are two of the most fundamental and important questions we can ask, and our answers are enormously consequential. In fact, our answers shape our lives because everything we say and do reflects who and what we think we are. The answers given by contemplative psychologies differ dramatically from everyday assumptions because meditation allows us to introspect and investigate ourselves deeply and precisely.

For example, under microscopic meditative examination, what was formerly assumed to be a relatively consistent, permanent self or ego is recognized as a continuously changing flux of thoughts, images, and emotions. This discovery is not unique to meditators and can occur whenever people introspect with sufficient care. For example, among Western philosophers, William James spoke of the "stream of consciousness," and David Hume concluded that the self is "nothing but a bundle or collection of different perceptions, which succeed each other with an inconceivable rapidity and are in a perpetual flux and movement" (Jones, 1975, p. 305).

A similar situation exists with psychoanalytic object relations theory. Comparing psychoanalytic and Buddhist systems, psychologist and meditation teacher Jack Engler (1983) found that in both psychologies:

> What we take to be our "self" and feel to be so present and real is actually an internalized image, a composite representation, constructed by a selective and imaginative "remembering" of past encounters with the object world. In fact, the self is viewed as being constructed anew from moment to moment. But both systems further agree that the self is not ordinarily experienced this way. (p. 33)

Hence both contemplative psychologies and some schools of Western psychology and philosophy conclude that our "self" is very different from our usual unexamined assumptions. The usual sense of the self as being who we "really are" and as being continuous and consistent over time seems to be an illusory construction of imprecise awareness. Closer examination reveals that this self-sense is continuously and selectively constructed from a flux of thoughts, images, and emotions. This is similar to the *flicker fusion phenomenon* by which still photographs projected successively on a movie screen give the illusion of continuity, vitality, and movement.

This bears out a crucial contemplative claim: *We suffer from a case of mistaken identity*. We are not who, or even what, we thought we were. What we usually take to be our real self is merely a mental construction—that is, merely a self-image, a self-concept, or a self-representation.

This recognition has enormous implications. We worry about our "self-concept" and obsess over our "self-image" but rarely appreciate the far-reaching significance of this language. If they are merely concepts or images we have constructed, then they are not who or what we really are. We have mistaken a concept for our self and an image for reality. Then we devote our lives to defending, changing, or trying to live up to these images. In doing so, we become the victims of our own creation. It is as though we painted an ugly picture of ourselves, mistook it for our self, and then cringed in horror. As a classic yoga text tells us, "Pain is caused by false identification" (Prabhavananda & Isherwood, 1972, p. 127). The result is unnecessary suffering.

When this false identification is recognized, we can become free from the limitations, compulsions, and suffering it produces. Whereas traditional Western therapies teach us to modify our self-image, contemplative therapies also teach us to do something far more profound and transformative: to recognize that our self-image is only a fabrication and to thereby disidentify from and become free of it.

Contemplative therapies do this by cultivating sensitive, precise awareness. This awareness can penetrate into the depths of the psyche, recognize the false self-image as merely an image and thereby loosen its hold. When one is no longer identified with and tied to an outdated self-image, the mind is free to grow (Walsh & Shapiro, 2006). The self-concept and its boundaries are increasingly recognized as constructed rather than given, fluid rather than rigid, and capable of considerable expansion. The sense of self can then expand to become transpersonal, identifying with others, and eventually identifying with all humankind and the world. This culminates in a sense of one's inherent interconnectedness and unity with all, and the result is a natural sense of love and compassion for all.

As refined meditative awareness penetrates past arbitrary self-boundaries, it also penetrates into the very depths of the psyche. Below the self-concept, below the thoughts and images that construct this concept, awareness uncovers our deep nature and discovers—itself! In other words, our deep nature is said to be not the contents of mind such as thoughts, images, and feelings with which we usually identify but that which underlies and is aware of them: pure awareness or consciousness. This pure awareness is described in different contemplative traditions as *Mind, original Mind, Spirit, Self, Atman, Buddha Nature,* and *Tao mind.* Western psychologists sometimes describe it, for example, as *self-as-context* (acceptance and commitment therapy, or ACT) or as the "observing self" or "transpersonal self" (Walsh & Vaughan, 1993).

Contemplative traditions agree that the experience of this pure awareness that is our true nature can be extremely ecstatic, in fact, more satisfying than any other pleasure. After his own discovery of this, Shankara, one of India's greatest yogis, exclaimed:

> What is this joy I feel? Who shall measure it?
> I know nothing but joy, limitless, unbounded! . . .
> I abide in the joy of the Atman. (Prabhavananda & Isherwood, 1978, p. 113)

As a survey of the world's yogas concluded, "This is indeed the great message of all forms of yoga: happiness is our essential nature, and our perpetual quest for happiness is fulfilled only when we realize who we truly are" (Feuerstein, 1996, p. 2).

In summary, contemplative training culminates in the recognition of our deep identity, a recognition of enormous importance. This deep identity or True Nature has three aspects. First, it is the recognition of oneself as blissful pure consciousness, aware of but no longer identified with (and therefore not controlled by) the thoughts, images, morals, and emotions that parade through the mind. Second is the recognition that all people—in fact, all conscious creatures—possess this same consciousness, that we are intimately united with them and naturally feel care for them. Third, as our self-concepts and images are seen through, so too are the artificial boundaries and divisions they constructed, and we recognize our underlying interconnection and unity with all people and the universe. The result is the classical unitive experience sought by contemplatives around the world, and it is experienced as the mind's natural, healthy, mature, and ecstatic condition (Wilber, 2000b).

Similar, although temporary, unitive ecstatic experiences can emerge under other circumstances. They can be deliberately induced with rituals, fasting, psychedelics, or during lovemaking in experiences of "transcendent sex" that advanced tantric yogis use for self-transformation (Feuerstein, 1996). They can also occur spontaneously in nature, in advanced psychotherapy, during intensive exercise, during childbirth, and near death (Maslow, 1971).

From a contemplative perspective, these are glimpses, or *peak experiences,* of the mind's potentials and our deeper nature, and they can produce significant insights and transformations. However, these experiences are almost always transient. Only mental training can sustain such experiences and thereby transform them into the higher developmental stages and enduring ways of life that are the goals of advanced contemplative practices.

Western psychologists periodically rediscover unitive experiences and their benefits. Classic examples include William James's *cosmic consciousness*, Carl Jung's *numinous experience*, Abraham Maslow's *peak experience*, Erich Fromm's *at-onement*, and *transpersonal experiences*. In fact, some Western researchers have reached conclusions strikingly similar to those of contemplatives. For example, Carl Jung (1968) argued that "the deeper layers of the psyche . . . become increasingly collective until they are universalized" (p. 291), and William James (1960) suggested that "there is a continuum of cosmic consciousness against which our individuality builds but accidental forces and into which our several minds plunge as into a mother sea" (p. 324). "It is chiefly our ignorance of the psyche if these experiences appear 'mystic,'" claimed Jung (1955, p. 535).

However, Western clinicians usually see ego boundaries dissolve in the ego disintegration of psychoses. Therefore, it is understandable that healthy ego transcendence was sometimes confused with pathological ego disintegration and therefore dismissed as regressive psychopathology. This unfortunate example of the pre- and post- fallacy is an outmoded pathologizing interpretation. In fact, unitive experiences occur most often in psychologically healthy individuals, and they further enhance health and maturity (Alexander, Rainforth, & Gelderloos, 1991; Maslow, 1971).

Motivation

Contemplative psychologies tend to see motives as organized hierarchically from strong to (initially) weak, from survival to self-transcendence. This ordering is most explicit in Hindu yoga and is similar to Abraham Maslow's (1971) hierarchy of needs. Yoga and Maslow agree that physiological and survival motives such as hunger and thirst are initially most powerful and predominant. When these needs are fulfilled, drives such as sexual and power strivings may emerge as effective motivators in their turn, and after them emerge "higher" motives such as love and the pull toward self-transcendence. *Self-transcendence* is the desire to transcend our usual false constricted identity, to awaken to the fullness of our being, and to recognize our true nature. Self-transcendence, lying beyond even self-actualization, was the highest motive recognized by Maslow, but some contemplative psychologies give equal importance to selfless service. Contemplative practices aim to transform motivation by weakening compulsive immature motives and strengthening mature beneficial ones.

According to contemplative psychologies, higher motives—what Abraham Maslow called *metamotives*—such as self-actualization, self-transcendence, and selfless service are part of our very nature. Overlooking or ignoring them therefore produces several kinds of pain and pathology.

First, we suffer from a shallow, distorted, and distorting view of ourselves. This has tragic consequences because self-images tend to operate as self-fulfilling prophecies. As Gordon Allport (1964) pointed out, "Debasing assumptions debase human beings" (p. 36).

Second, if metamotives are an essential part of our nature, then to overlook them is to starve ourselves of something vital to our well-being. We may need the good, the true, and the beautiful to thrive; we may need to express kindness, care, and compassion to live fully (Wilber, 1999). Therefore, if we don't recognize and express our higher motives, we will remain immature, inauthentic, and unfulfilled. This lack of fulfillment is doubly problematic because we will not recognize the real source of our dissatisfactions and are likely to blame our malaise on our circumstances. These metamotive frustrations can mushroom into what Maslow (1971) called *metapathologies,* such as a deep sense of meaninglessness, cynicism, and alienation.

Maslow worried that these metapathologies are rampant in Western society and represent a major threat to our culture. But that is exactly what one would expect given that our culture has focused obsessively on material motives and overlooked and starved higher motives. Contemplatives have long emphasized that the recognition and cultivation of metamotives are essential not only for individuals but also for cultures and civilization.

A third problem with metamotive blindness is that we then naturally assure that lesser motives—such as desires for money, sex, prestige, and power—are the only means to happiness. Then we fall for the seductive delusion that if we can just get enough of them, we will finally be fully and permanently happy.

Unfortunately, there are serious problems with this idea. First, when we believe these lower-order goals are the only means to attain happiness, we become addicted to them. Then whenever we don't have them, we suffer. Even if we do succeed in getting them, we inevitably habituate and want more. To get the same high, the drug addict needs a bigger dose, the miser more wealth, the consumer yet another shopping binge. This is what psychologists call the *hedonic treadmill,* and what the Buddha pointed to with his words "The rain could turn to gold, and still your thirst would not be slaked" (Byrom, 1976, p. 70). Finally, obsession with wealth and possessions can tranquilize us with trivia and distract us from what is truly important in life. As the Taoist sage Chuang Tzu put it, "you use up all your vital energy on external things and wear out your spirit" (Feng & English, 1974, p. 108).

Recent research supports these claims. For example, once our basic needs are met, further income and possessions add surprisingly little to well-being. In fact, "there is only a slight tendency for people who make lots of money to be more satisfied with what they make" (Myers, 1992, p. 39). In short, money can certainly relieve the suffering of deprivation, but it is curiously ineffective in buying further happiness. Therefore, many contemplatives have echoed Muhammad's words: "The richest among you is the one who is not entrapped by greed" (Angha, 1995, p. 21).

None of this is to suggest that pleasures such as possessions, sex, and prestige are necessarily bad or that seeking them noncompulsively is pathological. But contemplatives do say that when we believe these are the only (or even the most important) pleasures, then we become addicted to them, impoverish our lives pursuing them, and are doomed to suffer. Contemplative psychologies therefore provide a valuable antidote to the destructive misunderstandings about motivation that pervade contemporary culture, create so much suffering, and derail so many lives.

Development

A developmental perspective is crucial to understanding contemplative claims. Recall that development proceeds through three major stages: prepersonal, personal, and transpersonal (or preconventional, conventional, and postconventional). Whereas Western psychology focuses on the first two stages, contemplatives zero in on the third, and recognize several postconventional levels beyond most Western psychological maps. The highest levels merge into experiences that have traditionally been thought of as religious, spiritual, or mystical but can now also be understood psychologically.

Higher Capacities

Postconventional development can produce exceptional psychological capacities. These capacities, which are supposedly available to us all if we undertake the necessary contemplative training, include the following.

In the emotional domain, painful emotions such as anger and fear can be greatly reduced (Goleman, 2003). At the same time, positive emotions such as love and joy can mature to become stronger, unconditional, unwavering, and all-encompassing. Cognitive development can proceed beyond Piaget's highest level of linear formal operational thinking to *vision logic* or *network logic*, which sees interconnections between groups of ideas simultaneously (Wilber, 1999). Motivation can be redirected up the hierarchy of needs so that motives such as self-transcendence and selfless service grow stronger and eventually predominate. The mind's usual ceaseless agitation can be stilled so that unwavering concentration and profound peace prevail. Wisdom can develop through sustained reflection on existential issues such as death and the causes of happiness and suffering (Walsh, 1999). A growing body of research, which is reviewed later, now supports several of these claims. More and more, the contemplative view of personality and potentials is coming to seem like a natural extension and enrichment of traditional Western views.

Variety of Concepts

Types of Meditation

There are many kinds of meditation, and no fully adequate typology is available. However, one simple division recognizes two main categories: *concentration* practices and *awareness* practices.

Concentration meditations hold attention on a single stimulus, such as an image or the sensations of the breath. This especially develops the ability to focus and concentrate.

Awareness meditations carefully explore the ongoing flux of moment-to-moment experience. Their aim is to cultivate clear sensitive awareness and to use it to explore the nature of mind and experience. This exploration produces insight and self-understanding, and it fosters mental health and maturation.

Psychopathology

Contemplative views of health and pathology are best understood developmentally. Recall that contemplative practices were originally designed to help with personal and transpersonal levels of development and with existential and transpersonal issues. Consequently, contemplative approaches by themselves offer little help with prepersonal stages and with major psychopathologies such as psychosis. Rather, their focus is more on *normal pathology*, and they agree with Abraham Maslow (1968) that "what we call normal in psychology is really a psychopathology of the average, so undramatic and so widely spread that we don't even notice it ordinarily" (p. 60).

From a contemplative perspective, this "psychopathology of everyday life," as Freud called it, is a reflection of psychological immaturity. Development has proceeded from preconventional to conventional but has then ground to a premature halt far short of our true potentials. The mind is operating suboptimally, unhealthy qualities flourish, and beneficial qualities and capacities remain underdeveloped.

Each contemplative system describes a long list of unhealthy mental qualities. They include emotional factors such as hatred and envy, motivational forces such as addiction and selfishness, cognitive distortions such as conceit and mindlessness, and attentional difficulties such as agitation and distractibility. Indian contemplatives emphasize the fundamental role of three specific mental factors in causing psychopathology. These three causes—which Buddhism picturesquely calls the *three poisons*—consist of one cognitive factor (delusion) and two motivation factors (craving and aversion).

The term *delusion* refers here to an unrecognized mental dullness, mindlessness, or unconsciousness that misperceives and misunderstands the nature of mind, reality, and self. These subtle yet fundamental misunderstandings produce pathogenic beliefs, behaviors, and motives, and the most destructive motives are craving and aversion. Contemplatives therefore agree with Albert Ellis (1987) that "virtually all human beings often hold blatant irrational beliefs and therefore are far from being consistently sane and self-helping" (pp. 373–374). According to Zen, the result is that, "When the deep meaning of things is not understood, the mind's essential peace is disturbed to no avail" (Sengstan, 1975).

The mind clouded by delusion forgets its inherently blissful true nature and so feels deficient and dissatisfied. It then searches for substitute satisfactions, mistakenly believing that if it can just get enough possessions and experiences it will be fully and permanently satisfied. Naturally, this faulty belief leads to craving: the second root cause of pain and pathology.

Craving corresponds to our Western concept of addiction, or what Albert Ellis calls *childish demandingness*, and is regarded as a major cause of psychopathology and suffering. Western psychologists emphasize addiction to drugs and food. However, contemplatives argue that we can become addicted to almost anything, including people and possessions, our self-image and ideas, and even our ideals. In fact, addictions to material pleasures—such as the *physical foursome* of money, sex, power, and prestige—are described as *iron chains*, whereas addictions to ideals such as always being good or never getting angry are described as *golden chains* (Walsh, 1999). Being human, we all fall short of our ideals, and if we are addicted to them, then we suffer.

Of course, it is crucial to distinguish compulsive craving from simple desire. Desire is mere wanting, craving a compulsive necessity; unfulfilled desires have little impact, unfulfilled addictions yield pain and pathology. We are a slave of what we crave. No wonder yoga warns that "Cravings torment the heart" (Prabhavananda & Isherwood, 1972, p. 41).

Along with addiction come painful emotions such as fear, anger, jealousy, and depression. These feelings are intimately tied to craving and reflect how it operates. We fear that we will not get what we crave, boil with anger toward whoever stands in our way, writhe with jealousy toward people who get what we lust after, and fall into depression when we lose hope. The therapist who recognizes these relationships has an invaluable perspective to offer clients lost in these painful emotions.

Craving is also the basis for many pain-producing life games and lifestyles. These include the *if only game* ("If only I had . . . , then I could be happy") and what Transactional Analysis calls the *until game* ("I can't be happy until I get . . ."). The amount of suffering in our lives reflects the gap between what we crave and what we have. In fact, for Asian meditative traditions, there is an almost mathematical precision to the relationship between psychological suffering and craving, which we might express in the following formula:

$$\text{Suffering} \, \alpha \, \Sigma \, \text{Strength of craving} \times (\text{Reality} - \text{Craved})$$

What this says is that the amount of psychological suffering in our lives is related to the strength of each craving multiplied by the gap between reality and what is craved. In other words, the greater the number of cravings, the stronger the cravings; and the greater the gap between reality and what we crave, the more we suffer.

Contemplative traditions draw a crucial conclusion. It is possible to reduce psychological conflict and suffering by reducing the number and strength of cravings or addictions and by accepting reality as it is. In fact, this does more than just reduce suffering. It also allows healthy motives to act freely and effectively, thereby orienting us toward more healthy and fulfilling goals (Walsh, 1999). No wonder neo-Confucians claim that "The learning of the great [person] consists entirely in getting rid of the obscuration of selfish desires [addictions]" (Chan, 1963, p. 660) and that the founder of Taoism, Lao Tzu, wrote, "to a land where people cease from coveting, peace comes of course" (Bynner, 1944/1980, p. 48).

Addiction also creates its mirror image, *aversion,* the third of the three root causes of psychopathology. Whereas addiction is a compulsive need to experience and possess desirable stimuli, aversion is a compulsive need to avoid or escape undesirable ones. Like addiction, aversion produces pain and breeds destructive reactions such as anger, fear, and defensiveness. What you are unwilling to experience runs your life and shrinks its scope. The mind ruled by addiction and aversion is enslaved in an endless pain-produced and pain-perpetuating quest to get what it craves and avoid what it fears.

This perspective has enormously important implications. It suggests that psychological pain is no mere nuisance to be ignored, anesthetized, or repressed. Rather, it offers opportunities for learning and growth because psychological pain is an invaluable feedback signal, a mental alarm pointing to addiction and aversion and the need to relinquish them.

Contemplative traditions recognize two possible strategies for responding to addictions. The first is common but tragic, the second rare but beneficial.

The first strategy is to devote our lives to satisfying addictions—and thereby mindlessly reinforce and strengthen them. The result is temporary satisfaction and long-term suffering, as drug addicts demonstrate all too well.

The second strategy is to reduce and relinquish addictions. This can be difficult at first, but it enhances long-term well-being. This was the basis of Gandhi's recommendation to "renounce and rejoice"—that is, to renounce and relinquish addictions and to rejoice in the freedom that follows.

Psychological Health

The contemplative ideal of health extends beyond conventional adjustment and encompasses three shifts:

- relinquishment of unhealthy mental qualities such as delusion, craving, and aversion;
- development of specific healthy mental qualities and capacities; and
- maturation to postconventional, transpersonal levels.

Each contemplative tradition has its own list of healthy mental characteristics, but they concur on the crucial importance of seven specific qualities. They agree that psychological health and maturity involve cultivating ethicality, transforming emotions, redirecting motivation, developing concentration, refining awareness, fostering wisdom, and practicing altruism and service (Walsh, 1999). Developing these seven qualities is a central part of contemplative practice.

PSYCHOTHERAPY

Theory of Psychotherapy

The central assumption underlying contemplative therapies is that the mind can be trained so that unhealthy qualities diminish, healthy ones flourish, and development ensues. Many techniques can be used, but effective disciplines include seven central kinds of practices to cultivate seven corresponding qualities of mind and behavior.

1. *Ethics.* With rare exceptions such as existential therapy, Western therapists have usually shied away from introducing ethical issues because of understandable concerns about moralizing and advice giving. However, the contemplative understanding of ethics is very psychologically astute and very different from conventional views. "Rare are those who understand virtue," sighed Confucius (Lau, 1979, p. 132).

   Contemplative traditions view ethics not in terms of conventional morality but in postconventional terms as an essential discipline for training the mind. Meditative introspection soon makes it painfully apparent that unethical behavior—behavior intending to inflict harm—both stems from and strengthens destructive qualities of mind such as greed, anger, and jealousy. In Western terms, unethical behavior reinforces or conditions these destructive qualities; in Asian terms, it deepens their *karmic imprint* on the mind, karma being the psychological residue left by past behavior.

   Conversely, ethical behavior—behavior intended to enhance the well-being of others—does the opposite. It deconditions destructive mental factors while cultivating healthy ones such as kindness, calm, and compassion. From a yogic perspective, ethics is therefore not something imposed from without but rather something sought from within—not a sacrifice but a service to both self and others. The great secret of mature postconventional ethics is recognizing that, as the Buddha pointed out, "Whatever you do, you do to yourself" (Byrom, 1976, p. 118).

   At first, ethical behavior involves a struggle to reverse old habits. However, with practice, it becomes increasingly effortless and spontaneous until eventually "whatever is . . . necessary for sentient beings happens all the time of its own accord" (Gampopa, 1971, p. 271). These heights of contemplative ethics overlap with the highest stages of moral maturity suggested by Harvard researchers Lawrence Kohlberg and Carol Gilligan.

2. *Emotional transformation.* Both contemplative and traditional Western therapies agree on the importance of reducing problematic emotions such as fear, anger, and jealousy. However, contemplative approaches complement this by also cultivating positive emotions such as love, joy, and compassion. Contemplative therapies contain a wealth of practices for cultivating beneficial emotions to remarkable levels. For example, when Buddhist and Confucian compassion or the Christian contemplative's *agape* (love) flower fully, they encompass all creatures unconditionally and unwaveringly. Emotional transformation presumably fosters "emotional intelligence," which research suggests is associated with exceptional personal, interpersonal, and professional success (Goleman, 2003).

3. *Redirecting motivation.* Ethical behavior and emotional transformation work together, along with practices such as meditation, to redirect motivation along healthier paths. As contemplative practices work their effects, motivation becomes less compulsive and more focused on what really matters. There is less concern with material acquisition and more concern with metamotives, especially self-actualization, self-transcendence, and selfless service. Traditionally, this motivational shift was described as *purification*; in contemporary terms, it is analogous to movement up Maslow's (1971) hierarchy of needs.

4. *Training attention.* Contemplative traditions regard training attention and concentration as essential for psychological well-being. By contrast, Western psychology has long accepted William James's forlorn conclusion that "Attention cannot be continuously sustained" (James, 1899/1962, p. 51). Yet James went further to suggest that:

The faculty of voluntarily bringing back a wandering attention over and over again is the very root of judgment, character, and will. No one is *compos sui* [master of himself] if he have it not. An education which would improve this faculty would be the education par excellence. . . . It is easier to define this ideal than to give practical direction for bringing it about. (James, 1910/1950, p. 424)

Here, then, we have a stark contrast between traditional Western psychology, which says attention *cannot* be sustained, and contemplatives who argue that attention can be sustained, indeed *must* be sustained, if we are to mature and realize our potentials.

Developing concentration has many benefits. First, controlling attentional wanderlust is crucial for fostering calm and concentration. Second, the mind tends to take on the qualities of the objects to which it attends. Yoga summarizes this important principle as "Whatever we contemplate or place our attention on, that we become" (Feuerstein, 1996, p. 71).

We have all experienced this ourselves. For example, when we think of an angry person we feel anger, whereas contemplating a loving person elicits feelings of love. People who can control attention can choose what they focus on and can therefore choose and cultivate desired emotions. The primary tool for developing these capacities is meditation.

5. *Refining awareness.* The fifth contemplative practice refines awareness by making perception—both external and internal—more sensitive and accurate. This is necessary because our awareness is usually insensitive and fogged: fragmented by attentional instability, colored by clouding emotions, and distorted by scattered desires. Similar ideas echo through Western thought, which suggests that we mistake shadows for reality (Plato), because we see through *narrow chinks* (William Blake) or a *reducing valve* (Aldous Huxley).

Meditators report that perception becomes more sensitive and their inner world more available. Research indicates that meditators' perceptual processing becomes more sensitive and rapid, their empathy more accurate, and their introspection more refined (Sedlmeier et al., 2012; Walsh, 2008). Meditators claim that clear awareness can be healing and transformative, and they would agree with Fritz Perls (1969), the founder of Gestalt therapy, that "Awareness per se—by and of itself—can be curative" (p. 16).

6. *Wisdom.* Wisdom is deep understanding of oneself and the central existential issues of life plus practical skill in responding effectively and benevolently (Walsh, 2013). Existential issues are those crucial, universal concerns that all of us face simply because we are human. They include finding meaning and purpose in a universe vast beyond comprehension, living in inevitable uncertainty and mystery, managing relationships and facing aloneness, and dealing with sickness, suffering, and death (Walsh, 1999). A person who has developed deep insight into these issues plus skills for dealing with them is wise indeed.

Wisdom is considerably more than knowledge. Whereas knowledge is gained simply by acquiring information, wisdom requires understanding it. Knowledge is something we have; wisdom is something we must become. Knowledge informs us, whereas wisdom transforms us; knowledge empowers, wisdom enlightens.

Contemplative disciplines regard the cultivation of wisdom as a central goal of life. They particularly advise us to seek wisdom from the company of the wise, from studying their writings, from meditation, and from reflecting on the nature of life and death. Jewish contemplatives hold that "Wisdom comes from knowing reality" and urge us to "attend to reality with fullness of heart, mind, and action" (Shapiro, 1993, pp. 30, 84). Mature therapists—who have themselves reflected deeply on existential issues—can be of great assistance here and can offer wise company, recommend readings, encourage introspection, and facilitate reflection.

However, contemplative traditions suggest that social interaction is best balanced with periods of quiet and solitude, especially in nature. Both contemplatives and researchers agree that being in nature "can enhance both physical and mental health," including "greater cognitive, attentional, emotional, spiritual, and subjective well-being" (Walsh, 2011, p. 584).

7. *Altruism and service.* Contemplatives regard altruistic service as both a means to and an expression of psychological well-being. "Make it your guiding principle to do your best for others," urged Confucius, and "put service before the reward you get for it" (Lau, 1979, p. 116). Generosity transforms the mind. Giving inhibits harmful qualities such as craving, jealousy, and fear of loss while it strengthens positive emotions such as love and happiness.

In addition, what we intend others to experience we tend to experience ourselves. For example, if we plot revenge and pain for others, we tend to experience and reinforce emotions such as anger and hatred. Yet when we desire happiness for others, we feel it ourselves: an experience that Buddhists call *empathic joy*. This is why meditations designed to cultivate benevolent feelings such as love or compassion toward other people can produce remarkably ecstatic states in ourselves.

Western psychologists are reaching a similar conclusion: Altruism is correlated with psychological maturity and well-being. For example, Adler's *social interest* and Erikson's *generativity* are said to be essential expressions of successful adult development. Likewise, Maslow (1967, p. 280) claimed that "self-actualizing people, without one single exception, are involved in a cause outside their own skin."

Research shows that generous people tend to be happier, psychologically healthier, and to experience a *helper's high* (Myers, 1992). The so-called paradox of pleasure is that giving time to make others happy makes us happier than devoting all our efforts to our own pleasure (Myers, 1992). Abraham Maslow (1970) summarized the contemplative understanding well when he said, "the best way to become a better helper is to become a better person. But one necessary aspect of becoming a better person is via helping other people" (p. xii).

Some therapists use this principle in their work. For example, Alfred Adler sometimes advised clients to help someone each day. Properly understood, altruistic service to others is not self-sacrifice but enlightened self-interest.

Process of Psychotherapy

Most people who begin contemplative practices find them slow but cumulative, and it may be several weeks before the benefits of brief daily sessions are clearly evident. Meditation and yoga are skills; as with any skill, the initial phase can be the least rewarding, but perseverance usually brings increasing benefits. Because meditation is central to contemplative approaches, has been extensively researched, and is widely used by psychotherapists, we will focus on it here.

After instruction, practice usually starts with short sessions of perhaps 20 minutes once or twice a day. One of the first discoveries that beginners make is how little control they have over their own attentional and cognitive processes, and just how much their minds and lives run on unconscious, automatic pilot. The following exercises—one a visualization and one focusing on the breath—give a glimpse of this automaticity. Read the following paragraphs and then do the exercises.

Visualization.   Seat yourself comfortably and close your eyes. Then visualize an image of a black ring with a black dot in the middle on a white background. Make the image as clear as you can, and then try to hold the image clear and stable for one or two minutes. If you become distracted, re-create the image and continue to try to hold it steady. At the end of that period, open your eyes. Stop reading and do the visualization now.

Now take a moment to reflect on your experience. How much of the time were you able to hold the image clear and steady? How often were you distracted? What does this tell you about your ability to concentrate? About your mental clarity and calm? What else can you learn about your mind from this exercise?

Breath Meditation.   For this exercise, set an alarm on a timer for about 10 minutes, then take a comfortable seat and assume an erect but relaxed posture, with your back relatively straight and head erect. To reduce back strain and aid relaxation, you may wish to support your lumbar back with a pillow. Take a moment to relax.

Now close your eyes and turn your attention to the sensations of breathing in your abdomen. Focus your attention carefully and precisely on the sensations that arise and pass away each instant as the abdominal wall rises and falls. Try not to let your attention wander. If thoughts or feelings arise, just let them be there and continue to focus your awareness on the sensations.

While you attend to the sensations, start counting the breaths from 1 to 10. After you reach 10, go back to 1 again. However, if you lose count or if your mind wanders from the sensations of the breath, even for an instant, then go back to one and start again. If you get distracted or lost in thoughts or fantasy, just recognize what happened, then gently bring your mind back to the breath and start counting from one again. Continue until the alarm tells you to stop. Stop reading and do the exercise now.

At the end of the exercise, estimate how much of the time you were fully aware of the breath and how much you were lost in thoughts and fantasies. Then take a moment to reflect on what you learned about yourself and your mind from this brief concentration meditation.

Most people are shocked to discover that they could not hold the image of the circle stable or maintain awareness of the breath for more than a few seconds. The mind has a mind of its own. The untrained mind is largely uncontrolled and uncontrollable, and a thoughtful person who realizes the full implications of this has made a discovery with life-changing potentials. Thus begins the first stage of meditation practice.

Stages of Practice

Meditation practice can be divided into six overlapping stages. The first three are stages of recognition or insight: the stages of recognizing mental dyscontrol, habitual patterns, and cognitive insights. The three advanced stages include the development of exceptional capacities, the emergence of transpersonal experiences, and the stabilization of transpersonal development.

The *first stage* can be humbling. One of the first recognitions is how little control we have over our own mental processes and how much of our time is spent lost in thoughts and fantasies. After my own first meditation retreat, I wrote, "Shorn of all my props and distractions, it became clear that I had little more than the faintest inkling of self-control over either thoughts or feelings and that my mind had a mind of its own . . . my former state of mindlessness or ignorance of [this] staggered me" (Walsh, 2008, pp. 265, 266).

This recognition of our mindlessness and lack of mental control is an insight of enormous importance. To the extent that our minds are out of control, so too are our lives. This recognition can initially seem overwhelming. However, under the guidance of a good therapist it can also be a powerful incentive to continue practicing and to develop mindfulness and mental mastery.

Experiments support these observations. Sampling people's experiences during the day reveals that "a human mind is a wandering mind, and a wandering mind is an unhappy mind" (Killingsworth & Gilbert, 2010, p. 932). In other words, people spend much of their days lost in mindless thoughts and fantasies and are less happy at these times. Contemplative traditions would add that a contemplatively trained mind wanders less, is present more, and feels happier.

The *second stage* involves recognizing habitual patterns. Here one identifies repetitive mental and behavioral patterns similar to those that insight-oriented psychotherapy unveils.

The *third stage* begins as refined awareness unveils still deeper cognitive insights. Here one can microscopically investigate subtle psychological processes such as thought, motivation, and perception. For example, one sees the way a single thought can elicit emotions, color perception, and provoke muscle tension. One observes how craving evokes tension, grasps at the desired object, fears its loss, and generates anger toward competitors. Insight after insight emerges about how the mind works and how we can better relate to it and live more skillfully.

In advanced stages, which we can consider briefly, exceptional capacities and experiences first emerge and eventually stabilize. The *fourth stage* is marked by the emergence of a variety of exceptional abilities, which are discussed in detail in the research section. In the *fifth stage*, transpersonal experiences emerge, producing identification with others and compassionate concern for them.

The *sixth and final stage* is one of stabilization. Here peak experiences extend into plateau experiences and transient capacities mature into permanent abilities. For example, a practitioner might initially have brief tastes of calm and joy only during meditation sessions. However, with long-term practice, these may deepen into profound peace and joy and expand to pervade daily life. The remarkable nature of these advanced capacities can be sensed from Jack Kornfield's (2008) interview of a contemporary Buddhist meditation master:

> His mind stays completely steady, silent, and free throughout both his waking and sleeping hours. He says, "I haven't experienced a single moment of anger or frustration for over 20 years." He sleeps only one or two hours a night, and describes his inner life, "When I am alone, my mind rests in pure awareness, which has peace and equanimity. Then as I encounter people and experiences, the awareness automatically manifests as loving-kindness or compassion. This is the natural function of pure awareness." (n.p.)

Studies of master meditators reveal unique psychometric and EEG profiles consistent with some of their claims (Lutz, Dunne, & Davidson, 2007). Needless to say, these advanced experiences and developmental stages are rare and usually require long-term or intensive retreat practice. However, they suggest the remarkable potentials available to all of us and that contemplative practices can awaken.

Difficulties

As with any deep uncovering therapy, some experiences can be difficult. The most common are emotional lability, psychosomatic symptoms, unfamiliar perceptual changes, and existential challenges (Wilber et al., 1986).

Emotional lability is probably most frequent. Intense but usually short-lived emotions may surface such as anger, anxiety, or sadness, sometimes accompanied by psychosomatic symptoms such as muscle spasm. Often a therapist need only encourage the practitioner to accept and investigate these experiences—and thereby allow them to resolve by themselves in the healing light of awareness.

As perception becomes more sensitive, habitual perceptions and assumptions may be questioned, and unfamiliar experiences can emerge. One's sense of self and the world may change, resulting in a sense of unfamiliarity or even unreality that can produce confusion and fear. However, continued practice usually brings greater equanimity and comfort with an ever-widening range of experiences and insights.

Most profound and important are existential and spiritual challenges. Freed from external distractions and trivia, the mind naturally turns to what is most important and so ponders questions of deep personal and human significance. These include perennial questions about life's meaning and purpose, our inevitable suffering and death, whether one is living honestly and authentically, and the nature of one's mind, identity, and destiny. These are the deepest questions of life, and focusing on them can be unsettling at first. Yet they are the gateway to wisdom, and exploring them is essential for forging a mature, authentic, and well-lived life (Walsh, 1999; Yalom, 2002).

In many cases, meditative difficulties represent the emergence of previously repressed or incompletely processed memories and conflicts. The initial discomfort of experiencing them may therefore be a necessary price for processing and discharging them. This process is variously described as *karmic release* (yoga), *unstressing* (TM), *interior purification* (Christian contemplation), and *catharsis* and *working through* (psychology).

Like other uncovering therapies, contemplative practices can sometimes unveil underlying pathology. The most extreme result is a psychotic reaction, though fortunately these are very rare. They are most likely in individuals with prior psychotic breaks, who are not taking medication, and who do intensive, unsupervised practice (Wilber et al., 1986).

Therapists familiar with both contemplative and traditional Western therapies can be especially helpful with contemplative difficulties. They can recognize and treat common minor difficulties, as well as the less common but more severe underlying pathologies that occasionally surface. Because of their personal familiarity with common difficulties, meditatively experienced therapists can recognize them in their clients, empathize sincerely, and treat them effectively.

There are many useful strategies for treating common difficulties. In many cases, they resolve spontaneously with further practice, especially when a therapist provides reassurance and normalization (advice that these are normal, common challenges). *Reframing* and *reattribution* (reinterpreting experiences as potential opportunities for learning and growth) are especially valuable. Common problems can also be treated with standard Western therapeutic techniques such as relaxation or with specific remedies suggested by contemplative disciplines. It can be very valuable to explore the psychological and existential implications of contemplative experiences.

Medication is rarely necessary for contemplative difficulties, which are usually transient and better treated with psychological and contemplative strategies. However, medication may be entirely appropriate when contemplatives also suffer from severe psychological disorders such as depression.

Mechanisms of Psychotherapy

Explanations of how contemplative therapies work are of three main types: metaphorical, process, and mechanistic. All three are valuable because many factors are involved, and each type illuminates a facet of the rich growth process that contemplation catalyzes.

Traditional explanations are usually metaphorical. Common metaphors used to describe the meditative or yogic process include *awakening* from our collective trance, *freeing* us from illusions and conditioning, and *purifying* the mind of toxic qualities. Others include *unfolding* our innate potentials, *uncovering* our true identity, and *enlightening* us about our true identity. These metaphors offer several insights. They suggest that contemplative practices set in motion growth processes that are organic, healing, self-actualizing, and even enlightening. Some of the ways they do this are suggested by the following mechanisms.

Mechanisms Suggested by Contemplative Traditions

Calming the Mind.   The untrained mind is agitated and distracted, continuously leaping from past to future, from thought to fantasy. Contemplative techniques concentrate and calm the mind. As the opening lines of a classic yoga text state: "Yoga is the settling of the mind into silence. When the mind has settled, we are established in our essential nature, which is unbounded Consciousness" (Shearer, 1989, p. 49).

This process of calming and stilling is the basis for the Western suggestion that meditation works, in part, by producing a *relaxation response*. However, research shows that the effects of meditation are far larger than those of relaxation alone (Sedlmeier et al., 2012).

Enhanced Awareness.   Heightened awareness is emphasized across contemplative practices (Walsh, 1999). It is the primary focus in Buddhist mindfulness and Taoist *internal observation* and is also central to the Sufi practice of *watchfulness of the moment* and the Christian contemplative discipline of *guarding the intellect*.

Many clinicians also regard it as central to psychotherapy. In fact, "virtually all therapies endorse the expansion of consciousness . . ." (enhanced awareness) (Norcross & Beutler, 2013). Examples include Eugene Gendlin's "experiencing" and the Jungian claim that "therapeutic progress depends on awareness . . ." (Whitmont, 1969, p. 293). Refining awareness may therefore be a central process producing the benefits of both meditation and psychotherapy. It may also be a necessary precondition for a further important contemplative process—disidentification.

Disidentification.   This is the process by which awareness precisely observes and therefore ceases to unconsciously identify with mental content such as thoughts, feelings, and fantasies (Walsh & Shapiro, 2006). For example, if the thought "I'm scared" arises but is not carefully observed and recognized as just a thought, then it becomes a belief and is accepted as reality. One identifies with the thought, which is no longer something that is seen; rather, it is that from which, and through which, one sees. What was an *object* of awareness has become the *subject* of awareness; what was "it" has become "me."

The self is now identified with this thought, hypnotized by it, or "fused" with it as ACT practitioners would say. One's experiential reality is now "I'm scared." What was merely a thought now appears to be terrifying reality. As yoga points out, "The cause of suffering is the identification of the perceiver with the perceived" (Nisargadatta, 1973, p. 136).

However, if the meditator is sufficiently mindful when the thought "I'm scared" arises, then it is recognized as what it is: merely a thought. It is not mistaken for reality and has little effect on mind or body. Awareness has disidentified from the thought, is no longer hypnotized by it, and therefore not controlled by it. Of course, the meditator can still act on the thought if appropriate, but such action is now a conscious choice rather than an unconscious automaticity.

The general principle is that when we unconsciously identify with a part of the mind—say a thought or fantasy—we assume it to be true, and are hypnotized by it. When we consciously disidentify from it, we are free, and this freedom produces healing and growth.

Rebalancing Mental Elements.   Contemplative psychologies commonly divide mental contents into healthy and unhealthy categories. Naturally, a major contemplative goal is to increase healthy factors and decrease unhealthy ones. This can be seen as a process of rebalancing of mental elements and metaphorically as purification.

Buddhist psychology offers a particularly sophisticated map of mental elements and emphasizes the "seven factors of enlightenment." These are seven qualities of mind that, when cultivated and balanced one with another, are said to optimize health and growth. The first factor is *mindfulness,* a precise conscious awareness of each stimulus that can be regarded as a refinement of the psychoanalytic observing ego. The remaining six mental factors are divided into two groups: one composed of three energizing qualities and the other of three calming qualities. The three energizing factors are *effort, investigation* (active exploration of experience), and *rapture* (ecstasy that results from clear, concentrated awareness). The three calming factors are *concentration, calm,* and *equanimity.*

This model of mental health invites intriguing comparisons between contemplative and conventional Western therapies (Walsh & Vaughan, 1993). Western therapists recognize that the energizing factors of effort and investigation are essential. However, they are less aware of the potentiating effects of simultaneously developing the calming factors. When the mind is concentrated, calm, and equanimous, then awareness is clearer, insight is deeper, and growth is quicker. Cultivating and balancing all seven factors is said to be optimal for growth and to lead to the pinnacle of transpersonal maturity: enlightenment.

Mechanisms Suggested by Mental–Health Professionals

Western researchers have suggested a range of psychological and physiological mechanisms to account for the effects of meditation. Psychological possibilities include relaxation, desensitization to formerly stressful stimuli, counterconditioning, and catharsis. Automatic habits may undergo *deautomatization*, becoming less automatic and coming under greater voluntary control. Cognitive mechanisms include learning and insight, as well as self-acceptance, self-control, and self-understanding.

Probably the most encompassing explanation is developmental. Both contemplatives and psychologists suggest that meditation may work many of its effects by restarting and catalyzing development (Wilber, 1999). In fact, many traditions map progress in developmental terms. Classic examples include the Jewish *stages of ascent*, Sufi levels of identity, Taoism's *five periods* of increasing calm, and the Buddhist *stages of insight*. Research studies of TM are supportive and suggest that it fosters ego, cognitive, and moral development, as well as coping skills and self-actualization (Alexander et al., 1991). Practices that can foster maturation are obviously extraordinarily important. Figure 12.1 illustrates a variety of contemplative practices that are sometimes used in psychotherapy.

APPLICATIONS

Who Can We Help?

Considerable evidence suggests that contemplative practices can help with an exceptionally wide range of psychological, somatic, and spiritual issues, and we can divide the kinds of benefits into three categories. First are therapeutic applications for psychological and somatic disorders. Second is the enhancement of psychological capacities and well-being, and third are the classic goals involving transpersonal growth and spirituality.

Therapeutic Applications: Psychological Disorders

Stress Disorders.   Contemplative practices can benefit a wide array of psychological and psychosomatic disorders, and stress disorders have been the most extensively researched. For example, mindfulness-based therapies can ameliorate multiple anxiety disorders including generalized, social, panic, phobic, and posttraumatic stress disorders. Meta-analyses show large effect sizes compared to cognitive behavior therapy

FIGURE 12.1

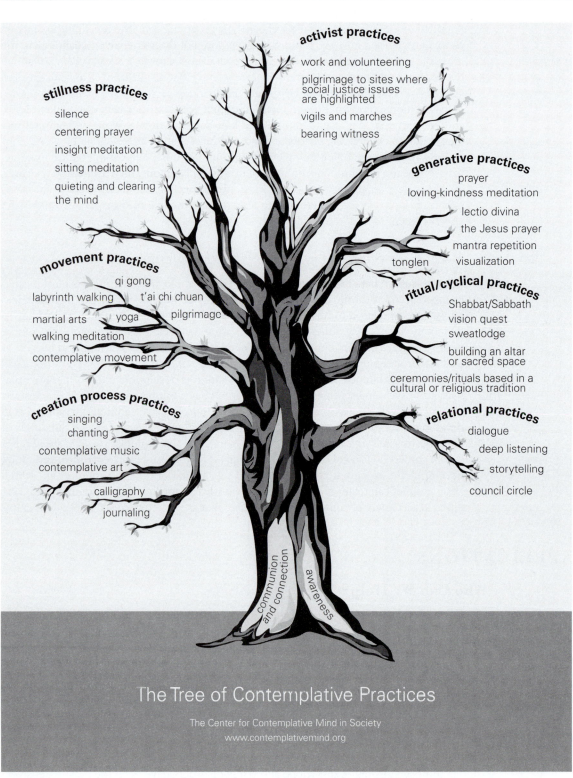

The Tree of Contemplative Practices

The Center for Contemplative Mind in Society
www.contemplativemind.org

© The Center for Contemplative Mind in Society Concept & design by Maia Duerr; illustration by Carrie Bergman. Reprinted with permission.

(CBT), and that multicomponent mindfulness-based therapies—such as MBSR, MBCT, and ACT—are more effective than mindfulness alone (Vøllestad, Nielson, & Nielson, 2011). In short, mindfulness-based therapies are effective treatments for stress disorders and may be even more effective when combined with therapeutic lifestyle changes (TLCs) such as exercise, pescovegetarian diet, and time in nature (Walsh, 2011).

Meditation also reduces anxiety in special populations. Examples include the dying and their caregivers, as well as prisoners who also display reduced aggression and recidivism. Given the many people languishing in prison, especially in the United States, and their tragically high recidivism rates, these findings are of considerable importance (Alexander, Walton, Orme-Johnson, Goodman, & Pallone, 2003).

Drugs are often used to manage stress, and TM reduces the use of both legal and illegal drugs. However, TM practitioners are required to stop using drugs for several days before their initial training, so they may be only mildly addicted and particularly responsive. A review of mindfulness-based treatments concluded that they are promising but not yet fully proven therapies for drug use disorders (Zgierska et al., 2009).

These stress-related benefits of meditation are consistent both with physiological studies of meditators and classic claims. Classically, "Relaxation is the alpha and omega of yoga" (Feuerstein, 1996, p. 51). However, as yet research support for yoga's effectiveness in reducing anxiety and depressive disorders is promising but inconclusive (Kirkwood, Rampes, Tuffrey, Richardson, & Pilkington, 2005).

Depression.   Depression is one of the most painful of all psychological disorders, is often chronic and relapsing, and exacts an enormous worldwide toll. Unfortunately, antidepressant medications help only some two-thirds of patients, often incompletely, and do not correct psychological and lifestyle causes of depression. Fortunately, MBCT as well as therapeutic lifestyle changes (TLCs) such as exercise and diet (especially fish oil supplements) can be helpful (Walsh, 2011). MBCT can reduce relapse rates as effectively as antidepressants with far fewer side effects (Chiesa & Serreti, 2011).

Attention Deficit Hyperactivity Disorder (ADHD).   Given meditation's dramatic effects on attention, could it benefit ADHD? The few studies to date suggest benefits but are inconclusive (Krisanaprakornkit, Ngamjarus, Witoonchart, & Piyavhatkul, 2010).

Contemplation for Children.   There is considerable enthusiasm for offering meditation and yoga to children as is often done in Asia. Positive anecdotes abound, school programs are expanding, and preliminary research suggests academic, social, and behavioral benefits (Greenberg & Harris, 2012).

Meditation Combination Therapies.   Many combination therapies that meld mindfulness with conventional Western psychotherapies are effective with additional disorders. The original approach, MBSR, has been applied to stress, chronic pain, and multiple other psychological and physical conditions. Mindfulness-based approaches targeting specific disorders include mindfulness-based eating awareness therapy (MB-EAT) for eating disorders, and mindfulness-based therapy for insomnia.

Combination therapies that incorporate a meditation component other than mindfulness include dialectical behavior therapy for borderline personality disorders and ACT. Both have strong research support (Vøllestad et al., 2011). Further combination therapies continue to appear and will doubtless be applied to more and more disorders.

Many therapists have observed a mutually beneficial interaction when clients engage in both conventional psychotherapy and contemplative practice. Conventional therapies can help clients deal with painful issues that emerge during meditation. They can also resolve defenses and other blocks inhibiting contemplative progress. Likewise, meditation and yoga can facilitate conventional psychotherapy by cultivating requisite skills, such as calm and introspection, and by allowing clients to work on issues outside the therapeutic hour.

Therapeutic Applications for Somatic Issues

Contemplative therapies can help treat some diseases and reduce the anxiety and distress that accompany many diseases. Considerable research suggests that many stress-related psychosomatic disorders benefit from meditation.

The Cardiovascular System

Meditation produces several cardiovascular benefits. It reduces both high blood pressure and cholesterol levels, but the effects dissipate if practice is discontinued (Anderson, Liu, & Kryscio, 2008).

Coronary artery disease offers a particularly dramatic demonstration of the power of contemplative and lifestyle treatments. Coronary artery disease is a leading cause of death and disability, was long thought to be irreversible, and was believed to require major surgery or cholesterol-lowering drugs. However, research demonstrates that far less dangerous and far healthier lifestyle changes—especially a combination of low-fat diet, exercise, interpersonal openness, plus meditation and yoga—can actually reverse the disorder. My 76-year-old mother went from being a "cardiac cripple" to an athletic jogger after going through this program. These lifestyle changes also seem to slow or perhaps even reverse the progression of prostate cancer (Ornish et al., 2008).

Hormonal and Immune Effects

The hormonal and immune systems are also affected by meditation. Partially responsive hormonal disorders include type II diabetes, primary dysmenorrhea, and premenstrual dysphoric disorder (Murphy & Donovan, 1997). Meditation can also enhance immune function in both healthy people and cancer patients (Kabat-Zinn, 2003). For example, meditators have an enhanced response to influenza immunization.

Further Adjuvant Treatments

Meditation has been shown to enhance the conventional treatment of many other physical disorders, including asthma, psoriasis, prostate cancer, and chronic pain disorders (Kabat-Zinn, 2003). It is not surprising that meditation, yoga, and tai chi can reduce secondary distress in a wide array of illnesses including cancer, fibromyalgia, rheumatoid arthritis, and gastrointestinal disorders (Lin, Hu, Chang, Lin, & Tsauo, 2011; Wang et al., 2010). Because anxiety and distress complicate so many illnesses, contemplative practices will likely prove useful adjuvant therapies for many psychological and somatic disorders.

Enhancing Well-Being

Contemplative practices were originally intended to enhance psychological and spiritual well-being. These ancient claims have been tested experimentally, and the results are clear. Considerable research now demonstrates that clients, therapists, and the general population may all show improvements on multiple measures of personality and performance, health and well-being, maturity and relationships. The clearest way of demonstrating these improvements is with a graph drawn from a massive meta-analysis of 163 studies of nonpatient populations (See Figure 12.2; Sedlmeier et al., 2012).

What do the results tell us? First, the overall effect of meditation on all variables combined was 0.28. (For comparison, an effect size of 0.1 is considered small, 0.3 is medium, and 0.5 or more is large.) The value 0.28 is therefore a medium-sized highly significant effect that lays to rest once and for all the question of whether meditation can be beneficial. The researchers concluded, "The present meta-analysis yields a clear answer: yes" (Sedlmeier et al., 2012, p. 20).

How does this effect size of 0.28 compare to other interventions? It was larger (by 0.16) than active control treatments and considerably larger than relaxation (0.21). It was even slightly larger than the combined effect size from thousands of studies of educational, psychological, and psychotherapeutic interventions. Clearly meditation can be powerful.

FIGURE 12.2   **The effect size of meditation practice on psychological variables.**

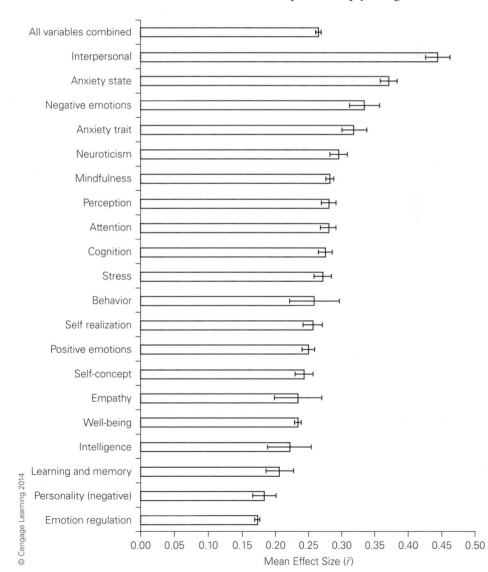

The findings are derived from a meta-analysis of 163 studies of non-patient populations done by Sedlmeier et al., 2012.

Does everyone benefit equally? Well, there were no age or gender differences. Longer practice did produce greater effects. However, the additional benefits tended to plateau eventually, possibly because the variables studied do not measure advanced psychological and spiritual states.

What Specific Benefits Does Meditation Produce?

The graph vividly demonstrates a wide array of benefits, but their size varies significantly.

Clearly, meditators can undergo major emotional transformations. Anxiety, negative emotions, and neuroticism show some of the largest reductions, whereas positive emotions and the ability to regulate emotions increase. In short, meditators tend to become happier, their stress levels fall, and their sense of well-being soars.

Strikingly, the largest impact of all was to improve the quality of relationships. These interpersonal changes make sense given the dramatic personal changes in emotions and empathy. For example, one mindfulness-based relationship enhancement program improved multiple measures of both individual and relationship satisfaction in couples. Individuals felt more relaxed and optimistic, and as a couple they felt closer, yet also more autonomous, accepting, and satisfied. Benefits persisted through a three-month follow-up period (Carson, Carson, Gil, & Baucom, 2004).

Because meditation trains perception, attention, and mindfulness, it is not surprising that these improve. Perceptual sensitivity, accuracy, and speed all increase. So does interpersonal empathy. For example, advanced meditators pick up subtle interpersonal cues, such as brief emotional facial expressions, that the rest of us overlook.

Likewise, meditation improves multiple measures of attention and concentration. This has practical benefits for students, who report that they notice mind wandering more quickly, and so can study more effectively. As expected, their academic performance also improves (Shapiro, Astin, Bishop, & Cordova, 2005).

Meditation benefits multiple cognitive capacities. Short- and long-term memory improve, as do measures of intelligence and creativity. The effect on short-term (working) memory is particularly intriguing because it appears to be a key determinant of intelligence and was thought to be largely hard wired and resistant to change.

Given that meditation is a self-regulation strategy it is understandable that practitioners report enhanced self-control, self-esteem, and self-compassion. The net effect of these changes, and the many others already discussed, is an improved self-concept. In short, meditators tend to feel better about themselves, and this improved self-concept appears to be grounded in multiple personal and interpersonal benefits.

Do Different Meditations Produce Different Effects?

The overall effect size for mindfulness, TM, and "other" meditations were similar. However, analysis of the individual variables unveiled a more nuanced picture. For example, TM appeared particularly effective for reducing negative emotions, trait anxiety, and neuroticism, as well as in improving memory and self-realization. On the other hand, mindfulness was more beneficial for reducing negative personality traits and improving self-concept. In short, specific meditations produce similar overall effects but somewhat different specific effects.

MBSR Versus Mindfulness Alone

MBSR is a multimodality program that centers on mindfulness training, but it also offers education, yoga, and social support. These additional components produce additional benefits because MBSR has a significantly larger effect size (0.31) than mindfulness alone (0.25). These benefits show up especially in heightened well-being and in reduced anxiety, stress, and negative emotions (Eberth & Sedlmeier, 2012).

Psychological Maturity

A classic contemplative goal is to encourage mental maturation, and research studies are supportive. Meditators tend to score higher on developmental measures such as ego, moral, and cognitive maturity, as well as in coping skills, defenses, and self-actualization (Alexander et al., 1991; Sedlmeier et al., 2012; Travis, Arenander, & DeBois, 2004). This suggests that meditation can restart or catalyze psychological development in adults.

Do Contemplative Practices Reduce the Effects of Aging?

Contemplative traditions, especially yogas, have long claimed to enhance not only natural and physical health but also even longevity. Is this a mere myth or might there be something to this dramatic claim? Remarkably, several studies are supportive.

Surveys of TM meditators suggest that they are healthier than normal and use approximately half the usual amounts of psychiatric and medical care. Practitioners also score significantly younger than control subjects on markers of biological age, and the extent of improvement correlates with amount of meditation (Alexander, Langer, Newman, Chandler, & Davies, 1989). However, it is unclear how much of this superior general health actually results from meditation and how much from associated factors such as prior good health and healthy lifestyles.

However, carefully controlled studies of meditators do demonstrate reduced psychological and neural effects of aging. Psychologically, meditators do not seem to suffer usual age-related losses of attention skills. Neurally, meditators show greater gray matter volume and density in areas such as the hippocampus and prefrontal cortex, greater connectivity within and between hemispheres, and less age-related loss of gray matter (Ott, Hölzel, & Vaitl, 2011).

One well-designed study demonstrated dramatic effects on elderly retirement home residents whose average age was 81. Those who learned TM performed better on several measures of cognitive function and mental health than did residents who were taught relaxation, were given other mental training, or were left untreated. However, the most striking finding was a highly significant ($p < 0.001$) difference in survival rates. Three years later, all the meditators were still alive, compared to only three-quarters of the untreated study subjects and only two-thirds of residents who did not participate in the study (Alexander et al., 1989). For thousands of years, yogis have claimed that contemplative practices increase longevity, and this claim now has initial experimental support.

Benefits for Health Professionals

Many of the benefits conferred by contemplative practices are both personally and professionally helpful for health professionals and especially for psychotherapists. For example, meditation can enhance essential therapist qualities such as Rogers's *accurate empathy*, Freud's *evenly hovering attention*, and Horney's *wholehearted attention*. Karen Horney (1952/1998) observed that, although "such wholeheartedness is a rare attainment," it is "commonplace in Zen" (p. 36). Other therapeutically useful capacities enhanced by meditation include self-actualization, self-acceptance, compassion, and calm (Germer, Siegel, & Fulton, 2005; Irving et al., 2009).

Shapiro and Carlson (2009) point out that learning to manage stress and enhance self-care should be a central part of clinical training and professional development. In fact, it rarely is. High stress levels are common challenges for health-care professionals, and both they and their patients pay a price. Fortunately, research suggests that a personal contemplative practice can reduce symptoms of stress—such as anxiety and depression—while enhancing life satisfaction in health-care professionals and students (Shapiro et al., 2005).

Therapists report that the deep insights into the workings of their own minds that contemplative practices provide also foster insight into and compassion for their clients. Many therapists feel that their skills are enhanced by these practices and recommend them as part of psychotherapists' training. A study of psychotherapists who were taught meditation during their training found that their patients had significantly better treatment outcomes than those of control-group therapists (Grepmair et al., 2007).

Not surprisingly, personal contemplative practice can enhance psychotherapists' ability to work with patients who practice contemplation. A personal practice deepens clinicians' understanding of contemplative experiences, increases their ability to diagnose and work with contemplative difficulties, and enhances empathy and therapeutic effectiveness (Germer et al., 2005).

Transpersonal Growth

Finally, contemplative disciplines are available for those who wish to practice more intensely to foster growth to transpersonal levels. Here they can be used to explore the depths of mind, probe existential questions, develop exceptional abilities and well-being, and seek advanced levels of psychological and spiritual maturity. Although deep insights can occur at any moment, these exceptional capacities and levels often require long-term practice reckoned in years rather than days or weeks. Of course, this is true of any mastery.

Specific Techniques and Skills

Our discussion so far has focused on general principles common to most contemplative practices. However, there are also hundreds of specific meditative and yogic techniques designed to elicit specific capacities and skills. The following are brief descriptions of two skills—the cultivation of love and lucid dreaming—that Western psychologists considered impossible until recently. Together, they point to the remarkable range of practices and powers of mind that contemplatives have discovered in their 3,000-year-long exploration of our inner universe.

The Cultivation of Love.   There are many specific practices for cultivating love. One such meditation begins by first calming the mind and then focusing attention unwaveringly on an image of someone you love. In a calm, concentrated mind, feelings of love can arise intensely. After they do, you gradually and successively substitute images of a friend, a stranger, and groups of people and thereby cultivate and condition the feelings of love to them. With continued practice, you can eventually visualize all people while embracing them in love.

Other practices cultivate related positive emotions such as *empathic joy* (happiness at the happiness of others, which is a superb antidote to jealousy) and *compassion* (the emotional basis for altruism). Western psychologists have recently recognized altruism as an independent drive but lament that they know so little about how to cultivate it. In contrast, contemplative disciplines contain literally dozens of practices to cultivate altruism.

Love and compassion practices can be powerful. They not only strengthen positive emotions but also reduce negative emotions such as anger and fear. Classic texts describe advanced benefits such as deep, encompassing, unwavering, and unconditional love for all people and compassion for all who suffer (Kornfield, 1993).

Contemporary research is beginning to agree. Studies of loving-kindness meditation suggest that students, patients, and therapists can all benefit. These benefits include reductions in negative emotions, as well as small but significant increases in people's daily experience of "a wide range of positive emotions, including love, joy, contentment, gratitude, pride, hope, interest, amusement and awe" (Hofmann, Grossman, & Hinton, 2011, p. 1129). It is no surprise that people's relationships also improve.

Lucid Dreaming.   Dream yoga is a 2,000-year-old technique for developing lucid dreaming: the ability to know one is dreaming while still asleep. Adepts are able to observe and modify their dreams so as to continue their explorations and learning during sleep. The most advanced practitioners maintain unbroken awareness throughout the night, during both dream and nondream sleep, thereby combining the benefits of clear awareness and the extreme peace of conscious sleep (Walsh & Vaughan, 1993). The result is continuous lucidity—or "ever-present wakefulness," as the contemplative Plotinus called it—throughout day and night. Western psychologists long dismissed lucid dreaming as impossible until sleep EEGs confirmed its existence.

Both classic lucid dream instructions and contemporary induction techniques are now freely available (Walsh & Vaughan, 1993). Consequently, people can now enjoy this ancient yogic skill and can explore and cultivate the mind in the comfort of their own beds. For Freud, dreams were a royal road to the unconscious. For contemplatives, lucid dreams are a royal road to consciousness.

Treatment

As contemplative therapies evolved across centuries, practitioners devised literally thousands of techniques ranging across somatic, psychological, and spiritual domains. These include everything from diet and breathing disciplines through ethical and lifestyle changes to visualizations and meditations (Feuerstein, 1996).

In general, novices begin with one or two simple meditative or yogic practices. Over time, they add related exercises and begin more demanding practices so that more and more of their experiences and lives are used for learning and growth. Tailoring the evolving program to the individual practitioner is the mark of a skilled therapist. The following are simple introductory exercises and meditations—from each of the seven practices common to contemplative therapies—that have proved valuable for both clients and therapists.

Ethical Behavior: Say Only What Is True and Helpful

Mark Twain is credited with the line "Truth is so very precious, man is naturally economical in its use." Contemplative disciplines take a different approach. Meditators cannot long escape recognizing the painful toll—for example, anxiety, agitation, and guilt—that unethical behavior such as deceit and aggression exacts on their own minds. As a result, the desire to live more truthfully and ethically grows stronger.

Truth telling does not imply blurting out everything that comes to mind or being insensitive to people's feelings. Rather, it means bringing careful awareness to each situation to find what we can say that is true to our experience and, wherever possible, helpful to others. When we don't know what is truthful or helpful, it is appropriate either to say we don't know or to remain silent. The Buddha's succinct recommendation was to say only what is true and helpful.

Exercise 1: Look for the Lie.   It is intriguing to see how much personal and interpersonal pain is a result of lying to either oneself or others. Consequently, a useful exercise in psychotherapy (and life) is to look for the lies that are causing and perpetuating suffering and then to explore how to end them.

Exercise 2: Say Only What Is True and Helpful for a Day.   An excellent way to begin the practice of truth telling is to commit to doing it for a day. This exercise becomes even more powerful if you carefully record any temptations to lie and take the time to identify the underlying motives and emotions. On hearing of this exercise, some people obsess over the question of what the "truth" is. However, the point is not to become lost in endless philosophical musings but to be honest about the only thing we ever know: our experience.

Transforming Emotions: Use Wise Attention to Cultivate Beneficial Emotions

By enhancing concentration, contemplative practices allow us to practice "wise attention." This is the practice of directing attention to people and situations that foster desired qualities (Walsh, 1999). The underlying principle is that we tend to strengthen those qualities to which we give attention. What we focus on, we become. For example, many studies show that watching violence on television can foster aggression. On the other hand, contemplative therapies suggest that when we attend to people who are kind and generous, we cultivate these qualities in ourselves (Kornfield, 1993). What we put into our minds is just as important as what we put into our mouths.

Exercise.   First, relax or meditate and be aware of how you feel. Notice the emotions you are experiencing. Next, visualize or think of someone who tends to be angry and aggressive. Notice any emotions that arise and how you feel. Then take a moment to relax or meditate again. Now visualize or think of someone who is kind and loving and observe the corresponding emotions. Note how differently you feel after visualizing these two people. What we meditate on, we cultivate. Put down the book and do the exercise now.

Transforming Motivation: Explore the Experience of Craving

Bringing clear awareness to experiences and behavior is crucial to transforming them. Yet when caught by an addiction, we usually focus on what we are trying to get rather than on the actual experience of craving and what it is doing to our mind.

Exercise.   For this exercise, take the opportunity to carefully explore craving. You can do this in two ways: You can wait for an addictive urge to arise spontaneously or you can choose to think of something you're attached to. For this exercise, it's best to work with a mild craving rather than one that may overwhelm you.

When you become aware of a craving, stop whatever you are doing. Then turn attention to your craving and explore it. Try to identify the experiential components that make it up: the underlying emotions, body sensations, thoughts, feelings, and tensions. Bringing careful awareness to the experience of craving rather than mindlessly acting it out gives insight into it and can also decondition and weaken it. In fact, contemplative disciplines suggest that weak addictions "can be removed by introspection and meditation" (Nisargadatta, 1973, p. 112).

Develop Concentration and Calm: Do One Thing at a Time

In our overly busy lives, distractions proliferate, electronic gadgets demand attention, and we often juggle several things simultaneously. New words are emerging to describe our jangled lives and minds. These words include *multitasking, technostress, digital fog, techno-brain burnout, frazzing* (frantic, inefficient multitasking), and *attention-deficit trait*, which is attention-deficit caused by information overload (Walsh, 2011).

Multitasking offers a seductive illusion of efficiency. Yet research now demonstrates what contemplative therapies have long argued: Multitasking and attentional fragmentation actually reduce efficiency and creativity while at the same time inflicting anxiety and agitation. Just as important, they also reduce clarity, thoughtful reflection, and introspection. Distracted fragmented lives create distracted fragmented minds.

Contemplative therapies counteract frenzy and fragmentation by fostering concentration and calm. Regular practice of concentration meditation—such as focusing attention on the breath as described earlier—is an excellent method. The following exercise is a useful addition.

Exercise: Do One Thing at a Time.   To begin, commit a specific time—a day might be good to begin with—to doing only one thing at a time. For this day, give up all multitasking. Give your full attention to each individual activity and each conversation. This very simple exercise can have dramatic effects.

Cultivate Awareness: Mindfulness Meditation and Mindful Eating

After a lifetime of therapeutic work, Jungian psychiatrist Edward Whitmont (1969) concluded that "Therapeutic progress depends upon awareness; in fact the attempt to become more conscious is the therapy" (p. 293). Contemplative traditions agree and have long emphasized the value of cultivating awareness and introspection. Buddhist meditators are told to observe each experience, whereas Jewish and Christian contemplatives respectively urge us to "Attend to each moment" and "Above all . . . be watchful" (Palmer, Sherrard, & Ware, 1993, p. 97; Shapiro, 1993, p. 17).

However, contemplatives recommend that awareness be cultivated not only during therapy sessions but also during every waking moment. The goal is to become what Carl Rogers described as "fully functioning people [who] are able to experience all their feelings, afraid of none of them, allowing awareness to flow freely in and through their experiences" (Raskin & Rogers, 1995, p. 141). For this, contemplative disciplines recommend mindfulness (awareness) meditation coupled with awareness exercises.

Mindfulness meditation is an art. Like any art, it is best learned via personal instruction, and mastery requires long-term practice. However, even brief experiences can sometimes offer valuable insights, and the following exercise offers a taste of the process. It is best done in quiet surroundings where you will not be disturbed.

Exercise 1: Mindfulness Meditation.   Set an alarm for a period of 10 to 15 minutes, find a comfortable sitting posture, and take a moment to relax. Then let your attention settle on the sensations of the breath and investigate these physical sensations as sensitively and carefully as you can. Continue to explore those sensations until another stimulus—perhaps a sound, emotion, or sensation—draws attention to it. Then simply explore this stimulus sensitively and carefully until it disappears or is no longer interesting. At this point, return attention to the breath until attracted by another stimulus.

Periodically, you will recognize that you have been lost in thoughts and fantasies. At that point, simply return to the breath and start again. Awareness meditation is a gentle dance of awareness in which you begin with the breath, allow attention to move to interesting stimuli, explore them, and then return to the breath.

Simply investigate experiences as carefully as you can, allowing them to come and go without interference, without judging or condemning, or struggling to change them. Not surprisingly, this cessation of struggle can eventually lead to deep peace, but most beginners are initially shocked to discover how agitated their minds are. Take a few minutes now to do the meditation and see for yourself.

Mindfulness meditation is a gentle exercise in cultivating awareness, insight, and acceptance. It is based on the recognition, recently popularized by acceptance and commitment therapy, that within the mind, whatever we bring awareness to and accept can begin to heal. Conversely, what we resist or attempt to suppress can rebound, producing an *ironic effect* opposite to what we want. Contemplative traditions, and especially mindfulness meditations, therefore emphasize that, to put it poetically:

Be kind to your mind
For what you resist will surely persist,
But what you befriend may come to an end.

Exercise 2: Mindful Eating.   More than 2,000 years ago, Confucius's grandson observed "Amongst people there are none who do not eat and drink but there are few who really appreciate the taste" (Yu-Lan, 1948, p. 175). Apparently, things have not changed much. Often we multitask distractedly, even as we eat. We sit down to a meal and also carry on a conversation, watch television, or read the newspaper. The next thing we notice is that our plate is empty. No wonder that mindful eating is an effective strategy for weight control.

For this exercise, choose a time when you can eat without distraction. Seat yourself comfortably and take a few mindful breaths to relax. Mindful eating involves attending to and enjoying each sensation and taste, so begin by enjoying the sight and smell of the food. Observe the sensations as you reach for it, the feelings of anticipation, and the touch as it enters the mouth. Then note experiences such as the temperature and texture of the food, subtle background flavors, and feelings of pleasure. Continue to eat each mouthful carefully, consciously, and as enjoyably as you can. Periodically, you will realize that you have been lost in thoughts or fantasies and were quite unaware of the last few mouthfuls. That is how we usually eat and live our lives: in semiconscious distraction. Simply return attention to the experience of eating again and enjoy your meal as fully as you can.

Of course, many meals are social occasions and celebrations, and here mindful eating is more difficult. But the basic issue is the same as with other meditations and therapies. It is the *challenge of generalization*: the challenge of generalizing the skills learned in therapy to other areas of life.

Developing Wisdom: Reflect on Our Mortality

Contemplative therapies offer many techniques for cultivating wisdom, and among them careful reflections on our life and inevitable death are deemed particularly powerful. Without recognizing our mortality, we tend to squander our lives in inauthentic petty pursuits, tranquilize ourselves with trivia, and forget what really matters. Contemplative disciplines emphasize that, as Muhammad stated, "Death is a good advisor" (Angha, 1995, p. 82). They therefore encourage us to recall that, as Taoists point out, our lives last "but a moment" and that, in Shankara's words, "Youth, wealth and the years of a [person's] life . . . roll quickly away like drops of water from a lotus leaf" (Prabhavananda & Isherwood, 1978, p. 136). When we remember that we don't know how long we and other people will live, we are inspired to live more fully, lovingly, boldly, and impeccably.

Mortality and Wisdom Reflections.   The following questions are common topics for reflection in contemplative disciplines and can be examined in several formats. One approach is to reflect on them in therapy sessions. However, they can also be pondered alone, written about in a journal, or discussed with a trusted friend. Advanced practitioners use the power of concentrated awareness to meditate on them. Consider using one of these formats to explore the following questions:

Given that we will all die, what is truly important in your life?

If you were to die tomorrow, what would you regret not having done?

What relationships remain unhealed in your life, and how could you begin healing them?

These reflections can motivate us to reorder our priorities, live more fully and authentically, and heal our relationships (Walsh, 1999).

Generosity and Service: Transform Pain into Compassion

Research shows that one effective strategy for combating sadness and grief is *downward comparison* in which we compare ourselves with others who are worse off (Myers, 1992). However, contemplative traditions suggest that it can be taken further and used as an effective strategy for cultivating compassion.

Compassion Exercise.   Traditionally, this exercise, like so many contemplative exercises, would be done after a period of meditation. The mind is then calm and concentrated, and this enhances the impacts of selected thoughts and images. Therefore, if you already know how to meditate, begin by doing so. Otherwise, simply relax for a moment.

Think of some difficulty you are having, either physical or psychological. Next, think of people who are suffering from related difficulties, perhaps even more than you are. If you know specific individuals suffering in this way, bring them to mind. Think of the pain your difficulty has brought you and of all the pain that others must be experiencing. Recognize that just as you want to be free of pain, so do they. Open yourself to the experience of their suffering and let concern and compassion for them arise. Stop reading and do the exercise now.

Defenseless awareness of the suffering of others arouses compassion and contribution. Contemplative traditions agree that compassionate service to others "clarifies the mind and purifies the heart" (Nisargadatta, 1973, p. 72) and is therefore both a means to, and an expression of, psychological maturity and well-being.

Contemplative therapies begin by presenting simple introductory meditations and exercises such as these. As skill develops, practitioners are encouraged to practice more deeply and intensely and to move on to more advanced disciplines.

Evidence

The classic approach to evaluating contemplative therapies is via personal experience. For thousands of years, the traditional answer to the question "Do these techniques work?" has been "Test them for yourself." However, more than a thousand studies now demonstrate their psychological effects on personality and performance, physiological effects on body and brain, biochemical impact on chemicals and hormones, and therapeutic benefits on mind and body for both patients and therapists.

Exceptional Aspects of the Research

The research on contemplative practices is exceptional in several ways.

First is the sheer amount. Studies of meditation appear daily, making it probably the most intensively and extensively researched of all therapies.

Second is the wide array of demonstrated effects. In addition to diverse psychological and psychotherapeutic benefits, research has demonstrated developmental, physiological, biochemical, and neural effects—far more than for any other psychotherapy.

The research demonstrates multiple exceptional abilities.

Research support is available for most applications (and has been summarized throughout the chapter as specific disorders have been discussed). Consequently, this section focuses on general research principles and on some additional psychological effects, especially exceptional abilities. Space precludes detailing the numerous physiological and biochemical findings.

Who Benefits?

A crucial question for all therapies is "What type of client is likely to benefit?" TM studies suggest that successful practitioners are likely to be interested in internal experiences, open to unusual ones, and willing to recognize unfavorable personal characteristics. They may also have a sense of self-control, have good concentration, and be less emotionally labile and psychologically disturbed (Alexander et al., 1991; Murphy & Donovan, 1997).

It is still unclear how durable various contemplative effects are. Some simple physiological changes (such as reduced blood pressure) tend to dissipate if practice is discontinued. However, other effects may persist long term, even if practice ceases, depending on factors such as the extent to which they are reinforced and incorporated into lifestyles.

Exceptional Abilities

A distinctive feature of contemplative therapies is their claim to be able to enhance psychological well-being, development, and abilities beyond normal levels (Walsh & Shapiro, 2006). This claim sounds less presumptuous than it once did because of the considerable evidence now available that, under favorable circumstances, development can proceed to postconventional levels. Examples include postconventional morality, Maslow's metamotives, and postformal operational cognition. Contemplative disciplines claim to facilitate development to these kinds of stages and beyond, and growing research offers initial support for exceptional abilities such as the following.

Attention and Concentration.   William James (1899/1962) famously concluded that "Attention cannot be continuously sustained . . ." (p. 51). However, contemplative disciplines insist that it can, even to the point of unbroken continuity over hours, as in advanced yogic *samadhi* and TM's *cosmic consciousness*. For example, in the Buddhist state of *calm abiding*, according to the Dalai Lama (2001), "your mind remains placed on its object effortlessly, for as long as you wish" (p. 144). Several studies now support these claims, demonstrating that meditation can enhance concentration and resultant perceptual capacities, even to levels previously though impossible (Walsh & Shapiro, 2006).

Emotional Maturity.   Like Western therapies, contemplative therapies aim to reduce destructive emotions. For Taoists, a goal is "emotions but no ensnarement," and for the Dalai Lama, "the true mark of a meditator is that he has disciplined his mind by freeing it from negative emotions" (Goleman, 2003, p. 26).

Going beyond most Western therapies, contemplative practices also aim to cultivate positive emotions such as joy, love, and compassion. Examples include the intense, unwavering, and all-encompassing love of Buddhist *metta,* yogic *bhakti,* and Christian contemplative *agape,* as well as the compassion of Confucian *jen.* Negative emotions can be reduced and positive ones strengthened far more than therapists usually assume possible.

Experiments demonstrate such shifts. Meditators tend to become happier whether practicing in daily life or more intensely in retreat. They report fewer negative emotions and more positive ones, and their EEG patterns shift accordingly. Advanced practitioners demonstrate EEG shifts associated with exceptionally high levels of well-being (Goleman, 2003; Lutz et al., 2007).

Equanimity.   Equanimity is the capacity for maintaining calm and mental equilibrium in the face of provocative stimuli. Equanimity is the opposite of reactivity, agitation, or emotional liability and is highly valued across contemplative traditions. It is, for example, a basis of the Sufi's *contented self,* yogic *evenness,* the Christian contemplative's *divine apatheia,* and Taoism's *principle of the equality of things.* Equanimity extends Western concepts of *stress resistance, emotional resilience,* and *affect tolerance* to include not only tolerance but also serenity in the face of provocative stimuli. Preliminary experimental support comes from measures of emotional stability and startle response (Goleman, 2003; Travis et al., 2004). Obviously, the cultivation of equanimity has considerable therapeutic potential.

Moral Maturity.   Can we foster moral maturity? This is one of humankind's most crucial questions, and the fate of our species and our planet may depend on how well we succeed in answering it. Unfortunately, traditional interventions—such as instruction in moral thinking—produce only modest gains.

Contemplative traditions claim to be able to enhance ethical motivation and behavior in several ways. These include emotional and motivational practices to reduce problematic motives and emotions (such as greed and anger) while strengthening morality-supporting emotions (such as love and compassion). Further practices include cultivating altruism, sensitizing awareness to the costs of unethical acts (costs such as guilt in oneself and pain in others), and identifying with others via transpersonal experience (Dalai Lama, 2001; Walsh, 1999).

Western research and theory offer partial support. Researcher Lawrence Kohlberg eventually grounded his highest stage of moral maturity in the kinds of transpersonal experiences that meditation induces. Likewise, Carol Gilligan concluded that women develop along a moral trajectory—maturing from *selfish* to *care* to *universal care*—similar to contemplative maturation (Wilber, 2000b). Experimental support comes from TM practitioners whose increased moral development scores correlate with duration of practice and with EEG measures (Travis et al., 2004).

Unique Abilities

Advanced meditators have now demonstrated more than a dozen abilities that psychologists once dismissed as impossible (Walsh & Shapiro, 2006). Some of these, such as lucid dream and lucid nondream sleep, have already been described. Other fascinating findings include a unique integrative cognitive style, control of the autonomic nervous system, dramatic reduction of drive conflicts, areas of increased cortical thickness, and the ability to detect fleeting facial expressions of emotion (even more effectively than CIA agents, the previous top scorers).

Initial studies of an advanced Tibetan Buddhist practitioner found two further unique capacities. The first was almost complete inhibition of the startle response. The second was an ability to respond with compassion and relaxation while observing a video of a severely burned patient that ordinarily elicits intense disgust. The astonished researcher conducting these studies stated that these were "findings that in 35 years of research I'd never seen before" (Goleman, 2003, p. 19).

Coupled with the research on postconventional development, these exceptional abilities hold remarkable implications. They suggest that what we long assumed to be "normality" and the ceiling of psychological development is not fixed. We have greatly underestimated our own potentials, and we are capable of further development. In fact, what we call *normality* is looking more and more like a kind of unrecognized collective developmental arrest. Both contemplative and conventional research now support Abraham Maslow's startling claim that "what we call 'normal' in psychology is really a psychopathology of the average, so undramatic and so widely spread that we don't even notice it ordinarily" (Maslow, 1968, p. 16).

There are still more potentials and mysteries within us than are dreamed of in our psychology.

Research Limitations

Clearly, there is now an enormous amount of exciting, groundbreaking research. Unfortunately, quantity does not always guarantee quality. The contemplatives studied are often only beginners; the studies usually brief, follow-up of long-term effects are insufficient; and control groups are not ideal.

A further problem is that most research has been *means oriented* rather than *goal oriented* (Maslow, 1971). In other words, researchers have focused on what is easy to measure (the means) rather than on the classic goals of contemplation. Consequently, we know more about effects on heart rate than on heart opening, love, wisdom, or enlightenment.

Of course, this general problem is not unique to contemplative practices. In fact, it is one of the major problems inherent in the quest for empirically supported therapies: What is easiest to measure is not necessarily what is most important. Changes in simple behaviors are relatively easy to study; deeper transformations, existential openings, and postconventional growth are much more difficult and much more important.

Psychotherapy in a Multicultural World

Cultural diversity and sensitivity are now topics of considerable discussion. Unfortunately, crucial factors are often overlooked—factors such as participants' level of psychological maturity and the creative positive potentials inherent in diversity situations.

A sophisticated approach that integrates such factors is *diversity dynamics*, which aims to study and foster *diversity maturity* (Gregory & Raffanti, 2009). Diversity dynamics points out the following:

Diversity occurs in *all* systems, including all (therapeutic) relationships.

All diversity creates *diversity tension*, which has both problematic and beneficial potentials.

Adults differ on their levels of psychological development, such as levels of ego, cognitive, and moral maturity. For example, research on moral development has identified three major stages—preconventional (egocentric), conventional (ethnocentric), and postconventional (worldcentric). As people mature through these three stages, they initially tend to identify with and focus their care and concern on themselves (egocentric), then on themselves and their community (ethnocentric), and finally on all people (worldcentric). In her studies of women's moral development, Carol

Gilligan described this as the maturation from *selfishness* to *care* to *universal care* (Wilber, 2000a).

People's (and therapists') developmental level influences what they observe and understand in any situation, the range of possible responses they recognize, and therefore how effectively they can respond and help.

A person's developmental stage will influence attitudes and responses to diversity. For example, consider the markedly different responses of people at three different stages: the conventional ethnocentric, the postconventional *pluralistic*, and the postconventional *integral* stages.

At the conventional ethnocentric stage, people (and therapists) simply assume that their own beliefs and values are basically correct and those of other peoples and cultures are not. Cultural and diversity sensitivity at this stage therefore means tolerating and accepting other people's (erroneous) beliefs and values.

However, when people mature to the early postconventional *pluralistic* stage, they increasingly question their own assumptions and come to recognize that all beliefs and values are largely personal and cultural constructions. Different beliefs and cultures are therefore considered valid by their own rights, and cultural sensitivity means honoring their validity. Key traps at this stage are cultural relativism and developmental denial. *Cultural relativism* assumes that all values and beliefs are *equally* valid, and that evaluating or ranking them amounts to judgmental cultural imperialism. *Developmental denial* either denies the existence of adult developmental stages or assumes that recognizing them amounts to an insidious elitism.

At the later postconventional *integral* stage, people are increasingly able to question and evaluate all beliefs and values—their own and other people's—from multiple perspectives. This allows them to remain open to the potential validity of diverse beliefs and values, yet simultaneously evaluate them according to such criteria as fairness, helpfulness, and maturity. Diversity-mature people tend to "always be in discovery mode" (Gregory & Raffanti, 2009, p. 52), constantly seeking ways to transform the challenges of diversity into opportunities for all participants.

> For people at certain development stages, the idea of developmental possibilities beyond their own can be threatening. However, developmental diversity is just one more kind of diversity that needs to be recognized, honored, and used to benefit everyone.
>
> All diversity situations contain creative potentials. As such, they offer participants, including both therapists and patients, opportunities for learning and maturing.
>
> Once these ideas and findings are recognized, a key concern for diversity training (and psychotherapy training) becomes fostering psychological maturity, including diversity maturity.

This is yet one more reason why all therapists should undergo their own personal psychotherapy—which ideally would include individual, group, and contemplative approaches.

CASE EXAMPLE

Clients who have a contemplative practice can sometimes make surprisingly rapid progress in psychotherapy for several reasons. For example, they have probably already done preliminary psychological work during their contemplative sessions. In addition, they may have developed helpful capacities such as introspective sensitivity, clarity, and concentration, and they can use these capacities during therapy sessions to explore their experiences sensitively and deeply. Contemplatives in therapy therefore often benefit from an enhanced ability to access feelings, recognize thoughts and images, plumb deep layers of the psyche, and work with difficult issues and emotions. Therapists who are themselves contemplatives are especially able to use these client abilities to deepen and speed the therapeutic process. These abilities, and the resultant facilitation of insight and healing, are evident in the following session with Jan, a 32-year-old female mental-health trainee, who was a long-term yoga practitioner, teacher, and meditator.

Jan requested a consultation to deal with intense feelings of dislike toward a fellow female trainee whom she perceived as not only exceptionally competent but also competitive and duplicitous. Jan literally writhed on the couch as she reported the underhanded actions of the co-worker, her own intense feelings of anger and fantasies of revenge, disappointment with herself at having such rage, and anguish over not knowing how to protect herself and others.

After listening to her account, I asked her where in her body she felt the conflict. "In my stomach" she replied, whereupon I asked her to carefully feel the body sensation and identify its size, shape, and texture. This is an excellent way to help someone explore the somatic representation of an emotion or conflict and to sustain attention on it.

Jan described the characteristics of the sensation and recognized it as an expression of anger, conflict, and confusion. I asked her to concentrate on the sensation and to notice any changes. Because of her contemplative training, Jan was able to keep her attention focused on the sensation, and over the next few minutes she reported that it was becoming smaller, smoother, and fainter. As it did, she noticed herself becoming less angry and agitated, and another sensation becoming prominent in her chest. This she identified as feelings of sadness at her reactivity and at her inability to protect the other people affected by her co-worker. I asked her to simply hold attention on the feeling of sadness and to notice any thoughts or images associated with it. Jan reported a stream of images of herself looking helpless and anxiety- and guilt-provoking thoughts such as, "I should be able to do something. I should know what to do. What's wrong with me?"

I encouraged her to simply observe the stream of thoughts and images without trying to change them in any way. As she did so, she found that she was becoming less identified with the thoughts and feelings and less reactive to them. She reported that she could feel her mind and body relaxing, and tears came to her eyes as she described feelings of relief welling up inside her along with thoughts such as "I'm only human. It's OK not to know what to do. I don't have to feel responsible for everyone." This spontaneous self-transformation and self-healing of thoughts, images, and emotions as they are observed mindfully—without attempting to change them deliberately—is a frequent finding in meditation and one of the distinctive differences between many contemplative and traditional psychotherapeutic approaches.

At this stage, I simply encouraged Jan to bring a sensitive awareness to the feelings of calm and relief and to see what emerged next. After a pause of perhaps two minutes, she began to describe several insights about how she could handle the situation more effectively. These were accompanied by greater acceptance of her limitations and what she could realistically expect to accomplish, as well as by an initial sense of empathy and compassion for her colleague. As we reviewed the session, Jan concluded, "I can see how she's driven by a need to be in control just like I am, and I want to work on feeling more compassion for her." In subsequent meditation and psychotherapy sessions she did just that. Two years later, I heard from a colleague that Jan and her former nemesis had become friends.

SUMMARY

Contemplative disciplines include many techniques, of which the best known in the West are meditation, contemplation, tai chi, and yoga. Across centuries and cultures, they have been used to plumb the depths of the psyche and the heights of human possibility, and after 3,000 years they remain the world's most widely used therapies.

The Future of Psychotherapy

Most discussions of the future of psychotherapy focus on local issues such as novel techniques, empirical validation, and insurance reimbursement. Yet the fact is that the future of psychotherapy will primarily be determined by larger forces at work in the world, forces that will shape not only the future of therapy but also the future of our society and planet.

We have catapulted ourselves into what Nobel laureate chemist Paul Crutzen calls the "anthropocene epoch," a new phase in Earth's history defined by human effects on the planet, in which the next few decades will determine our collective fate. It is a time of paradox. On the one hand, we possess unprecedented scientific, psychological, and technological resources. On the other hand, millions of people starve, our ecosystem is near collapse, weapons multiply, and our survival is in question.

What is striking is that each major threat to humankind is now human created. For example, overpopulation, pollution, poverty, and conflicts all stem directly from our own behavior. Our global problems are therefore actually global symptoms: symptoms of our individual and collective psychological dysfunctions. The state of the world reflects the state of our minds. This means that to heal our social and global problems, we must also understand and heal the psychological forces within us and between us that spawned them in the first place.

Will our growth in psychological understanding and wisdom be sufficient? This is one of the great questions of our times. The challenge of how to foster widespread psychological and social healing and maturation is no longer an academic question but a collective challenge. Clearly, we are in a race between consciousness and catastrophe, the outcome remains uncertain, and mental-health professionals are called to contribute. What *is* certain is that if we don't solve these problems, there will be little future for psychotherapy or psychotherapists.

Limits of Psychotherapy Training

Unfortunately, most training of psychotherapists and other mental-health professionals is woefully unsuited to deal with many major causes of psychological suffering and pathology, let alone with larger social and global issues. Much psychological suffering has roots in social, educational, and economic factors such as poverty, ignorance, faulty collective beliefs, and inequality. Yet as numerous critiques point out, most psychotherapy training focuses on treating individuals or, at most, families.

Likewise, mental-health professionals have seriously underestimated the importance of lifestyle factors for mental health. More specifically, mental-health professionals have underestimated the importance of lifestyle factors in the causation and treatment of multiple psychopathologies, the enhancement of psychological and social well-being, and the optimization and maintenance of cognitive capacities. Yet lifestyle factors—such as diet, exercise, relationships, recreation, relaxation, time in nature, religion or spirituality, and service to others—can sometimes be as therapeutically effective as either psychotherapy or pharmacotherapy, for example, in treating several forms of depression (Walsh, 2011). In the 21st century, therapeutic lifestyles will need to be a central focus of mental, medical, and public health, and psychotherapists have much to contribute.

Compounding this neglect of social and lifestyle factors is an almost exclusive emphasis on tertiary treatment rather than primary prevention. In other words, most resources are dedicated to treating illnesses and their complications after they arise rather than preventing them from arising in the first place. Yet primary prevention is far more effective and efficient than later tertiary treatment. Of course, this bias contaminates not only individual psychotherapists and training institutions but also the economic and insurance systems that emphasize individual treatment over large-scale prevention, especially in the United States.

Like other professionals, psychotherapists are subject to "professional deformation." This is the harmful distortion of perception, personality, and behavior that results from professional and social forces. Biases and blind spots such as those cited are examples of widespread professional deformation.

Questions for Contemplative Approaches

As contemplative practices become increasingly popular in the West, new opportunities and questions are emerging. These questions include:

What role should contemplative approaches play in medical and mental-health systems?

How are contemplative methods best combined with conventional psychotherapies?

Should contemplative training become part of psychotherapy training? Psychotherapy's effectiveness depends on the personal and interpersonal qualities of the therapist. However, meditation is one of the very few methods that have been demonstrated to cultivate effective therapist qualities such as empathy and to specifically enhance therapeutic effectiveness (Grepmair et al., 2007). Accordingly, contemplative practices could be a valuable element of training.

How can contemplative practices be made more widely available in society—for example, in educational, professional, and penal systems?

Will contemplative therapies prove prophylactic for disorders for which they have already proved therapeutic? If so, how can they be made available for this purpose—for example, within the educational system?

Can contemplative practices contribute to cultivating the psychological qualities, maturity, and values that our society and times require? If so, how can we foster these contributions?

Will our views of human nature, capacities, and potentials expand to encompass the heights long suggested by contemplative therapies and now increasingly supported by research? This is a crucial question because, as Gordon Allport (1964) pointed out, "By their own theories of human nature psychologists have the power of elevating or degrading that same nature. Debasing assumptions debase human beings; generous assumptions exalt them" (p. 36). Contemplative practices offer a generous view of human nature and a means to foster those qualities that exalt it.

Counseling CourseMate Website:

See this text's Counseling CourseMate website at www.cengagebrain.com for learning tools such as chapter quizzing, videos, glossary flashcards, and more.

ANNOTATED BIBLIOGRAPHY

Baer, R. (Ed.). (2005). *Mindfulness-based treatment approaches.* St. Louis: Academic Press.
This comprehensive collection offers a summary of many mindfulness-based therapies, their applications, and the research on them.

Feuerstein, G. (1996). *The Shambhala guide to yoga.* Boston: Shambhala.
Certain traditional philosophical and metaphysical assumptions are accepted uncritically, but otherwise the book is solid and provides a concise, readable overview.

Shapiro, S., & Carlson, L. (2009). *The art and science of mindfulness.* Washington, DC: American Psychological Association.
This book offers an excellent introduction to the field. It clearly introduces the art of practicing and using meditation, surveys the scientific research, and summarizes the benefits that therapists themselves can gain from meditation.

Walsh, R. (1999). *Essential spirituality: The seven central practices.* New York: Wiley.
This practical book introduces contemplative practices of both Asia and the West and emphasizes integrating them into daily life.

Walsh, R. (2011). Lifestyle and mental health. *American Psychologist, 66*(7), 579–592.
This article reviews contemplative and other therapeutic lifestyles.

Wilber, K. (1999). *No boundary.* Boston: Shambhala.
Ken Wilber is an encyclopedic integrator of multiple contemplative and conventional schools of psychology and psychotherapy. *No Boundary* is an easily readable but somewhat dated introduction to his ideas. A more expanded treatment, including related social and philosophical issues, is *A Brief History of Everything.* In the rather dense *Integral Psychology: Consciousness, Spirit, Psychology, Therapy,* Wilber summarizes his psychological theory. An overview of Wilber's writings appears at http://www.drrogerwalsh.com/topics/integral-studies/.

Books by contemplative teachers that offer a rich array of insights into the mind, life, wisdom, and well-being include Kornfield (1993), *A Path with Heart*; Adyashanti (2011), *Falling Into Grace*; Tolle (1999), *The Power of Now*; and Laird (2006), *Into the Silent Land*, which offers an excellent introduction to Christian contemplation. For summaries of contemplative practices from multiple traditions see J. Shear (Ed.), *The Experience of Meditation* (St. Paul, MN: Paragon Press).

WEB SITES AND OTHER RESOURCES

Mindfulness Research Guide (www.mindfulexperience.org/newsletter.php)
This valuable Web site lists meditation research and treatment centers, and it publishes the excellent *Mindfulness Research Monthly*, which reviews recent research.

Guided meditation instructions are available at:
www.mindfulness-solution.com/DownloadMeditations.html
www.drrogerwalsh.com/topics/meditation

the Insight Meditation Society and Spirit Rock Meditation Center for mindfulness meditation,

the transcendental meditation program, and

the Integrative Restoration Institution (iRest), founded by psychologist and yoga teacher Richard Miller, which offers trainings that many therapists have found valuable.

Contemplative Training Centers

There are now numerous training centers around the world. In the United States some of the most recognized include:

CASE READINGS

Eisenlohr-Moul, T. A., Peters, J. R., & Baer, R. A. Using mindfulness effectively in clinical practice: Two case studies. In D. Wedding & R. J. Corsini (Eds.). (2013). *Case studies in psychotherapy* (7th ed.). Belmont, CA: Cengage.
Two brief cases are presented to illustrate the use of mindfulness-based interventions. The case of Rachel demonstrates awareness-based behavior therapy (ABBT), whereas the case of Miranda is used to illustrate the application of dialectical behavior therapy (DBT).

Germer, C., Siegel, R., & Fulton, P. (Eds.). (2005). *Mindfulness and psychotherapy.* New York: Guilford Press.
This practical book focuses especially on mindfulness meditation in psychotherapy. Good case histories are also available in R. Baer's *Mindfulness-Based Treatment Approaches.*

Shapiro, D. (1980). Meditation as a self-regulation strategy: Case study–James Sidney. In *Meditation: Self-regulation strategy and altered states of consciousness* (pp. 55–84).

Hawthorne, NY: Aldine. [Also in D. Wedding & R. J. Corsini (Eds.). (2011). *Case studies in psychotherapy* (6th ed.). Belmont, CA: Cengage.]

> This case provides an excellent example of combining contemplative and other approaches. The therapist uses meditation, together with behavior therapy techniques and careful behavioral assessment, to treat insomnia and interpersonal difficulties.

Tart, C. (2001). *Mind science: Meditation training for practical people.* Novato, CA: Wisdom Press.

A clear, simple guide to meditation practice written by a psychologist. Other practical introductions to learning meditation include S. Bodian (2006). *Meditation for Dummies,* New York: IDG Books Worldwide. For mindfulness meditation, see J. Goldstein (1987), *The Experience of Insight.* For Christian contemplation, see Laird (2006), *Into the Silent Land.* For children, see Greenland (2010) *The Mindful Child.*

REFERENCES

Adyashanti. (2011). *Falling into grace.* Boulder, CO: Sounds True.

Alexander, C., Langer, E., Newman, R., Chandler, H., & Davies, J. (1989). Transcendental meditation, mindfulness, and longevity. *Journal of Personality and Social Psychology, 57,* 950–964.

Alexander, C. N., Rainforth, M. V., & Gelderloos, P. (1991). Transcendental Meditation, self-actualization, and psychological health. *Journal of Social Behavior and Personality, 6,* 189–247.

Alexander, F., & Selesnich, S. (1966). *The history of psychiatry.* New York: New American Library.

Alexander, C., Walton, K., Orme-Johnson, D., Goodman, R., & Pallone, N. (Eds.). (2003). *Transcendental Meditation in criminal rehabilitation and crime prevention.* New York: Haworth Press.

Allport, G. (1964). The fruits of eclecticism: Bitter or sweet? *Acta Psychologica, 23,* 27–44.

Anderson, J. W., Liu, C., & Kryscio, R. J. (2008). Blood pressure response to transcendental meditation: A meta-analysis. *American Journal of Hypertension, 21*(3), 310–316.

Angha, N. (Trans.). (1995). *Deliverance: Words from the Prophet Mohammad.* San Rafael, CA: International Association of Sufism.

Arlow, J. (1995). Psychoanalysis. In R. J. Corsini & D. Wedding (Eds.), *Current psychotherapies* (5th ed., pp. 15–50). Itasca, IL: F.E. Peacock.

Armstrong, K. (2006). *The great transformation: The beginning of our religious traditions.* New York: Knopf.

Bynner, W. (Trans.). (1980). *The way of life according to Lao Tzu.* New York: Vintage. (Original work published 1944)

Byrom, T. (Trans.). (1976). *The Dhammapada: The sayings of the Buddha.* New York: Vintage.

Carson, J., Carson, K., Gil, K., & Baucom, D. (2004). Mindfulness-based relationship enhancement. *Behavior Therapy, 35,* 471–494.

Chan, W. (Ed.). (1963). *A sourcebook in Chinese philosophy.* Princeton, NJ: Princeton University Press.

Chiesa, A., & Serretti, A. (2011). Mindfulness based cognitive therapy for psychiatric disorders: A systematic review & meta-analysis. *Psychiatry Research,* 187, 441–453.

Dalai Lama. (2001). *An open heart: Practicing compassion in everyday life.* Boston: Little, Brown.

Duncan, B., Miller, S., & Sparks, J. (2004). *The heroic client: A revolutionary way to improve effectiveness through client-directed, outcome-informed therapy* (Rev. ed.). San Francisco: Jossey-Bass.

Eberth, J., & Sedlmeier, P. (2012). The effects of mindfulness meditation: a meta-analysis. *Mindfulness, 3,* 174–189, DOI 10. 1007/s12671-012-0101-x

Ellis, A. (1987). The impossibility of achieving consistently good mental health. *American Psychologist, 42,* 364–575.

Engler, J. H. (1983). Vicissitudes of the self according to psychoanalysis and Buddhism: A spectrum model of objects relations development. *Psychoanalysis and Contemporary Thought, 6,* 29–72.

Feng, G., & English, J. (Trans.). (1974). *Chuang Tsu: Inner chapters.* New York: Vintage Books.

Fjorback, L., & Walach, H. (2012). Meditation based therapies—A systematic review and some critical observations. *Religions, 3,* 1–18.

Feuerstein, G. (1996). *The Shambhala guide to yoga.* Boston: Shambhala.

Fischer, L. (1954). *Gandhi.* New York: New American Library.

Frank, J. (1982). *Sanity and survival in the nuclear age.* New York: Random House.

Freud, S. (1943). *A general introduction to psychoanalysis.* Garden City, NY: Garden City Publishers. (Original work published 1917)

Freud, S. (1965). *New introductory lectures on psychoanalysis* (J. Strachey, Trans.). New York: Norton. (Original work published 1933)

Gabbard, G. (1995). Psychoanalysis. In H. Kaplan & B. Saddock (Eds.), *Comprehensive textbook of psychiatry* (6th ed., Vol. 1, pp. 431–478). Baltimore: Williams & Wilkins.

Gampopa. (1971). *The jewel ornament of liberation* (H. Guenther, Trans.). Boston: Shambhala.

Germer, C., Siegel, R., & Fulton, P. (Eds.). (2005). *Mindfulness and psychotherapy.* New York: Guilford Press.

Giles, H. (Trans.). (1969). *Chuang-tzu: Mystic, moralist, and social reformer* (Rev. ed.). Taipei: Ch'eng Wen. (Original work published 1926)

Goleman, D. (Ed.). (2003). *Destructive emotions*. New York: Bantam Books.

Greenberg, M. T., & Harris, A. R. (2012). Nurturing mindfulness in children and youth: Current state of research. *Child Development Perspectives, 6,* 2, 161–166.

Greenland, S. (2010). *The mindful child*. New York: Free Press.

Gregory, T., & Raffanti, M. (2009). Integral diversity maturity: Toward a postconventional understanding of diversity dynamics. *Journal of Integral Theory and Practice, 4,* 41–58.

Grepmair, L., Mittelehner, F., Loew, T., Bachler, E., Rother, W., & Nickel, M. (2007). Promoting mindfulness in psychotherapists in training influences the treatment results of their patients. *Psychotherapy and Psychosomatics, 76*(6), 332–338.

Harvey, A. (1996). *The essential mystics*. San Francisco: Harper.

Helminski, K. (Ed.). (2000). *The Rumi collection*. Boston: Shambhala.

Hofmann, S., Grossman, P., & Hinton, D. (2011). Loving-kindness and compassion meditation. *Clinical Psychology Review, 31,* 1126–1132.

Hoffman, E. (1985). *The heavenly ladder: A Jewish guide to inner growth*. San Francisco: Harper & Row.

Horney, K. (1998). *Neurosis and human growth*. New York: Norton. (Original work published 1952)

Irving, J., Dobkin, P., & Park, J. (2009). Cultivating mindfulness in health care practitioners. *Complementary Therapies in Clinical Practice, 15,* 16–66.

James, W. (1924). *Memories and studies.* New York: Longmans, Green. (Original work published 1911)

James, W. (1950). *The principles of psychology*. New York: Dover. (Original work published 1910)

James, W. (1958). *The varieties of religious experience*. New York: New American Library.

James, W. (1960). *William James on psychical research* (G. Murphy & R. Ballou, Eds.). New York: Viking.

James, W. (1962). *Talks to teachers on psychology and to students on some of life's ideals*. New York: Dover. (Original work published 1899)

Jones, W. (1975). *A history of western philosophy* (Vols. 1–5, 2nd ed.). New York: Harcourt, Brace, Jovanovich.

Jung, C. (1955). *Mysterium conjunctionis: Collected works of Carl Jung* (Vol. 14). Princeton, NJ: Princeton University.

Jung, C. (1968). *The psychology of the child archetype, in collected works of C. J. Jung* (Vol. 9, Part I), Bollingen Series (2nd ed.). Princeton, NJ: Princeton University.

Jung, C. (1973). *Letters* (G. Adler, Ed.). Princeton, NJ: Princeton University Press.

Kabat-Zinn, J. (2003). Mindfulness-based interventions in context: Past, present, and future. *Clinical Psychology: Science and Practice, 10,* 144–156.

Kaplan, A. (1985). *Jewish meditation*. New York: Schocken Books.

Killingsworth, M., & Gilbert, D. (2010). A wandering mind is an unhappy mind. *Science, 330,* 932.

Kirkwood, G., Rampes, H., Tuffrey, V., Richardson, J., Pilkington, K. (2005). Yoga for anxiety: A systematic review of the research evidence. *British Journal of Sports Medicine, 39*(12), 884–891.

Kornfield, J. (1993). *A path with heart*. New York: Bantam.

Kornfield, J. (2008). Unpublished interview.

Krisanaprakornkit, T., Ngamjarus, C. Witoonchart, C., & Piyavhatkul, N. (2010, June 16). Meditation therapies for attention-deficit/hyperactivity disorder (ADHD). *Cochrane Database Systematic Reviews,* 6: CD 006507.

Laird, M. (2006). *Into the silent land*. New York: Oxford University Press.

Lau, D. (Trans.). (1979). *Confucius: The analects*. New York: Penguin.

Lin, K., Hu, Y., Chang, K., Lin, H., & Tsauo, J. (2011). Effects of yoga on psychological health, quality of life, and physical health of patients with cancer: A meta-analysis. *Evidence Based Complementary & Alternative Medicine*. New York: Hindawi Publishing Corporation.

Lutz, A., Dunne, J., & Davidson, R. (2007). Meditation and neuroscience of consciousness. In P. Zelag, M. Moscoritch, & E. Thompson (Eds.), *Cambridge handbook of consciousness*. (pp. 497–550), New York: Cambridge University Press.

Maslow, A. (1967). Self-actualization and beyond. In J. Bugental (Ed.), *Challenges of humanistic psychology* (pp. 279–286). New York: McGraw-Hill.

Maslow, A. (1968). *Toward a psychology of being* (2nd ed.). Princeton, NJ: Van Nostrand.

Maslow, A. (1970). *Religions, values and peak experiences*. New York: Viking.

Maslow, A. (1971). *The farther reaches of human nature*. New York: Viking.

Miller, S., Hubble, M., & Duncan, B. (2007, November–December). Supershrinks: What's the secret of their success? *Psychology Networker,* 26–35.

Murphy, M., & Donovan, S. (1997). *The physical and psychological effects of meditation* (2nd ed.). Petaluma, CA: Institute of Noetic Sciences.

Myers, D. (1992). *The pursuit of happiness*. New York: Avon.

Needleman, J. (1980). *Lost Christianity*. Garden City, NY: Doubleday.

Nisargadatta, S. (1973). *I am that: Conversations with Sri Nisargadatta Maharaj, Vol. II* (M. Frydman, Trans.). Bombay, India: Cheltana.

Norcross, J., & Beutler, L. (2013). Integrative psychotherapies. In R. J. Corsini & D. Wedding (Eds.), *Current psychotherapies* (10th ed., pp. 499–532). Belmont, CA: Brooks/Cole.

O'Brien, E. (Trans.). (1964). *The essential Plotinus*. Indianapolis: Hackett.

Ornish, D., Lin, J., Daubenmier, J., Weidner, G., Epel, E., Kemp, C., Magbanua, M. J. M., . . . Blackburn, E. H. (2008). Increased telomerase activity and comprehensive lifestyle changes: A pilot study. *Lancet Oncology, 9,* 11, 1048–1057.

Ott, U., Hölzel, B., & Vaitl, D. (2011). Brain structure & meditation. In H. Walach, S. Schmidt & W. Jones (Eds.). *Neuroscience consciousness and spirituality* (pp. 119–128). New York: Springer.

Palmer, G., Sherrard, P., & Ware, K. (Trans.). (1993). *Prayer of the heart: Writings from the Philokalia.* Boston: Shambhala.

Perls, F. (1969). *Gestalt therapy verbatim.* Lafayette, CA: Real People Press.

Prabhavananda, S., & Isherwood, C. (Trans.). (1972). *The song of God: Bhagavad Gita* (3rd ed.). Hollywood, CA: Vedanta Society.

Prabhavananda, S., & Isherwood, C. (Trans.). (1978). *Shankara's crest-jewel of discrimination.* Hollywood, CA: Vedanta Press.

Raskin, N., & Rogers, C. (1995). Person-centered therapy. In R. Corsini & D. Wedding (Eds.), *Current Psychotherapies* (5th ed., pp. 128–161). Itasca, IL: F.E. Peacock.

Savin, O. (Trans.). (1991). *The way of a pilgrim.* Boston: Shambhala.

Sedlmeier, P., Eberth, J., Schwarz, M., Zimmerman, D., Haarig, F., Jaeger, S., & Kunze, S. (2012). The psychological effects of meditation: A meta-analysis. *Psychological Bulletin.* Advance online publication. doi: 10. 1037/a0028168

Sengstan. (1975). *Verses on the faith mind* (R. Clarke, Trans.). Sharon Springs, NY: Zen Center.

Shapiro, R. (Trans.). (1993). *Wisdom of the Jewish sages: A modern reading of Pirke Avot.* New York: Bell Tower.

Shapiro, S., & Carlson, L. (2009). *The art and science of mindfulness.* Washington, DC: American Psychological Association.

Shapiro, S., Astin, J., Bishop, S., & Cordova, M. (2005). Mindfulness-based stress reduction and health care professionals. *International Journal of Stress Management, 12,* 164–176.

Shearer, P. (Trans.). (1989). *Effortless being: The yoga sutras of Patanjali.* London: Unwin.

Swan, L. (2001). *The forgotten Desert Mothers.* Mahaw, NJ: Paulist Press.

Tart, C. (1986). *Waking up.* Boston: New Science Library/Shambhala.

Tolle, E. (1999). *The power of now.* Novato, CA: New World Library.

Travis, F., Arenander, A., & DuBois, D. (2004). Psychological and physiological characteristics of a proposed object-referral/self-referral continuum of self-awareness. *Consciousness and Cognition, 13,* 401–420.

Vøllestad, J., Nielsen, M., & Nielsen, G. (2011). Mindfulness- and acceptance-based interventions for anxiety disorders: A systematic review and meta-analysis. *British Journal of Clinical Psychology, 59,* 239–260.

Walsh, R. (1999). *Essential spirituality: The seven central practices.* New York: Wiley.

Walsh, R. (2007). *The world of shamanism.* Woodbury, MN: Llewellyn Press.

Walsh, R. (2008). Initial meditative experiences. In D. Shapiro and R. Walsh (Eds.). *Meditation: Classic and Contemporary Perspectives* (pp. 265–270). New York; Aldine.

Walsh, R. (2011). Lifestyle and mental health. *American Psychologist, 66*(7), 579–592.

Walsh, R. (Ed.). (2013). *The world's great wisdom.* Albany: SUNY Press.

Walsh, R., & Shapiro, S. (2006). The meeting of meditative disciplines and Western psychology: A mutually enriching dialogue. *American Psychologist, 61*(3), 227–239.

Walsh, R., & Vaughan, F. (Eds.). (1993). *Paths beyond ego.* New York: Tarcher/Putnam.

Wang, C., Bannuru, R., Ramel, J. Kupelnick, B., Scott, T., & Schmid, C. (2010). Tai chi on psychological well-being: A systematic review and meta-analysis. *BMC Complementary & Alternative Medicine. 10*(23), 1–16.

Whitmont, E. (1969). *The symbolic quest.* Princeton, NJ: Princeton University Press.

Wilber, K. (1999). *The collected works of Ken Wilber: The Atman project.* Boston: Shambhala.

Wilber, K. (2000a). *A brief theory of everything.* Boston: Shambhala.

Wilber, K. (2000b). *Integral psychology.* Boston: Shambhala.

Wilber, K., Engler, J., & Brown, D. (Eds.). (1986). *Transformations of consciousness: Conventional and contemplative perspectives on development* (2nd. ed.). Boston: Shambhala.

Yalom, I. (2002). *The gift of therapy.* New York: Harper Collins.

Yalom, I., & Josselson, R. (2013). Existential psychotherapy. In R. Corsini & D. Wedding (Eds.), *Current Psychotherapies* (10th ed., pp. 265–298). Belmont, CA: Cengage.

Yu-Lan, F. (1948). *A short history of Chinese philosophy* (D. Bodde, Trans.). New York: Free Press/Macmillan.

Zgierska, A., Rabago, D., Chalwa, N., Kushner, K., Koehler, R., & Marlatt, A. (2009). Mindfulness meditation for substance use disorders: A systematic review. *Substance Abuse, 30,* 266–294.

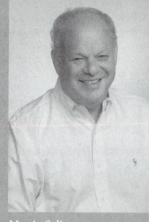

Martin Seligman
Courtesy of Marty Seligman

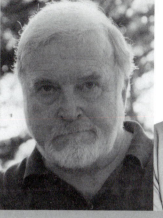

Mihaly Csikszentmihalyi
Courtesy of Mihaly Csikszentmihalyi

Chris Peterson (1950–2012)
Courtesy of University of Michigan

13 | POSITIVE PSYCHOTHERAPY

Tayyab Rashid and Martin Seligman

OVERVIEW

Basic Concepts

For more than a century, psychotherapy has been viewed as a setting in which clients discuss their *troubles*. Likewise, thousands of people each year attend motivational lectures, workshops, and courses, and they go to retreats and makeover camps where the focus is nearly always on repairing *negatives*—wounds, symptoms, deficits, and disorders. These therapeutic ventures are based on the bold—but largely untested—assumption that uncovering childhood traumas, untwisting faulty thinking, or restoring dysfunctional relationships is curative.

This propensity to attend to negatives in psychotherapy makes intuitive sense, but we believe clinicians have lost sight of the importance of the positive. Most psychotherapists hear—but do not heed—a simple plea from clients: "Doc, I just want to be happy." Therapists employ one or more of the techniques and methods discussed in this book to make clients less miserable, assuming that doing so will automatically promote well-being. However, we believe clients with some of the heaviest psychological baggage care about much more than simply relief from their distress. Psychologically troubled clients desire more joy, satisfaction, zest, and courage in their lives, not simply less sadness, fear, anger, or boredom. They want to explore, express, and enhance their strengths, not just remediate their weaknesses and guard against their vulnerabilities. They want lives that are imbued with purpose and meaning. However, these states do not come about spontaneously and are highly unlikely if the therapeutic focus is primarily on symptom alleviation.

Many therapists believe simply helping clients to get rid of their misery will leave them happy. But it does not. Instead, what results are *empty clients* because psychotherapy often ends—or at least is suspended—when the symptoms of suffering are no longer present. Teaching clients about *flourishing*—a state characterized by positive emotions, a strong sense of personal meaning, good work, and positive relationships—requires far more than simply relieving the symptoms of psychological distress. To foster these skills, systematic and sustained therapeutic effort is essential. Therefore, in our view, psychotherapy is a partnership between client and therapist in which the building of positive resources should get every bit as much attention as the amelioration of symptoms.

Positive psychotherapy (PPT) is a therapeutic approach within the broader field of Positive Psychology that aims to expand and enhance the scope of traditional psychotherapy. Closely aligned with the Positive Psychology movement, PPT scientifically studies those experiences, traits, and processes that facilitate individual and group well-being and flourishing within a clinical and counseling context. Its basic premise is that psychologically distressed clients can be better understood and served if they are taught to employ their highest and intact resources—both personal and interpersonal—to meet life's toughest challenges. For psychologically distressed clients, knowing their personal strengths, learning the skills necessary to cultivate positive emotions, strengthening positive relationships, and imbuing their lives with meaning and purpose can be tremendously motivating, empowering, and therapeutic.

The term *positive psychotherapy* may suggest that the rest of the existing psychotherapies are negative. However, PPT is not intended to replace traditional therapeutic approaches—instead, it is simply an approach that seeks to balance the attention given to negative and positive life events in psychotherapy. For example, a therapist may balance discussion of some perceived slight or personal injustice with a discussion of recent acts of kindness shown to a client. Similarly, along with insults, hubris, and hate, experiences of genuine praise, humility, and harmony are deliberately elicited. Without dismissing or minimizing the client's concerns, the pain associated with trauma is empathetically understood and recognized while the potential for growth is simultaneously explored. We do not consider positive psychotherapy a new genre of psychotherapy, but a therapeutic reorientation to a *build-what's-strong* model that supplements the traditional *fix-what's-wrong* approach (Duckworth, Steen, & Seligman, 2005).

Other Systems

Almost all other psychotherapy systems—and almost all of those described and discussed in this book—aim to address basic human deficiencies, and all of them focus on what can be called *negative* thoughts, feelings, and behavior. Psychotherapy's historic skew toward the negative is understandable because human beings spend a disproportionate amount of time thinking about what goes wrong and not nearly enough time thinking about what goes right in their lives. Evolution has endowed us with brains that are oriented toward and more strongly responsive to negative experiences than positive ones. This in-built propensity for negativity is a critical factor in shaping human experience. It gave a clear evolutionary advantage for human beings by helping people keep themselves and their kin safe (e.g., fighting fires and attacking trespassers) while attending to their critical survival needs (competing for and securing food, shelter, and mates). Indeed, those ancestors who only basked in sunshine while ignoring storms perished. Despite securing a steady food supply chain and making our environment safer and livable, the human brain continues to function as if life is a Darwinian test of survival of the fittest. To this day, our evolutionary endowment arouses curiosity about stories of evil, deceit, conflict, and conspiracy more than about accounts of virtue, integrity, cooperation, altruism, or humility.

Negatives are pervasive as well as potent. Negative impressions and stereotypes are quicker to form and are massively more resistant to disconfirmation than are positive ones. Negative memories stay with us for days, months, or even years, whereas positive memories tend to be transient (Baumeister, Bratslavsky, Finkenauer, & Vohs, 2001). People tend to over think negative emotions for months or even years, and the result is often depression, anxiety, suspicion, and anger. Responding to this inherent propensity for negativity, thinkers such as Arthur Schopenhauer and Sigmund Freud convinced us that the best humans could ever achieve was minimizing their own misery. Freud posited that negatives were an indispensable element of human existence, especially conflicts associated with infantile sexuality and aggression. We build defenses to repress these conflicts and manage the unbearable anxiety they cause. Freud even thought that this anxiety was transmuted into a compensatory mechanism that was fundamental to the development of civilization. However, when repression fails, symptoms of psychopathology surface.

This core Freudian view is still widely prevalent and pervasive, and it has influenced art, literature, and academia. Contemporary media is a vivid illustration of this phenomenon. It creatively juxtaposes violence, apprehension, greed, deceit, and sexual infidelity in cyberspace, digital media, news, film, music, theatre, and reality TV shows. The in-built bent toward negativity has made us good at capturing negative events and experiences but not nearly as good at dwelling on positive events in life. To overcome our brain's natural catastrophic tendency, we need to learn to develop and practice skills that allow us to think about what has gone well in our lives.

Psychotherapy can help us understand the adverse outcomes of our in-built negativity by dissecting catastrophic thinking and unpacking maladjusted behavior. Furthermore, it can incorporate the behavioral implications of dopaminergic and serotonergic activity and of gene interactions.

Psychotherapy significantly outperforms placebos and is longer lasting than medication used alone (Leykin & DeRubeis, 2009). Empirically validated psychotherapies are available for dozens of mental ailments such as depression, schizophrenia, posttraumatic stress disorder, obsessive–compulsive disorder, phobias, panic disorder, and eating disorders (Barlow, 2008; Seligman, 1995). Finer aspects of psychotherapy such as the therapeutic alliance, nuances of therapeutic communication, nonverbal language, therapist effects, treatment process, and the feedback process to and from the client have all been studied (Wampold, 2001). Although the focus on psychopathology has resulted in treatments that reduce symptoms for many disorders, most psychotherapists don't have the skills and strategies necessary to help clients focus on what has gone well in their lives. In addition, we believe psychotherapists' exclusive focus on negatives has reached a dead end. About 30% to 40% of clients see no benefits, and a small group of clients—between 5% and 10%—actually deteriorate during therapy (Lambert, 2007). Psychotherapy, in our view, faces a high and significant barrier: the 65% barrier.

The 65-Percent Barrier

It is illustrative to describe this barrier as it applies to the most prevalent form of psychopathology—depression—a disorder sometimes called "the common cold of mental illness." Consider two treatments that we know are efficacious: cognitive therapy of depression and selective serotonin reuptake inhibitors (SSRIs) such as Prozac, Zoloft, and Lexapro. Each produces about a 65% response rate, and we know *that this response incorporates a placebo effect that ranges from 45% to 55%* (Rief et al., 2009). The more valid and realistic the placebo, the greater the placebo response. These numbers crop up over and over. A recent 30-year meta-analytic review of randomized placebo-controlled trials of antidepressants documented a high percentage of variance in responding that can be attributed to the placebo response (Undurraga, & Baldessarini, 2012; Kirsch et al., 2008). But why is there a 65-percent barrier, and why are the specific effects of therapy so small? We believe this is because behavioral change is difficult for people in general, and it is especially difficult for clients seeking therapy. They may lack motivation, have co-morbid issues, or live in unhealthy environments that are not amenable to change. As a result, many clients continue to behave in entrenched and maladaptive ways, and the notion of change, which can be overwhelming, is threatening, ill advised, and believed to be impossible. Indeed, large-scale trials of psychotherapy delivered to clients with a broad range of presenting problems show that approximately 10% to 15% of adult clients deteriorate and another 25% to 35% show no improvements (Lambert, 2007).

Psychotherapy faces another serious problem: About 40% of clients terminate therapy prematurely (Sharf, Primavera, & Diener, 2010). Often, clients only make superficial changes as a result of therapy, partly because *traditional psychotherapy takes a palliative approach*. Palliation is not a bad thing, but it is—and should be—only a way station on the way to cure. In the context of psychotherapy, *cure* entails deep transformative change across multiple domains of personality, character, and behavior. If psychotherapy is effective, then these changes persist even after the termination of therapy.

Many psychotherapists, much like biological psychiatrists, have given up the notion of cure. Managed care and limited-treatment budgets have resulted in a situation in which biological psychiatrists and most mental-health professionals devote their time and talents to firefighting rather than fire prevention. Their focus is almost entirely about crisis management and the rendering of cosmetic treatments. The fact that treatment is often only cosmetic partly explains the 65% barrier and the unacceptably high early termination rate.

In traditional deficit-oriented psychotherapy, many therapists believe one way to minimize negative emotions is to express them, especially bottled-up anger. Clients are encouraged to express anger with an assumption that if it is not expressed, it will simply manifest itself through other symptoms. The self-help therapeutic literature abounds with phrases such as *hit a pillow, blow off the steam*, and *let it out* that illustrate this kind of hydraulic thinking. However, this approach has left current psychotherapy as largely a science of victimology, one that portrays clients as passive respondents to life and life circumstances. Drive, instinct, and need create inevitable conflicts, which at best can be partially relieved through venting. In our view, venting is at best a cosmetic remedy and at worse a treatment that may trigger both resentment and heart disease (Chida & Steptoe, 2009). There is an alternative approach: learning to function well in face of dysphoria or psychological distress.

Depression, anxiety, and anger often result from heritable personality traits that can be ameliorated but not eliminated. All negative emotions and negative personality traits have strong biological boundaries, and it is unrealistic to expect that psychotherapy can overcome these limits. The best that traditional psychotherapy with its palliative approach can do is to help clients live in the upper most part of these set ranges of depression or anxiety or anger. Consider Abraham Lincoln and Winston Churchill, two historical figures who clearly suffered from unipolar clinical depression. They were both enormously high-functioning human beings who dealt with the "black dog of depression" and functioned admirably, even when depressed. One thing psychotherapy needs is to develop interventions that train clients to function well despite the presence of these dominant dysphorias. We are convinced PPT can help clients function well in the presence of dysphorias—and possibly break the 65% barrier.

There is another critical reason to challenge and change traditional approaches to psychotherapy (such as those described in every other chapter in this book). A good life, the ultimate goal of psychotherapy, cannot be fully explained through the traditional deficit-oriented therapeutic framework. For example, the *absence* of normal and positive characteristics predicts the onset of depression far better than the *presence* of negative factors such as a history of depression, neuroticism, or physical illness. One study controlled for these negative characteristics and found that people who had few positive characteristics had twice the risk of developing depression (Wood & Joseph, 2010). Likewise, the presence of character strengths (e.g., hope, appreciation of beauty and excellence, and spirituality) has been shown to make a significant incremental contribution toward recovery from depression (Huta & Hawley, 2010). Hope and optimism (Carver, Scheier, & Segerstrom, 2010) and gratitude (Flinchbaugh, Moore, Chang, & May, 2012) clearly lead to lower levels of stress and depression.

Psychotherapy outcome researchers have emphasized that indicators of quality of life need to be included in the evaluation of treatment outcome (Crits-Christoph et al., 2008) and that psychological well-being needs to be incorporated into the definition of recovery (Fava & Ruini, 2003). Larry Davidson and his colleagues (Davidson, Shahar, Lawless, Sells, & Tondora, 2006) have used the term *recovery-oriented care* to describe treatment that elicits and cultivates the positive elements of a person's life—such as his or her assets, aspirations, hopes, and interests—at least as much as it attempts to ameliorate and decrease symptoms.

HISTORY

Precursors

For ages, sages and scientists have attempted to define happiness, well-being, and flourishing. Confucius believed that the meaning of life lies in the ordinary human existence harnessed through discipline, education, and harmonious social relationships. Socrates, Plato, and Aristotle all saw the pursuit of a virtuous life as a necessary condition for happiness.

Before World War II, psychology had three clear missions: curing psychopathology, making the lives of all people more productive and fulfilling, and identifying and nurturing high talent (Seligman & Csikszentmihalyi, 2000). Immediately after the war, largely because of economic and political exigencies, the assessment and treatment of psychopathology became virtually the exclusive mission of psychology. However, humanistic psychologists and others continued to advocate for positive approaches to psychotherapy. Carl Rogers, Abraham Maslow, Henry Murray, Gordon Allport, and Rollo May all tried to describe the good life and to identify ways our inherent tendency toward growth can facilitate this life. Maslow (1970) pointed out:

> The science of psychology has been far more successful on the negative than on the positive side. It has revealed to us much about man's shortcomings, his illness, his sins, but little about his potentiates, his virtues, his achievable aspirations, or his fully psychological height. It is as if psychology has voluntarily restricted itself to only half its rightful jurisdiction, and that, the darker, meaner half. (p. 354)

Beginnings

Jahoda (1958), in her book *Current Concepts of Positive Mental Health,* made a persuasive argument that well-being should be appreciated in its own right. Frankl (1963) noted that the primary human drive was not pleasure, but the pursuit of meaning. These ideas, as important as they are, nonetheless did not change the landscape of psychotherapy, which from the time of World War II until very recently, uncritically accepted the medical model of psychotherapy and embraced the concepts, language, and organic explanations of mental disorders associated with psychiatric hegemony (Albee, 2000).

To illustrate this hegemony, an electronic search of *Psychological Abstracts* since 1887 turned up 8,072 articles on anger, 57,800 on anxiety, and 70,856 on depression. Only 5,701 addressed life satisfaction, 2,958 happiness, and fewer than 860 mentioned the word *joy*. In this sampling, negative emotions trounced positive emotions by a 14-to-1 ratio (Myers, 2000).

Another illustration comes from the *Handbook of Psychotherapy and Change* by Bergin and Garfield (Lambert, 2013). It is one of the most important overviews of psychotherapy research findings, and *The Handbook* is considered a standard reference in the field. However, the fourth edition (Bergin & Garfield, 1994) does not even include words such as *well-being* or *happiness* in the subject index.

It appears that psychotherapists have learned a lot about damage, deficits, and dysfunction, but almost nothing about the good life and how it can be encouraged. Since 1952, five editions of the *Diagnostic Statistical Manual* (DSM-5; American Psychiatric Association, 2013) have catalogued hundreds of symptoms associated with psychiatric disorders, but there was not a single and coherent classification of strengths until 2004 (Peterson & Seligman, 2004).

Only a handful of interventions during the last quarter of the previous century explicitly attended to the positive resources of clients. One important example is the work of Fordyce (1983), who focused on increasing happiness for college students through 14 strategies, including being active, socializing, engaging in meaningful work, and forming closer and deeper relationships with loved ones.

Well-being therapy (WBT) integrates CBT and elements of well-being and has been shown to be effective in treating affective and anxiety disorders (Ruini & Fava, 2009). Similarly, Frisch's *quality-of-life therapy* (QOLT) integrates cognitive therapy with Positive Psychology ideas and has been shown to be effective with depressed clients (Grant, Salcedo, Hynan, Frisch, & Puster, 1995). However, these interventions only dot the vast landscape of deficit-oriented psychological treatments.

Positive interventions have been making steady progress (Rashid, 2009) over the past decade. The May 2009 issue of the *Journal of Clinical Psychology* focused exclusively on positive interventions for a variety of clinical disorders. This issue included a meta-analysis by Sin and Lyubomirsky (2009) of 51 positive interventions, and it documented that positive interventions are effective in significantly enhancing well-being and decreasing symptoms of depression.

Many other Positive Psychology interventions are being explored in clinical settings. For example, Flückiger and Grosse Holtforth (2008) found that focusing on client's strengths before each therapy session improved therapy outcome. Positive Psychology interventions have also been found effective as adjunct to traditional clinical work (e.g., Edwards & Pedrotti, 2004; Karwoski, Garratt, & Ilardi, 2006; Perlman et al., 2010).

In addition to packaged treatments, interventions focusing one or two positive attributes have been conducted to examine their relevance to clinical conditions such as gratitude in countering the pernicious effects of depression (Wood, Maltby, Gillett, Linley, & Joseph, 2008), hope as a change mechanism in treatment of posttraumatic stress disorder (Gilman, Schumm, & Chard, 2012), the therapeutic role of spirituality and meaning in psychotherapy (Steger & Shin, 2010; Worthington, Hook, Davis, & McDaniel, 2011) and forgiveness as a way of slowly letting go of anger (Harris et al., 2006; Worthington, 2005). Other studies have documented the relationship between creativity and bipolar disorder (Murray & Johnson, 2010), positive emotions and social anxiety (Kashdan, Julian, Merritt, & Uswatte, 2006), and social relationships and depression (Oksanen, Kouvonen, Vahtera, Virtanen, & Kivimäki, 2010). Fitzpatrick and Stalikas (2008) suggest that positive emotions powerfully predict therapeutic change. Other convincing and converging scientific evidence shows that positive emotions simply don't reflect success and health; they also produce success and health by adaptively changing attitudes (Fredrickson, 2009). After a slow start, Positive Psychology interventions, with an equally weighted focus on both the negative and positive aspects of human experience, are advancing the knowledge base of psychotherapy.

Current Status

I (MS) have spent most of my life working on psychology's venerable goal of relieving misery and uprooting the disabling conditions of life. In 1998, as president of the American Psychological Association (APA), I urged psychology to supplement this historical goal with a new goal: Exploring what makes life worth living and building the enabling conditions of a life worth living. I did not realize at the time that my call would usher in a tectonic upheaval in psychology. The scale of this upheaval can be assessed by following developments:

- Between 2000 and 2010, more than a thousand articles related to Positive Psychology were published in peer-reviewed journals establishing both causal and correlational links between constructs such as optimism, gratitude, zest, courage kindness, forgiveness, happiness, well-being, and psychological and physical well-being (Azar, 2011). Peer-reviewed journals include the *Journal of Positive Psychology, Journal of Happiness Studies*, and two recently launched journals, *International Journal of Well-being* and *Applied Psychology: Health & Wellbeing.* They regularly publish scholarly articles about the latest findings regarding well-being and happiness. This scholarship is increasingly focused on developing sophisticated interventions that boost well-being.

- Positive Psychology exercises have been taught internationally through several innovative approaches. First, along with Dr. Ben Dean, I taught four live telephone courses to more than 800 professionals. Each course was 2 hours per week for 6 months. Each week I gave a live lecture and assigned dozens of Positive Psychology exercises for participating therapists to introduce to their patients and clients as well as practice in their own lives. Second, the Positive Psychology Center (PPC) at the University of Pennsylvania has developed a train-the-trainer training program to enable large-scale dissemination of Positive Psychology interventions in schools and workplaces. Third, the University of Pennsylvania has established a Master of Applied Positive Psychology (MAPP) program to combine cutting-edge scholarship with the application of the knowledge to the real world as its mission. Furthermore, several graduate-level training programs in Positive Psychology have been established (e.g., Claremont Graduate University, University of East London, UK). At the undergraduate level, hundreds of Positive Psychology courses are currently being taught, and a Positive Psychology course at Harvard University in 2006 enrolled a record 855 undergraduates (Goldberg, 2006). Harvard University affiliated McLean Hospital has also recently launched the Institute of Coaching which, according to director and practicing positive psychologist Dr. Carol Kauffman, will advance applied Positive Psychology in health-care and public service.

- Several online Positive Psychology resources are available that offer valuable information on positive interventions. Among them are the following.

    www.authentichappiness.com. With more than 2 million users from around the world, this Web site offers valuable resources including a number of free online Positive Psychology measures, which are also available in Chinese and Spanish.

www.ppc.com. This is the home page of the Positive Psychology Center, University of Pennsylvania. The Web site offers valuable information regarding opportunities to participate in Positive Psychology endeavors, provides information about education programs, and lists resources for teachers and researchers. It also contains list of faculty at various universities who are affiliated with Positive Psychology.

www.viacharacter.org. This is the Web site of the Values in Action Institute. The site offers free scientifically validated character strengths assessment (Values in Action–Inventory of Strengths, VIA-IS; Peterson & Seligman, 2004) of adults and youth. The VIA-IS is available in more than 18 languages. This Web site also lists useful resources for applying strengths in several settings, including psychotherapy.

www.positivepsychologynews.com. This site offers regular updates from the world of research. Its interactive component allows registered users to exchange their ideas. Web-site content is available in Spanish, Chinese, and Portuguese.

- Through several large grants, PPC is exploring longitudinal indicators of positive health, positive neuroscience, the mechanisms of self-regulation, and retention among college students. Robert Emmons, who studies gratitude, recently received a $5.6 million grant from the John Templeton Foundation to continue his research on gratitude. Emmons is leading the charge to find evidence-based ways to help people incorporate gratitude into their daily lives.

- Founded in 2007, the International Positive Psychology Association (IPPA; www.ippa.org) is the flagship organization of the discipline with a healthy membership of more than 4,000 people from more than 80 countries. Governed through a board, IPPA has 6 divisions: basic research, clinical, coaching, education, health, and organization. Benefits of paid membership include online access to two Positive Psychology journals, online membership directory, the *IPPA Newsletter* and participation in quarterly webinars with renowned positive psychologists.

- Positive Psychology holds several international level scientific gatherings, including biennial International Positive Psychology Association (IPPA) congresses; an annual Positive Psychology Summit hosted by the Gallup Organization in Washington, D.C.; and several regional conferences, including the European Positive Psychology Conference, Canadian Positive Psychology Association Conference, and Chinese, Asian, and South African Positive Psychology conferences.

- With rates of combat fatigue and suicide at all-time highs, the U.S. Army has become interested in Positive Psychology. There was a clear need to take a protective approach to help soldiers become more psychologically resilient rather than continuing to follow the traditional model that required waiting until soldiers, sailors, and airmen begin to flounder. Positive Psychology exercises under the Comprehensive Soldier Fitness Program (Cornum, Matthews, & Seligman, 2011) are now being taught to more than 3,100 sergeants who in turn will provide this training for soldiers. A recent report from the Army suggests that the program has significantly improved resilience and psychological health compared relative to a control group who had not received this Positive Psychology training (Lester, Harm, Herian, Kraiskova, & Beal, 2011).

- Positive Psychology has received considerable popular press attention including a cover story in *Time* magazine (January 17, 2005) and feature articles in the *Washington Post* (2002), the *London Sunday Times Magazine* (2005), *The New York Times Magazine* (2006), and *U.S. News & World Report* (2009), as well as a six-part BBC series, *The Happiness Formula* (2006).

PERSONALITY

Theory of Personality

Positive Psychology strongly challenges the notion that childhood determines adult personality and that we spend rest of our lives futilely attempting to resolve sexual or aggressive impulses. Before the advent of cognitive behavioral therapy, the great bulk of therapy time in consulting room of psychiatrists and psychologists was often devoted to minute exploration of childhood memories. Likewise, the *inner-child* movement told us that the trauma of childhood, not our own misguided decisions, was responsible for the mess we found ourselves in as adults and that we could recover from our "victimization" only by coming to grips with this early trauma.

In our view, most events of childhood are relatively insignificant. It has turned out to be difficult to find even small effects of childhood events on adult personality, and there is no evidence at all for large effects (Ferguson, 2010; Horwitz, Widom, McLaughlin, & White, 2001). Major trauma in childhood (e.g., sexual abuse) may have some influence on adult personality, but these experiences don't necessarily condemn their victim to a life of unhappiness. Bad childhood events, in short, do not determine adult personality. There is no justification in these studies for blaming the client's depression, anxiety, bad marriage, drug use, sexual problems, unemployment, aggression, alcoholism, or anger on what happened to him or her as a child.

Many studies of the effects of childhood trauma are methodologically inadequate, and these studies often fail to control for genetic effects. However, our genes have a tremendous influence on adult personality, in contrast to negligible effects from adverse childhood events. Hundreds of studies investigating the effects of genetics on personality document that roughly 50% of all adult personality traits are directly attributable to one's genetic inheritance. But heritability does not determine how unchangeable a trait will be. Some highly heritably traits (such as sexual orientation and body weight) do not change much at all, whereas other highly heritable traits (such as pessimism and fearfulness) are very malleable. *We believe happiness is one of those personality traits that can be changed.*

A growing body of research suggests that roughly 40% to 50% of happiness is accounted for by genetics (Bartels & Boomsma, 2009). A counterintuitive finding from this body of research is that only 10% to 15% of happiness is explained by life circumstances—that is, whether one is affluent or poor, healthy or unhealthy, attractive or homely, married or single. In fact, much of the variance in happiness is under volitional control. This can conceptualized as:

H (enduring level of happiness) = S (personal set range) + C (circumstances) + V (factors under personal volitional control)

It is not the job of Positive Psychotherapy to promulgate the belief that one should be optimistic or spiritual, or kind or good humored; however, PPT therapists can describe the consequence of these traits. For example, being optimistic is associated with less depression, better physical health, and higher achievement. Similarly, gratitude is linked with a host of psychological and physical benefits. What one does with this information depends on one's individual values.

Variety of Concepts

Positive Psychology focuses on character strengths. Whereas symptoms and their severity help us understand the stress, sadness, anger, and anxiety of clients, character strengths such as gratitude, hope, love, kindness, and curiosity help us understand the ways in which clients can be good, sane, and high functioning. Just as psychology has shown that individuals who experience negative emotions such as anger, hostility, vengeance, or narcissistic traits are more likely to develop a host of psychological problems, individuals who experience gratitude, forgiveness, humility, love, and kindness are more likely to report being happier and more satisfied with life. Hence, assessing strengths along with symptoms is critical for a balanced and holistic clinical practice, as well as understanding that *psychotherapy is as much about cultivation of wellness as it is about alleviation of distress*. We argue that psychotherapy is one of the most important venues to build strengths because of the following:

- Fixing weaknesses yields remediation, whereas nurturing strengths produces growth and more well-being.

- Repairing or fixing weakness does not necessarily make clients stronger or happier.

- Using strengths increases clients' self-efficacy and confidence in ways focusing on weakness cannot.

- Strengths offer ways to facilitate being good, being kind, humorous, industrious, curious, creative, and grateful.

- Strengths essentially come from being good, not feeling good. Trite feel good statements such as "You can do anything if you work hard enough" and "The sky's the limit" are ineffectual stratagems; in contrast, strengths are built through specific, realistic actions.

Christopher Peterson and Martin Seligman, along with two dozen prominent scholars and scientists from a number of fields, read Aristotle, Plato, Aquinas and Augustine; the Old Testament and the Talmud; Confucius, Buddha, and Lao Tze; the Bushido (the samurai code), the Koran, Benjamin Franklin, and the Upanishads; and some 200 virtue catalogues, including popular songs, greeting cards, bumper stickers, obituaries; and testimonials, mottoes, and credos; and personal ads in newspapers to assemble an exhaustive list of character strengths referred as the Values in Action Classification of Character Strengths and Virtues (Peterson & Seligman, 2004). The classification consists of 24 core human character strengths, subsumed under six overarching virtues, which are valued in every culture. According to Peterson and Seligman (2004), character strengths are ubiquitous traits that are valued in their own right and not necessarily tied to tangible outcomes. Character strengths, for the most part, do not diminish others; rather, they elevate those who witness the strength, producing admiration rather than jealousy.

There are tremendous individual variations in the patterns of strengths individuals possess. Societal institutions, through rituals, attempt to cultivate these character strengths, which are morally desired traits of human existence. However, the VIA classification is descriptive rather than prescriptive, and character strengths can be studies like other behavioral variables. Character strengths are expressed in combinations (rather than singularly), and viewed within the context. The 24 character strengths in the VIA Classification are subsumed under six broader categories called virtues. Table 13.1 lists and describes the 24 core character strengths and virtues.

Character strengths (e.g., kindness, teamwork, zest) are distinguished from talents and abilities. Athletic prowess, photographic memory, perfect pitch, manual dexterity, and physical agility are examples of talents and abilities. Strengths have moral features, whereas talents and abilities do not.

Psychology has placed a predominant emphasis on weaknesses, which has led clinicians as well as clients to think of psychological disorders primarily in terms of the presence of symptoms. Taking a similar categorical approach, disorders can also be conceptualized as overuse or underuse of multiple character strengths. However, a dimensional approach makes more sense in attempting to understand the complexities of the strength–symptom relationship (McGrath, Rashid, Park, & Peterson, 2010). A

TABLE 13.1   Values in Action Classification of Character Strengths

Wisdom and Knowledge. Cognitive strengths that involve acquiring and using knowledge.
Creativity (Ingenuity, Originality). Thinking of novel and productive ways to do things.
Curiosity (Interest, Novelty Seeking, Openness to Experience). Taking an interest in all of ongoing experience.
Judgment (Critical Thinking). Thinking things through and examining them from all sides.
Love of Learning. Mastering new skills, topics, and bodies of knowledge.
Perspective (Wisdom). Being able to provide wise counsel to others; taking the "big picture" view.
Courage. Emotional strengths that involve exercise of will to accomplish goals in the face of opposition, whether external or internal.
Bravery (Valor). Not shrinking from threat, challenge, or pain.
Perseverance (Persistence, Industry, Diligence). Finishing what one starts; completing a course of action in spite of obstacles.
Honesty (Authenticity and Integrity). Speaking the truth and presenting oneself in a genuine way.
Zest (Vitality). Approaching life with excitement and energy; not doing things halfway or halfheartedly; living life as an adventure; feeling alive and activated.
Humanity. Interpersonal strengths that involve tending and befriending others.
Love (Capacity to Give and Receive Love). Valuing close relations with others, in particular those in which sharing and caring are reciprocated; being close to people.
Kindness (Compassion, Altruism, Generosity, Care). Doing favors and good deeds for others; helping them; taking care of them.
Social Intelligence. Being aware of the motives and feelings of self and others; knowing what to do to fit into different social situations; knowing what makes other people tick.
Justice. Strengths that underlie healthy community life.
Teamwork (Citizenship, Social Responsibility, Loyalty). Working well as member of a group or team; being loyal to the group; doing one's share.
Fairness (Equity). Treating all people the same according to notions of fairness and justice; not letting personal feelings bias decisions about others; giving everyone a fair chance.
Leadership. Encouraging a group of which one is a member to get things done and at the same time maintain good relations within the group; organizing group activities and seeing that they happen.
Temperance. Strengths that protect against excess and vices.
Forgiveness (Mercy). Forgiving those who have done wrong; accepting the shortcomings of others; giving people a second chance; not being vengeful.
Humility (Modesty). Letting one's accomplishments speak for themselves; not seeking the spotlight; not regarding oneself as more special than one is.
Prudence. Being careful about one's choices; not taking undue risks; not saying or doing things that might later be regretted.
Self-Regulation (Self-Control). Regulating what one feels and does; being disciplined; controlling one's appetites and emotions.
Transcendence. Strengths that forge connections to the larger universe and provide meaning.
Appreciation of Beauty and Excellence (Awe, Wonder, Elevation). Noticing and appreciating beauty, excellence, or skilled performance in all domains of life, from nature to arts to mathematics to science.
Gratitude. Being aware of and thankful for the good things; taking time to express thanks.
Hope (Optimism, Future Mindedness). Expecting the best in the future and working to achieve it; believing that a good future is something that can be brought about.
Humor (Playfulness). Liking to laugh and tease; bringing smiles to other people; seeing the light side; making (not necessarily telling) jokes.
Spirituality (Sense of Purpose, Faith, Meaning, Religiousness). Knowing where one fits within the larger scheme; having coherent beliefs about the higher purpose and meaning of life that shape conduct and provide comfort.

dimensional approach views strengths in terms of their overuse and underuse, and their expression is assumed to exist in degrees.

Strength use varies by context, so there is no perfect mean; however, positive psychologists accept what Aristotle referred as the *golden mean*—the right combination of strengths applied to the right degree in the right situation. From this perspective, depression might be viewed as an underuse of the character strengths of hope or optimism, humor or playfulness, and zest; it also can be conceptualized as the overuse of the character strengths of judgment and critical thinking as well as of perseverance as reflected in thought rumination. Likewise, anxiety nearly always involves the underuse of bravery or courage, whereas attention deficit disorders reflect an underuse of the character strength of perspective.

Chris Peterson (2006) has proposed a model for evaluating psychological disorders, and he addresses each of the 24 VIA strengths by asking: (1) What psychological state or trait reflects absence of character strength? (2) What state or trait signifies its opposite? (3) What state or trait displays its exaggeration? A disorder may result from the absence of a given character strength, but it can also result from its presence in extreme forms.

Peterson (2006) argues that if *psychology as usual* uses a lens of abnormality to view normality, "then why not use the lens of normality or even super normality to view abnormality?" (p. 35). In other words, if the presence of character strengths implies optimal functioning, then why not use the absence of character strengths as the hallmarks of "real" psychological disorder such as depression. Peterson acknowledges that the absence of character strengths may not necessarily apply to disorders such as schizophrenia and bipolar disorder that have clear biological markers. However, many psychologically based disorders (e.g., depression, anxiety, attention and conduct problems, and personality disorders) may be more holistically understood in terms of presence of symptoms as well as the absence character strengths. Extending Peterson's argument, we have listed the symptoms of major psychological disorders in terms of underdeveloped strengths (Table 13.2). For example, depression can result, in part, because of lack of hope, optimism and zest, among other variables; likewise, a lack of grit and patience can explain some aspects of anxiety and a lack of fairness, equity and justice might underscore conduct disorders.

TABLE 13.2   **Major Psychology Disorders and Dysregulation of Strengths**

	Presence of Symptoms	Lack and Excess of Strengths
1. Major depressive disorder	Depressed mood, feeling sad, hopeless, helpless, slow, fidgety, bored	Lack of joy, amusement, hope, optimism, and playfulness Excess: eccentricity, Pollyannaism, buffoonery
	Diminished pleasure	Lack of pursuing and appreciating positive experiences, lack of a sense of wonder Excess: self-indulgence, sensation seeking
	Fatigued, slow	Lack of alertness, diligence Excess: overexcitement
	Indecision	Lack of determination, resolution, and winnowing Excess: overanalytical, inflexible

TABLE 13.2 **Continued**

	Presence of Symptoms	Lack of Excess of Strengths
2. Bipolar disorder	Manic or hypomanic phase	
	Elevated, expensive, irritable mood	Lack of equanimity, even-temperedness, and level headedness Excess: inhibition, caginess
	Inflated self-esteem or grandiosity	Lack of humility Excess: self-scorning
	More talkative than usual	Lack of reflection Excess: rumination
	Excessive involvement in pleasurable activities: e.g., unrestrained buying sprees, sexual indiscretions, thoughtless business or career choices	Lack of moderation, prudence, simplicity Excess: denunciation
3. Generalized anxiety disorder	Worrying excessively about real or perceived danger	Lack of gratitude, inability to let go, and inability to see alternative side of things Excess: detachment
	Feeling restless, fidgety, jittery, edgy	Lack of relaxation, mindfulness Excess: lenience
5. Obsessive–compulsive disorder	Repeated intrusive thoughts	Lack of mindfulness and letting go Excess: reflection without action
6. Panic disorder	Intense fear and discomfort	Lack of composure Excess: apathy and insensitivity
7. Social phobia	Fear of social or performance situation	Lack of courage, preparedness Excess: unreserved, gullible
8. Attention hyperactivity deficit disorder	Failing to give close attention to details; does not seem to listen when spoken to directly	Lack of vigilance and social intelligence Excess: excessive watchfulness
	Difficulty organizing tasks and activities	Lack of discipline and managing Excess: strictness
	Avoiding or disliking tasks requiring sustained attention or mental effort	Lack of grit and patience Excess: doggedness and tedious
	Excessive fidgeting, motor activity, running, pacing	Lack of calmness and composure Excess: unenthusiastic, lazy
	Talking excessively, interrupting, or intruding others; difficulty awaiting turn	Lack of social intelligence, self-awareness Excess: reticence, bashfulness
9. Oppositional defiant disorder	Annoying people deliberately	Lack of kindness, lack of empathy, and fairness Excess: clemency, subjugated

(*Continue*)

TABLE 13.2   Continued

	Presence of Symptoms	Lack of Excess of Strengths
	Often being angry, resentful, spiteful, or vindictive	Lack of forgiveness, gratitude, and level-headedness Excess: leniency
10. Conduct disorder, antisocial personality disorder	Bullying, threatening, intimidating others	Lack of kindness and citizenship Excess: acquiescence
	Stealing, destroying other's property	Lack of honesty, fairness, and justice Excess: inflexible righteousness
Personality Disorders		
a. Borderline	Pervasive relationship instability; imagined or real abandonment	Lack of capacity to love and be loved in one-to-one relationships; lack of emotional intimacy and reciprocity in relationships Excess: dependency, promiscuity
	Idealization and devaluation	Lack of authenticity and trust in close relationships Excess: offensive, impolite
	Self-damaging impulsivity (e.g., spending, reckless driving, binge eating, spending) and anger outburst	Lack of self-regulation, prudence, and gratitude Excess: denunciation, inhibition
b. Narcissistic	Pattern of grandiosity, arrogance, need for admiration, sense of self-importance	Lack of modesty and authenticity Excess: self-deprecation, criticism
	Lack of empathy	Lack of kindness and social intelligence Excess: pity or overidentifying
	Fantasies of unlimited success, power, brilliance, beauty, or ideal love	Lack of perspective and critical thinking Excess: rationalizing, intellectualizing
	Sense of entitlement, expectations of unreasonably favorable treatment	Lack of gratitude, citizenship, and fairness Excess: self-criticism, inflexibility, righteousness
	Interpersonal exploitation	Lack of fairness, equity, and justice Excess: rigidity
	Envious of others	Lack of generosity and appreciation Excess: self-deprecation
c. Histrionic	Excessive emotionality and attention seeking	Lack of equanimity and modesty Excess: detachment

TABLE 13.2 Continued

	Presence of Symptoms	Lack of Excess of Strengths
	Inappropriate sexual seduction, overemphasis on physical appearance	Lack of discretion and self-regulation Excess: denunciation, disinterest
	Shallow and hasty emotional expression	Lack of mindfulness and social intelligence Excess: grimness and excessive analysis
	Overvaluing relationships	Lack of critical appraisal in relationship Excess: excessive scrutiny and analysis
d. Obsessive–compulsive	Preoccupation with orderliness and perfectionism	Lack of perspective as what is more important; lack of spontaneity Excess: chaos and confusion
	Interpersonal control at the expense of flexibility, openness, and efficiency	Lack of kindness, empathy, and ability to follow Excess: submission and leniency
	Preoccupation with details, rules, lists, organizations, or schedules to the extent that primary aim of the activity is overshadowed; perfectionism	Lack of flexibility and creativity in thinking of novel and productive ways to do things Excess: disarray and instability
	Working excessively at the expense of leisure and friendships	Lack of balance and savoring and lack of appreciation for relationships Excess: self-indulgence
	Rigidity and stubbornness	Lack of adaptability, flexibility, creative problem solving Excess: frenzy, chaos
e. Avoidant	Social isolation, avoiding people	Lack of interpersonal strengths and intimacy Excess: overreliance, promiscuity
	Feeling of inadequacy, perceiving oneself as socially inept, fear of being criticized	Lack of self-assurance, self-efficacy, hope, and optimism Excess: egotism, haughtiness
	Reluctance to take risks to engage in any new activities	Lack of bravery and curiosity Excess: risk taking, prying
f. Dependent	Excessive need to be taken care of, fear of being left alone	Lack of independence, initiative, and leadership Excess: seclusion
	Difficulty making everyday decisions, lack of perspective	Lack of determination and perspective Excess: rigid and unyielding

(Continue)

TABLE 13.2 Continued

Presence of Symptoms	Lack of Excess of Strengths
Difficulty expressing disagreements with others	Lack of bravery, not being able to speak up for what is right; lack of judgment Excess: uncompromising
Difficulty initiating	Lack of self-efficacy, optimism, and curiosity Excess: complacency

© Cengage Learning 2014

PSYCHOTHERAPY

Theory of Psychotherapy

Most therapies espouse a belief system based on assumptions about the nature, cause, course, and treatment of problematic behavior. However, a distressed client seeking psychotherapy is unlikely to ask a therapist about his or her assumptions regarding the nature and cause of human distress. The deficit-oriented psychotherapy model assumes that psychopathology is result of conflictual relationships or faulty cognitions, and these assumptions shape treatment planning and the therapeutic relationship. Just as surely, the fundamental assumptions in PPT will influence the course of treatment.

PPT is based on **three primary assumptions**. First, like many other humanistic psychotherapies, *PPT rests on the fundamental belief that psychopathology results when clients' inherent capacities for growth, fulfillment, and happiness are thwarted by sociocultural factors*. Positive psychotherapists do not believe that happiness and psychopathology somehow reside "inside" the person; instead, it is the interaction between the clients and their environment that engenders both happiness and psychopathology. Whenever people become "damaged" by these interactions, psychotherapy offers a viable option for restoring clients' growth tendencies.

Second, *positive emotions and strengths are authentic and as real as symptoms and disorders*, and they are valued in their own right. They are not merely byproducts resulting from the absence of negative traits. When a psychotherapist actively works to restore and nurture courage, kindness, modesty, perseverance, and emotional and social intelligence, the lives of clients become fulfilling; in contrast, when a psychotherapist primarily focuses on amelioration of symptoms, client lives only become less miserable. Focusing on strengths takes added importance in PPT as a distressed client is likely to accept unconditionally whatever diagnosis a therapist makes. Some clients may even define themselves in terms of these diagnostic labels. Incorporating strengths along with symptoms widens the views and expands therapeutic options for both clients and therapists.

The final assumption is that *effective therapeutic relationships can be built on exploration and analysis of positive personal characteristics and experiences* (e.g., positive emotions, strengths, and virtues). This opposes the traditional approach in which the psychotherapist analyzes and explains the presenting problems of clients. The unsophisticated portrayal of psychotherapy in the popular media leads clients to believe that therapy exclusively entails talking about troubles, ventilating bottled-up emotions, and recovering lost or tattered self-esteem. These stereotypes perpetuate the stigma of mental illness and reinforce the clients' belief that they are somehow deeply flawed or damaged, with the only way "out" being protracted and painful discussions of one's childhood traumas, dissatisfactions, unmet needs, and so forth. It is not that these problems are not worth discussing, but this discussion cannot be the *sine qua non* for the therapeutic relationship.

Powerful therapeutic bonds can also be built, and more effectively be built, by working hard to identify and cultivate positive emotions as well as other positive experiences.

Explicitly focusing on positive emotions in therapy has been found to be effective in enhancing hope (Cheavens, Feldman, Gum, Michael, & Snyder, 2006). In addition, Fitzpatrick and Stalikas (2008) posit that engendering positive emotions, particularly in the early part of therapy, opens clients up to the therapeutic process. When a therapist asks a client, "What strengths do you bring to deal with your troubles?" it is likely to result in a very different discussion than the pathology-oriented question, "What weaknesses have contributed to your troubles?"

Theoretical Foundations

PPT is primarily based on Seligman's (2002) conceptualization of happiness and well-being. Seligman deconstructs the vague and fuzzy notion of "happiness" into three more scientifically measurable and manageable components: *positive emotion* (the pleasant life), *engagement* (the engaged life), and *meaning* (the meaningful life). Fulfillment in these three areas is associated with lower rates of depression and higher life satisfaction (Headey, Schupp, Tucci, & Wagner, 2010; Lamont, 2011; Sirgy & Wu, 2007).

The Pleasant Life

This is the dimension of human experience endorsed by hedonic theories of happiness. It consists of experiencing positive emotions about the present, past, and future and learning new skills to amplify the intensity and duration of these emotions. Positive emotions about the past include satisfaction, contentment, fulfillment, pride, and serenity. Positive emotions about the future include hope and optimism, faith, trust, and confidence. Positive emotions about the present include savoring and mindfulness. Unlike negative emotions, positive emotions tend to be transitory, yet they play a key role in making thought processes more flexible, creative, and efficient. Positive emotions build resilience by "undoing" the effects of negative emotions, and they predict longevity, marital satisfaction, friendship, income, and resilience (for reviews, see Fredrickson, 2009; Lyubomirsky, King, & Diener, 2005).

Schwartz, Reynolds, Thase, Frank, Fasiczka, and Haaga (2002) found that depressed clients seeking psychotherapy experience a lower than 0.5 to 1 ratio of positive to negative emotion, while Fredrickson (2009) found that *experiencing three positive emotions for every single negative emotion may be a threshold for flourishing*. It appears, then, that the absence of positive emotions and pleasure may be *causes* of psychopathology as well as *symptoms* of psychopathology. Enhancing the pleasant life can be one goal of psychotherapy.

The Engaged Life

This dimension of happiness relates to the pursuit of engagement, involvement, and absorption in work, intimate relations, and leisure. The notion of engagement stems from Csikszentmihalyi's (1990) work on *flow*, which is the psychological state brought about by intense concentration. Flow typically results in temporal distortion (i.e., a lost sense of time) for the performer. Provided one's skill levels are sufficient to meet the challenge of the task, individuals are likely to become deeply absorbed or "at one" with the experience. Seligman (2002) proposes that one way to enhance engagement is to identify clients' salient character or *signature strengths* and then help them find opportunities to use them more. Every client possesses signature strengths that are self-consciously owned and celebrated and that feel authentic when used. In PPT, clients learn about undertaking intentional activities that use their signature strengths to create engagement.

These activities are relatively more time intensive and might include rock climbing, chess, basketball, dancing, creating or experiencing art, music, literature, spiritual activities, social interactions, and other creative pursuits such as baking, gardening, or playing with a child. Compared with sensory pleasures, which fade quickly, these activities last longer, involve more thinking and interpretation, and do not habituate easily.

Engagement can be an important antidote to boredom, anxiety, and depression. Anhedonia, apathy, boredom, multitasking, and restlessness—hallmarks of many psychological disorders—are largely manifestations of disrupted attention (McCormick, Funderburk, Youngkhill, & Hale-Fought, 2005). Intense engagement typically eliminates boredom and rumination because, in seeking to successfully complete a challenging task, attentional resources must be activated and directed toward the task at hand (leaving less attentional capacity for processing self-relevant, threat-related information). Character strengths have been shown to meaningfully relate with mindfulness, a practice that harnesses attention (Niemiec, Rashid, & Spinella, 2012). In addition, the sense of accomplishment that follows in the aftermath of engaged activity often leaves one reminiscing and basking, which are two forms of positive rumination (Feldman, Joormann, & Johnson, 2008). Detailed therapeutic interventions have been developed based on the principles of engagement (Grafanaki, Brennan, Holmes, Tang, & Alvarez, 2007).

The Meaningful Life

The third dimension of Seligman's model of happiness is the pursuit of meaning. This consists of using signature strengths to belong to and serve something bigger than oneself. Frankl (1963), a pioneer in the study of meaning, emphasized that happiness cannot be attained by desiring happiness. Rather, it must "ensue" as the unintended consequence of working for a goal greater than oneself. People who successfully pursue activities that connect them to such larger goals achieve a meaningful life. This can be achieved in many ways: close interpersonal relationships; pursuing artistic, intellectual, or scientific innovations; philosophical or religious contemplation; social or environmental activism; careers experienced as callings; and spirituality or other potentially solitary pursuits such as meditation (Stillman & Baumeister, 2009). It doesn't matter *how* a person establishes a meaningful life; simply doing so produces a sense of satisfaction and the belief that one has lived well (Hicks & King, 2009).

Meaning and purpose can motivate psychologically distressed clients to set and then steadily pursue goals. Therapy can be a useful venture to help clients define and set concrete goals and clarify the overarching meaning associated with such goals in ways that increase the likelihood of goal attainment (McKnight & Kashdan, 2009). There is also good evidence that having a sense of meaning and purpose helps individuals recover or rebound quickly from adversity and buffers against feelings of hopelessness and uncontrollability (Graham, Lobel, Glass, & Lokshina, 2008). Furthermore, clients whose lives are imbued with meaning are more likely to persist rather than quit in the face of difficult circumstances. PPT asserts that a lack of meaning is not just a symptom but also a *cause* of depression and various psychological disorders.

The theory of happiness has recently been revised, and two new elements—positive relationships and accomplishment—have been added. **Positive relationships** are important because very little that is positive is solitary. Traditional deficit-oriented psychotherapy mostly locates problems within the client, underestimating the huge influence of the interpersonal landscape that envelops clients. Ask any client, when did he laugh uproariously? The last time she felt indescribable joy? The last time he sensed profound meaning and purpose? The last time she felt enormously proud of an accomplishment? The evidence is clear: *All of these experiences probably involved other people.* Other people are the best antidotes to discouragement in the face of life's challenges.

Accomplishment (or achievement) is sometimes pursued for its own sake. People who lead the achieving life are often absorbed in what they do, pursue pleasure avidly, and feel positive emotion when they win—and they win in the service of something larger than themselves.

The Full Life

The full life entails happiness and life satisfaction and is much more than the sum of its components—pleasure, engagement, and meaning. These components are neither exclusive nor exhaustive. Peterson, Park, and Seligman (2005) found that pleasure, engagement, and meaning were empirically distinguishable routes to happiness, but they are not at all incompatible. As a result, all can be pursued simultaneously, with each individually associated with life satisfaction. Peterson et al. (2005) also found that engagement and meaning were highly correlated with life satisfaction, whereas pleasure was only marginally correlated (Vella-Brodrick, Park, & Peterson, 2009). These findings suggest that pleasure is not a strong predictor of happiness and life satisfaction, although it is still relevant to happiness. Indeed, pathological loss or pathological excess of pleasure is a devastating feature of affective disorders such as major depression and mania. Many psychologically distressed individuals try to quash their unhappiness by experiencing more and more pleasure. However, because of genetic limitations, we cannot dramatically alter our ability to experience pleasure (Kahneman, Krueger, Schkade, Schwarz, & Stone, 2006). In addition, we adapt quickly to pleasure, and pleasure per se, especially sensory pleasure, clearly does not lead to happiness. In contrast, we adapt slowly to those activities that deeply engage us and are imbued with meaning. This is because during engaging experiences we are *completely absorbed*, and we are required to continually adjust our relationship with the environment and with the challenge or task at hand. As we master the challenge in an activity, we strive for increasingly complex goals. Over time, a sense of meaning and purpose may evolve from this engagement, elevating engagement in artistic pursuits, for example, from being absorbing in the short term to being highly meaningful in the long term. A full life entails pleasure, engagement, meaning, positive relationships, and accomplishment through separate activities or through a single activity. In contrast, an empty life lacks these features, particularly engagement and meaning, and results in psychological problems.

Process of Psychotherapy

As shown in Table 13.3, from the outset of PPT clients deeply explore their strengths and positive attributes. The therapist first focuses on building a congenial relationship by mindfully listening to the concerns of clients and encouraging them to introduce themselves through a real-life story that shows them at their best or an experience when clients successfully coped with some challenging situation. The positive introduction is discussed in detail and often runs as a dynamic narrative throughout the course of therapy. Therapists encourage clients to describe strengths illustrated in their positive introduction. Clients are then provided a handout that briefly describes the 24 core character strengths, without their labels. Next clients are asked to complete an online Values in Action–Inventory of Strengths (VIA-IS; Peterson & Seligman, 2004) to identify their *Signature Strengths*. According to Seligman (2002), signature strengths are authentic strengths that an individual self-consciously owns and celebrates, thinking *this is the real me;* the individual feels excited while displaying these signature strengths, learns quickly as they are practiced, feels more invigorated than exhausted when using them, and creates and pursues projects that revolve around them.

TABLE 13.3   **An Overview of the 14-Session Model of PPT**

Session	Topic and Homework	Description
1	Orientation to PPT Positive introduction	Confidentiality and its limits; rules, roles, and responsibilities are discussed; importance of completing homework is also underscored. Presenting problems are discussed in the context of a lack of positive resources such as positive emotions, engagement, positive relationship, meaning, character strengths, positive relationships, and meaning. Client writes one-page (about 300 words) "positive introduction" in which she tells a concrete story showing her at her best.
2	Character strengths Dynamic strengths assessment Blessing journal	Client identifies his character strengths, also those illustrated in his positive introduction; character strengths are discussed to cultivate engagement and flow. Client completes online 72-item character strengths inventory; two significant others (family member and friend) identify his top character strengths, also known as *signature strengths*. (optional) Benefits of positive emotions are discussed. The client starts a journal to record three good things every night (big or small). Each subsequent session begins with processing weekly blessing journal and identifying benefits, patterns, and challenges.
3	Signature strengths Signature strength action plan	Signature strengths are identified integrating various perspectives. The client and therapist discuss specific, measurable, and achievable goals targeting specific problems or to cultivate more engagement. Client completes and frames goals into a concrete signature strengths action plan (SSAP).
4	Good vs. bad memories Writing memories	The role of bad and bitter memories is discussed in terms of how they perpetuate psychological distress. Positive cognitive reappraisal strategies are discussed to rewrite and repack bad and bitter memories The benefits of good memories are also highlighted. The client writes bad memories and about feelings of anger and bitterness and their impact in perpetuating emotional distress.
5	Forgiveness Forgiveness letter	Forgiveness is explored as a potential option to transform feelings of anger and bitterness associated with a specific transgression into neutral or even positive emotions. The client describes a transgression and its related emotions and pledges to forgive the transgressor. Does not necessarily deliver the letter.
6	Gratitude Gratitude letter and visit	Gratitude is discussed as an enduring thankfulness. The roles of good and bad memories are discussed again, with an emphasis on gratitude. The client writes and delivers in person a gratitude letter to someone he never properly thanked.

TABLE 13.3 Continued

Session	Topic and Homework	Description
7	Midtherapy feedback session	Signature strengths action plan: the forgiveness and gratitude assignments are followed up. Therapeutic progress is discussed. Feedback to and from client is discussed, and necessary changes are made.
8	Satisficing vs. maximizing Satisficing	Concepts of satisficing (good enough) and maximizing are discussed. Client identifies and plans areas where he could benefit from satisficing.
9	Hope, optimism, and posttraumatic growth One door closes, one door opens	Optimism and hope are discussed in detail. The client is helped to think of times when important things were lost but other opportunities opened up. Potential growth from trauma is also explored. Client writes about the three doors that closed and then asks, what doors opened?
10	Positive communication Active constructive	Discussion about active-constructive, a technique of positive communication. The client self-monitors for active-constructive opportunities.
11	Signature strengths of others Family strengths tree	The significance of recognizing and associating through character strengths of family members is discussed. Client asks family members to take the signature strengths online measure and then draws a family tree of strengths and arranges an in-person or virtual gathering to discuss family members' signature strengths.
12	Savoring Planned savoring activity	Savoring is discussed, along with techniques and strategies to safeguard against adaptation. Client plans a savoring activity using specific techniques.
13	Altruism Gift of time	The therapeutic benefits of helping others are discussed. Client plans to give the gift of time doing something that also uses her signature strengths.
14	The full life	Full life is discussed as the integration of positive emotions, engagement, positive relationships, meaning, and accomplishment. Therapeutic gains and experiences are discussed, and ways to sustain positive changes are devised.

Generally the top five VIA-IS scores are identified as a client's signature strengths. Clients are then asked to find new ways to use these signature strengths. This approach, although useful and effective in nonclinical setting, may not meet critical clinical needs. For example, exclusive focus on top-ranked strength scores could give an inadvertent message to clients that weaknesses, deficits, and challenges—which are equally real and inevitable—do not deserve clinical attention. Thus, a unique opportunity to integrate strengths with symptoms could be missed. To avoid this shortcoming, PPT follows a comprehensive approach known as *dynamic strength-assessment* (Rashid & Ostermann,

TABLE 13.4 **An Example of a Dynamic Strength Assessment**

	Strength	Self	Other	VIA	Tonic/ Phasic	Under/ Over	Desired	Composite
1	Appreciation of beauty and excellence							
2	Authenticity and honesty							
3	Bravery and valor							
4	Creativity							
5	Curiosity							

© Cengage Learning 2014

2009). Using the Values in Action classification model (Peterson & Seligman, 2004; Table 13.3), the client is first provided a sheet with brief descriptions (approximately 20–25 words per strength) of 24 core strengths without their titles. Clients identify (but *don't* rank) five strengths that best illustrate their personality. Identical collateral data is collected from a friend or family member. Clients then complete an online self-report measure of strengths: the 72-item Signature Strengths Questionnaire (SSQ; Rashid & Uliaszeck, 2012) or the 240-item Values in Action-Inventory of Strengths (VIA-IS; Peterson & Seligman, 2004). Next, clients are provided a worksheet with names of all 24 strengths to compute their strengths. Through a worksheet, clients sum up all perspectives to derive a composite score (see Table 13.4). The top five strengths scores across rows are generally regarded as signature strengths. Ties are resolved through mutual discussion in terms of their relevance in addressing presenting concerns. In other words, if kindness and love of learning are tied, then kindness will be given precedence if it is more applicable to the resolution of the presenting concern.

Next, clients share memories, experiences, real-life stories, anecdotes, accomplishments, and skills that illustrate development and use of these strengths. Obviously, not all strengths can be readily used in all situations. PPT employs a calibrated and flexible use of strengths that could adaptively meet the dynamics of each individual in various situations (Schwartz & Sharpe, 2006). This leads to discussion of character strengths identified from various perspective. In terms of their usage, strengths are discussed as *tonic* (kindness is displayed in nearly all situations) or *phasic* (kindness is displayed only at work but not at home, fairness only in a few situations, or teamwork only with preferred group, etc.).

Clients also identify under- or overuse of strengths (e.g., underuse of kindness in close relationships). After exploring the nuances and subtleties of strengths, clients are asked to identify five desired strengths that could be deployed adaptively to solve presenting concerns. The synergistic impact of signature strengths is also discussed. For example, a client can use both kindness and social intelligence to deal with a troubling social relationship or self-regulation can be combined with perseverance to achieve a personal goal such as quitting smoking or incorporating exercise in one's daily schedule.

Character strengths can easily be incorporated into therapeutic work throughout treatment. Even therapists trained and experienced in the deficit model can find a balanced approach to explore if their clients are able to reflect on their challenges and strengths (emotional intelligence); identify troubling negative memories (e.g., holding grudges); access positive memories of specific people, situations, or experiences (savoring); and develop skills in using their strengths to overcome their problems (e.g., self-regulation, persistence, and courage).

Most therapists can incorporate strengths in therapy without significantly changing their therapeutic framework. The following vignettes illustrate how specific strengths can be linked to presenting problems:

- An anxious 29-year-old female reported doing things halfway or halfheartedly, not feeling alive, and being unable to approach life with excitement and energy. Eliciting cheerful anecdotes and experiences from this client helped her build zest and enthusiasm.

- A 19-year-old second-year college student, despite a solid academic achievement record, expected the worst in the future and believed he would not be able to achieve his goal of getting into a graduate school no matter how hard he tried. He lacked, among other strengths, hope and optimism. Having him reappraise the situation, realistically and optimistically, based on his previous accomplishments, helped reorient his expectations, and he started reassuring himself that as long as he worked hard, he would be able to accomplish his goal (persistence, optimism).

- A 29-year-old ethnic female could not appreciate that good things do happen in her life, and she could only focus on the negative aspects of her life. Recording three good things in her gratitude journal and discussing them with her therapist helped her to notice and deeply acknowledge the good things that already existed in her life.

- A 33-year-old female gave up the moment any task became challenging, and she was never able to complete things that she started. PPT helped her to slow down (savor), and break down the task in concrete steps and monitor her activity level (self-regulation and persistence). Furthermore, she elicited support of a close friend to help her complete some tasks that had been left undone because of her lack of specific skills.

- A 38-year-old single mother, depressed and going back to school, stated that most PPT exercises helped initially, but then the effects of the intervention tapered off. Creativity was one of her top strengths. She was asked to introduce variety in specific exercises (e.g., choosing a domain to express gratitude, work, or family). Eventually, she was able to create a variety of ways to do the exercises without adapting to them so quickly.

These five vignettes illustrate how clients can be helped to devise personalized strength-based pathways to solve life's problems. These pathways often are hidden from clients because of symptomatic distress. However, clients are encouraged to develop their practical intelligence through the careful consideration of which signature strength is relevant to the problem, whether it conflicts with other strengths (e.g., should one be honest or kind if one cannot be both?), and how to translate abstract signature strengths into concrete actions (Schwartz & Sharpe, 2006). In using strengths, clients are encouraged to adopt a flexible approach. It is almost always necessary to do so in complex and dynamic interpersonal contexts. For example, clients are helped to contextualize the use of strengths but are also encouraged to self-monitor the process, learning how and when to recalibrate or reallocate mental and physical resources in using specific strengths so that a healthy and optimal state can be achieved.

Clients seek psychotherapy because they are often troubled by negative emotions and negative memories and feel trapped by these memories. This infrastructure, coupled with ever-thinning social support, reinforces a victim mindset. This mindset, in turn, encourages abdication of personal responsibility. PPT exercises such as *positive reappraisal* help clients unpack these bitter memories. Additional strategies include the following:

1. Clients create *psychological space* between themselves and the negative memory. One way to do so is to describe the bitter memory from a third person's perspective—this is obviously less personal and more neutral.

2. Clients devise an *inventory of both negative and positive aspects of the bitter memory*. The purpose is to recollect positive or adaptive aspects of the bitter memory that might have been overlooked because of the mind's penchant for negativity.

3. Clients *recognize cues that activate the recall of a bitter memory* and are helped to immediately engage in an adaptive and alternative activity (diversion) to stop the full recollection of a bitter memory. Densely interconnected, the bitter memories of depressed clients are often triggered by external cues. Engagement into an alternative activity diverts the attentional resources and helps clients to eventually forget aspects of the bitter memories.

4. Finally, clients engage in *mindfulness*. Meditation helps to quiet anxious and depressed clients. In addition, mindfulness naturally engenders positive emotions. It emphasizes the self-regulation of emotions and actions with appreciation for the fact that emotions are transitory and impermanent.

Clients are also invited to consider the option of *forgiveness*. Research shows that personal written disclosures often ease the cognitive and emotional constrictions associated with painful memories and experiences and enhance well-being (Bauer, McAdams, & Pals, 2006). It is not uncommon for exercises employed in PPT to generate negative and uncomfortable emotions. Despite what might be implied by the name, the focus of Positive Psychotherapy is not exclusively on the positive aspects of human experience. It would be naive to conceive of a life without negative experiences. As such, PPT does not deny negative emotions or encourage clients to see the world through rose-colored glasses. Instead, it aims to validate these experiences while at the same time gently encouraging clients to explore their effects and seek out potential positives from their difficult and traumatic experiences. This is encouraged because research has shown that doing so tends to yield health benefits and promote psychological growth (Bonanno & Mancini, 2012). However, during these explorations it is important that the therapist not trivialize such experiences by, for instance, too quickly pointing out the positive opportunities that trauma, loss, or adversity may present for personal growth and development. Amidst the warmth, understanding, and goodwill created in PPT, a therapist who listens mindfully and can facilitate affective expression will be able to help the client explore and reflect on these uncomfortable experiences in a way (and at a pace) that leads to positive outcomes. In so doing, clients can learn how to encounter negative experiences with a more positive mindset and reframe and label those experiences in ways that are helpful. PPT therapists work diligently to articulate the positive aspects of a client's experience; however, they are careful not to engender a Pollyannaish or panglossian view of happiness. They build a warm, authentic, and collaborative relationship so they can enter a client's world wearing magnifying glasses that focus on the identification of strengths and the capacity for building strengths. They need to know where and how to look for strengths and how to align these strengths with the client's personality, goals, values, resources, interpersonal world, and life circumstances. We believe this process creates a more egalitarian therapeutic relationship than a traditional deficit-oriented approach.

PPT also explicitly focuses on cultivating positive emotions such as gratitude. Throughout the course of therapy, clients are asked to write down daily three good things that happened to them and why they happened. This becomes an ongoing journal of blessings large and small. Most clients find this helpful not only in coping with negative experiences but also in cementing relationships through explicitly noticing (in a gratitude journal) the kind acts and gestures of friends and family. Thus, a new sense of appreciation develops for existing relationships. Clients are also asked to think of someone to whom they are grateful but who they have never properly thanked. They compose a letter to this person describing their gratitude and are asked to read the letter to that person by phone or in person. This exercise, when done in person, produces deep and profound positive emotions.

Clinical experience suggests most clients seek therapy as a means of managing the stressors associated with living in fast-paced, highly complex environments. PPT exercises such as *satisficing versus maximizing* (Schwartz, Ward, Monterosso, Lyubomirsky, White, & Lehman, 2002) and *savoring* teach clients to deliberately slow down and enjoy experiences they would normally hurry through (e.g., eating a meal, taking a shower, walking to work). When the experience is over, clients reflect and write down what they did and how they felt differently compared to when they rushed through it. The last few exercises focus on close relationships because a meaningful life cannot be fostered without nurturing relationships, whether with significant others, at work, or within communities (Stillman & Baumeister, 2009). Exercises that focus on the strengthening of interpersonal relationships include getting clients to explore the signature strengths of others, learning about active and constructive communication styles (Gable, Reis, Impett, & Asher, 2004), and participating in acts of generosity that involve devoting time to the concerns of others. A potentially daunting task for a clinician practicing PPT is to ensure that what he or she purports to be "positive" is not perceived by clients as prescriptive. PPT has an empirical base that clearly documents the benefits of positive attributes. Just as medical research shows that eating vegetables and exercising are beneficial, research also shows that the adoption of specific habits and behaviors is associated with happiness and well-being (Gable & Haidt, 2005). PPT exercises are custom-tailored to meet a client's immediate clinical needs (e.g., conflict with significant others, a romantic breakup, or career-related issues), and the length of therapy and order of the exercises can be varied to suit each client's circumstances and the likelihood he or she will complete the exercises.

Mechanisms of Psychotherapy

There are several mechanism of change in PPT.

1. PPT *broadens and builds* therapeutic resources, as do all other approaches to psychotherapy. For example, in traditional psychodynamic psychotherapy, a client opens up her subjective world, which is interpreted solely by the therapist. The therapist will interpret these associations to help the client achieve insight, thereby producing a broader perspective. Cognitive and behavioral therapies do the same by widening the client's behavioral and cognitive repertoires. PPT broadens the client's perspective by having him or her undertake activities that generate positive emotions. Although fleeting in nature, positive emotions broaden meaning, expand behavioral repertoires, help clients generate new ideas, and facilitate reinterpretation of old and bitter memories. This broadening occurs at cognitive, affective, and behavioral levels. Therefore, positive emotions in PPT are not only simply indications of joy or happiness but also more and importantly generate cognitive, behavioral, and affective changes. For example, writing a gratitude journal helped a 23-year-old depressed female client feel much better, and she began appreciating the small acts of kindness by her mother. This led her to change her view about her mother from being dominating, pushy, and anxious to a more realistic view of a caring mother who could at times be somewhat overbearing.

2. Clients seek psychotherapy because they are often troubled by negative emotions and negative memories. PPT exercises (e.g., bitter memories) help clients unpack negative memories and do a careful and thorough positive reappraisal using the specific strategies described in this chapter. The aim is to increase behavioral, cognitive, and affective flexibility. This is usually done after clients complete their positive introductions and identify their character strengths—exercises that often produce positive emotions.

3. Experiential and skill-building PPT exercises allow clients to develop their signature strengths. Symptomatic distress keeps these assets hidden, and clients coming for therapy are often aware of their specific strengths.

Unlike hedonic activities, which are shortcuts and rely on modern gadgets, PPT exercises are intentional activities which are time intensive (e.g., first writing about and then completing a gratitude visit, devising a plan to use signature strengths, writing three good things in the journal daily, arranging a savoring date, giving a gift of time). Compared to sensory pleasures that fade quickly, these activities last longer, involve quite a lot of thinking and interpretation, and do not habituate easily. Clients from the onset of the therapy are instructed that happiness does not simply happen but is something that they must *make* happen. In the PPT paradigm, happiness is not just feeling good, it is about doing good, which often leads to feeling good (Steger, Kashdan, & Oishi, 2008).

PPT exercises change because any activity that taps clients' signature strengths can be engaging. For example, a client with the signature strength of creativity was asked to think of something that would use her creativity. She selected pottery—something she always wanted to do but was never motivated enough to do.

4. PPT is about dealing with problems head on. Some psychotherapies may be effective in bringing about therapeutic changes through venting of bottled-up emotions or providing a place to vent anger or resentment. PPT empathically attends to the concerns of clients, but it also actively teaches clients to function well despite their depressive symptoms. Exercises such as positive appraisal and using signature strengths to solve problems can ultimately help clients learn to be comfortable with some unavoidable uncomfortable aspects of their personality or environment. Furthermore, the systematic and thorough identification of signature strengths allows clients to think more deeply about their positive qualities. If thinking about our weaknesses is likely to make them feel vulnerable, then thinking about strengths in a realistic way is likely to bolster their self-confidence and prepare them to deal more effectively with their problems.

5. Finally, an overarching mechanism that helps clients change is *reeducation of attention*. Most clients presenting for psychotherapy experience an elevated natural negative tendency, and they have learned to exaggerate it by focusing on and recalling negative aspects of their experience. Several PPT exercises aim to reeducate attention, memory, and expectations away from the negative and catastrophic and toward the positive and hopeful. For example, keeping a *gratitude journal* can counteract the tendency to ruminate on the dissatisfying aspects of one's life (e.g., obstacles, disappointments) and orient clients toward events that enrich life and are vitalizing (e.g., caring acts, goal attainment). Similarly, the gratitude visit may shift a client's memory away from the unfavorable aspects of past relationships to savoring the good things about interactions with friends and family. This reeducation of attention, memory, and expectation is accomplished verbally via journal writing. Participating in time-intensive positive activities does not leave clients time to brood over their misery.

Effective psychotherapy requires the generation of ideas and actions to solve problems. However, this cannot be done unless the therapist establishes a strong therapeutic alliance. All major approaches to psychotherapy emphasize that therapist–client interaction should be positive and characterized by empathy, warmth, and genuineness. Although this is achieved primarily through discussion of weaknesses within traditional psychotherapy, the PPT client and therapist talk about instances in which the parents meet the needs of the child, when the client transgressed but was forgiven, and when criticism was balanced by genuine appreciation. When this occurs, the focus on personal strengths is likely to be a more potent generator of change than a focus on personal weaknesses would have been. For example, low mood and a loss of interest in previously enjoyed activities were hallmark characteristics of one client who spent hours each day ruminating on her problems. Through PPT, she discovered that an appreciation of beauty and curiosity were among her signature strengths and, with the help of her therapist, she was able to design activities that tapped these strengths. After engaging in these activities, she reported a decrease in levels of unhelpful rumination.

Who Doesn't Benefit?

PPT is not prescriptive. Instead, it is a descriptive approach based on converging scientific evidence documenting that certain benefits accrue when individuals attend to the positive aspects of their experience. Still, some clients may feel that character has no place in therapeutic discourse because it may invoke judgment by the therapist. Our stance is that *responsibility and free will are essential processes in PPT*. If life's circumstances are blamed for a client's problems, then that client's responsibility will be minimized, if not completely ignored. Therefore, a client with deeply entrenched self-perception of being victim may not benefit from PPT initially. Also, identification of character strengths may exaggerate the inflated self-view of someone with narcissistic characteristics. Therefore, it is important to have a thorough discussion about the features associated with each character strength.

PPT is not a panacea and will not be appropriate for all clients in all situations. For example, clients who have experienced trauma may not benefit from a PPT approach initially and may respond better to a treatment specifically targeting their trauma and its aftermath. It is important that the therapist does not dismiss or minimize the debilitating impact of trauma and rush toward *posttraumatic growth* (PTG). Knowing that PTG is a built-in process can be reassuring to clients, but clinical judgment and collaborative decision making are needed to determine the suitability, timing, and completion of all PPT exercises.

Both therapists and clients expecting a linear progression of improvement may not do well with PPT, in part because the motivation to change long-standing behavioral and emotional patterns fluctuates during the course of therapy. It is clear that behavioral change is hard and requires sustained effort. Moreover, clients benefit differentially from variously PPT exercises. The progress of one client should not bias the therapist about the likely progress of another client. Finally, although pilot studies have reported promising findings, these should be viewed cautiously and will need to be replicated on a large scale before any firm conclusions can be made about the efficacy of PPT with specific clinical condition, its generalizability, or the role of possible mediating variables.

APPLICATIONS

Who Can We Help?

In addition to clinical samples, the core exercises that constitute PPT (e.g., exploring and using signature strengths, three blessings journal, the gratitude letter or visit, and active-constructive responding) have been widely used with nonclinical samples in life and executive coaching, education, and organizations (see Seligman, 2011, for a review). Furthermore, randomized controlled intervention studies completed online using these exercises have also shown promising results (Mitchell, Stanimirovic, Klein, & Vella-Brodrick, 2009). The Internet offers the potential to disseminate information about Positive Psychology and PPT exercises to a broad audience in an accessible and affordable manner. Because PPT both alleviates suffering and builds well-being, it offers tremendous potential for expanding the horizons of psychotherapy.

One way to expand this influence of PPT is to reach out to "normal" people who may not have exhibited clinical symptomology but who do need help to develop skills to improve their well-being. Positive Psychology interventions, with their emphasis on development of personal resources toward well-being, have been widely used in personal, life, and executive coaching with executives from corporate, health-care, education, and public administration sectors. Similarly, artists and individual working in a variety of creative fields have benefitted from Positive Psychology interventions that focus on creative optimal experience—flow (Csikszentmihalyi's, 1990).

PPT can also help a wide range of psychologically disturbed individuals. For example, depressed clients who were raised on a steady diet of criticism can be helped to name and believe in their strengths. This seemingly simple exercise, along with a realistic appraisal of weaknesses, can instill hope in clients.

Treatment

Clients with symptoms of depression appear to benefit most from PPT exercises because these exercises explicitly generate positive emotions and experiences that counteract the client's depressed mood and feelings of sadness, hopelessness, and helplessness. In addition to depression, clients with co-occurring disorders (e.g., depression and anxiety, depression and adjustment issues) can benefit from PPT exercises that teach them to explore, develop, and use their character strengths such as hope, optimism, perseverance, and self-regulation. This process can be helpful for any psychologically distressed person. For example, consider a client with low hope. This client is also likely to lack motivation, and she may have to struggle to clearly articulate her therapeutic goals. The process of identifying, labeling, and acknowledging her strengths through real-life narratives (positive introduction; Table 13.3) is likely to boost her self-confidence and self-efficacy to collaboratively create specific goals that will move her in the direction of well-being. Group PPT has also been shown to be effective with a range of psychological disorders, including depression (Bay, 2012), addiction (Akhtar & Boniwell, 2009), borderline personality disorder (Rashid & Uliaszek, 2012), and schizophrenia (Meyer, Johnson, Parks, Iwanski, & Penn, 2012).

The PPT treatment protocol shown in Table 13.3 may appear structured and sequential. However, PPT is actually a flexible psychoeducational approach. Its exercises can be adapted to address individual concerns, and they can be used in any sequence that meets a particular client's clinical needs. Moreover, sometimes one or two exercises will be sufficient to produce a therapeutic response. For example, I (TR) recently worked with a young male adult who experienced symptoms of social anxiety marked by perceived fears of negative evaluation by others. The PPT exercise of positive introduction was adapted, and the client was asked to describe a real-life situation when he overcame the actual or perceived negative evaluation. He wrote a moving story in which he mustered up all his courage to play only last three minutes of a crucial basket ball game and scored the winning three points. He stated he did so, "without caring for the piercing eyes of audience—I only focused on the game." We discussed the internal resources he used to accomplish the feat and how can he use these resources now. Identification of his signature strengths, especially by others, helped him tremendously to regain a sense of self-confidence that proved to be a crucial element in his therapeutic progress. Only two exercises were used: positive introduction and dynamic assessment of strengths, and these exercises only took about six sessions. However, they were sufficient to produce enough therapeutic progress that therapy was terminated by mutual consent.

Group PPT is more structured and more powerful than individual PPT because listening to group members' strength-based narratives and their ways of creating positive emotions and engagement often creates a therapeutic synergy that helps group members bond together in supporting each others' well-being.

PPT exercises can also be adopted for other treatment modalities. For example, Kaufman and Silberman (2009) describe a case study in which they used a modified version of the gratitude journal by asking each partner what the other did that was positive when things went wrong. Over time, the couple was able to notice a number of day-to-day things that each partner did for the other, gradually improving the quality of their relationship. Similarly, we have adapted the generic genogram to a PPT exercise (family strengths tree; Table 13.3) that helps family members acknowledge, discuss, own, and value the character strengths they see in their families and themselves. PPT can be done as a stand-alone treatment, or its exercises can be used through a dismantling approach or easily integrated into well-established protocols such as cognitive behavior therapy (Karwoski et al., 2006).

When conducting treatment, especially with clients from diverse cultural backgrounds, the therapist must remember that treatment is neither presented as prescriptive nor enveloped within Eurocentric confines. For example, curing mental health primarily through talk therapy and applying formal logic (e.g., positive cognitive appraisal in PPT) may be more amenable to Westerners who prefer to verbalize their reasoning and categorize emotions and experiences, and who can easily overlook the influence of context. Easterners, on the other hand, are more willing to entertain apparently contradictory propositions, reflect more, and are better able to see relationships between events (Nisbett, 2008). A skillful therapist must always be cognizant of the cultural lens through which he or she views the world.

Evidence

Two randomized controlled-intervention studies—by Seligman, Steen, Park, and Peterson (2005) and Seligman, Rashid, and Parks (2006)—demonstrated that PPT exercises, delivered singularly or packaged into comprehensive treatment package, are effective in undoing symptoms of depression as well as in amplifying well-being. An outcome measure of PPT, the Positive Psychotherapy Inventory (PPTI), has been created and validated to assess the specific active ingredients of the treatment such as pleasure, engagement, and meaning. Three studies have demonstrated its validity and reliability (Bertisch, 2012; Guney, 2011; Seligman et al., 2006). Moreover, four independent replications of these studies with minor variations, with clinical and nonclinical samples by Mongrain and Anselmo-Matthews (2012), Meyer et al. (2012), Bay (2012), and Mitchell et al. (2009), have further demonstrated that PPT exercises improve psychological well-being, boost hope, enhance savoring, promote psychological recovery and self-esteem, and ameliorate psychiatric symptoms. Rashid and Uliaszek (2012) integrated PPT with dialectical behavioral therapy (DBT) exercises in a 12-session group therapy program called *skills and strengths group* (SSG) with clients who experienced symptoms associated with borderline personality disorder. Compared to the comparison group (treatment as usual), participants in the intervention group (SSG) improved more on several measures, including well-being, emotional regulation, and overall symptom reduction (assessed by structured interviews).

PPT exercises have also been applied with adolescents and children. In the United Kingdom, Akhtar and Boniwell (2010) found that PPT exercises were effective with adolescents seeking treatment for drug addiction and behavioral challenges. In a randomized control trial with grade six students, Rashid and Anjum (2008) found that PPT exercises were effective in increasing well-being and improving social skills, as reported by teachers and parents. More recently, the first author trained eight psychologists in administering PPT in school settings. Three of them delivered PPT through a group intervention at the Toronto District School Board. Participants were teachers who completed PPT exercises over a period of one academic year. Despite experiencing a high dropout rate (33%), participants in the intervention group, compared to the comparison group, showed significant changes in well-being. No significant changes in depressive symptoms were found. This was expected because the overall sample was nonclinical. The year-long intervention allowed participants to engage in detailed discussion regarding their usefulness of each exercise. Schueller (2011) found that individual's preference for one Positive Psychology exercise was linked to increased adherence for the match exercise. Clients benefit differentially from different exercises, and a sense of autonomy increases the efficacy of each exercise. Taken together across samples and settings, the findings about the effectiveness of PPT are encouraging. However, more research is needed to evaluate PPT's effectiveness with a variety of psychological disorders, including comparisons with traditional symptom-targeted treatments.

A range of useful books on positive interventions and clinical practice has also emerged (e.g., Conoley & Conoley, 2009; Fredrickson, 2009; Joseph & Linley, 2006; Lyubomirsky, 2008; Magyar-Moe, 2009), as have many theoretical advances that incorporate strengths in traditional clinical practices (e.g., Dick-Niederhauser, 2009; Lent, 2004; Smith, 2006; Wong, 2006). Taken together, this burgeoning body of work suggests that positive clinical interventions will be a significant therapeutic pillar that complements advances already made in psychotherapy.

Psychotherapy in a Multicultural World

Happiness, at least in Western culture, has become synonymous with feeling good (hedonism). However, we believe that PPT's approach, largely based on the notion of pursuit of good life (*eudemonia*), is more conducive to multicultural clients because it includes a broader notion of happiness through multiple routes, positive emotions, character strengths, positive relationship, and meaning. Therefore, it accommodates cultural sensitivities more than a traditional deficit-oriented psychotherapy framework largely based on Western notions of psychopathology. The traditional psychotherapy model tends to exaggerate daily life's difficulties and turn them into psychiatric disorders. When viewed within a specific cultural context, these difficulties, instead of being pathologized within DSM-based categories, could simply be viewed as the challenges associated with being human. For example, a relaxed style of communication, characteristic of many cultures, might be viewed as pathological slow speech and a sign of depression. In contrast, rapid and emotive style of speech, characteristic of many cultures, might be perceived as a symptom of mania. Similarly, duty to family may be perceived as a sign of dependency by a deficit-oriented therapist and parents' decision to sleep with their young children—a common practice in many non-Western countries—might be interpreted as enmeshment.

In PPT, not all idiosyncratic patterns of behaving, thinking, feeling, or desiring qualify for medical labels. Pathologizing culturally relevant behavior may discourage minorities from seeking psychotherapy, and these individuals may believe therapy, as portrayed in popular media, only involves discussing weaknesses in minuscule detail or identifying childhood resentments or monitoring distorted thoughts. PPT, on the other hand, starts with a positive introduction, and through stories, anecdotes, and experiences of resilience, it elicits meaning, relationship, engagement, and accomplishment. These can all be examined and discussed within a cultural context. We believe balancing the negative with the positive will make psychotherapy more attractive and empowering for clients from diverse backgrounds.

Melanie Bay (2012), working in France, compared group PPT with CBT and with medication and found clients in PPT experienced greater therapeutic benefits on measures of depression, optimism, life satisfaction, and emotional intelligence. In Iran, Moeenizadeh and Salagame (2010) found that well-being therapy faired better than CBT. That said, the therapist in PPT needs to be cognizant that manifestation of strengths may differ from culture to culture. For example, courage in the North American context may entail taking an active stand on an unpopular issue or voicing an unpopular opinion, whereas courage in a Southeast Asian culture may be reflected in one's ability to endure. It is important to discuss cultural values with the clients and their expectations about the meaning of specific strengths in their particular culture.

CASE EXAMPLE

Introduction

Lindsey, a 43-year-old, married woman, presented with significant symptoms of depression that severely affected her ability to function at home and work. She lived with her husband and a 9-year-old son and 7-year-old daughter. Lindsey worked for an accountant. At the time she entered treatment, she reported being sad, empty, and slow. She had diminished appetite, low libido, and sleep disturbance. She constantly worried and was chronically anxious. These symptoms had been present for 5 months, and they became severe enough that Lindsey was unable to continue her job and had to take sick leave. Lindsey described her marriage as stable but somewhat "empty and lacking intimacy." She often felt lonely because her husband traveled frequently for his work. She sometimes worried about her son's academic performance, although her son was earning good grades. Lindsey had actually stopped socializing with her close friends. Her health was generally good, and she was not taking any medications. This was the first time Lindsey had sought psychotherapy

Course of Assessment and Treatment

From a deficit-oriented model, Lindsey was administered the Minnesota Multiphasic Personality Inventory–2 (MMPI-2) and Beck Depression Inventory (BDI-II; Beck, Steer, Ball & Ranieri, 1996). Her scores on MMPI-2's depression scale and the BDI were significantly elevated. She did not endorse any thoughts of suicide. Based on clinical interview and the test results, the clinician (TR) determined that Lindsey's mood was consistent with a DSM-IV diagnosis of major depressive disorder. On PPTI, her scores suggested a lack of positive emotions, engagement, and meaning.

Our first two sessions were devoted to establishing rapport, exploring Lindsey's history of depression, understanding the family dynamics, and assessing her perception of her problems and her reasons for seeking therapy. In the third session, the clinician and Lindsey discussed her clinical profile from a deficit-oriented perspective, underscoring patterns of symptoms and the natural course of depression and its consequences. Speaking in a soft tone and making little eye contact, Lindsey endorsed her profile and expressed feelings of hopelessness about her ability to get better. Toward the end of this session, Lindsey was gently asked to introduce herself through a real-life story, which would show her at her best. Initially reluctant, Lindsey agreed to give it a try. In the next session, she brought in her story. She was encouraged to read it. Lindsey read:

> I was in tenth grade when my family moved across the country. I loved my previous high school and had a lot of friends. I missed it greatly and felt like not going to my new school, but I had to. Class work was less painful, but the lunch period was the worst because I didn't have anyone to eat with and I felt like a lonely dork. During the second week, sitting alone, I was staring at my salad and almost believing that onions curls formed the word "loser" when I heard some students laughing hysterically at the next table. At first, I thought, they must have read what was written on my salad. I hunkered down and dared not to look at them but soon I figured out

that their laugh was not directed at me or my salad. I turned and looked and discovered that the laughter came from a bunch of kids who seemed quite cool. Soon, I noticed that they were all laughing at this boy who was sitting alone at an adjacent table and there seemed something not alright with him. I didn't know it then, but Harris had a neurological disorder that made him jerk his head involuntarily. It was quite obvious that he was not doing this on his own. He was embarrassed and confused. I thought it was very mean of these kids to make fun of him. I felt very sad. For a moment I thought I should stop them but then I thought, they are the "cool" kids and if I did that I will never be able to make any friend at this school. But this selfish impulse passed quickly, and I started feeling angry. Without thinking much, I just got up and walked to them and in a single breath I almost shouted, "I don't know you—and I don't know him—but what you are doing is sick. I thought I was a loser here for not having any friends, but I think you are much bigger losers." I came back to my table and felt good.

Lindsey finished the story with misty eyes but with her face lit up. On prompting, Lindsey identified courage and fairness as salient strengths displayed in her story. She was then asked to complete the online VIA Inventory of Strengths and bring the printout of her feedback to the next session.

In the following week, Lindsey brought the printed feedback from the VIA-IS. Interestingly, neither courage nor fairness was included as one of her top strengths. However, from a list of 24 core strengths, the capacity to love and be loved, creativity, social intelligence, appreciation of beauty, and spirituality were her top strengths. Courage and fairness were in the middle of the pack, and zest and self-regulation were placed toward the end. During next three sessions, Lindsey completed a dynamic strength assessment (see Table 13.4), and the therapist and Lindsey discussed her wholeness—integrating her symptoms of depression and her profile of strengths. We also discussed how her self-identified strengths of courage and fairness might still serve her during tough times. We discussed the notion of using her top strengths and working on her lesser developed strengths such as zest and self-regulation to help her confront and overcome her depressive symptoms.

The idea of combining Lindsey's strengths was discussed using the metaphor of an *orchestra of strengths*, an orchestra that was constantly changing and adapting its tempo and tune in accordance with changing circumstances. The concepts of change and adaptation were particularly highlighted because strengths have their shadow sides. In Lindsey's case, one of her top strengths (social intelligence) helped her at work as she used her acute awareness of emotions and intentions of others to make her co-workers and customers feel comfortable. However, at the same time, in making everyone feel comfortable, she took on too much responsibility and had trouble saying no. She believed that she understood everyone, but almost no one understood her. This belief saddened her and left her feeling helpless.

After thorough discussions of the integration of strengths, Lindsey selected those strengths she would work on to decrease her depression. Lindsey began with appreciation of beauty: She actively sought out glimpses of natural and artistic beauty on a daily basis, and she journaled about the beauty around her. She also decided to use her creativity to experience flow. For example, Lindsey loved cooking. Every Sunday, she started enjoying the long, slow dance of chopping, grating, stirring, simmering, tasting, seasoning, and sharing her culinary creations with her family. She also decided to work on self-regulation and joined a gym and worked out three times a week.

During this process, Lindsey's symptoms were not ignored. She had good and bad days. Whenever she brought forth her struggles with depression, her concerns were validated, but her attention was gently guided away from her problems so she could mindfully work on her strengths.

Outcome and Prognosis

Assessing and leveraging her strengths helped Lindsey shift her focus from deficits and helplessness to what was right about her. She learned ways to use her deepest psychological resources to manage her depressed moods. Using strengths through concrete actions helped her reeducate her attention and memory so she could attend to and notice the genuinely good aspects of her life. After about 20 sessions, both measures of psychopathology and strengths were administered again. Lindsey's scores on depression decreased significantly, and she no longer met criteria for major depressive disorder. Her strengths profile remained largely unchanged, with the exception of self-regulation, which moved from bottom of the pack to the middle. In addition, Lindsey was able to return to work.

In many ways, Lindsey represents a typical depressed client whose symptoms might have been ameliorated but not eliminated if she was only treated with deficit-oriented psychotherapy. However, in the early sessions of therapy, the therapist identified Lindsey's core strengths, and this helped enhance the doctor–patient relationship. The identification and promotion of Lindsey's strengths made it possible for her to internalize the notion that she was a worthy person who had the character strengths necessary to establish a life of pleasure, engagement, and meaning.

SUMMARY

Positive Psychotherapy treats negative emotions and experiences head-on by identifying the client's psychological assets such as character strengths, engagement, meaning, and positive relationships. PPT requires systematic and sustained therapeutic work to identify and amplify these resources, opening a client's mindsets beyond the innate propensity for negativity with the ultimate goal of helping him or her establish a life worth living. PPT's initial promising results—with both clinical and nonclinical clients—demonstrate that human beings not only want to be less miserable but also want to live lives filled with pleasure, engagement, and meaning.

 Counseling CourseMate Website:

See this text's Counseling CourseMate website at www.cengagebrain.com for learning tools such as chapter quizzing, videos, glossary flashcards, and more.

ANNOTATED BIBLIOGRAPHY AND WEB RESOURCES

Burns, G. W. (Ed.). (2010). *Happiness, healing and enhancement: Your casebook collection for applying Positive Psychology in therapy*. New York: John Wiley & Sons.
This 27-chapter volume, written by leading practitioners of Positive Psychology, provides compelling case illustrations regarding the clinical use of Positive Psychology exercises with clients in distress. Many of the chapters offer step-by-step strategies, most of which are empirically based.

Magyar-Moe, J. L. (2009). *Therapist's guide to positive psychological interventions*. New York: Elsevier Academic Press.
This five-part book introduces and integrates Positive Psychology with counseling and psychotherapy. It has a good section on positive psychological tests and measures and a comprehensive chapter on several Positive Psychol-

ogy interventions, each described in detail. The final part of the book discusses ways of carrying out a treatment plan infused with Positive Psychology.

Fluckinger, C., Wusten, G., Zinbarg, R., & Wampold, B. (2009). *Resource activation: Using client's own strengths in psychotherapy and counseling*. Boston: Hogrefe.
This brief (68-page) guide offers practical clinical strategies that will help clinicians ask meaningful questions to help clients identify their character strengths. The book emphasizes that the activation of client resources by focusing on strengths is not incompatible with distress remediation: It is simply a very positive and effective way to increase client well-being and reduce distress.

Stephen, J. & Linley, A. (2006). *Positive therapy: A meta-theory for positive psychological practice*. London: Routledge.

From two leading voices in the applied Positive Psychology field, this book argues that therapy is not so much about what you do as how you do it, emphasizing the influence of the views clinicians hold about human nature. While discussing the meta-therapy of Positive Psychology, the authors provide insights about how to reframe client beliefs using a positive psychological perspective.

Niemiec, R., & Wedding, D. (2013). *Positive Psychology at the movies: Using films to build virtues and character strengths* (2nd ed.). Boston: Hogrefe.
This book uses films as a vehicle to introduce students to the core principles of Positive Psychology, and an exhaustive appendix lists hundreds of films that offer particularly good examples of virtues and character strengths.

ADDITIONAL CLINICAL BOOKS

O'Hanlon, B., & Bertolino, B. (2012). *The therapist's notebook on Positive Psychology activities, exercises, and handouts*. London: Routledge.

Levak, R. W., Siegel, L., & Nichols, S. N. (2011). *Therapeutic feedback with the MMPI-2: A Positive Psychology approach*. New York: Taylor & Francis.

SPECIAL ISSUES, SECTIONS ON POSITIVE CLINICAL PSYCHOLOGY, AND GUEST EDITORS

Journal of Clinical Psychology. In Session, May 2009: T. Rashid

The Psychologist, 16, 2003: A. P. Linley, S. Joseph, & I. Boniwell

Journal of Cognitive Psychotherapy, 20(2), 2006: R. Ingram

The Counseling Psychologist, 34(2), 2006: S. J. Lopez, J. L. Magyar-Moe, S. E. Petersen, J. A. Ryder, T. S. Krieshok, K. K. O'Byrne, J. W. Lichtenberg, & A. N. Fry

American Psychologist, 55, 2000: M. E. P. Seligman & M. Csikszentmihalyi

NONCLINICAL BOOKS WITH PRACTICAL RESOURCES

Flourish by Martin Seligman (2011): Free Press.

Authentic Happiness by Martin Seligman (2002): Free Press.

Happier by Tal Ben-Shahar (2007): McGraw Hill.

The How of Happiness by Sonja Lyubomirsky, (2008): Penguin Press.

A Primer in Positive Psychology by Christopher Peterson (2007): Oxford.

Positive Psychology: The Scientific and Practical Explorations of Human Strengths by C. R. Snyder & Shane J. Lopez (2006): Sage.

Happiness: Unlocking the Mysteries of Psychological Wealth by Ed Diener & Robert Biswas-Diener (2009): Blackwell.

Positivity: Discover the Ratio That Tips Your Life Toward Flourishing by Barbara Fredrickson (2009): Crown.

Flow by Csikszentmihalyi (1991): Harper Perennial/ HarperCollins.

The Happiness Hypothesis by Jon Haidt (2006): Basic Books.

DOCUMENTARIES

The Happiness Formula: Six-part BBC documentary, aired April 2006 (news.bbc.co.uk/2/hi/programmes /happiness_formula/).

"Happiness—How to Find It, Understand It, and Achieve It": *20/20* (ABC), first aired January 2008 (www.abcnews-store.go.com).

In Pursuit of Happiness: Find Happiest Canadian: documentary by Sarah Spinks (www.spinfree.ca).

Introducing Positive Psychology: MontanaPBS.

CASE READINGS

Burns, G. W. (Ed.) (2010). *Happiness, healing, enhancement: Your casebook collection for applying Positive Psychology in therapy*. Hoboken, NJ: Wiley.
George Burns describes a case of a woman being treated for major depression. Burn treats the client using the PPT

theoretical model. Treatment involves facilitating a therapeutic process that helped a client turn her life around by being open to, and willing to explore, the possibility that life could hold greater pleasure, greater engagement, and greater meaning.

Journal of Clinical Psychology (2009, May), *65*(2)

This special issue on positive interventions contains six case studies. The first case study by Rashid and Ostermann (2009) focuses on strength-based assessment of a middle-age female depressed client. At the onset of psychotherapy, many clients experience a diminished sense of worth and feel overwhelmed by their problems. This case illustrates that when weaknesses and strengths are assessed and discussed in an integrative manner, clients are more likely to find psychotherapy to be affirming and empowering. This improves their motivation as they view themselves beyond a diagnostic label.

Kauffman, C., & Silberman, J. (2009). Finding and fostering the positive in relationships: Positive interventions in couples therapy. *Journal of Clinical Psychology, 65*(5), 520–531. doi:10.1002/jclp.20594

Carol Kaufman and Jordan Silberman describe a case that illustrates use of positive interventions to foster a positive and healthier relationship. In this case, a couple in their early 40s, married for 10 years and deeply unhappy in their relationship, use several PPT exercises—including three good things, grudge, acknowledging, and nurturing of each other's strengths—to better harness their own strengths.

Rashid, T., & Ostermann, R. F. (2009). Strength-based assessment in clinical practice. *Journal of Clinical Psychology: In Session, 65* (5), 488–498. [Reprinted in D. Wedding & R. J. Corsini. (2013). *Case studies in psychotherapy.* Belmont, CA: Cengage.]

This case illustrates how a strength-based assessment can "enhance clinical clarity, improve the range of informa-tion, and provide amore complete picture of clients and their circumstances." The case was specifically selected by Rashid and Seligman to complement their chapter in *Current Psychotherapies.*

Ruini, C., & Fava, G. A. (2009). Well-being therapy for generalized anxiety disorder. *Journal of Clinical Psychology, 65*(5), 510–519. doi:10.1002/jclp.20592

Chiara Ruini and Giovanni Fava describe a case of a 29-year-old single woman with symptoms of anxiety disorder, complicated by other subclinical syndromes. This clinical case illustrates the use of standard cognitive-behavioral therapy followed by well-being therapy (WBT). Similar to PPT, WBT focused on core six positive dimensions of well-being: autonomy, environmental mastery, purpose in life, positive relations, and self-acceptance. This case illustrates how CBT can be used to change beliefs and attitudes detrimental to well-being and stimulate personal growth.

Seligman, M. E. P. (2002). *Authentic happiness: Using the new Positive Psychology to realize your potential for lasting fulfillment.* New York: Free Press.

This book describes the treatment of Len, a man who was handsome, articulate, bright, and a very eligible bachelor; however, when it came to love, he was a total failure. PPT helped this man live a fuller life and learn to love. Len's story highlights that there are various routes to happiness and sometimes clients get struck. PPT can help clients find other routes and detours that lead to resolution of their problems.

REFERENCES

Akhtar, M., & Boniwell, I. (2010). Applying Positive Psychology to alcohol-misusing adolescents: A group intervention. *Groupwork, 20*(3), 6–31.

Albee, G. W. (2000). The Boulder model's fatal flaw. *American Psychologist, 55*(2), 247–248. doi:10.1037/0003-066X.55.2.247

American Psychiatric Association. (2013). *Diagnostic and statistical manual of mental disorders* (DSM-5). Retrieved from www.dsm5.org.

Azar, B. (2011). Positive Psychology advances, with growing pains. *APA Monitor, 42*(4), 32. Retrieved from www.apa.org/monitor/2011/04/positive-psychology.aspx.

Barlow, D. H. (2008). *Clinical handbook of psychological disorders: A step-by-step treatment manual* (4th ed.). New York: Guilford Press.

Bartels, M., & Boomsma, D. I. (2009). Born to be happy? The etiology of subjective well-being. *Behavior Genetics, 39*(6), 605–615. doi:10.1007/s10519-009-9294-8.

Bauer, J. J., McAdams, D. P., & Pals, J. L. (2006). Narrative identity and eudaimonic well-being. *Journal of Happiness Studies, 9*(1), 81–104. doi:10.1007/s10902-006-9021-6.

Baumeister, R. F., Bratslavsky, E., Finkenauer, C., & Vohs, K. D. (2001). Bad is stronger than good. *Review of General Psychology, 5*(4), 323–370. doi:10.1037/1089-2680.5.4.323.

Bay, M. (2012). *Comparing Positive Psychotherapy with cognitive behavioral therapy in treating depression.* Unpublished manuscript. Paris West University Nanterre La Défense (Université Paris Ouest Nanterre La Défense).

Beck, A. T., Steer, R. A., Ball, R., & Ranieri, W. (1996). Comparison of Beck Depression Inventories -IA and -II in psychiatric outpatients. *Journal of Personality Assessment, 67*(3), 588–97. doi:10.1207/s15327752jpa6703_13.

Bergin & Garfield, 1994.

Bertisch, H. (2012). Positive Psychology and resilience in rehabilitation medicine. *Achieves of Physical Medicine and Rehabilitation, 93*(10), p. 48e.

Bonanno, G. A., & Mancini, A. D. (2012). Beyond resilience and PTSD: Mapping the heterogeneity of responses to potential trauma. *Psychological Trauma, 4,* 74–83.

Carver, C. S., Scheier, M. F., & Segerstrom, S. C. (2010). Optimism. *Clinical Psychology Review, 30*(7), 879–889. doi:10.1016/j.cpr.2010.01.006.

Cheavens, J. S., Feldman, D. B., Gum, A., Michael, S. T., & Snyder, C. R. (2006). Hope therapy in a community sample: A pilot investigation. *Social Indicators Research. Special Issue: Subjective Well-Being in Mental Health and Human Development Research Worldwide, 77*(1), 61–78. doi:10.1007/s11205-005-5553-0.

Chida, Y., & Steptoe, A. (2009). The association of anger and hostility with future coronary heart disease: A meta-analytic review of prospective evidence. *Journal of the American College of Cardiology, 53*(11), 936–946. doi:10.1016/j.jacc.2008.11.044.

Conoley, C. W., & Conoley, J. C. (2009). *Positive Psychology and family therapy.* Hoboken, NJ: Wiley.

Cornum, R., Matthews, M. D., & Seligman, M. E. P. (2011). Comprehensive soldier fitness: Building resilience in a challenging institutional context. *The American Psychologist, 66*(1), 4–9. doi:10.1037/a0021420.

Crits-Christoph, P., Connolly Gibbons, M. B., Ring-Kurtz, S., Gallop, R., Stirman, S., Present, J., Temes, C., et al. (2008). Changes in positive quality of life over the course of psychotherapy. *Psychotherapy, 45*(4), 419–430. doi:10.1037/a0014340.

Csikszentmihalyi, M. (1990). *Flow: The psychology of optimal experience.* New York: HarperCollins.

Davidson, L., Shahar, G., Lawless, M. S., Sell, D. & Tondora, J. (2006). Play, pleasure, and other positive life events: "Non-specific" factors in recovery from mental illness? *Psychiatry, 2*(69), 151–163.

Dick-Niederhauser, A. (2009). Therapeutic change and the experience of joy: Toward a theory of curative processes. *Journal of Psychotherapy Integration.19,* 187–211.

Duckworth, A. L., Steen, T. A., & Seligman, M. E. P. (2005). Positive Psychology in clinical practice. *Annual Review of Clinical Psychology, 1*(1), 629–651. doi:10.1146/annurev.clinpsy.1.102803.144154.

Edwards, L. M., & Pedrotti, J. T. (2004). Utilizing the strengths of our cultures. *Women & Therapy, 27*(1-2), 33–43. doi:10.1300/J015v27n01_03.

Fava, G. A., & Ruini, C. (2003). Development and characteristics of a well-being enhancing psychotherapeutic strategy: Well-being therapy. *Journal of Behavior Therapy and Experimental Psychiatry, 34*(1), 45–63. doi:10.1016/S0005-7916(03)00019-3.

Feldman, G. C., Joormann, J., & Johnson, S. L. (2008). Responses to positive affect: A self-report measure of rumination and dampening. *Cognitive Therapy and Research, 32,* 507–525.

Ferguson, C. J. (2010). A meta-analysis of normal and disordered personality across the life span. *Journal of personality and social psychology, 98*(4), 659–667. doi:10.1037/a0018770.

Fitzpatrick, M. R., & Stalikas, A. (2008). Integrating positive emotions into theory, research, and practice: A new challenge for psychotherapy. *Journal of Psychotherapy Integration, 18*(2), 248–258. doi:10.1037/1053-0479.18.2.248.

Flinchbaugh, C. L., Moore, E. W. G., Chang, Y. K., & May, D. R. (2012). Student well-being interventions: The effects of stress management techniques and gratitude journaling in the management education classroom. *Journal of Management Education, 36*(2), 191–219. doi:10.1177/1052562911430062.

Flückiger, C., & Grosse Holtforth, M. (2008). Focusing the therapist's attention on the patient's strengths: A preliminary study to foster a mechanism of change in outpatient psychotherapy. *Journal of Clinical Psychology, 64*(7), 876–890. doi:10.1002/jclp.20493.

Fordyce, M. W. (1983). A program to increase happiness: Further studies. *Journal of Consulting Psychology, 30,* 483–498.

Frankl, V. E. (1963). *Man's search for meaning: An introduction to logotherapy.* New York: Washington Square Press.

Fredrickson, B. L. (2009) *Positivity: Discover the ratio that tips your life toward flourishing.* New York: Crown.

Gable, S. L., & Haidt, J. (2005). What (and why) is Positive Psychology? *Review of General Psychology, 9,* 103–110.

Gable, S. L, Reis, H. T., Impett, E. A., & Asher, E. R. (2004). What do you do when things go right? The intrapersonal and interpersonal benefits of sharing positive events. *Journal of Personality and Social Psychology. 87,* 228–245.

Gilman, R., Schumm, J. A., & Chard, K. M. (2012). Hope as a change mechanism in the treatment of posttraumatic stress disorder. *Psychological Trauma: Theory, Research, Practice, and Policy, 4*(3), 270–277. doi:10.1037/a0024252.

Goldberg, C. (2006, March 10). Harvard's crowded course to happiness: "Positive Psychology" draws students in droves. *The Boston Globe.* Retrieved from www.boston.com/news/local/articles/2006/03/10/harvards_crowded_course_to happiness/

Grafanaki, S., Brennan, M., Holmes, S., Tang, K., & Alvarez, S. (2007). "In search of flow" in counseling and psychotherapy: Identifying the necessary ingredients of peak moments of therapy interaction, person-centered, and experiential psychotherapies. *International Journal of Person-Centered and Experiential Psychotherapies, 6,* 239–255.

Graham, J. E., Lobel, M., Glass, P., & Lokshina, I. (2008). Effects of written constructive anger expression in chronic pain patients: Making meaning from pain. *Journal of Behavioral Medicine, 31,* 201–212.

Grant, G. M., Salcedo, V., Hynan, L. S., Frisch, M. B., & Puster, K. (1995). Effectiveness of quality of life therapy for depression. *Psychological Reports, 76*(3, part 2), 1203–1208. Retrieved from www.ncbi.nlm.nih.gov/pubmed/7480486.

Guney, S. (2011). The Positive Psychotherapy Inventory (PPTI): Reliability and validity study in Turkish population. *Social and Behavioral Sciences, 29,* 81–86.

Harris, A. H. S., Luskin, F., Norman, S. B., Standard, S., Bruning, J., Evans, S., &Thoresen, C. E. (2006). Effects of a group forgiveness intervention on forgiveness, perceived stress, and trait-anger. *Journal of Clinical Psychology, 62*(6), 715–733. doi:10.1002/jclp.20264.

Headey, B., Schupp, J., T., Ingrid, T. & Wagner, G. G. (2010). Authentic happiness theory supported by impact of religion on life satisfaction: A longitudinal analysis with data for Germany. *The Journal of Positive Psychology, 5,* 73–82.

Hicks, J. A., & King, L. A. (2009). Meaning in life as a subjective judgment and lived experience. *Social and Personality Psychology Compass, 3*(4), 638–658.

Horwitz, A. V., Widom, C. S., McLaughlin, J., & White, H. R. (2001). The impact of childhood abuse and neglect on adult mental health: A prospective study. *Journal of Health and Social Behavior, 42*(2), 184–201.

Huta, V., & Hawley, L. (2010). Psychological strengths and cognitive vulnerabilities: Are they two ends of the same continuum or do they have independent relationships with well-being and ill-being? *Journal of Happiness Studies*, *11*(1), 71–93. doi:10.1007/s10902-008-9123-4.

Jahoda, M. (1958). *Current concepts of positive mental health.* New York: Basic Books.

Joseph, S., & Linley, A. P. (2006). *Positive Therapy: A meta-theory for positive psychological practice.* New York: Rutledge.

Kahneman, D., Krueger, A. B., Schkade, D., Schwartz, N., & Stone, A. A. (2006). Would you be happier if you were richer? A focusing illusion. *Science, 312*, 1908–1910.

Karwoski, L., Garratt, G. M., & Ilardi, S. S. (2006). On the integration of cognitive-behavioral therapy for depression and Positive Psychology. *Journal of Cognitive Psychotherapy*, *20*(2), 159–170. doi:10.1891/jcop.20.2.159.

Kashdan, T. B., Julian, T., Merritt, K., & Uswatte, G. (2006). Social anxiety and posttraumatic stress in combat veterans: Relations to well-being and character strengths. *Behaviour Research and Therapy, 44*, 561–583.

Kauffman, C., & Silberman, J. (2009). Finding and fostering the positive in relationships: positive interventions in couples therapy. *Journal of Clinical Psychology*, 65(5), 520–31. doi:10.1002/jclp.20594.

Lambert, M. J. (2007). Presidential address: What we have learned from a decade of research aimed at improving psychotherapy outcome in routine care. *Psychotherapy Research*, *17*(1), 1–14. doi:10.1080/10503300601032506.

Lambert, M. J. (2013). *Bergin and Garfield's handbook of psychotherapy and behavior change* (6th ed.). New York: Wiley.

Lamont, A. (2011). University students' strong experiences of music: Pleasure, engagement, and meaning. *Music and Emotion, 15*, 229–249.

Lent, R. W. (2004). Towards a unifying theoretical and practical perspective on well-being and psychosocial adjustment. *Journal of Counseling Psychology, 5*, 482–509.

Lester, B. P., Harm, P. D., Herian, M. N., Kraiskova, D. V. & Beal, S. J. (2011). The Comprehensive Soldier Fitness Program Evaluation. Retrieved from http://dma.wi.gov/dma/news/2012news/csf-tech-report.pdf on October 3, 2012.

Leykin, Y., & DeRubeis, R. J. (2009). Allegiance in psychotherapy outcome research: Separating association from bias. *Clinical Psychology: Science and Practice*, *16*(1), 54–65. doi:10.1111/j.1468-2850.2009.01143.x.

Lyubomirsky, S. (2008). *The how of happiness.* London: Sphere.

Lyubomirsky, S., King, L. A., & Diener, E. (2005). The benefits of frequent positive affect: Does happiness lead to success? *Psychological Bulletin, 131*, 803–855.

Kirsch, I., Deacon B. J., Huedo-Medina T.B., Scoboria A., Moore T. J., et al. (2008). Initial severity and antidepressant benefits: A meta-analysis of data submitted to the Food and Drug Administration. *PLoS Med, 5*(2): e45. doi:10.1371/journal.pmed.0050045.

Magyar-Moe, J. L. (2009). *Therapist's guide to positive psychological interventions.* New York: Elsevier Academic Press.

Maslow, A. H. (1970). *Motivation and personality* (2nd ed.). New York: Harper & Row.

McCormick, B. P., Funderburk, J. A., Lee, Y. & Hale-Fought, M. (2005). Activity characteristics and emotional experience: Predicting boredom and anxiety in the daily life of community mental health clients. *Journal of Leisure Research, 37*, 236–253.

McGrath, R. E., Rashid, T., Park, N., & Peterson, C. (2010). Is optimal functioning a distinct state? *The Humanistic Psychologist, 38*(2), 159–169. doi:10.1080/08873261003635781.

McKnight, P. E., & Kashdan, T. B. (2009). Purpose in life as a system that creates and sustains health and well-being: An integrative, testable theory. *Review of General Psychology, 13*, 242–251.

Meyer, P. S., Johnson, D. P., Parks, A. C., Iwanski, C. & Penn, D. L. (2012). Positive living: A pilot study of group Positive Psychotherapy for people with schizophrenia. *Journal of Positive Psychology, 7*, 239–248.

Mitchell, J., Stanimirovic, R., Klein, B., & Vella-Brodrick, D. (2009). A randomized controlled trial of a self-guided internet intervention promoting well-being. *Computers in Human Behavior, 25*, 749–760.

Moeenizadeh, M., & Salagame, K. K. K. (2010). Well-being therapy (WBT) for depression. *International Journal of Psychological Studies, 2*(1), 107–115.

Murray, G., & Johnson, S. L. (2010). The clinical significance of creativity in bipolar disorder. *Clinical Psychology Review, 30*(6), 721–732. doi:10.1016/j.cpr.2010.05.006.

Myers, D. G. (2000). The funds, friends, and faith of happy people. *American Psychologist 55*(1), 56–67. doi:10.1037//0003-066X.55.1.56.

Niemiec, R. M., Rashid, T., & Spinella, M. (2012). Strong mindfulness: Integrating mindfulness and character strengths. *Journal of Mental Health Counseling, 34*, 240–253.

Nisbett, R. E. (2008). Eastern and Western ways of perceiving the world. In Y. Shoda, D. Cervone, & G. Downey (Eds.), *Persons in context: Constructing a science of the individual* (pp. 62–83). New York: Guilford Press.

Oksanen, T., Kouvonen, A., Vahtera, J., Virtanen, M., & Kivimäki, M. (2010). Prospective study of workplace social capital and depression: Are vertical and horizontal components equally important? *Journal of Epidemiology and Community Health, 64*(8), 684–689. doi:10.1136/jech.2008.086074.

Perlman, L. M., Cohen, J. L., Altiere, M. J., Brennan, J. A., Brown, S. R., Mainka, J. B., & Diroff, C. R. (2010). A multidimensional wellness group therapy program for veterans with comorbid psychiatric and medical conditions. *Professional Psychology: Research and Practice, 41*(2), 120–127. doi:10.1037/a0018800.

Peterson, C. (2006). The Values in Action (VIA) classification of strengths. In M. Csikszentmihalyi & I. S. Csikszentmihalyi (Eds.), *A life worth living: Contributions to Positive Psychology* (pp. 29–48). New York: Oxford.

Peterson, C., Park, N., & Seligman, M. E. (2005). Orientations to happiness and life satisfaction: The full life versus the empty life. *Journal of Happiness Studies, 6*, 25–41.

Peterson, C., & Seligman, M. E. P. (2004). *Character strengths and virtues: A handbook and classification.* New York: Oxford University Press; Washington, DC: American Psychological Association.

Rashid, T. (2009). Positive interventions in clinical practice, *Journal of Clinical Psychology, 65,* 461–466.

Rashid, T., & Anjum. A (2008). Positive psychotherapy for children and adolescents. In J. R. Z. Abela & B. L. Hankin (Eds.), *Depression in children and adolescents: Causes, treatment and prevention.* New York: Guilford Press.

Rashid, T., & Ostermann, R. F. O. (2009). Strength-based assessment in clinical practice. *Journal of Clinical Psychology: In Session, 65,* 488–498.

Rashid, T., & Uliaszeck, A. (2012). *Skills and strengths group: Integrating skills from dialectical behavioral therapy skills with Positive Psychotherapy (PPT) skills.* Unpublished manuscript, University of Toronto, Scarborough, Canada.

Rashid, T., Anjum, A., Stevanovski, S., Chu, R., Zanjani, A. & Love, A. P. (2013). Strength-based resilience: Integrating risk and resources towards holistic well-being. In A. G. Fava & C. Ruini (Eds.), *Increasing psychological well-being across cultures.* The Netherlands: Springer.

Rief, W., Nestoriuc, Y., von Lilienfeld-Toal, A., Dogan, I., Schreiber, F., Hofmann, S. G., Barsky, A. J., et al. (2009). Differences in adverse effect reporting in placebo groups in SSRI and tricyclic antidepressant trials: A systematic review and meta-analysis. *Drug Safety: An International Journal of Medical Toxicology and Drug Experience, 32*(11), 1041–1056. doi:10.2165/11316580-000000000-00000.

Ruini, C., & Fava, G. A. (2009). Well-being therapy for generalized anxiety disorder. *Journal of clinical psychology, 65*(5), 510–519. doi:10.1002/jclp.20592.

Schwartz, B., & Sharpe, K. E. (2006). Practical wisdom: Aristotle meets Positive Psychology. *Journal of Happiness Studies, 7,* 377–395.

Schwartz, B., Ward, A., Monterosso, J., Lyubomirsky, S., White, K., & Lehman, D. R. (2002). Maximizing versus satisficing: happiness is a matter of choice. *Journal of Personality and Social Psychology, 83*(5), 1178–1197. doi:10.1037/0022-3514.83.5.1178.

Schwartz, R. M., Reynolds, C. F., III, Thase, M. E., Frank, E., Fasiczka, A. L., & Haaga, D. A. F. (2002). Optimal and normal affect balance in psychotherapy of major depression: Evaluation of the balanced states of mind model. *Behavioral and Cognitive Psychotherapy, 30,* 439–450.

Seligman, M. E. P. (1995). The effectiveness of psychotherapy: The Consumer Reports study. *American Psychologist, 50*(12), 965–974. doi:10.1037/0003-066X.50.12.965.

Seligman, M. E. P. (2002). *Authentic happiness: Using the new Positive Psychology to realize your potential for lasting fulfillment.* New York: Free Press.

Seligman, M. E. P., (2011). *Flourish: A visionary new understanding of happiness and well-being.* New York: Simon & Schuster.

Seligman, M. E. P. & Csikszentmihalyi, M. (2000). Positive Psychology: An introduction. *American Psychologist, 55*(1), 5–14. doi:10.1037/0003-066X.55.1.5.

Seligman, M. E. P., Rashid, T., & Parks, A. C. (2006). Positive psychotherapy. *American Psychologist, 61,* 774–788.

Seligman, M. E. P., Steen, T. A., Park, N., & Peterson, C. (2005). Positive Psychology progress: Empirical validation of interventions. *American Psychologist, 60,* 410–421.

Sharf, J., Primavera, L. H., & Diener, M. J. (2010). Dropout and therapeutic alliance: A meta-analysis of adult individual psychotherapy. *Psychotherapy: Theory, Research, Practice, Training, 47*(4), 637–645. doi:10.1037/a0021175.

Sin, N. L., & Lyubomirsky, S. (2009). Enhancing well-being and alleviating depressive symptoms with Positive Psychology interventions: A practice-friendly meta-analysis. *Journal of Clinical Psychology, 65*(5), 467–487. doi:10.1002/jclp.20593.

Sirgy, M. J., & Wu, J. (2009). The pleasant life, the engaged life, and the meaningful life: What about the balanced life? *Journal of Happiness Studies, 10,* 183–196.

Smith, E. J. (2006). The strength-based counseling model. *The Counseling Psychologist, 34,* 13–79.

Steger, M. F., Kashdan, T. B., & Oishi, S. (2008). Being good by doing good: Daily eudaimonic activity and well-being. *Journal of Research in Personality, 42,* 22–42.

Steger, M. F., & Shin, J. Y. (2010). The relevance of the meaning in life questionnaire to therapeutic practice: A look at the initial evidence. *International Forum for Logotherapy, 33*(2), 95–104.

Stillman, T. F. & Baumeister, R. F. (2009). Uncertainty, belongingness, and four needs for meaning. *Psychological Inquiry, 20,* 249–251.

Undurraga, J., & Baldessarini, R. J. (2012). Randomized, placebo-controlled trials of antidepressants for acute major depression: Thirty-year meta-analytic review. *Neuropsychopharmacology, 37*(4), 851–864. doi:10.1038/npp.2011.306.

Vella-Brodrick, D. A., Park, N. & Peterson, C. (2009). Three ways to be happy: Pleasure, engagement, and meaning: Findings from Australian and U.S. samples. *Social Indicators Research, 90,* 165–179.

Wampold, B. E. (2001). *The great psychotherapy debate: Models, methods, and findings.* Mahwah, NJ: Lawrence Erlbaum Associates.

Wong, W.J. (2006). Strength-centered therapy: A social constructionist, virtue-based psychotherapy. *Psychotherapy, 43,* 133–146.

Wood, A. M., & Joseph, S. (2010). The absence of positive psychological (eudemonic) well-being as a risk factor for depression: A ten-year cohort study. *Journal of Affective Disorders, 122*(3), 213–217. doi:10.1016/j.jad.2009.06.032.

Wood, A. M., Maltby, J., Gillett, R., Linley, P. A., & Joseph, S. (2008). The role of gratitude in the development of social support, stress, and depression: Two longitudinal studies. *Journal of Research in Personality, 42,* 854–871.

Worthington, E. L., Jr. (Ed.). (2005). *Handbook of forgiveness.* New York: Brunner-Routledge.

Worthington, E. L., Hook, J. N., Davis, D. E., & McDaniel, M. A. (2011). Religion and spirituality. *Journal of Clinical Psychology, 67*(2), 204–214. doi:10.1002/jclp.20760.

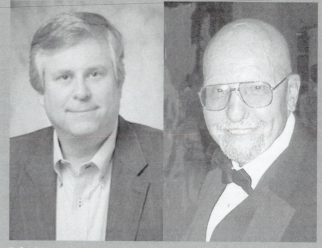

John Norcross
Courtesy of John Norcross

Larry Beutler
Courtesy of Larry Beutler

14 | INTEGRATIVE PSYCHOTHERAPIES

John C. Norcross and Larry E. Beutler

OVERVIEW

Rivalry among theoretical orientations has a long and undistinguished history in psychotherapy dating back to Freud. In the infancy of the field, therapy systems, like battling siblings, competed for attention, affection, and adherents. Clinicians traditionally operated from within their own theoretical frameworks, often to the point of being blind to alternative conceptualizations and potentially superior interventions. An ideological "cold war" reigned as clinicians were separated into rival schools of psychotherapy.

As the field of psychotherapy has matured, integration has emerged as a mainstay. We have witnessed both a decline in ideological struggle and a movement toward rapprochement. Clinicians now acknowledge the inadequacies and potential value in every theoretical system. In fact, many young students of psychotherapy express surprise when they learn about the ideological cold war of the preceding generations.

Psychotherapy integration is characterized by dissatisfaction with single-school approaches and a concomitant desire to look across school boundaries to see how patients can benefit from other ways of conducting psychotherapy. Although various labels are applied to this movement—integration, eclecticism, treatment adaptation, responsiveness, prescriptive therapy, matching—the goals are similar. The ultimate goal is to enhance the efficacy and applicability of psychotherapy.

Applying identical psychosocial treatments to all patients is now recognized as inappropriate and probably impossible. Different folks require different strokes. The efficacy and applicability of psychotherapy will be enhanced by tailoring it to the unique needs of the client, not by imposing procrustean methods on unwitting consumers of psychological services. The integrative mandate is embodied in Gordon Paul's (1967) famous question: *What* treatment, by *whom,* is most effective for *this* individual with *that* specific problem and under *which* set of circumstances?

Any number of indicators attest to the popularity of psychotherapy integration. *Eclecticism,* or the increasingly favored term *integration,* is the most popular theoretical orientation of English-speaking psychotherapists. Leading psychotherapy textbooks routinely identify their theoretical persuasion as integrative, and an integrative chapter is regularly included in compendia of treatment approaches. The publication of books that synthesize various therapeutic concepts and methods continues unabated; they now number in the hundreds. Handbooks on psychotherapy integration have been published in at least a dozen countries. This integrative fervor will apparently persist well into the 21st century: A recent panel of psychotherapy experts predicted the escalating popularity of integrative treatments (Norcross, Pfund, & Prochaska, 2013).

Basic Concepts

There are numerous pathways toward integrative psychotherapies; many roads lead to an integrative Rome. The four most popular routes are *technical eclecticism, theoretical integration, common factors,* and *assimilative integration.* Research (Norcross, Karpiak, & Lister, 2005) reveals that each is embraced by a considerable number of self-identified eclectics and integrationists (19% to 28% each). All four routes are characterized by a desire to increase therapeutic efficacy and applicability. All look beyond the confines of single approaches, but each is distinctive and focuses on a different level of the patient–therapy process.

Technical eclecticism seeks to improve our ability to select the best treatment techniques or procedures for the person and the problem. This search is guided primarily by research on what specific methods have worked best in the past with similar problems and patient characteristics. Eclecticism focuses on predicting for whom interventions will work; its foundation is actuarial rather than theoretical.

Technical eclectics use procedures drawn from different therapeutic systems without necessarily subscribing to the theories that spawned them, whereas theoretical integrationists draw their concepts and techniques from diverse systems that may be epistemologically or ontologically incompatible. For technical eclectics, no necessary connection exists between conceptual foundations and techniques. "To attempt a theoretical rapprochement is as futile as trying to picture the edge of the universe. But to read through the vast amount of literature on psychotherapy, *in search of techniques,* can be clinically enriching and therapeutically rewarding" (Lazarus, 1967, p. 416).

In *theoretical integration,* two or more therapies are united with the hope that the result will be better than the constituent therapies alone. As the name implies, there is an emphasis on integrating the underlying theories of psychotherapy along with the techniques from each. Treatment models that integrate psychoanalytic and interpersonal theories, cognitive and behavioral theories, or systems and humanistic theories illustrate this path.

Theoretical integration involves a commitment to a conceptual or theoretical creation beyond a technical blend of methods. The goal is to create a conceptual framework that synthesizes the best elements of two or more therapies. Integration aspires to more than a simple combination; it seeks an emergent theory that is more than the sum of its parts.

The *common factors* approach seeks to identify core ingredients shared by different therapies with the eventual goal of creating more parsimonious and efficacious treatments based on those commonalities. This search is predicated on the belief that commonalities are more important in accounting for therapy success than the unique factors that differentiate among them. The common factors most frequently proposed are the development of a therapeutic alliance, opportunity for catharsis, acquisition and practice of new behaviors, and clients' positive expectancies (Grencavage & Norcross, 1990; Tracey, Lichtenberg, Goodyear, Claiborn, & Wampold, 2003).

Assimilative integration entails a firm grounding in one system of psychotherapy but with a willingness to selectively incorporate (assimilate) practices and views from other systems (Messer, 2001). In doing so, assimilative integration combines the advantages of a single, coherent theoretical system with the flexibility of a broader range of technical interventions from multiple systems. A cognitive therapist, for example, might use the gestalt two-chair dialogue in an otherwise cognitive course of treatment.

To its proponents, assimilative integration is a realistic way station on the path to a sophisticated integration; to its detractors, it is a waste station of people unwilling to commit themselves to a full evidence-based eclecticism. Both camps agree that assimilation is a tentative step toward full integration: Most therapists gradually incorporate parts and methods of other approaches once they discover the limitations of their original approach. Inevitably, therapists gradually integrate new methods into their home theory.

Of course, these four integrative pathways are not mutually exclusive. No technical eclectic can disregard theory, and no theoretical integrationist can ignore technique. Without some commonalities among different schools of psychotherapy, theoretical integration would be impossible. Assimilative integrationists and technical eclectics both believe that synthesis should occur at the level of practice, rather than theory, by incorporating therapeutic methods from multiple schools. And even the most ardent proponent of common factors cannot practice "nonspecifically" or "commonly" on their own; specific methods must be applied.

In some circles, the terms *integrative* and *eclectic* have become synonymous and collectively have acquired emotionally ambivalent connotations because of their alleged disorganized and indecisive nature. However, much of this opposition should be properly redirected to *syncretism*—uncritical and unsystematic combinations. This haphazard approach is primarily an outgrowth of pet techniques and inadequate training. It is an arbitrary blend of methods without systematic rationale or empirical verification (Eysenck, 1970).

Integration, by contrast, is the product of years of painstaking training, research, and experience. It is integration by design, not default; that is, clinicians competent in several therapeutic systems who systematically select treatment methods and therapeutic relationships on the basis of outcome research and patient need. The strengths of systematic integration lie in its ability to be taught, replicated, and evaluated.

Our own approach to psychotherapy is broadly characterized as integrative and is specifically labeled *systematic eclectic, systematic treatment selection*, or *prescriptive.* We intentionally blend several of the four paths toward integration. Concisely put, we attempt to customize psychological treatments and therapeutic relationships to the specific and varied needs of individual patients as defined by a multitude of diagnostic and particularly nondiagnostic considerations. We do so by drawing on effective methods across theoretical schools (eclecticism), by matching those methods to particular clients on the basis of evidence-based principles (treatment selection), and by adhering to an explicit and orderly (systematic) model.

Although some integrative therapies, particularly those identified with technical eclecticism, provide menus of specific methods, we are committed to defining broader change principles, leaving the selection of specific methods that comply with these principles to the proclivities of the individual therapist. Accordingly, our integrative therapy is expressly designed to transcend the limited applicability of single-theory or "school-bound" psychotherapies. This is accomplished by building the therapeutic interventions around research-based change principles rather than around a closed theory or a limited set of techniques.

In other words, our integrative therapy ascertains the treatments (and therapeutic relationships) of choice for individual patients rather than restricting itself to a single view of psychopathology or change mechanisms. We believe that no theory is uniformly valid and no mechanism of therapeutic action is applicable to all individuals. Thus, we strive to create a new therapy for each patient. We believe that the purpose of integrative psychotherapy is *not* to create a single system or a unitary treatment. Rather, we select different methods according to the patient and the context. The result is a more efficient and efficacious therapy—and one that fits both the client and the clinician.

On the face of it, virtually all clinicians endorse matching the therapy to the individual client. After all, who can seriously dispute the notion that psychological treatment should be tailored to the needs of the individual patient in order to improve its success? However, integrative therapy goes beyond this simple acknowledgment in at least five ways.

1. Our integrative therapy is derived directly from outcome research rather than from an idiosyncratic theory. In our view, empirical knowledge and scientific research are the best arbiters of theoretical differences when it comes to health care.

2. We embrace the potential contributions of multiple systems of psychotherapy rather than working from within a single system. All psychotherapies have a place—but a specific and differential place.

3. Our treatment selection is predicated on many diagnostic and nondiagnostic client characteristics, in contrast to relying on patient diagnosis alone. It is frequently more important to know the patient who has the disorder than to know the disorder the patient has.

4. Our aim is to offer the optimal treatment methods *and* healing relationships, whereas most theorists focus narrowly on selecting methods. Both interventions and relationships, both the instrumental and the interpersonal—intertwined as they are—are required in effective psychotherapy.

5. Selecting and matching methods to the client occur throughout the course of therapy, not only at pretreatment as a case formulation. As clients evolve and progress, integrative therapy tracks their progress and evolves with them through termination.

Other Systems

Integrative psychotherapies gratefully acknowledge the contributions of the traditional, single-school therapy systems, such as psychoanalytic, behavioral, cognitive, and experiential. Such pure-form therapies are part and parcel of the foundation for integrative approaches. Integration, in fact, could not occur without the constituent elements provided by these respective therapies—their theoretical systems and clinical methods. Integration gathers, in the words of Abraham Lincoln, "strange, discordant, and even, hostile elements from the four winds."

In a narrow sense, pure-form or single-school therapies do not contribute to integration because, by definition, they have no provisions for synthesizing various interventions and conceptualizations. But in a broader and more important sense, they add to the therapeutic armamentarium, enrich our understanding of the clinical process, and produce the process and outcome research from which integration draws. One cannot integrate what one does not know.

The goal of integration, as we have repeatedly emphasized, is to improve the efficacy and applicability of psychotherapy. Toward this end, we must collegially recognize the valuable contributions of pure-form therapies and collaboratively enlist their respective strengths.

Even so, it is important to remember that most single-school therapies also manifest several weaknesses. First, the creation of most psychotherapies was more rational than empirical. Originators developed their therapies without, or with little regard to, the research evidence on their effectiveness. In an era of accountability demanding *evidence-based practice*, psychotherapies without controlled outcome research will not last long. Second, single-school therapies tend to favor the strong personal opinions, if not pathological conflicts, of their originators. Sigmund Freud found psychosexual conflicts in practically all his patients, Carl Rogers found compromised conditions of worth in practically all his patients, Joseph Wolpe found conditioned anxiety in practically all his patients, and Albert Ellis found maladaptive thinking in practically all his patients. However, patients do not routinely suffer from the favorite problems of famous theorists. It strikes us as far more probable that patients suffer from a multitude of specific problems that should be remedied with a similar multitude of methods.

Third and relatedly, most pure-form systems of psychotherapy recommend their treasured treatment for virtually every patient and problem they encounter. Of course, this simplifies treatment selection—give every patient the same brand of psychotherapy!—but it flies in the face of what we know about individual differences, patient preferences, and disparate cultures. It is akin to seeking the remedy for all ills in a hardware store, simply because it is a "good store." The clinical reality is that no single psychotherapy is effective for all patients and situations, no matter how good it is for some; relational-sensitive, evidence-based practice demands a flexible, if not integrative, perspective. Psychotherapy should be flexibly tailored to the unique needs and contexts of the individual client, not universally applied as one size fits all.

Imposing a parallel situation onto other health-care professions drives the point home. To take a medical metaphor, would you entrust your health to a physician who prescribed the identical treatment (say, antibiotics or neurosurgery) for every patient and illness encountered? Or, to take an educational analogy, would you prize instructors who employed the same pedagogical method (say, a lecture) for every educational opportunity? Or would you entrust your child to a child-care worker who delivers the identical response (say, a nondirective attitude or a slap on the bottom) to every child and every misbehavior? "No" is probably your resounding answer. Psychotherapy clients deserve no less consideration.

A fourth weakness of unitary therapies is that they largely consist of descriptions of psychopathology and personality rather than of mechanisms that promote change. They are actually theories of personality rather than theories of psychotherapy; they offer lots of information on the content of therapy but little on the change process. We believe integrative theory should explain how people change. (Specific criticisms of 16 therapy systems from an integrative perspective can be found in Prochaska and Norcross, 2013).

We are convinced of the clinical superiority of a pluralistic or integrative psychotherapy. Among the advantages of integrative psychotherapies are those inferred from the foregoing criticisms of pure-form therapies: Integrative therapies tend to be more empirical in creation and more evidence based in revision; case conceptualization is predicated more on the actual patient than on an abstruse theory; therapy is more likely to be adapted or responsive to the unique patient and the singular situation; and treatment is more focused on the process of change than on the content of personality. In other words, integration promises more evidence, flexibility, responsiveness, and change.

HISTORY

Precursors

Integration as a point of view has probably existed as long as philosophy and psychotherapy. In philosophy, the third-century biographer Diogenes Laertius referred to an eclectic school that flourished in Alexandria in the second century (Lunde, 1974). In psychotherapy, Freud consciously struggled with the selection and integration of diverse methods. As early as 1919, he introduced psychoanalytic psychotherapy as an alternative to classical psychoanalysis in recognition that the more rarified approach lacked universal applicability (Liff, 1992).

More formal ideas on synthesizing the psychotherapies appeared in the literature as early as the 1930s (Goldfried, Pachankis, & Bell, 2005). For example, Thomas French (1933) stood before the 1932 meeting of the American Psychiatric Association and drew parallels between certain concepts of Freud and of Pavlov. In 1936, Sol Rosenzweig published an article that highlighted commonalities among various systems of psychotherapy. These and other early attempts at integration, however, were largely theory driven and empirically untested.

If not conspiratorially ignored altogether, these precursors to integration appeared only as a latent theme in a field organized around discrete theoretical orientations. Although psychotherapists secretly recognized that their orientations did not adequately assist them in all they encountered in practice, a host of political, social, and economic forces—such as professional organizations, training institutes, and referral networks—kept them penned within their own theoretical school yards and typically led them to avoid clinical contributions from alternative orientations.

Beginnings

Systematic integration was probably inaugurated in the modern era by Frederick Thorne (1957, 1967), who is credited with being the grandfather of eclecticism in psychotherapy. Persuasively arguing that any skilled professional should come prepared with more than one tool, Thorne emphasized the need for clinicians to fill their toolboxes with methods drawn from many different theoretical orientations. He likened contemporary psychotherapy to a plumber who used only a screwdriver. Like such a plumber, inveterate psychotherapists applied the same treatment to all people, regardless of individual differences, and expected the patient to adapt to the therapist rather than vice versa.

Thorne's admonitions went largely ignored, as did a book published more than a decade later by Goldstein and Stein (1976) that first identified the *Prescriptive Psychotherapies* of its title. This book, far ahead of its time, outlined treatments for different people based on the nature of their problems and on aspects of their living situations.

Since the late 1960s, Arnold Lazarus (1967, 1989) has emerged as the most prominent spokesperson for eclecticism. His influential *multimodal therapy* inspired a generation of mental-health professionals to think and behave more broadly. He was joined by the two of us and others soon thereafter (e.g., Beutler, 1983; Frances, Clarkin, & Perry, 1984; Norcross, 1986, 1987).

Simultaneously, efforts were under way to advance common factors. In his classic *Persuasion and Healing,* Jerome Frank (1973) posited that all psychotherapeutic methods are elaborations and variations of age-old procedures of psychological healing. Frank argued that therapeutic change is predominantly a function of four factors common to all therapies: an emotionally charged, confiding relationship; a healing setting; a rationale or conceptual scheme; and a therapeutic ritual. Nonetheless, the features that distinguish psychotherapies from each other receive special emphasis in the pluralistic, competitive American society. Little glory has traditionally been accorded to common factors.

In 1980, Sol Garfield introduced an eclectic psychotherapy predicated on common factors, and Marvin Goldfried published an influential article in the *American Psychologist* calling for the delineation of therapeutic change principles. Goldfried (1980), a leader of the integration movement, argued,

> [to] the extent that clinicians of varying orientations are able to arrive at a common set of strategies, it is likely that what emerges will consist of robust phenomena, as they have managed to survive the distortions imposed by the therapists' varying theoretical biases. (p. 996)

In specifying what is common across orientations, we may also be selecting what works best among them.

In the late 1970s and the 1980s, several attempts at theoretical integration were introduced. Paul Wachtel authored the classic *Psychoanalysis and Behavior Therapy: Toward an Integration*, which attempted to bridge the chasm between the two systems. His integrative book began, ironically, in an effort to write an article portraying behavior therapy as "foolish, superficial, and possibly even immoral" (Wachtel, 1977, p. xv). But in preparing his article, he was forced for the first time to look closely at what behavior therapy was and to think carefully about the issues. When he observed some of the leading behavior therapists of the day, he was astonished to discover that the particular version of psychodynamic therapy toward which he had been gravitating dovetailed considerably with what many behavior therapists were doing. Wachtel's experience should remind us that isolated theoretical schools perpetuate caricatures of other schools, thereby foreclosing basic changes in viewpoint and preventing expansion in practice.

The transtheoretical (across theories) approach of James Prochaska and Carlo DiClemente was also introduced in the late 1970s with the publication of one of the first integrative textbooks, *Systems of Psychotherapy: A Transtheoretical Analysis* (Prochaska, 1979). This book reviewed different theoretical orientations from the standpoint of common change principles and the stages of change. The transtheoretical approach in general, and the stages of change in particular, are the most extensively researched integrative therapies (Schottenbauer, Glass, & Arnkoff, 2005).

Only within the past 30 years, then, has psychotherapy integration developed into a clearly delineated area of interest. The temporal course of interest in psychotherapy integration, as indexed by both the number of publications and the development of organizations and journals (Goldfried et al., 2005), reveals occasional stirrings before 1970, a growing interest during the 1970s, and rapidly accelerating interest from 1980 to the present. To put it differently, integrative psychotherapy has a long past but a short history as a systematic movement.

Current Status

Between one-quarter and one-half of contemporary clinicians disavow an affiliation with a particular school of psychotherapy, preferring instead the label of *integrative* or *eclectic*. Some variant of integration is routinely the modal orientation of responding psychotherapists. A review of 25 studies performed in the United States between 1953 and 1990 (Jensen, Bergin, & Greaves, 1990) reported a range from 19% to 68%. A review of a dozen studies published during the past decade (Norcross, 2005) found that integration was still the most common orientation in the United States but that cognitive therapy was rapidly challenging it and might soon become the modal theory. That same review also determined that integration receives robust but lower endorsement outside of the United States and Western Europe. Thus, integration is typically the modal orientation in the United States but not in other countries around the world.

The prevalence of integration can be ascertained directly by assessing endorsement of the integrative orientation (as noted) or gleaned indirectly by determining endorsement of multiple orientations. For example, in a study of Great Britain counselors, 87% did *not* take a pure-form approach to psychotherapy (Hollanders & McLeod, 1999). In a study of clinical psychologists in the United States, for another example, fully 90% embraced several orientations (Norcross & Karpiak, 2012). Very few therapists adhere exclusively to a single therapeutic tradition.

The establishment of several international organizations both reflects and reinforces the popularity of integrative psychotherapies. Two interdisciplinary societies, the Society for the Exploration of Psychotherapy Integration (SEPI) and the Society of Psychotherapy Research (SPR), hold annual conferences devoted to the pluralistic practice and ecumenical research of psychotherapy. Both societies also publish international scientific journals: SEPI's *Journal of Psychotherapy Integration* and SPR's *Psychotherapy Research.*

Psychotherapy integration, then, has taken earliest and strongest root in the United States. Nonetheless, it is steadily spreading throughout the world and is becoming an international movement. Both SPR and SEPI now have multiple international chapters and regularly hold their annual meetings outside the United States.

In past years, psychotherapists were typically trained in a single theoretical orientation. The ideological singularity of this training did not always result in clinical competence, but it did reduce clinical complexity and theoretical confusion (Schultz-Ross, 1995). In recent years, psychotherapists have come to recognize that single orientations are theoretically incomplete and clinically inadequate for the variety of patients, contexts, and problems they confront in practice. They are receiving training in several theoretical orientations—or at least are exposed to multiple theories, as evidenced in this book.

The evolution of psychotherapy training has moved the field further toward integration, but this may be a mixed blessing. On the one hand, integrative training addresses the daily needs of clinical practice, satisfies the intellectual quest for an informed pluralism, and responds to the growing research evidence that different patients prosper under different treatments and relationships. On the other hand, integrative training increases the pressure for students to obtain clinical competence in multiple methods and formats and, in addition, challenges the faculty to create a coordinated training enterprise (Norcross & Halgin, 2005).

Studies indicate that training directors are committed to psychotherapy integration but disagree on the best route toward it. Approximately 80% to 90% of directors of psychology programs and internship programs agree that knowing one therapy system is not sufficient; instead, training in a variety of models is needed. However, their views on the optimal integrative training process differ. About one-third believe that students should be trained first to be proficient in one therapeutic system; about half believe that students should be trained to be at *least* minimally competent in a variety of systems; and the remainder believe that students should be trained in a specific integrative system from the outset (Lampropoulos & Dixon, 2007).

Computerized multimedia may increase the effectiveness of training in integrative psychotherapies. A pilot study using a virtual patient reported case-by-case success in training clinicians to recognize cues suggesting which treatment is likely to be most effective for the patient (Beutler & Harwood, 2004). A free online program has been developed (www.innerlife.com) to guide patients in selecting an optimal treatment and finding a clinician who can best implement that integrative treatment. A companion program is available to clinicians (at the same Web site) for a modest cost to help them plan a research-informed treatment that is both broad and flexible in applying fundamental principles of change. Completing the Innerlife STS requires approximately 15 minutes and takes the person through a series of item-branching questions. At completion, the Innerlife STS renders a report to the patient that addresses crucial treatment issues tailored to the person:

- potential areas of concern,
- treatments to consider,
- treatments to avoid,
- compatible therapist styles,
- picking a psychotherapist, and
- self-help resources.

A similar set of treatment issues are addressed in the parallel report directed to the clinician. This more detailed report also addresses programmatic considerations that should be addressed in structuring the environment and directing the staff of treatment centers in what is needed for effective change.

The ensuing treatment recommendations in this system are governed by 30 years of research on identifying evidence-based principles that point to optimal relations among patient characteristics (including diagnosis), treatment methods, and therapeutic relationships.

Integrative training is both a product and a process. As a product, psychotherapy integration will be increasingly disseminated through books, videotapes, courses, seminars, curricula, workshops, conferences, supervision, postdoctoral programs, and institutional changes. The hope is that educators will develop and deliver integrative products that are less parochial, more pluralistic, and more effective than traditional single-theory products.

Our more fervent hope is that, as a process, psychotherapy integration will be disseminated in a manner that is consistent with the pluralism and openness of integration itself. The intention of integrative training is not necessarily to produce card-carrying, flag-waving "integrative" psychotherapists. This scenario would simply replace enforced conversion to a single orientation with enforced conversion to an integrative orientation, a change that may be more liberating in content but certainly not in process. Instead, the goal is to educate therapists to think (and perhaps to behave) integratively—openly, flexibly, synthetically, but critically—in their clinical pursuits (Norcross & Halgin, 2005).

Integrative therapies respond to the mounting demands for short-term and evidence-based treatments in mental health. With 90% of all patients in the United States covered by some variant of managed care, short-term therapy has become the de facto treatment imperative. Integration, particularly in the form of technical eclecticism, responds to the pragmatic injunction of "whatever therapy works better—and quicker—for this patient with this problem."

The international juggernaut of evidence-based practice (EBP) lends increased urgency to the task of using the best of research and experience to tailor psychological treatment to the client (Norcross, Beutler, & Levant, 2006). Data-based clinical decision making will become the norm. Evidence-based practice has sped the breakdown of traditional schools and the escalation of informed pluralism (Norcross, Hogan, & Koocher, 2008). The particular decision rules for what qualifies as evidence remain controversial, but EBP reflects a pragmatic commitment to "what works for whom." The clear emphasis is on what works, not on what theory applies. Integrative therapies stand ready to meet this challenge.

PERSONALITY

Theory of Personality

Beginning with Freud, most psychotherapy systems have consisted primarily of theories of personality and psychopathology (*what* to change). This is not true of most integrative therapies, which instead emphasize the process of change (*how* to change). The integration is directly focused on the selection of therapy methods and relationships as opposed to theoretical constructs of how people and psychopathology develop. Although a latent theory necessarily underpins any treatment, integrative therapy is relatively personality-less and immediately change-ful.

Our integrative conceptualization makes no specific assumptions about how personality and psychopathology occur. Such a determination is relatively unimportant if one knows what therapy methods and relationships are likely to evoke a positive response in a specific patient. Effective treatment can be applied from a wide number of theories or from no theoretical framework at all.

To the limited extent that they exist, integrative theories of personality are predictably broad and inclusive. They embrace life-span approaches of developmental psychology. They reflect that humans are, whether functional or dysfunctional, the products of a complex interplay of our genetic endowment, learning history, sociocultural context, and physical environment.

Variety of Concepts

To say that integrative therapies do not rely on a theory of personality is not to say that they pay no heed to personality characteristics. Indeed they do. As detailed in the next section, the patient's personality is a key determinant in integrative therapy, as are the therapist's personality and their mutual match. However, personality characteristics are not separated out into a broader theory of human development and motivation. Like all other patient characteristics in integrative therapy, personality traits are incorporated to the extent that the research evidence has consistently demonstrated that identifying them contributes to effective treatment.

Our data-based therapy eschews the view that one needs to know how a problem developed in order to solve it. Instead, we assert that when one encounters particular behavior patterns or environmental characteristics, it is more important to know what treatment is likely to promote change.

In the next section, we will describe several personality characteristics that the research indicates are useful in helping the clinician improve the efficacy of psychotherapy. To anticipate ourselves, we will present here an example of how personality concepts differ between conventional psychotherapies and integrative therapies.

A patient's coping style is a vital personality characteristic to consider when deciding to conduct insight-oriented or symptom-change methods. Coping style is an enduring quality defined by what one does when confronted with new experience or stress. A person may engage in a cluster of behaviors that disrupt social relationships such as impulsivity, blaming, and rebellion (externalizing) on the one hand, or in a cluster of behaviors that increase personal distress such as self-blame, withdrawal, and emotional constriction (internalizing) on the other. These clusters are relatively enduring, cut across situations, and distinguish among people. Thus, they are personality traits. But integrative therapy makes little effort to understand why they occur; we concentrate on how they impact psychotherapy and improve its success.

Our integrative approach is principally concerned with tailoring psychotherapy to the patient's personality, not with developing a theory about that personality. We are committed to the remediation of psychopathology, not preoccupied with its explanation. Let us now move on to the practice of integrative psychotherapy.

PSYCHOTHERAPY

Theory of Psychotherapy

In contrast to the absence of a cohesive theory of personality and psychopathology, integrative psychotherapy strongly values clinical assessment that guides effective treatment. Such assessment is conducted early in psychotherapy to select treatment methods and therapy relationships that are most likely to be effective, throughout therapy to monitor the patient's response and to make mid-course adjustments as needed, and toward the end of psychotherapy to evaluate the outcomes of the entire enterprise. Thus, assessment is continuous, collaborative, and invaluable.

In this section, we begin with an extensive discussion of clinical assessment that fuels and guides treatment selection. This account then segues naturally into the process of psychotherapy, just as it does in actual practice.

Clinical Assessment

Clinical assessment of the patient in integrative therapy is relatively traditional, with one major exception. The assessment interview(s) entail collecting information on presenting problems, relevant histories, and treatment expectations and goals, as well as building a working alliance. As psychologists, we also typically use formal psychological testing as a means of securing additional data and identifying Axis I and Axis II disorders. We recommend both symptomatic rating forms (e.g., Beck Depression Inventory II, Symptom Checklist–90R) and broader measures of pathology and personality (e.g., Minnesota Multiphasic Personality Inventory-II, Millon Clinical Multiaxial Inventory-III).

The one way in which assessment in integrative therapy departs from the usual is that we collect, from the outset, information on multiple patient characteristics that will guide treatment selection. In fact, the Innerlife STS Web-based assessments for both clinicians and clients described earlier enhance the development of treatment plans within the integrative tradition (Beutler & Groth-Marnat, 2003; Harwood & Williams, 2003).

To apply treatment-focused assessment, integrative therapy is faced with the central challenge of identifying those patient characteristics and corresponding treatment qualities that will improve our treatments. There are tens of thousands of potential permutations and combinations of patient, therapist, method, relationship, and setting variables that could contribute. We rely primarily on the available empirical research to identify a limited number of patient dimensions that influence therapy success, and we use focused assessments to target those dimensions that are most predictive of differential treatment response (Castonguay & Beutler, 2006; Beutler, Clarkin, & Bongar, 2000).

This assessment tactic is not without several problems. The main problem has always been the sheer number of potentially valuable patient characteristics that have been researched. Even if all were effective predictors of change, there are far too many of them for clinicians to organize and use consistently. Moreover, researchers may disagree about which characteristics of patients and therapies are the most important. Both of these problems must be overcome before it is possible to prioritize what works best for a particular individual.

Fortunately, our programmatic research over the years (Beutler et al., 2000; Castonguay & Beutler, 2006; Norcross, 2011) addressed these problems by identifying the most potent patient contributors to change and the most powerful means to adapt treatment to those patient characteristics. Reviews of outcome studies, cross-validation studies, sophisticated statistical analyses (structural equation modeling), and a series of meta-analyses led to a manageable number of patient and treatment qualities that demonstrably improve the effectiveness of psychotherapy.

Six Patient Characteristics

In this chapter, we present six patient characteristics commonly used by integrative psychotherapists. These patient characteristics guide us in identifying a beneficial fit between patient and treatment. Of course, integrative therapists are not confined to these six considerations, but they do illustrate the process of clinical assessment and treatment matching in integrative psychotherapies.

Diagnosis.   We organize our treatment planning in part around the disorders as described in the DSM and ICD. Although diagnosis alone is never sufficient, there are practical reasons why diagnosis is necessary. First, insurance companies demand a diagnosis, and utilization review is done in reference to diagnosis. Second, outcome research is usually organized around determining what is helpful to specific diagnostic groups, and the major symptoms comprising a diagnosis make a suitable way of evaluating the effectiveness of treatment. In order to profit from this research, one must know the patient's diagnosis. Third, specialized and manualized treatments have been developed for many disorders.

At the same time, there are many reasons why diagnosis alone is insufficient for treatment planning. Diagnoses are pathology oriented and neglect a patient's strengths. The criteria established for disorders are multiple, change continually, and select different groups of patients. Axis I patients may also suffer from co-morbid Axis I disorders, in addition to one or more Axis II disorders. Few treatments exert effects that are restricted or specific to a particular diagnostic group. It is for these reasons that one must formulate treatment plans for entire individuals, not for isolated disorders.

The combination of all DSM-IV axes—a large array of possibilities—must be considered in treatment planning. Diagnosis is not limited to Axis I (symptoms) and Axis II (personality disorders) but includes physical conditions (Axis III), environmental stressors (Axis IV), and overall functioning (Axis V). (As we write, we do not know for certain the final structure of DSM-V.) This is why it should be no surprise that patients sharing the same Axis I disorder could and should receive quite different treatments. The Axis V or Global Assessment of Functioning rating may be of particular importance in treatment planning, serving as a simple index of the patient's level of functional impairment.

Stages of Change.   The stages represent a person's readiness to change, defined as a period of time as well as a set of tasks needed for movement to the next stage. The stages are behavior and time specific, not enduring personality traits. *Precontemplation* is the stage at which there is no intention to change behavior in the foreseeable future. Most individuals in this stage are unaware or underaware of their problems; however, their families, friends, and employers are often well aware that the precontemplators have problems. When precontemplators present for psychotherapy, they often do so because of pressure or coercion from others. Resistance to recognizing a problem is the hallmark of precontemplation (or denial, as it is sometimes unhelpfully known).

Contemplation is the stage in which people are aware that a problem exists and are seriously thinking about overcoming it but have not yet made a commitment to take action. Contemplators struggle with their positive evaluations of their dysfunctional behavior and the amount of effort, energy, and loss it will cost to overcome it. Serious consideration of problem resolution is the central element of contemplation.

Preparation is the stage that combines intention and behavioral criteria. Individuals in this stage intend to take action in the near future and have unsuccessfully taken action in the past year. Individuals who are prepared for action report small behavioral changes, such as drinking less or contacting health-care professionals. Although they have reduced their problem, they have not yet reached a threshold for effective action, such as abstinence from alcohol abuse. They are intending, however, to take such action in the very near future.

Action is the stage in which individuals modify their behavior, experiences, or environment to overcome their problems. Action involves the most overt behavioral changes and requires considerable commitment of time and energy. Behavioral changes in the action stage tend to be most visible and externally recognized. Actual modification of the target behavior is the hallmark of action.

Maintenance is the stage in which people work to prevent relapse and consolidate the gains attained during action. For addictive behaviors, this stage extends from 6 months to an indeterminate period past the initial action. For some behaviors, maintenance can be considered to last a lifetime. The ability to remain free of the problem and to consistently engage in a new, incompatible behavior for more than 6 months are the criteria for maintenance.

A patient's stage of change recommends the use of certain treatment methods and relationships. Table 14.1 illustrates where leading systems of therapy are probably most effective in the stages of change. Methods associated with psychoanalytic and insight-oriented psychotherapies are most useful during the earlier precontemplation and contemplation stages. Existential, cognitive, and interpersonal therapies are particularly well suited to the preparation and action stages. Behavioral, exposure, and solution-focused therapies are most useful during action and maintenance. Each therapy system has a place, a differential place, in the big picture of behavior change.

The therapist's relational stance is also matched to the patient's stage of change (Norcross, Krebs, & Prochaska, 2011). With precontemplators, often the therapist's stance is like that of a nurturing parent joining with the resistant youngster who is both drawn to and repelled by the prospect of independence. With contemplators, the therapist's role is akin to that of a Socratic teacher who encourages clients to develop their own insights and ideas about their condition. With clients who are preparing for action, the therapist is like an experienced coach who has been through many crucial matches and can provide a fine game plan or can review the person's own action plan. With

TABLE 14.1   **Integration of Psychotherapy Systems within the Stages of Change**

Stages of Change

Precontemplation	Contemplation	Preparation	Action	Maintenance
Motivational interviewing				
Strategic family therapy				
Psychoanalytic therapy				
	Analytical therapy			
	Adlerian therapy			
		Existential therapy		
		Rational emotive behavior therapy (REBT)		
		Cognitive therapy		
		Interpersonal therapy (IPT)		
		Gestalt and experiential therapyy		
			Behavior therapy	
			Solution-focused therapy	
			EMDR and exposure	

clients who are progressing into maintenance, the integrative psychotherapist becomes more of a consultant who is available to provide expert advice and support when progress is not smooth.

Coping Style.   The client's coping style consists of his or her habitual behavior when confronting new or problematic situations. Patients tend to adopt a style of coping that places them somewhere between two extreme but relatively stable types. Simply, they tend either toward *externalizing* coping (impulsive, stimulation seeking, extroverted) or *internalizing* coping (self-critical, inhibited, introverted).

Coping style is a marker for whether the psychotherapy should ideally focus on symptomatic reduction or broader thematic objectives. Symptom-focused and skill-building therapies are more effective among externalizing patients. Acting-out children and impulsive adults, for example, are usually best served by reducing their problems via skill development methods. By contrast, the use of insight and awareness-enhancing therapies is typically most effective among internalizing patients. Methods here vary from therapist to therapist but may well include interpretations of the parent–child linkage, analysis of transference and resistance, review of recurrent themes, and exercises to enhance awareness of feelings (Beutler et al., 2000; Beutler, Harwood, Kimpara, & Blau, 2011).

Reactance Level.   Patient reactance is a variation of behaviors that are often described as *resistance*. A reactant patient is easily provoked by and responds oppositionally to external demands. The propensity to engage in reactance is a reliable marker for the amount of therapist directiveness: High reactance indicates the need for nondirective, self-directed, or paradoxical techniques, whereas low client reactance calls for more directive techniques. In other words, the use of nondirective and client-directed methods improves outcomes with highly resistant patients. By contrast, directive and structured techniques, such as cognitive restructuring, advice, and behavior contracting, improve outcomes with less-resistant patients (Beutler, Harwood, Michelson, Song, & Holman, 2011). How directive should a therapist be? It depends on the patient—specifically, his or her level of reactance.

Patient Preferences.   When ethically and clinically appropriate, we accommodate a client's preferences in psychotherapy. These preferences may be heavily influenced by the client's personality, values, attachment style, and previous experiences in psychotherapy. These preferences may be related to the person of the therapist (age, gender), the therapeutic relationship (how warm or tepid, how active or passive), therapy methods (preference for against homework, dream analysis, two-chair dialogues), or treatment formats (refusing group therapy or medication).

We work diligently in the beginning sessions to identify our patients' strong preferences and subsequently to accommodate these preferences when feasible. Controlled research and clinical experience demonstrate that attending to what the patient desires decreases misunderstandings, strengthens the alliance, decreases dropouts, and establishes collaboration—all relationship qualities connected to therapy success (Norcross, 2011). It would be naïve to assume that patients always know what they want and what is best for them. But if clinicians had more respect for the notion that their clients often sense how they can best be served, fewer relational mismatches might occur (Lazarus, 1993).

Culture.   Related to patient preferences is the client's culture—defined broadly to include ethnicity, race, gender, sexual orientation, disability status, and age. Multicultural competence is not simply an ethical or political ideal but also a clinical necessity in integrative therapy. Both treatment methods and healing relationships are fit to the patient's culture(s), as they are to the patient's stage of change, coping style, and reactance level. Therapy can be culturally adapted by responsive use of language, therapist attributes, metaphors, methods, goals, and content.

As with any of the transdiagnostic patient characteristic that guide treatment selection, it is essential not to assume that a single or visible culture defines the person's experience. We respectfully discuss with the client which cultures—or intersections of cultures—are fundamental to tailoring psychotherapy. Automatically presuming that a client's gender or ethnicity or sexual orientation should be the primary determinant of treatment selection is probably as hurtful as ignoring them altogether.

Summary.   The six client characteristics previously listed serve as reliable markers to systematically adapt psychotherapy to the individual patient, problem, and context. Although this list is likely to evolve as research progresses, these have emerged from extensive reviews and meta-analyses. These client characteristics, including but not limited to diagnosis, can be applied independently of a specific theoretical orientation. All of this is to say that psychotherapy has progressed to the point where readily assessable patient characteristics call for specific treatment methods and healing relationships that demonstrably increase the effectiveness of our clinical work.

Process of Psychotherapy

The integrative imperative to match or tailor psychotherapy to the patient can be (and has been) misconstrued as an authority-figure therapist prescribing a particular form of psychotherapy for a passive client. The clinical reality is precisely the opposite. Our goal is for an empathic therapist to work toward an optimal relationship that both enhances collaboration and secures the patient's sense of safety and commitment. The nature of such an optimal relationship is determined by patient preferences, culture, and personality. If a client frequently resists, for example, then the therapist considers whether she is pushing something that the client finds incompatible (preferences), or the client is not ready to make changes (stage of change), or the client is uncomfortable with a directive style (reactance). Integrative psychotherapy leads by following the client (Norcross, 2010).

Change takes place through interrelated processes: the nature of the patient–therapist relationship, the treatments that are used, and the way the patient avoids relapse (Beutler, Forrester, Gallagher-Thompson, Thompson, & Tomlins, 2012). A comprehensive treatment involves defining the setting in which treatment will be applied, the format of its delivery, its intensity, the role of pharmacotherapy (medications), and the particular therapeutic strategies and techniques.

Therapeutic Relationship

All psychotherapy occurs within the sensitive and curative context of the human relationship. Empirically speaking, therapy success can best be predicted by the properties of the patient and of the therapy relationship (see Norcross, 2011, for reviews); only 10% of outcome is generally accounted for by any particular treatment method.

It is a colossal misunderstanding to view treatment selection as a disembodied, technique-oriented process. Integrative psychotherapies attempt to customize not only therapy techniques but also relationship stances to individual clients. One way to conceptualize the matter, paralleling the notion of *treatments of choice* in terms of techniques, is how clinicians determine *therapeutic relationships of choice* in terms of interpersonal stances (Norcross & Beutler, 1997).

In creating and cultivating the therapy relationship, we rely heavily on clinical experience and empirical research on what works. Meta-analyses of thousands of studies indicate that the therapeutic alliance, empathy, goal consensus, collaboration, positive regard/support, congruence, modest self-disclosure, and management of countertansfernce are effective (Norcross, 2011). Collecting real-time feedback from the client about his or her progress throughout psychotherapy (Lambert & Shimokawa, 2011) and repairing ruptures in the alliance (Safran, Muran, & Eubanks-Carter, 2011) also improve success. Conducting the best of evidence-based treatment all comes to naught unless the client feels safe, connected, and cared for.

Early on, then, we strive to develop a working alliance and to demonstrate empathy for the client's experiences and concerns. We proceed collaboratively in establishing treatment goals, in securing the patient's preferences, in allaying the initially expected distrust and fear, and in presenting ourselves as caring and supportive. Of course, the therapy relationship must also be matched or tailored to the individual patient and his or her cultures.

Treatment Planning

Treatment planning invariably involves the interrelated decisions about setting, format, intensity, pharmacotherapy, and strategies and techniques. The important point here is that each client will respond best to a different configuration or mix of components. We cannot and should not assume that the treatment will automatically be outpatient individual therapy on a weekly basis. In the following, we consider each of these decisions, devoting more time to the strategies and methods.

Treatment Setting.   The setting is where the treatment occurs: a psychotherapist's office, a psychiatric hospital, a halfway house, an outpatient clinic, a secondary school, a medical ward, and so on. The choice of setting depends primarily on the relative need for restricting and supporting the patient, given the severity of psychopathology and the support in the patient's environment.

Each treatment decision is related to the other treatment decisions, as well as to certain patient characteristics. The optimal setting, for example, is partially determined by symptomatic impairment and partially reflects reactance level. Those clients who are most impaired and resistant have the greatest need for a restrictive environment. Outpatient treatment is always preferred over a restrictive setting; indeed, preference is nearly always for the least-restrictive setting.

Treatment Format.   The format indicates who directly participates in the treatment. It is the interpersonal context within which the therapy is conducted. The typical treatment formats—individual, group, couples, and family—are characterized by a set of treatment parameters, all determined largely by the number and identities of the participants. (See "Treatment" in this chapter for additional remarks on treatment formats.)

Treatment Intensity.   The intensity of psychotherapy is the product of the *duration* of the treatment episode, the *length* of a session, and the *frequency* of contact. It may also involve the use of multiple formats, such as both group and individual therapy or both pharmacotherapy and psychotherapy.

Intensity should be gauged as a function of problem complexity and severity, also taking into account the patient's resources. For example, a patient with a multiplicity of treatment goals, severe functional impairment, few social supports, and a personality disorder is likely to require substantially longer, more intense, and more varied treatment than a patient with a simpler problem. Brief treatments are obviously not for everyone; many patients will need long-term treatment or lifetime care.

Pharmacotherapy.   Decades of clinical research and experience have demonstrated that psychotropic medications are particularly indicated for more severe and chronic disorders. If pharmacotherapy is indicated, then the question becomes how it should be prescribed: Which medication in which dosage and for how long?

Unlike some systems of psychotherapy, integrative psychotherapies are well suited to the integration of pharmacotherapy and psychotherapy. This position, of course, is consistent with the pluralism underlying treatment selection.

At the same time, we would offer a cautionary note here. Tightening insurance reimbursements and restrictions on mental-health care are unduly favoring pharmacotherapy at the expense of psychotherapy. This situation is clinically and empirically appalling to us because research indicates that, in fact, there is frequently no stronger medicine than psychotherapy (e.g., Antonuccio, 1995; DeRubeis et al., 2005). The preponderance of scientific evidence shows that psychotherapy is generally as effective as medications in treating nonpsychotic disorders, especially when patient-rated measures and long-term follow-ups are considered. This is not to devalue the salutary impact of pharmacotherapy; rather, it is to underscore the reliable potency of psychotherapy. In addition, we believe that combined treatments should be carefully coordinated and entail psychoeducation for patients and their support system. Medication alone is not an integrative treatment.

Strategies and Techniques.   When clinicians first meet clients, they are tempted to focus immediately and intensely on particular therapy strategies and techniques. However, as we have noted, treatment selection always involves a cascading series of interrelated decisions. A truly integrated treatment will recursively consider these other decisions before jumping to therapy strategies.

The selection of techniques and strategies is the most controversial component of integrative therapies. Proponents of disparate theoretical orientations endorse decidedly different views of what appear to be the same techniques. Moreover, any given technique can be used in different ways. Thus, rather than focusing on specific techniques per se, we prefer prescribing change principles. These principles can be implemented in a number of ways and with diverse techniques. By mixing and matching procedures from different therapy systems, we tailor the treatment to the particular patient.

Humans, including psychotherapists, cannot process more than a handful of matching dimensions at once (Halford, Baker, McCredden, & Bain, 2005). As illustrated above, we principally consider six patient characteristics (diagnosis, stage of change, coping style, reactance level, preferences, and culture) that have a proven empirical track record as prescriptive guidelines.

Relapse Prevention.   Tailoring psychotherapy to the individual patient, as we have described, enhances the effectiveness of psychotherapy. But even when psychotherapy is effective, relapse is the rule rather than the exception in many behavioral disorders, particularly the addictive, mood, and psychotic disorders. Thus, teaching relapse prevention to clients toward the end of psychotherapy is strongly advisable in practically all cases.

Relapse prevention helps clients identify "high risks" for regression, makes plans for avoiding such situations, and builds maintenance skills (Marlatt & Donovan, 2007). The patient and therapist examine the environment in which the patient lives, works, and recreates and then pinpoint those locations, people, and situational demands that have characteristically provoked dysfunction. This analysis is coupled with teaching the patient to identify cues that signal when he or she is beginning to experience the depression, anxiety, or even euphoria that has typically triggered the problem. These cues are linked to alternative behaviors that involve help seeking, self-control practice, and avoidance of overwhelming situational stress. Finally, in most circumstances, we try to overcome obstacles that may prevent the patient from seeking help from us or other mental-health professionals once again.

Maintenance sessions are indicated when the problem is complex, the patient is highly impaired, and a personality disorder is present. Maintenance work may also be indicated when the course of treatment is erratic and when symptom resolution is not consistently obtained within a period of six months. These features are particularly strong indicators of the tendency to relapse, and maintenance sessions can address emerging problems before they are recognized by the patient.

Mechanisms of Psychotherapy

Integrative psychotherapies do not presume single or universal change mechanisms. The mechanism of action may be very different for different individuals, even though they all may manifest similar symptoms. To an individual who is defensive, the mechanism may be the benevolent, corrective modeling of trust and collaboration offered by an empathic therapist, but for an individual who is trusting and self-reflective, the mechanism of action may be insight and reconceptualization. Similarly, the change mechanism for helping an anxious patient may be exposure to feared events and supportive reassurance. The point is that there are multiple pathways of change.

Table 14.2 presents nine mechanisms of action or, as we would prefer to call them, *change processes*. These processes have received the most empirical support to

TABLE 14.2   Nine Change Processes and Representative Therapy Methods

Change Process	Definition: Representative Methods
Consciousness raising	Increasing awareness about self and problem: observations, reflections, challenges, interpretations, bibliotherapy
Self-reevaluation	Assessing how one feels and thinks about oneself with respect to a problem: value clarification, imagery, corrective emotional experience
Emotional arousal	Experiencing and expressing feelings about one's problems: expressive exercises, psychodrama, grieving losses, role playing
Social liberation	Increasing alternatives in society: advocating for rights of oppressed, empowering, policy interventions
Self-liberation	Choosing and committing to act or belief in ability to change: decision-making therapy, logotherapy techniques, commitment-enhancing techniques
Counterconditioning	Substituting incompatible healthy alternatives for problem behaviors: relaxation, desensitization, assertion, acceptance, cognitive restructuring
Environmental control	Reengineering environmental stimuli that elicit problem behaviors: adding positive reminders, restructuring the environment, avoiding high-risk cues, fading
Contingency management	Rewarding oneself or being rewarded by others for making changes: contingency contracts, overt and covert reinforcement, self-reward, behavioral incentives
Helping relationships	Being understood, validated, and supported by a significant other: empathy, collaboration, positive regard, feedback, self-disclosure

Source: Adapted from Prochaska, Norcross, & DiClemente, 1995.

date in our research. The change processes most often used by psychotherapists are consciousness raising and the helping relationship. Virtually all therapies endorse the expansion of consciousness and the therapeutic relationship as potent mechanisms of action or change processes. The least frequently used processes are environmental control and social liberation; the former is seen by some therapists as unduly emphasizing the power of the environment, the latter as improperly bordering on political advocacy.

Integrative therapists experience no hesitation in employing any or all of these change processes; we have no ideological axe to grind. Like therapists from single-school systems, integrative therapists rely heavily on consciousness raising and the therapeutic relationship. But unlike many therapists from single-school approaches, integrative therapists have at their disposal the full range of these change processes, ready to choose among them depending on the specific situation. Some cases call for building skills and implementing environmental control; addicts, in particular, need to learn to avoid people, places, and things that trigger their substance abuse. Other cases call for social liberation; oppressed and minority clients, in particular, profit from a therapist's modeling political advocacy and encouraging liberation strategies.

Moreover, these change processes are differentially effective at different stages of change. In general terms, change processes traditionally associated with the experiential and psychoanalytic persuasions are most useful during the earlier precontemplation and contemplation stages. Change processes traditionally associated with the existential, cognitive, and behavioral traditions, by contrast, are most useful during action and maintenance.

This pattern serves as an important guide. Once a patient's stage of change is evident, the integrative psychotherapist knows which change processes to apply in order to help that patient progress to the next stage of change. Rather than apply the change processes in a haphazard or trial-and-error manner, therapists can begin to use them in a much more systematic and effective way. It is not enough simply to declare that multiple change processes operate in psychotherapy; we must know how they can be selected and sequenced in ways that accelerate psychotherapy and improve its outcome.

We have observed two frequent mismatches in this respect. First, some therapists rely primarily on change processes most indicated for the contemplation stage, such as consciousness raising and self-reevaluation, when clients are moving into the action stage. They try to modify behavior by helping clients become more aware. This is a common criticism of psychoanalysis: Insight alone does not necessarily bring about behavior change. Second, other therapists rely primarily on change processes most indicated for the action stage, such as contingency management, environmental control, and counterconditioning, when clients are still in the precontemplation or contemplation stage. They try to modify behavior by pushing clients into action without the requisite awareness and commitment. This is a common criticism of behaviorism: Overt action without insight is likely to lead only to temporary change.

APPLICATIONS

Who Can We Help?

By virtue of its flexibility, integrative psychotherapy is applicable to practically all patient populations and clinical disorders. Children, adolescents, adults, and older adults; diagnosable disorders and growth experiences; private pay or managed care. Avoiding one-size-fits-all treatment and tailoring therapy to the unique individual make it adaptable to a wide range of problems. In fact, we cannot envision a client or a disorder for whom integrative psychotherapy would be contraindicated.

Integrative psychotherapy is particularly indicated for (1) complex patients and presentations, such as clients with multiple diagnoses and co-morbid disorders; (2) disorders that have not historically responded favorably to conventional, pure-form psychotherapies, such as personality disorders, eating disorders, PTSD, and chronic mental illness; (3) disorders in which the controlled treatment outcome research is scant; and (4) clients for whom pure-form therapies have failed or have been only partially successful.

The research indicates that patients who are functionally impaired respond best to a comprehensive and integrated treatment. Specifically, more impaired or disabled patients call for more treatment, lengthier treatment, psychoactive medication, multiple therapy formats (individual, couples, group), and explicit efforts to strengthen their social support networks (Beutler, Harwood, Alimohamed, & Malik, 2002). Schizophrenia, borderline personality disorder, and multiple addictions are cases in point; to put it simply, complex problems require complex treatments.

No therapy or therapist is immune to failure. It is at such times that experienced clinicians often wonder whether therapy methods from orientations other than their own might more appropriately have been included in the treatment or whether another orientation's strength in dealing with the particular problems might complement the therapist's own orientational weakness. Integrative therapies assume that each orientation has its particular domain of expertise and that these domains can be linked to maximize their effectiveness (Pinsof, 1995).

When integrative therapy fails, it may be a result of a failure to follow the guiding integrative principles, a lack of skill in implementing a particular treatment, or a poor fit between the particular patient and the particular therapist. Each alternative should be considered when a patient is not accomplishing his or her goals at a rate expected among similar patients.

One clear strength of mixing and matching therapy methods is the ability to address clients' multiple goals. Most clients desire both insight and action; they seek awareness into themselves and their problems, as well as reduction of their distressing symptoms. The integrative therapist can focus on one or both broad goals, depending on the client's preferences. Similarly, integrative therapists can simultaneously tackle improvement in several domains of a client's life: symptoms, cognitions, emotions, relationships, and intrapsychic conflicts. Change in one domain or on a single level nearly always generates synergistic change in another.

Treatment

The term *integration* refers typically to the synthesis of diverse systems of psychotherapy, but it also has a host of other meanings. One is the combination of therapy formats—individual, couples, family, and group. Another is the combination of medication and psychotherapy, also known as combined treatment. Still another meaning—and one of our favorites—is the integration of practice and research (Beutler, 2009).

In practice, integrative psychotherapies are committed to the synthesis of practically all effective, ethical change methods. These include integrating self-help and psychotherapy, integrating Western and Eastern perspectives, integrating social advocacy with psychotherapy, integrating spirituality into psychotherapy, and so on. All are compatible with a comprehensive treatment, but we have restricted ourselves in this chapter to the traditional meaning of integration as the blending of diverse theoretical orientations.

We are impressed by the effectiveness of group, couples, and family therapy. Therapy conducted in these formats is generally as effective as individual therapy, but patients and therapists usually prefer the individual format. Even so, a multiperson format is indicated if social support systems are low and if one or more of the major problems involves a specific other person.

Integrative psychotherapy embraces both long-term and short-term treatments. The length of therapy should be determined not by the therapist's preference or theoretical orientation but by the patient's needs. Virtually every form of brief therapy advertises itself, in comparison to its original long version, as active in nature, collaborative in relationship, and integrative in orientation (Hoyt, 1995). Brief therapy and integrative therapy share a pragmatic and flexible outlook that is contrary to the ideological one that characterized the earlier school domination in the field.

Evidence

The empirical evidence on integrative treatments has grown considerably in recent years, and controlled research has been undertaken on several specific integrative therapies, including our own.

The outcome research supporting integrative psychotherapies comes in several guises. First and most generally, the entire body of psychotherapy research has provided the foundation for the key principles on which integrative treatment rests. This is the basis from which we have systematized the process of treatment selection. A genuine advantage of being integrative is the vast amount of research attesting to the efficacy of psychotherapy and pointing to its differential effectiveness with certain types of patients. Integration tries to incorporate state-of-the-art research findings into its open framework, in contrast to becoming yet another "system" of psychotherapy.

A second source of research evidence is that conducted on specific integrative treatments. A review of integrative therapies (Schottenbauer et al., 2005) determined substantial empirical support (defined as four or more randomized controlled studies) for

- acceptance and commitment therapy,
- cognitive analytic therapy,
- dialectical behavior therapy,
- emotionally focused couple therapy,
- eye movement desensitization and reprocessing (EMDR),
- mindfulness-based cognitive therapy,
- systematic treatment selection (STS), and
- transtheoretical psychotherapy (stages of change).

Integrative therapists can use these treatments for a particular patient—say, dialectical behavior therapy for a patient suffering from borderline personality disorder. Or integrative therapists can use parts of these treatments for many patients—say, teaching mindfulness or employing EMDR when indicated. These treatments and their elements are optimally employed with patients and in situations for which research has found evidence of effectiveness. We hasten to add that the incorporation of these treatments and their parts should occur within a systematic process and an integrative perspective—that is, be integrative, not syncretic.

Another dozen self-identified integrative therapies have garnered some empirical support, defined as between one and four randomized controlled studies. These include behavioral family systems therapy, integrative cognitive therapy, process-experiential therapy, and Lazarus's multimodal therapy.

A third and specific source of research evidence supporting our integrative psychotherapy is our ongoing programmatic research on treatment selection according to client characteristics (for details, see Castonguay & Beutler, 2006; and Norcross, 2011). In the following we summarize the reviews of research evidence underpinning our approach in terms of transdiagnostic patient characteristics.

Stages of Change

The amount of progress clients make in treatment tends to be a direct function of their pretreatment stage of change (Norcross, Krebs, & Prochaska, 2011). This strong effect has been found to be true for patients suffering from dozens of mental and medical disorders immediately following intervention as well as 12 months afterward. In one representative study of 570 smokers (Prochaska & DiClemente, 1983), for example, only 3% of precontemplators took action by 6 months; 20% of contemplators took action; and, of those in preparation, 41% attempted to quit by 6 months. These data demonstrate that treatment designed to help people progress just one stage can double the chances of their taking action in the near future.

One of the most powerful findings to emerge from our research is that particular processes of change are more effective during particular stages of change. Thirty years of research in behavioral medicine and psychotherapy converge in showing that different processes of change are differentially effective in certain stages of change. A meta-analysis (Rosen, 2000) of 47 cross-sectional studies examining the relationships among the stages and the processes of change showed large effect sizes ($d = 0.70$ and 0.80). In other words, adapting psychotherapy to the client's stage of change significantly improves outcome across disorders. This stage matching has been demonstrated in large controlled trials for depression, stress management, smoking cessation, bullying violence, and health behaviors (see Prochaska & Norcross, 2013, for review).

In sum, hundreds of studies have demonstrated the effectiveness of tailoring treatment to the client's stage of change. Longitudinal studies affirm the relevance of these constructs for predicting premature termination and treatment outcome. Comparative outcome studies attest to the value of stage-matched treatments and relationships. Population-based studies support the importance of developing interventions that match the needs of individuals at all stages of change.

Coping Style

The research has been devoted primarily to the externalizing (impulsive, stimulation seeking, extroverted) and internalizing coping styles (self-critical, inhibited, introverted). Approximately 80% of the studies investigating this dimension have demonstrated differential effects of the type of treatment as a function of patient coping style. A meta-analysis of 12 of those studies, involving more than a thousand patients, revealed a medium effect ($d = 0.55$) for matching therapist method to patient coping style (Beutler, Harwood, Michelson, Song, & Holman, 2011). Specifically, interpersonal and insight-oriented therapies are more effective among internalizing patients, whereas symptom-focused and skill-building therapies are more effective among externalizing patients.

Reactance Level

Research confirms what one would expect: High patient reactance is consistently associated with poorer therapy outcomes (in 82% of studies). But matching therapist directiveness to client reactance mightily improves therapy outcome. Specifically, clients presenting with high reactance benefited more from self-control methods, minimal therapist directiveness, and paradoxical interventions. By contrast, clients with low reactance benefited more from therapist directiveness and explicit guidance. This strong, consistent finding can be expressed as a large effect size (d) averaging 0.76 (Beutler, Harwood, Michelson, Song, & Holman, 2011).

These client markers provide prescriptive as well as proscriptive guidance to the psychotherapist. In reactance, the prescriptive implication is to match the therapist's amount of directiveness to the patient's reactance, and the proscriptive implication is to avoid meeting high client reactance with high therapist direction. In stages of change, action-oriented therapies are quite effective with individuals who are in the preparation or action stage. However, these same therapies tend to be less effective and even detrimental with individuals in the precontemplation and contemplation stages.

Preferences

Client preferences and goals are frequently direct indicators of the best therapeutic method and healing relationship for that person. Decades of empirical evidence attest to the benefit of seriously considering, and at least beginning with, the relational preferences and treatment goals of the client. A meta-analysis of 35 studies compared the treatment outcomes of clients matched to their preferred treatment to those clients not matched to their preference. The findings indicated a medium positive effect ($d = 0.31$) in favor of clients matched to preferences. But, more important, clients who were matched to their preference were a third less likely to drop out of psychotherapy—a powerful effect indeed (Swift, Callahan, & Vollmer, 2011).

Culture

A meta-analysis of 65 studies, encompassing 8,620 clients, evaluated the effectiveness of culturally adapted therapies versus traditional, nonadapted therapies. The most frequent methods of adaptation in the studies involved incorporating cultural content and values, using the client's preferred language, and matching therapists of similar ethnicity. The results revealed a positive effect ($d = 0.46$) in favor of clients receiving culturally adapted treatments (Smith, Rodriguez, & Bernal, 2011). Cultural "fit" works.

Diagnosis

Of the patient characteristics considered here, diagnosis is the one with the least evidence of differential treatment effects. Although we cannot match with certainty, some marriages of disorder and treatment are probably better than others. For example, behavior therapy and parent training seem to be the treatments of choice for most externalizing child conduct disorders. Some form of exposure seems best for obsessive–compulsive disorders and posttraumatic stress disorder (PTSD). Conjoint treatments seem best suited for sibling rivalry and couples distress. At the same time, we would reiterate that excessive reliance on diagnosis alone to select a treatment is empirically questionable and clinically suspect.

Psychotherapy in a Multicultural World

The integrative maxim of "Different strokes for different folks" converges naturally with multiculturalism. And by *culture*, we do not refer solely to race, but more broadly to the wonderful diversity of humanity: age and generational influences, disability status, religion, ethnicity, social status, sexual orientation, indigenous heritage, national origin, gender, and so on (Hays, 1996).

Single-school therapies, particularly those born of a dominant "father" and rooted in a culture-bound theory of personality, tend to subtly maintain white, androcentric (male-centered), Western European, heterosexual norms. Many of the single-school "universal" principles are now rightfully perceived as examples of clinical myopia or cultural imperialism. Integrative therapies, by contrast, rely on neither a particular founder nor a theory of personality. Our sole "universal" principle is that people and cultures differ and should be treated as such. Evidence-based pluralism reigns as integration infuses diversity and flexibility into psychotherapy. No wonder that virtually every feminist, multicultural, and cultural-responsive theory describes itself as eclectic or integrative in practice.

Integrative psychotherapies have been applied cross-culturally and internationally with equal success. As offered to clients, integrative psychotherapies manifest as culturally sensitive or culturally adapted—modified to improve utilization, retention, and outcome. Psychotherapy can be adapted in many ways, such as incorporating the cultural values of the client into therapy, collaborating with indigenous healers, and matching clients with therapists of the same culture who literally speak the same language.

As in all practical matters in integrative psychotherapy, incorporating culture should be informed by the cumulative research. As summarized above, adapting psychotherapy to the patient's culture is demonstrably effective. Particularly effective are orienting treatment to a specific cultural group (instead of a variety of cultural backgrounds) and conducting therapy in the client's native language (Smith et al., 2011). Moreover, avoid translators in sessions whenever possible because their use is associated with weak alliances, more misdiagnoses (usually more severe than necessary), and higher dropout rates (Paniagua, 2005).

The upshot is for psychotherapists of all persuasions to mutually explore the singular needs and unique cultures of clients from the inception of psychotherapy. One effective practice, especially for historically marginalized populations, is to acquaint beginning clients with the respective roles of patient and therapist. Many patients hold divergent expectations about the process of psychotherapy and may be uncomfortable with mental-health treatment. Pretherapy orientation is designed to clarify these expectations and to collaboratively define a more comfortable role for the client.

Another effective practice entails augmenting an individualistic position with a collectivistic orientation to clinical work. The optimal treatment format and therapist team, for example, may well depend on the culture of the particular client. In some cultures, clients will automatically enlist the support of friends, family members, neighbors, clergy, and perhaps traditional healers as part of their treatment and perhaps in their sessions. The culture-sensitive relationship, for another example, may well demand more than ordinary therapist empathy; it may require cultural empathy (Pederson, Crethar, & Carlson, 2008). As defined in the Western culture, empathy takes on an individualistic interpretation of human desire and distress. "I understand your personal feelings." Cultural empathy takes on a more inclusive orientation by placing cultural responsiveness at the center. It is a learned ability to accurately understand the client's self-experience from another culture and then express that understanding back to the client. "I understand your personal feelings *and* your cultural context."

We enthusiastically embrace multiculturalism in psychotherapy. It's called *integration*, diversity within unity. Integrative therapy posits that the context for every individual—African, Asian, Latino, or Anglo; straight, gay, bisexual, or transgendered; Muslim, Christian, Jew, or atheist—is unique. And each psychotherapy needs to be individually constructed to match the needs of a particular person. In some cases, this involves helping individuals become free from social oppression. In other cases, it means helping them become free from mental obsessions. In yet other cases, it involves treatment of biological depression (Prochaska & Norcross, 2013).

CASE EXAMPLE

Ms. A is a 72-year-old Euro-American widow who was referred for psychotherapy by her son, a psychiatrist in her neighborhood. She sought treatment for anxiety and agoraphobia.

History and Background

Ms. A was raised in Boston as the daughter of a modestly wealthy family. She was the only child of middle-aged and quite rigid parents. She related a poor relationship with her family and especially experienced difficulties with her mother, whom she described as "bossy and unreasonable."

Ms. A related that her first experience of panic when going out of the house occurred when she was 12. At the time, she was staying with a girlfriend while her mother shopped. As they were playing with dolls, Ms. A suddenly experienced a full-blown panic attack. She was overcome with a fear of dying, experienced heart palpitations, and felt short of breath to the point of fearing suffocation. Ms. A ran into the street and tried to yell for help, but she couldn't communicate, and no one heard her or offered assistance. She gradually calmed herself through self-control and forced breath control. She experienced periodic but relatively mild and spontaneous panic attacks through the next 2 years.

At about age 16, Ms. A began suffering from panic attacks more frequently and more severely. This resulted in her sleeping with her parents for several months and increasingly confining herself to known places and locations. She denied knowing what precipitated the increase in her panic attacks, but they occurred during a developing relationship with a young man. He pursued her, but she found him unattractive and had no interest in a long-term relationship. He was insistent, and as a result, Ms. A began to see him socially; however, they had a tumultuous relationship punctuated by many separations and reunions. She finally succumbed to his insistence on marriage when she was 17, partially in response to the persuasion of her mother. The couple subsequently moved to Rhode Island to live close to his family.

Throughout the courtship and early years of marriage, the patient endured periodic panic attacks and bouts of agoraphobia. Ms. A's symptoms increased and necessitated their moving back to Boston to be close to her family, where she could get the care that she felt she needed. She contemplated divorce and, indeed, separated and moved back with her parents, only to discover that she was pregnant. Ms. A reunited with her husband briefly after the baby's birth, but her panic became so extreme that she called and begged her mother to allow her to return home, claiming the situation to be a matter of life or death. She subsequently filed for divorce, but her husband fought the marital dissolution and successfully prevailed on the court to disallow the divorce.

Ms. A blamed her parents for her marital difficulties, and when she was unable to obtain a divorce, she left home, leaving the baby in the care of her mother, whom she despised. The patient successfully escaped the pursuit of her husband and her parents for several years. During that time, she experimented with homosexual relationships and came to think of herself as a lesbian. Concomitantly, her panic and agoraphobia abated, and she recalled having no panic attacks for a period of about three years. The attacks began again, however, shortly after her parents, who had hired a private investigator to find her, reinitiated contact with her through an attorney. She was forced to negotiate an arrangement for the care of her daughter because her parents were getting too old to take care of the girl.

As plans for the future progressed, Ms. A was forced to meet with her estranged husband. For some time before and following these visits, the patient's panic episodes escalated. The patient acceded to her husband's demand that they reconcile and take the child and move away from her parents to "start over." They moved to Oregon.

Ms. A's effort to reestablish her marriage was successful for only a short period of time. In Oregon, she first sought medical treatment for panic and was briefly hospitalized. She was discharged with medication but stopped taking it after a couple of months. She reported no long-term benefit from the hospitalization. After discharge from the hospital, Ms. A initiated several lesbian affairs, which finally provoked her husband to leave. He subsequently returned to his family on the East Coast and left her to raise the child on her own. He successfully filed for divorce. She struggled to find work and to support her daughter, yet despite this turmoil, the intensity of her panic and agoraphobia abated once again. Nonetheless, she worried about the effect of her lesbian relationships on her daughter.

Soon, Ms. A met a wealthy man who fell in love with her in spite of her "secret" lesbian lifestyle. He proposed marriage to her and vowed to support her and her daughter, to adopt the daughter, and even to tolerate her lovers, on the condition that she would attempt to have children with him. Her daughter and any children that they produced would then be his heirs. After much thought, Ms. A agreed. The marriage lasted 25 years and produced two more children, a boy and a girl. Her husband died of cancer shortly after her youngest daughter graduated from high school. Following her husband's death, she began to live openly as a lesbian, and she has remained unmarried for the past 16 years.

About 10 years ago, Ms. A met a woman with whom she fell in love. They have maintained an ongoing, supportive relationship. During this time, even dating back to the end of her second marriage, Ms. experienced only occasional mild anxiety and no panic. She continued to fear the prospect of panic—"the fear of fear"—and described a general "distaste" for travel, as well as what she called a "tendency to put off" going out for fear of becoming anxious. Ms. A also described "being uncomfortable" when she is away from home, but she had not had any clinical symptoms of panic or phobia for more than a decade and a half. Even the most dominant and disturbing feeling that plagued her through most of her life, the sense of being smothered and unable to breathe, disappeared. However, Ms. A did feel despondent and lethargic, had difficulty staying asleep, and had suffered other troubling symptoms of dysphoria and avoidance.

One event was particularly troubling. Approximately five years ago, while Ms. A and her lover were on vacation in another country, she awoke disoriented after having sex. She characterized this state as "disassociation" and "amnesia." She was unable to recall where she was, why she was there, and who her lover or her parents were. These symptoms passed within hours, but they recurred several more times, all immediately after having an intense sexual encounter.

It was at this time that Ms. A sought psychotherapy for the first time. She saw a psychiatrist who found no medical reason for her dissociative experience and diagnosed it as a "transitory histrionic conversion." The psychiatrist followed Ms. A for about a year and prescribed antidepressants. This work was somewhat helpful, and as a result, Ms. A and her lover decided to cease further sexual contact for fear of triggering another "dissociation" attack. She terminated psychotherapy shortly thereafter but continued to get a variety of tranquilizers from her family physician because she felt the need for them. Ms. A and her female partner continue to maintain a loving platonic relationship.

Clinical Assessment and Formulation

The integrative therapist took the preceding history, developed a positive alliance with Ms. A, and secured consensus on her treatment goals in the first session. The patient was asked to complete several self-report instruments to evaluate her mental status and to identify those characteristics important in treatment planning. These instruments included the Stages of Change Questionnaire, the Minnesota Multiphasic Personality Inventory–2 (MMPI-2), the Innerlife STS Self-Report Form, the Symptom Checklist 90R (SCL 90-R), and the Beck Depression Inventory–2 (BDI-2).

The results revealed Ms. A to be at the contemplation stage—aware of her problems but uncertain, conflicted, and anxious about how to solve them. She was worried and ruminative, with fears about her continuing ability to take care of herself and with guilt over her past mistakes. Ms. A was especially concerned that she might have harmed her children through ambivalence and neglect. She was, in addition, remorseful over not being able to provide the sexual gratification that her partner desired. These results suggested that the patient would be receptive to exploring her motivations and plans and to seeking understanding about the options that faced her in resolving her concerns.

Diagnostically, Ms. A had suffered from relatively severe panic in the past, but at the time she sought treatment it was considered to be largely in remission. Her agoraphobia, also severe in the past, was only mild to moderate. Like many anxious and agoraphobic patients, Ms. A was suffering from concurrent depression.

Her STS/innerlife and the MMPI-2 results both suggested relatively mild impairment of daily activities, cognitive focus, and emotional control. Ms. A was able to carry on basic life tasks, maintain intimate and social relationships, and provide for her care and comfort. She denied any suicidal ideation and intention. Although driving and traveling caused her some discomfort, she did both on a regular basis. The fear of fear seemed to be more disabling than her actual symptoms. The patient did not warrant an Axis II diagnosis.

The chronicity of Ms. A's problem suggested a guarded prognosis, but she possessed many intellectual strengths and insights that would improve her prognosis. With a mild level of current impairment, a nonintensive treatment was considered sufficient. She agreed to weekly sessions of individual psychotherapy, entailing neither medication nor more frequent sessions.

After some discussion of her "dissociative" experiences, the psychotherapist talked to the patient's family physician, who could not explain the symptoms. The therapist contacted a neurologist and found that a similar, relatively obscure condition had been observed, primarily among older males, to occur following strong exertion, including sexual activity. This condition, known as *sudden transient amnesia*, had rarely been noted among women, and even among men it was typically experienced only once or twice. It was not thought to be a continuing condition and was probably occasioned by exertion, hyperventilation, and the pattern of entering deep or delta sleep very shortly after the exertion.

Ms. A favored a predominantly internalizing style of coping (versus an externalizing style). Although she had some externalizing qualities, her test scores and interpersonal patterns indicated that her contemplative and ruminative style of functioning was dominant. These results were consistent with her contemplation stage of change and generally favored the use of insight-oriented and awareness-increasing methods.

At the same time, insight-based work should be preceded by efforts to reduce symptoms. This was especially a valued determination, given the patient's history of anxiety disorders and of angry, panic-driven behaviors. Thus, the therapist combined both action and insight with Ms. A. We began by using desensitization and exposure to address her fear of panic and her fear of fear. This was followed by stress-management methods derived from cognitive analyses of stress. It was necessary to ensure that her panic and fear behaviors were under control before proceeding to insight-based themes.

The therapist examined Ms. A's theme of wishes and avoidance in the insight work and inspected her persistent phobic response when she was pushed into heterosexual relationships. The hypothesis was that such relationships may have induced guilt and fear that exacerbated and maintained panic. The therapist hypothesized that the first panic attack may have occurred during sexual play with her playmate at age 12. Based on the strength of this interplay of heterosexual pressure and panic, we explored ways in which Ms. A had been smothered and pressured into these relationships by her parents. Both Ms. A and the therapist believed that the key to insight was understanding her marriages and feelings of being pressured sexually.

In cultural terms, Ms. A's personal values and sexual orientation were rejected by her controlling parents, invalidated by her first domineering husband, and discouraged by a heterosexist society. The anxiety of "fitting in" as a heterosexual wife and mother seems natural in retrospect. The panic of "losing herself" strikes us as almost inevitable. Ms. A was, in fact, suffocated and oppressed. The patient's reactance level was assessed by her interpersonal history and her test results on the MMPI-2 and STS/innerlife Ms. A's family history was characterized by conflict, mistrust, and forced control. It was associated with her response of moderate to severe rebelliousness. This pattern continued through her first marriage but dropped significantly in later relationships. The test results, on the other hand, suggested that Ms. A was reasonably responsive and nonresistant to therapist directiveness. She was willing to take direction and exhibited compliance with structure, as well as the ability to work collaboratively with the therapist. Accordingly, the therapist opted to employ moderate levels of guidance and direction to accomplish both her action goals and insight goals.

In the early stages of treatment, therefore, the integrative therapist guided Ms. A into exposure situations and suggested direct contact with feared and avoided activities (e.g., driving, leaving home). Later in treatment, the therapist used interpretations and suggestions about areas of emotional avoidance and thematic patterns in childhood related to the development of panic and agoraphobia. In particular, the therapist focused on the patient's symptoms of "suffocating" within a restricted environment and her subsequent symptom reduction during times when she was less restricted and scrutinized.

In terms of treatment goals, Ms. A expressed a preference for both symptom relief and psychological insight. After a life of fear and avoidance, she sought and was prepared for a therapy that exposed her to her anxiety symptoms associated with driving and traveling and then gradually confronted her thematic conflicts of relationship demands.

In terms of the therapeutic relationship, Ms. A was comfortable with the prospect of a male, heterosexual therapist, declining when asked whether she might be more comfortable with a female therapist. She sought an active collaborator in her growth who would provide direction for her, would be a sounding board, and who would help her discover the origins of her anxiety. Ms. A was eager to engage in homework assignments to facilitate her progress, and although she balked when these assignments required her to drive, she always complied with the therapist's recommendations. On one occasion, she drove 50 miles in a heavy rainstorm to attend psychotherapy, surpassing any accomplishment she thought she would ever achieve.

Treatment Course

The first goal of any psychotherapy is the creation of an empathic, trusting relationship between patient and therapist. Two sessions were spent exploring the patient's feelings and trying to uncover her ambivalence and fear associated with self-expression. We explored feelings of guilt about her children and fears of aging.

The next four sessions were devoted to in vivo work on Ms. A's avoidance patterns. Because her panic and agoraphobia symptoms were not obvious in the initial evaluation, we tried to produce some of those symptoms through rapid breathing, exposure training, and homework assignments. As we contacted areas of anxiety and fear, we introduced breathing control and cognitive restructuring to help her cope and to provide reassurance. For example, we walked around the neighborhood, spent time doing imagery to evoke arousal, and discussed matters about which she thought she might have anxiety. Interestingly, only momentary and mild anxiety was provoked. Relatively soon (within the first 8 sessions), we began exploring her relationships with parents and children that were associated with her guilt and fear.

Ms. A identified her fears of having become like her mother, an authoritarian tyrant. She blamed herself for having injured her oldest daughter by her demands and abandonment, and she expressed guilt for having "made" her oldest son gay by not being a good role model. With encouragement and supportive advice, Ms. A spoke to these children and was surprised to discover that they were accepting and acknowledging of her difficulties. They also reassured her that they did not feel pressured or smothered by her—the metaphorical symptoms that she loathed as an agoraphobic.

Ms. A's guilt led to discussions of her belief in God. She had been raised in a reformed Jewish family, but her first husband was an orthodox Jew. She found religion troubling and had, she said, largely left her belief in God behind, except in her sense of being punished for neglecting her children. Try as she might, she still found herself praying to God for forgiveness whenever she thought about her children.

To address these concerns, Ms. A kept a log of her religious thoughts and then used bibliotherapy materials to help her evaluate these thoughts. Specifically, she selected a cognitive therapy self-help book to work on her anxiety and depression. She kept track of thoughts and tried ways of changing those that were most hurtful to her. She kept notes about her progress, and we discussed these at each session.

In these sessions, we also discussed Ms. A's negative reaction to having sex with her partner. One session was held with the two of them together, largely because Ms. A's difficulty had never been experienced outside this relationship. The therapist and Ms. A explored her relationship and discussed their mutual sexual desires. Discovering that Ms. A's symptoms of acute amnesia had been described in the medical literature as sudden transient amnesia gave her some relief, but she was still reluctant to go through the experience again. The patient's partner remained devoted and supportive of her decisions, whether or not they could ever restore sexual contact. On one occasion they initiated a sexual encounter, but it was suspended when the patient began having anticipatory fears. They agreed not to try sexual relations again. Although this was not an entirely satisfactory conclusion, the therapist chose to honor the couple's informed decision to seek their own resolution in time.

Outcome and Follow-up

Over the course of 12 sessions, Ms. A impressively reduced her anxiety, minimized her avoidance of driving and traveling, and decreased her concurrent depression. The SCL-90R and BDI-2 were repeated at the end of treatment. Both her anxiety and her depression had dropped substantially (the BDI from 24 to 14 and the SCL-90R from 75T to 54T). Symptomatically, she was better than ever.

Interpersonally, Ms. A courageously approached and apologized to her grown children for her potentially neglectful actions and negotiated a more satisfying relationship with her partner. She mourned her losses and was moving forward. Despite all of these positive outcomes, as with most cases in psychotherapy, not all of her goals were realized. Her anticipatory fear of sexual relations led her not to attempt sex again.

Ms. A called the psychotherapist approximately one year after she had ended treatment "just to check in." She indicated that she had made several trips to the East Coast during the year and had experienced only one mild episode of panic. Nonetheless, she was thinking of returning to therapy for a few sessions to work on some "family issues." An appointment was made, but Ms. A called and cancelled, indicating that she would call again if she couldn't resolve the problem herself. An inadvertent contact with the patient's family some months later suggested that she was doing very well and had experienced no further difficulties.

Case Commentary

We have deliberately chosen to illustrate our integrative approach with a patient that psychotherapy has historically neglected: elderly and lesbian. Although we live in an in increasingly multicultural world, much of psychotherapy is still developed for and researched on the young and heterosexual. Let Ms. A remind us all of the clinical and re-search imperative to extend psychotherapy to the marginalized and oppressed in society.

The integrative therapist can share some credit for the salubrious outcome in this case, but Ms. A deserves the lion's share. She intentionally exposed herself to anxiety-provoking situations and topics. She was a bright, brave, and hard-working client who progressed from the contemplation stage to the action stage and ultimately to the maintenance stage.

Where the integrative therapist was probably most effective was in tailoring the therapeutic relationship and treatment methods specifically to Ms. A. The treatment proceeded stepwise in accordance with the research evidence, the patient's preferences, and her other nondiagnostic characteristics. The therapist combined several treatment goals (action and insight), therapy methods (those traditionally associated with behavioral, cognitive, psychodynamic, experiential, and systemic approaches), healing resources (psychotherapy, self-help, and spirituality), and treatment formats (individual, couples, and family) in a seamless and responsive manner.

Would a psychotherapist endorsing a single, brand-name therapy have achieved such impressive and comprehensive changes in the same number of sessions as the integrative therapist? We immodestly think not.

SUMMARY

Integrative psychotherapies are intellectually vibrant, clinically popular, and demonstrably effective. Integration converges with the evidence-based movement in emphasizing that different problems require different solutions and that these solutions increasingly can be selected on the basis of outcome research. Integrative therapies offer the evidence, flexibility, and responsiveness to meet the multifarious needs of individual patients and their unique contexts. For these reasons, integration will assuredly be a therapeutic mainstay of the 21st century.

Integration can take several different paths—theoretical integration, technical eclecticism, common factors, and assimilative integration—but it consistently searches for new ways of conceptualizing and conducting psychotherapy that go beyond the confines of single schools. Integration encourages practitioners and researchers to examine what other therapies have to offer, particularly when confronted with difficult cases and therapeutic failures. Rival therapy systems are increasingly viewed not as adversaries, but as welcome partners (Landsman, 1974); not as contradictory, but as complementary.

Integration is a meta-psychotherapy. It neither offers a model of psychopathology nor a theory of personality nor limits the mechanisms through which psychotherapy works. Instead, integration embraces the therapeutic value of many systems of psychotherapy and can be superimposed on whichever psychopathology model or therapy system a clinician endorses.

This chapter outlined our integrative therapy and its process of systematic treatment selection. This process applies empirical knowledge from multiple theoretical orientations on both diagnostic and nondiagnostic patient characteristics to the optimal choice of technical and relational methods. Such a therapy posits that many treatment methods and interpersonal stances have a valuable place in the repertoire of the contemporary psychotherapist. Their particular and differential place can be determined through outcome research, seasoned experience, and positioning the individual client at the center of the clinical enterprise. In the future, psychotherapy will be defined not by its brand names but by its effectiveness and applicability.

Counseling CourseMate Website:

See this text's Counseling CourseMate website at www.cengagebrain.com for learning tools such as chapter quizzing, videos, glossary flashcards, and more.

ANNOTATED BIBLIOGRAPHY AND WEB RESOURCES

Beutler, L. E., & Harwood, T. M. (2000). *Prescriptive psychotherapy: A practical guide to systematic treatment selection.* New York: Oxford University Press.
This book translates the principles of systematic treatment selection into a treatment manual that has been used in randomized controlled trials of integrative psychotherapy. It includes methods of assessing patients and their progress and outcome.

Harwood, T. M., Beutler, L. E., & Groth-Marnat, G. (Eds.). (2011). *Integrated assessment of adult personality* (3rd ed.). New York: Guilford Press.
This work identifies psychological assessment procedures and tests that evaluate the dimensions that predict psychotherapy outcome. The book reveals the relationships among patient variables and treatment effects and describes computer systems for helping the clinician develop treatment plans.

Castonguay, L. G., & Beutler, L. E. (Eds.). (2006). *Principles of therapeutic change that work.* New York: Oxford University Press.
This text reports the results of a joint task force of the Society of Clinical Psychology and the Society for Psychotherapy Research that identified research-informed principles that account for therapeutic change.

Norcross, J. C. (Ed.). (2011). *Psychotherapy relationships that work* (2nd ed.). New York: Oxford University Press.
This work is a compilation of the empirical research on what works in the therapy relationship in two ways: effective elements of therapy relationships (what works in general) and effective methods of adapting or tailoring therapy to the individual patient (what works in particular).

Norcross, J. C. (2013). *Changeology: Five steps to realizing your goals and resolutions.* New York: Simon & Schuster.
This self-help book provides the most recent and accessible summary of the stages of change. Written for laypersons and accompanied by an interactive Web site (www.ChangeologyBook.com).

Norcross, J. C., & Goldfried, M. R. (Eds.). (2005). *Handbook of psychotherapy integration* (2nd ed.). New York: Oxford University Press.
This handbook offers a state-of-the-art, comprehensive description of psychotherapy integration and its clinical practices by leading proponents. Along with integrative therapies, the book addresses the concepts, history, training, research, and future of psychotherapy integration.

Prochaska, J. O., & Norcross, J. C. (2013). *Systems of psychotherapy: A transtheoretical analysis* (8th ed.). Pacific Grove, CA: Cengage-Brooks/Cole.
This textbook presents a systematic and balanced survey of 16 systems of psychotherapy from an integrative perspective. The comparative analysis demonstrates how much psychotherapy systems agree on the processes producing change while disagreeing on the content that needs to be changed.

Society for the Exploration of Psychotherapy Integration: sepiweb.org/
The homepage of SEPI, the foremost integration organization, provides information on membership, conferences, the *Journal of Psychotherapy Integration,* and training opportunities.

InnerLife: Systematic Treatment Selection: www.innerlife.com/
This Web site provides an online assessment and treatment matching system for use by patients and professionals that is based on 30 years of research on systematic treatment. It can generate an individualized yet comprehensive report for treatment planning.

Transtheoretical Model: www.uri.edu/research/cprc/
Loads of resources on the stages of change and transtheoretical model, including publications, measures, and research studies, are available on this site.

CASE READINGS AND VIDEOTAPES

Beutler, L. E. (2008). *Evidence-based treatment.* DVD. Washington, DC: American Psychological Association.
Dr. Beutler demonstrates his research-directed systematic treatment. He uses a presession assessment to tailor his approach to working with a young man suffering with depression who wants to enjoy life again.

Beutler, L. E., Consoli, A. J., & Lane, G. (2005). Systematic treatment selection and prescriptive psychotherapy. In J. C. Norcross & M. R. Goldfried (Eds.), *Handbook of psychotherapy integration* (2nd ed., pp. 121–143). New York: Oxford University Press.
This chapter summarizes the research and practice of systematic treatment selection. A case study illustrates the use of principles rather than models to guide treatment.

Beutler, L. E., Harwood, T. M., Bertoni, M., & Thomann, J. (2006). Systematic treatment selection and prescriptive therapy. In D. Wedding & R. J. Corsini (Eds.), *Case studies in psychotherapy.* Belmont, CA: Cengage.
This chapter describes the systematic treatment model for planning and integrating psychotherapy.

Norcross, J. C. (Ed.). (1987). *Casebook of eclectic psychotherapy.* New York: Brunner/Mazel.
This volume presents 13 cases that concretely illustrate the practice of eclectic and integrative psychotherapy. Each case presents extensive transcripts, therapist remarks, and written patient impressions, followed by two invited commentaries on the case.

Norcross, J. C. (2011). An integrative therapist's perspective on Ruth. In G. Corey (Ed.), *Case approach to counseling and psychotherapy* (8th ed.). Belmont, CA; Brooks/Cole.
In this work, a dozen therapeutic approaches are applied to the same client, Ruth. In the concluding

chapter, Dr. Norcross presents an integrative perspective on the case and demonstrates both the intriguing similarities and the fundamental differences among theoretical orientations.

Norcross, J. C. (2013). *Integrative psychotherapy*. DVD. Washington, DC: American Psychological Association.

Dr. Norcross demonstrates his adaptable, client-focused approach that tailors the therapy to the client's unique goals, preferences, and stages of change. In this session, he works with a young man who presents with several goals in different stages of change.

Norcross, J. C., Beutler, L. E., & Caldwell, R. (2002). Integrative conceptualization and treatment of depression. In M. A. Reinecke & M. R. Davison (Eds.), *Comparative treatments of depression*. New York: Springer.

This book reviews the major treatments for clinical depression; our chapter presents the integrative perspective and applies it to the case of Ms. Nancy T., who suffers from unipolar depression and a mixed personality disorder.

Norcross, J. C., & Beutler, L. E. (2013). Evidence-based relationships and responsiveness for depression with substance abuse. In D. H. Barlow (Ed.), *Clinical handbook of psychological disorders* (5th ed.). New York: Guilford.

This chapter illustrates integrative therapy with a complex and challenging woman, who suffers from multiple mental disorders, and demonstrates the process of customizing psychological treatments and therapeutic relationships to her specific needs as defined by diagnostic and nondiagnostic considerations.

Stricker, G., & Gold, J. (Eds.). (2006). *Casebook of psychotherapy integration*. Washington, DC: American Psychological Association.

Prominent practitioners describe their respective integrative psychotherapies and then demonstrate them in brief cases.

REFERENCES

Antonuccio, D. O. (1995). Psychotherapy for depression: No stronger medicine. *American Psychologist, 50*, 450–452.

Beutler, L. E. (1983). *Eclectic psychotherapy: A systematic approach*. New York: Pergamon.

Beutler, L. E. (2009). Making science matter in clinical practice; Redefining psychotherapy. *Clinical Psychology: Science and Practice, 16*, 301–317.

Beutler, L. E., Clarkin, J., & Bongar, B. (2000). *Guidelines for the systematic treatment of the depressed patient*. New York: Oxford University Press.

Beutler, L. E., Forrester, B., Gallagher-Thompson, D., Thompson, L., & Tomlins, J. B., 2012. Common, specific and treatment fit variables in psychotherapy outcome. *Journal of Psychotherapy Integration 22, 255-281.*

Beutler, L. E., & Groth-Marnat, G. (2003). *Integrative assessment of adult personality* (2nd ed.). New York: Guilford.

Beutler, L. E., & Harwood, T. M. (2004). Virtual reality in psychotherapy training. *Journal of Clinical Psychology, 60*, 317–330.

Beutler, L. E., Harwood, T. M., Alimohamed, S., & Malik, M. (2002). Functional impairment. In J. C. Norcross (Ed.), *Psychotherapy relationships that work* (pp. 145–170). New York: Oxford University Press.

Beutler, L. E., Harwood, T. M., Kimpara, S., Verdirame, & Blau, K. (2011). Coping style. In J. C. Norcross (Ed.), *Psychotherapy relationships that work* (2nd ed., pp. 336–353). New York: Oxford University Press.

Beutler, L. E., Harwood, T. M., Michelson, A., Song, X., & Holman, J. (2011). Reactance/resistance. In J. C. Norcross (Ed.), *Psychotherapy relationships that work* (2nd ed., pp. 261–278). New York: Oxford University Press.

Castonguay, L. G., & Beutler, L. E. (Eds.). (2006). *Principles of therapeutic change that work*. New York: Oxford University Press.

DeRubeis, R. J., Hollon, S. D., Amsterdam, J. D., et al. (2005). Cognitive therapy vs. medications in the treatment of moderate to severe depression. *Archives of General Psychiatry, 62*, 409–416.

Eysenck, H. J. (1970). A mish-mash of theories. *International Journal of Psychiatry, 9*, 140–146.

Frances, A., Clarkin, J., & Perry, S. (1984). *Differential therapeutics in psychiatry*. New York: Brunner/Mazel.

Frank, J. D. (1973). *Persuasion and healing* (2nd ed.). Baltimore: Johns Hopkins University.

French, T. M. (1933). Interrelations between psychoanalysis and the experimental work of Pavlov. *American Journal of Psychiatry, 89*, 1165–1203.

Garfield, S. L. (1980). *Psychotherapy: An eclectic approach*. New York: Wiley.

Goldfried, M. R. (1980). Toward the delineation of therapeutic change principles. *American Psychologist, 35*, 991–999.

Goldfried, M. R., Pachankis, J. E., & Bell, A. C. (2005). History of psychotherapy integration. In J. C. Norcross & M. R. Goldfried (Eds.), *Handbook of psychotherapy integration* (2nd ed., pp. 24–60). New York: Oxford University Press.

Goldstein, A. P., & Stein, N. (1976). *Prescriptive psychotherapies*. New York: Pergamon.

Grencavage, L. M., & Norcross, J. C. (1990). Where are the commonalities among the therapeutic common factors? *Professional Psychology: Research and Practice, 21*, 372–378.

Halford, G. S., Baker, R., McCredden, J. E., & Bain, J. D. (2005). How many variables can humans process? *Psychological Science, 16*, 70–76.

Harwood, T. M., Beutler, L. E., & Groth-Marnat, G. (Eds.). (2011). *Integrated assessment of adult personality* (3rd ed.). New York: Guilford Press.

Harwood, T. M., & Williams, O. B. (2003). Identifying treatment relevant assessment: Systematic treatment selection. In *Integrative assessment of adult personality* (pp. 65–81). New York: Guilford.

Hays, P. A. (1996). Culturally responsive assessment with diverse older clients. *Professional Psychology: Research and Practice, 27*, 188–193.

Hollanders, H., & McLeod, J. (1999). Theoretical orientation and reported practice: A survey of eclecticism among counsellors in Britain. *British Journal of Guidance & Counselling, 27*, 405–414.

Hoyt, M. F. (1995). *Brief therapy and managed care.* San Francisco: Jossey-Bass.

Jensen, J. P., Bergin, A. E., & Greaves, D. W. (1990). The meaning of eclecticism: New survey and analysis of components. *Professional Psychology: Research and Practice, 21*, 124–130.

Lambert, M. J., & Shimokawa, K. (2011). Collecting client feedback. In J. C. Norcross (Ed.), *Psychotherapy relationships that work* (2nd ed., pp. 203–223). New York: Oxford University Press.

Lampropoulos, G. K., & Dixon, D. N. (2007). Psychotherapy integration in internships and counseling psychology doctoral programs. *Journal of Psychotherapy Integration, 17*, 185–208.

Landsman, J. T. (1974, August). *Not an adversity but a welcome diversity.* Paper presented at the meeting of the American Psychological Association, New Orleans, Louisiana.

Lazarus, A. A. (1967). In support of technical eclecticism. *Psychological Reports, 21*, 415–416.

Lazarus, A. A. (1989). *The practice of multimodal therapy.* Baltimore: Johns Hopkins University.

Lazarus, A. A. (1993). Tailoring the therapeutic relationship, or being an authentic chameleon. *Psychotherapy, 30*, 404–407.

Liff, Z. A. (1992). Psychoanalysis and dynamic techniques. In D. K. Freedheim (Ed.), *History of psychotherapy* (pp. 571–586). Washington DC: American Psychological Association.

Lunde, D. T. (1974). Eclectic and integrated theory: Gordon Allport and others. In A. Burton (Ed.), *Operational theories of personality* (pp. 381–404). New York: Brunner/Mazel.

Marlatt, G. A., & Donovan, D. M. (Eds.). (2007). *Relapse prevention: Maintenance strategies in the treatment of addictive behaviors* (2nd ed.). New York: Guilford.

Messer, S. B. (2001). Introduction to the special issue on assimilative integration. *Journal of Psychotherapy Integration, 11*, 1–4.

Norcross, J. C. (Ed.). (1986). *Handbook of eclectic psychotherapy.* New York: Brunner/Mazel.

Norcross, J. C. (Ed.). (1987). *Casebook of eclectic psychotherapy.* New York: Brunner/Mazel.

Norcross, J. C. (2005). The psychotherapist's own psychotherapy: Educating and developing psychologists. *American Psychologist, 60*, 840–850.

Norcross, J. C. (2010). The therapeutic relationship. In B. L. Duncan et al. (Eds.), *Heart and soul of change* (2nd ed.). Washington, DC: American Psychological Association.

Norcross, J. C. (Ed.). (2011). *Psychotherapy relationships that work* (2nd ed.). New York: Oxford University Press.

Norcross, J. C. (2013). *Changeology: Five steps to realizing your goals and resolutions.* New York: Simon & Schuster.

Norcross, J. C., & Beutler, L. E. (1997). Determining the therapeutic relationship of choice in brief therapy. In J. N. Butcher (Ed.), *Personality assessment in managed health care: A practitioner's guide* (pp. 42–60). New York: Oxford University Press.

Norcross, J. C., & Beutler, L. E. (2013). Evidence-based relationships and responsiveness for depression with substance abuse. In D. H. Barlow (Ed.)., *Clinical handbook of psychological disorders* (5th ed.). New York: Guilford.

Norcross, J. C., Beutler, L. E., & Caldwell, R. (2002). Integrative conceptualization and treatment of depression. In M. A. Reinecke & M. R. Davison (Eds.), *Comparative treatments of depression.* New York: Springer.

Norcross, J. C., Beutler, L. E., & Levant, R. F. (Eds.). (2006). *Evidence-based practices in mental health: Debate and dialogue on the fundamental questions.* Washington, DC: American Psychological Association.

Norcross, J. C., & Caldwell, N. A. (2000). Prescriptive eclectic approach with Ms. Katrina. *Cognitive and Behavioral Practice, 7*, 514–519.

Norcross, J. C., & Goldfried, M. R. (Eds.). (2005). *Handbook of psychotherapy integration* (2nd ed.). New York: Oxford University Press.

Norcross, J. C., & Halgin, R. P. (2005). In J. C. Norcross & M. R. Goldfried (Eds.), *Handbook of psychotherapy integration* (pp. 459–493). New York: Oxford University Press.

Norcross, J. C., Hogan, T. P., & Koocher, G. P. (2008). *Clinician's guide to evidence-based practice: Mental health and the addictions.* New York: Oxford University Press.

Norcross, J. C., & Karpiak, C. P. (2012). Clinical psychologists in the 2010s: Fifty years of the APA Division of Clinical Psychology. *Clinical Psychology: Science and Practice, 19*, 1–12.

Norcross, J. C., Karpiak, C. P., & Lister, K. M. (2005). What's an integrationist? A study of self-identified integrative and (occasionally) eclectic psychologists. *Journal of Clinical Psychology, 61*, 1587–1594.

Norcross, J. C., Krebs, P. M., & Prochaska, J. O. (2011). Stages of change. In J. C. Norcross (Ed.), *Psychotherapy relationships that work* (2nd ed., pp. 279–300). New York: Oxford University Press.

Norcross, J. C., Pfund, R. A., & Prochaska, J. O. (2013). *A Delphi poll on the future of psychotherapy.* Manuscript under review.

Paniagua, F. A. (2005). *Assessing and treating culturally diverse clients: A practical guide* (3rd ed.). Thousand Oaks, CA: Sage.

Paul, G. L. (1967). Strategy of outcome research in psychotherapy. *Journal of Consulting Psychology, 31*, 109–118.

Pederson, P. B., Crethar, H. C., & Carlson, J. (2008). *Inclusive cultural empathy.* Washington, DC: American Psychological Association.

Pinsof, W. M. (1995). *Integrative IPCT: A synthesis of biological, individual, and family therapies.* New York: Basic Books.

Prochaska, J. O. (1979). *Systems of psychotherapy: A transtheoretical analysis.* Homewood, IL: Dorsey.

Prochaska, J. O., & DiClemente, C. C. (1983). Stages and processes of self-change of smoking: Toward an integrative model of change. *Journal of Consulting and Clinical Psychology, 51,* 390–395.

Prochaska, J. O., & Norcross, J. C. (2013). *Systems of psychotherapy: A transtheoretical analysis* (8th ed.). Pacific Grove, CA: Brooks/Cole.

Prochaska, J. O., Norcross, J. C., & DiClemente, C. C. (1995). *Changing for good.* New York: Avon.

Rosen, C. S. (2000). Is the sequencing of change processes by stage consistent across health problems? A meta-analysis. *Health Psychology, 19,* 593–604.

Rosenzweig, S. (1936). Some implicit common factors in diverse methods in psychotherapy. *American Journal of Orthopsychiatry, 6,* 412–415.

Safran, J. D., Muran, J. C., & Eubanks-Carter, C. (2011). Repairing alliance ruptures. In J. C. Norcross (Ed.), *Psychotherapy relationships that work* (2nd ed., pp. 224–238). New York: Oxford University Press.

Schultz-Ross, R. A. (1995). Ideological insularity as a defense against clinical complexity. *American Journal of Psychotherapy, 49,* 540–547.

Schottenbauer, M. A., Glass, C. R., & Arnkoff, D. B. (2005). Outcome research on psychotherapy integration In J. C. Norcross & M. R. Goldfried (Eds.), *Handbook of psychotherapy integration* (2nd ed., pp. 459–493). New York: Oxford University Press.

Smith, T. B., Rodriguez, M. D., & Bernal, G. (2011). Culture. In J. C. Norcross (Ed.), *Psychotherapy relationships that work* (2nd ed., pp. 316–335). New York: Oxford University Press.

Stricker, G., & Gold, J. (Eds.). (2006). *Casebook of psychotherapy integration.* Washington, DC: American Psychological Association.

Swift, J. K., Callahan, J. L., & Vollmer, B. M. (2011). Preferences. In J. C. Norcross (Ed.), *Psychotherapy relationships that work* (2nd ed., pp. 301–315). New York: Oxford University Press.

Thorne, F. C. (1957). Critique of recent developments in personality counseling theory. *Journal of Clinical Psychology, 13,* 234–244.

Thorne, F. C. (1967). The structure of integrative psychology. *Journal of Clinical Psychology, 23,* 3–11.

Tracey, T. J. G., Lichtenberg, J. W., Goodyear, R. K., Claiborn, C. D., & Wampold, B. E. (2003). Concept mapping of therapeutic common factors. *Psychotherapy Research, 13,* 401–413.

Wachtel, P. L. (1977). *Psychoanalysis and behavior therapy: Toward an integration.* New York: Basic Books.

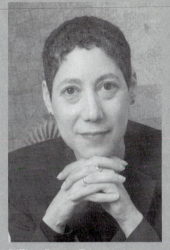
Lillian Comas-Díaz
Courtesy of Lillian Comas-Díaz

15 | MULTICULTURAL THEORIES OF PSYCHOTHERAPY

Lillian Comas–Díaz

OVERVIEW

Are the prevailing systems of psychotherapy relevant to culturally diverse individuals? Most therapeutic orientations recognize that individual differences must be respected and accepted. However, as products of Western society, the dominant models of psychotherapy tend to be grounded in a monocultural perspective. As such, they support mainstream cultural values that neglect multicultural worldviews. Unfortunately, a monocultural psychotherapy frequently promotes *ethnocentrism*, or the belief that one's worldview is inherently superior and desirable to others (Leininger, 1978). Ethnocentrism compromises psychotherapy when therapists project their values and attitudes onto their culturally different clients. As a result, scholars and practitioners questioned the multicultural applicability of mainstream psychotherapy (Bernal, Bonilla & Bellido, 1995; Sue, Bingham, Porche-Burke, & Vasquez, 1999). Multicultural psychotherapies emerged as a response to these concerns.

Proponents of multicultural psychotherapies advocate for cultural sensitivity—that is, awareness, respect, and appreciation for cultural diversity. Valuing diversity promotes a critical examination of established psychotherapeutic models and assumptions because definitions of health, illness, healing, normality, and abnormality are culturally embedded. Thus, multicultural psychotherapists examine their clients' as well as their own worldviews. The concept of *worldview* refers to people's systematized ideas and beliefs about the universe. When multicultural psychotherapists engage in self-examination, they explore their professional socialization and potential bias. They also examine the cultural applicability of their interventions and promote culturally relevant therapeutic strategies.

Monocultural, dominant psychotherapies tend to be decontextualized, ahistorical, and apolitical. When they fail to examine the historical and sociopolitical contexts, mainstream psychotherapies ignore the role of power and privilege in people's lives.

Conversely, multicultural psychotherapists consider power differences based on diversity characteristics such as ethnicity, race, gender, social class, sexual orientation, age, religion, national origin, ability or disability, language, ideology, and membership in other marginalized groups. They believe that ethnocentric psychotherapy paradigms resist change because they preserve the status quo. To embrace change, multicultural psychotherapists promote empowerment and social justice. Instead of focusing on deficits, they affirm strengths. The emphasis on diversity leads multiculturalists to endorse interdisciplinary approaches. Indeed, *unity through diversity* is a multicultural maxim. Consequently, multicultural psychotherapists benefit from the contributions of sociology, anthropology, cultural and ethnic studies, humanities, arts, history, politics, law, philosophy, religion and spirituality, neuroscience, and many other disciplines. Accordingly, multicultural psychotherapists also are represented in diverse theoretical schools, including psychodynamic, cognitive-behavioral, rational-emotive, humanistic-existential, Jungian, and various other combinations of dominant psychotherapies. Regardless of preferred theoretical approach, multicultural psychotherapists work to develop *cultural competence*. A basic concept in multicultural psychotherapies, cultural competence refers to the set of knowledge, behaviors, attitudes, skills, and policies that enables a practitioner to work effectively in a multicultural situation (Cross, Bazron, Dennis, & Isaacs, 1989).

Basic Concepts

Demographic changes in the United States signal the increasing number of culturally diverse individuals in need of psychotherapy. Multiculturalism acknowledges the presence of diverse worldviews where each culture is unique and dynamic, needing to be understood within its own context. Notably, multiculturalism embodies cultural constructionism—a process whereby individuals construct their world through social processes that contain cultural symbols and metaphors (Gergen & Gergen, 1997; Sue & Sue, 2008). In the United States, the term *multicultural* refers to the interaction between culturally diverse individuals such as people of color, internationals, immigrants, temporary workers, and the dominant European American culture.

Notwithstanding its increasing presence in society, multiculturalism has not fully reached dominant psychotherapy. Accordingly, the lack of cultural relevance in dominant psychotherapies has given birth to multicultural psychotherapies. This chapter defines multicultural psychotherapy as a culture-centered holistic approach that offers practical methods designed to enhance healing and liberation. Simply put, *multicultural psychotherapies infuse cultural competence into clinical practice.* Regardless of theoretical orientation, psychotherapists can incorporate a multicultural perspective into their practice. Indeed, a survey of psychotherapists predicted that in the future most mainstream psychotherapists will incorporate a multicultural dimension in their approach (Norcross, Hedges, & Prochaska, 2002). A multicultural dimension is crucial to psychotherapy because cultural misunderstandings and communication problems between psychotherapists and clients interfere with treatment effectiveness. This observation illustrates how psychotherapists' ethnocentric worldviews interfere with psychotherapy's usefulness.

Worldviews

Harry Triandis (1995) classified worldviews according to how individuals define themselves and how they relate to others. Those cultures where individuals' identity is associated with their relationships to others are called *collectivistic*. In contrast, members who frequently view themselves independently from others are denominated *individualistic* (Triandis, 1995). Western societies tend to be identified as individualistic because their members define themselves primarily in terms of internal features such as traits, attitudes, abilities, and agencies. In other words, their ideal personal characteristics include being direct, assertive, competitive, self-assured, self sufficient, and efficient. On the other hand, collectivistic members endorse relational values, prefer interdependence, encourage sharing resources, value harmony, tolerate the views of significant others, and prefer communication that minimizes conflicts (Triandis, 1995). Valuing connection, collectivistic persons frequently contextualize and have a holistic orientation. In reality, most people's worldviews can be placed within an individualist–collectivist spectrum. For instance, many African Americans have a combined collectivistic and individualist worldview.

The negotiation of client–therapist worldviews is crucial for effective psychotherapy. Regrettably, because of their individualistic worldview, mainstream psychotherapists tend to interpret multicultural clients' normative cultural behaviors as resistance, inferiority, or deviance (Young, 1990). For example, when collectivist members tolerate the limitations of significant others, individualist psychotherapists may misinterpret such behavior as poor judgment, instead of viewing it as a culturally accepted norm. Moreover, individualistic psychotherapists can violate personal and family norms by asking collectivistic clients to reveal intimate personal information, soliciting the expression of emotion and affect, and requesting individuals to air family disputes, all before earning their clients' trust and establishing a positive therapeutic alliance (Varma, 1988). Because the notion of being understood is an important aspect in healing, effective psychotherapy depends on the therapist's understanding of his or her client's worldview. The development of cultural competence helps therapists to appreciate and manage diverse worldviews.

Cultural Competence

Differences in therapists and clients' worldviews frequently lead to communication problems, misdiagnosis, or client premature treatment termination. However, cultural competence enhances adherence to psychotherapy and the completion of treatment. *Cultural competence* involves a set of congruent behaviors, attitudes, and policies that reflect an understanding of how cultural and sociopolitical influences shape individuals' worldviews and related health behaviors (Betancourt, Green, Carrillo, & Ananch-Firempong, 2003). Specifically, to become culturally competent, you need to:

1. become aware of your worldview,
2. examine your attitude toward cultural differences,
3. learn about different worldviews, and
4. develop multicultural skills (Sue et al., 1995).

Likewise, culturally competent therapists develop the capacity to:

1. value diversity,
2. manage the dynamics of difference,
3. acquire and incorporate cultural knowledge into their interventions and interactions,

4. increase their multicultural skills,

5. conduct self-reflection and assessment, and

6. adapt to diversity and to the cultural contexts of their clients.

Because all therapeutic encounters are multicultural—everyone belongs to diverse cultures and subcultures—cultural competence enables psychotherapists to work effectively in most treatment situations. Moreover, we can substitute the construct of clinical competence with cultural competence because cultural competence is superordinate over the traditional notion of clinical competence (Sue & Sue, 2008). For the purpose of this chapter, *culture* is defined as individuals' total environment. It includes beliefs, values, practices, institutions, and psychological processes, including language, cognition, and perception.

The American Psychological Association (APA) highlighted the importance of cultural competence by formulating a series of multicultural guidelines. The first set of principles—*Guidelines for Providers of Psychological Services to Ethnic, Linguistic, and Culturally Diverse Clients*—exhorted practitioners to:

1. recognize cultural diversity;

2. understand the central role that culture, ethnicity, and race play in culturally diverse individuals;

3. appreciate the significant impact of socioeconomic and political factors on mental health; and

4. help clients understand their cultural identification (APA, 1990).

Afterward, the APA (2003) published a second set of principles—*Guidelines on Multicultural Education, Training, Research, Practice and Organizations*—and encouraged psychologists to:

1. recognize that we are cultural beings,

2. value cultural sensitivity and awareness,

3. use multicultural constructs in education,

4. conduct culture-centered and ethical psychological research with culturally diverse individuals,

5. use culturally appropriate skills in applied psychological practices, and

6. implement organizational change processes to support culturally informed organizational practices and policy (APA, 2003).

The six specific multicultural guidelines follow here.

Commitment to Cultural Awareness and Knowledge of Self and Others

1. Psychologists are encouraged to recognize that, as cultural beings, they may hold attitudes and beliefs that can detrimentally influence their perceptions of and interactions with individuals who are ethnically and racially different from themselves.

2. Psychologists are encouraged to recognize the importance of multicultural sensitivity and responsiveness, knowledge, and understanding about ethnically and racially different individuals.

Education

3. As educators, psychologists are encouraged to employ the constructs of multiculturalism and diversity in psychological education.

Research

4. Culturally sensitive psychological researchers are encouraged to recognize the importance of conducting culture-centered and ethical psychological research among persons from ethnic, linguistic, and racial minority backgrounds.

Practice

5. Psychologists strive to apply culturally appropriate skills in clinical and other applied psychological practices.

Organizational Change and Policy Development

6. Psychologists are encouraged to use organizational change processes to support culturally informed organizational (policy) development and practices.

The interested reader can access the complete document at www.apa.org/pi/oema /resources/policy/provider-guidelines.aspx.

All multicultural guidelines provide a context for multicultural psychotherapies. Nonetheless, three areas are of particular relevance to multicultural psychotherapies. These are the commitment to cultural awareness and knowledge of self and others, guidelines related to psychological practice, and organizational change and policy development. Multicultural psychotherapists respond to their ethics code (APA, 2010) regardless of the purview of practice and setting.

The development of cultural competence is a lifelong process that requires acknowledging the need for ongoing learning. Cross and his colleagues (1989) identified the development of cultural competence across the following spectrum.

1. *Cultural destructiveness* is characterized by attitudes, policies, and practices that are destructive to cultures and to individuals within cultures (e.g., English-only mandates).

2. In *cultural incapacity*, individuals believe in the racial superiority of the dominant group and assume a paternalistic and ignorant position toward culturally diverse people.

3. In *cultural blindness*, individuals believe that culture makes no difference and thus the values of the dominant culture are universally applicable and beneficial.

4. In *cultural precompetence*, individuals desire to provide an equitable and fair treatment with cultural sensitivity but do not know exactly how to proceed.

5. In *cultural competence*, individuals value and respect cultural differences, engage in continuing self-assessment regarding culture, pay attention to the dynamics of difference, continue expanding their knowledge and resources, and endorse a variety of adaptations to belief systems, policies, and practices.

Multicultural psychotherapies' emphasis on context nurtured the emergence of cultural competence guidelines for organizations. Because many psychotherapists function within formal organizations, the APA formulated multicultural guidelines for psychologists within organizations through its multicultural guideline number 6. Addressing this problem, Howard-Hamilton and colleagues (1998) outlined principles for those counselors working with multicultural clients. They exhorted therapists to:

1. evaluate their institution's mission statement and policies to determine whether they include diversity issues,

2. assess policies with regards to diversity,

3. evaluate how people of color may perceive specific policies,

4. acknowledge within group diversity,

5. be aware that diversity requires examination from both the individual and the institutional levels, and

6. recognize that multicultural sensitivity may mean advocating for culturally diverse people.

Similarly, Wu and Martinez (2006) asked multicultural practitioners to help their organizations achieve cultural competence by:

1. including community representation and input at all stages of implementation;
2. integrating all systems of the health-care organization;
3. ensuring that changes made are manageable, measurable, and sustainable;
4. making the business case for implementation of cultural competency polices;
5. requiring commitment from leadership; and
6. helping to establish staff training on an ongoing basis.

Empowerment

In addition to promulgating cultural competence, multicultural psychotherapists challenged dominant approaches with conceptual, methodological, ethical, and sociopolitical concerns. Dominant psychotherapists' ignorance of the historical and sociopolitical contexts further disempowered marginalized individuals. This disempowering effect is detrimental for visible people of color, who, unlike majority group members, experience individual and collective oppression. A specific example of such disempowerment is dominant psychotherapists' inattention to racial microaggressions. *Racial microaggresions* refer to the assaults that individuals receive on a regular basis solely because of their race, color, or ethnicity (Pierce, 1995). Some illustrations of racial microaggressions include being harassed in public places, being ignored by clerks who favor white customers, being accused of being "affirmative action babies" (racial favoritism), being targeted for racial profiling, and so forth. Besides racial microaggressions, many people of color are exposed to other kinds of microaggressions based on elitism, sexism, heterosexism ageism, ableism, homophobia, and various combinations thereof. The constant and cumulative exposure to microaggressions drains people of color of their survivalist energy (Essed, 1991). As an illustration, racial microaggressions have been correlated with health problems among people of color (Comas-Díaz, 2012a).

Sadly, microaggressions also occur in therapy and include therapists' cultural blindness, denial of racism and other forms of oppression, adherence to the myth of meritocracy (without acknowledging the roles of oppression and privilege), misdiagnosis, and pathologizing culturally diverse behaviors (Sue et al., 2007). Moreover, these therapists' behaviors promote distress among culturally diverse clients. In contrast, multicultural psychotherapists emphasize empowerment because many people of color tend to internalize their disempowerment as helplessness. Therapeutic empowerment helps clients increase their access to resources, develop options to exercise choice, improve self- and collective esteem, implement culturally relevant assertiveness, augment agency, affirm cultural strengths, overcome internalized oppression, and engage in transformative actions.

Within their empowerment focus, multicultural psychotherapies frequently subscribe to the following assumptions:

1. Reality is constructed in a context.
2. Experience is valuable knowledge.
3. Learning and healing results from sharing multiple perspectives.
4. Learning and healing is anchored in meaningful and relevant contexts.

Along these lines, several multicultural practitioners espouse a liberation model, helping clients critically analyze their situations, affirm ethno-racial-cultural strengths, promote personal transformation, and foster sociopolitical change.

Indeed, the emphasis on empowerment frequently leads psychotherapists to commit to social justice. The history of human rights violations against many minorities has resulted in a *cultural trauma*, a legacy of adversity, pain, and suffering among many minority group members. Duran (2006) called this legacy a *soul wound*—the product of sociohistorical oppression, ungrieved losses, internalized oppression, and learned helplessness. Certainly, microaggressions and other types of oppression aggravate the cultural trauma of people of color. Moreover, group membership dynamics seem to reinforce oppression and privilege.

For example, research has identified a human tendency to categorize individuals into in-group and out-group members (Allport, 1954). Membership in one group helps to shape individuals' perceptions about their own group and other groups. When people belong to one group, they tend to prefer members of their own identity classification. Indeed, some studies have documented the existence of unconscious negative racial feelings and beliefs. By using cognitive psychology techniques (e.g., response latency as measure of bias), Dovidio and Gaertner (1986, 1998) demonstrated that people who appeared nonprejudiced in self-report measures often have generally negative attitudes toward blacks. Known as *aversive racism*, this phenomenon showed that both liberal and conservative whites discriminate against African Americans (and probably against other visible people of color) in situations that do not implicate racial prejudice as a basis for their actions (Whaley, 1998). Likewise, the expression of unintentional or symbolic racism can take subtle forms and thus is harder to identify. As a result, white individuals who grow up as members of a majority group may have either covertly or overtly racist attitudes (Brown, 1997). As an illustration, in-group favoritism—the informal networks that provide contacts, support, mentoring, rewards, and benefits to same-group members—tends to exclude people of color in predominantly white work environments (Rhode & Williams, 2007).

Psychotherapy will be unsuccessful if clients feel that their therapist is unconsciously racist, ethnocentric, sexist, elitist, xenophobic, homophobic, or the like. To counteract bias, multicultural psychotherapists explore their beliefs, values, and attitudes toward their in-group members as well as their attitudes toward out-group members. In other words, they become aware of and sensitive to their own attitudes toward others because they may be unconscious of how culturally biased these attitudes may be. Besides becoming familiar with different worldviews, multicultural psychotherapists understand the stigmatizing effects of being a member of an oppressed group. More specifically, they recognize how minority members' history with the dominant society—such as African American slavery, concentration camps for Japanese Americans, the American Indian holocaust, and the colonization of major Latino groups, including the forceful annexation of Mexican territories—can create cultural trauma and thus influence the worldview of people of color. An appreciation of such history requires awareness of how racism interacts with other types of discrimination such as sexism, classism, xenophobia, ageism, neocolonialism, homophobia, and heterosexism.

To undertake this appreciation, therapists engage in cultural self-awareness. Therapists' cultural self-awareness includes learning about one's position in relation to societal power and privilege. Understanding power dynamics is an important part of appreciating the relationship between oneself and others. To achieve this goal, multicultural psychotherapists analyze the power differences between their life experiences and those of their clients. Different from most dominant therapies' analyses, a power analysis goes beyond the power differential inherent in the therapist–client dyad. Multicultural psychotherapists compare their clients' cultural groups' social statuses with their own. This comparison entails the identification and challenge of internalized privilege and oppression because most individuals with power are unaware of its pervasive influence in their life. To increase awareness of power, Peggy McIntosh (1988) defined white privilege as unacknowledged systems that give power to European Americans and male individuals. She exhorted individuals to "unpack the invisible knapsack" by becoming aware of white privilege. Examples of the invisible knapsack include those situations when European Americans and men can do the following:

1. Go shopping alone most of the time, pretty well assured they will not be followed or harassed.
2. Turn on the television or open to the front page of the paper and see European American people widely represented.
3. Count on their skin color not to work against the appearance of financial reliability whenever they use checks, credit cards, or cash.
4. Be pretty sure of renting or purchasing housing in an area that they can afford and in which they would want to live.
5. Avoid the need to educate their children to be aware of systemic racism for their own daily physical protection.
6. Remain oblivious of the language and customs of persons of color who constitute the world's majority without feeling any penalty for such oblivion.
7. Exist with little fear about the consequences of ignoring the perspectives and powers of people of other races.
8. Confront a person of their own race if they ask to talk to the "person in charge."
9. Be confident that if a state trooper pulls them over, they haven't been singled out because of their race.
10. Take jobs with affirmative action employers without having co-workers suspect that they were hired because of their race.

The illustrations of white privilege reflect the importance of recognizing the effects of institutionalized power disparities on people's lives because such disparities favor members of dominant groups while disenfranchising members of minority groups. The denial of the unacknowledged privilege protects the status quo.

To summarize, multicultural psychotherapies' underlying assumptions include the following:

Culture is complex and dynamic.

Every encounter is multicultural.

Reality is constructed and embedded in context.

A Western worldview has dominated mainstream psychotherapy and has minimized the contributions of non-Western healing practices.

Multicultural psychotherapies are relevant to all individuals.

Cultural competence is crucial for effective psychotherapy.

Multicultural psychotherapists engage in self-awareness.

Healing entails empowering individuals and groups.

Healing involves multiple perspectives.

Healing is holistic and liberatory.

Other Systems

Multiculturalism draws on the benefits and perspectives of many disciplines, and multicultural psychotherapists acknowledge the contributions of diverse psychotherapeutic orientations. Although many multicultural therapists self-identify as adherents to one or another theoretical orientations, they also impart multicultural values into their specific therapeutic schools. Indeed, partly because of multicultural-ism's criticisms, mainstream clinicians are revising psychotherapy's basic tenets with respect to their applicability to culturally diverse clients. Psychoanalysts, for instance, are including the experiences of culturally diverse individuals to incorporate their social, communal, and spiritual orientations into treatment. For example, object relations theory focuses on how individuals internalize significant interpersonal relationships and how these internalizations become central to their interactions with the world. Within this perspective, Altman (1995, 2010) uses a modified psychoanalytic object relations framework, examining his clients' progress by their ability to use relationships to grow rather than by the insight they gain. In addition to the cultural adaptations of dominant psychotherapies, the specific influence of multicultural approaches is increasing. Research has reported inconsistent findings regarding the cultural sensitivity of mainstream psychological services. Although some studies found evidence-based practice (EBP) to be effective for many culturally diverse populations (CIEBP, 2008), other findings indicated that clients of color tend to drop out of cognitive-behavioral therapy (CBT) at a higher rate than their European American counterparts (Miranda et al., 2005). Research findings suggest that, to be effective, EBP needs to be culturally adapted to client's contexts (Morales & Norcross, 2010). These findings are consistent with the results of a study that showed African American clients who expressed positive expectations about seeking mental-health services found treatment less positive than their European American counterparts after using such services (Diala et al., 2000).

Indeed, after reviewing the research on dominant psychotherapies' cultural adaptations, Whaley and Davis (2007) concluded that culture affects psychotherapeutic process more than it affects treatment outcome. Dominant psychotherapies' ethnocentrism could partly explain Whaley and Davis's conclusion. To illustrate, a major area of discontent among people of color is their history of medical experimentation and abuse. Called *medical apartheid*, this history included the Tuskegee project—a research project in which African American men with syphilis were given a placebo instead of medication (penicillin), despite the fact that a cure for syphilis was found during the course of the research and administered to white men—and the involuntary sterilization of Puerto Rican women during routine medical examinations (Comas-Diaz, 2008). As many culturally diverse individuals endorse a collectivistic orientation, they situate themselves in context and time. Therefore, personal and collective history is an important element in the lives of people of color.

HISTORY

Precursors

Attention to the *other* dates from the beginning of time. Frequently, such attention has been in the form of concern, awareness, and even fascination. Diverse religious and spiritual traditions assigned an important role to the other. For instance, in Judaism the *other* is associated with sacred because *otherness* means *holy* in Hebrew. In Christianity, the concept of the *necessary other* facilitates the recovery of the divided self. Furthermore, a Buddhist view on the *other* as enemy entails that enemies are our best teachers because we learn the most from them. In accordance with spiritual traditions, multicultural psychotherapies aim to enhance the relationship between self and other.

542   LILLIAN COMAS-DÍAZ

Beginnings

Multicultural psychotherapies have interdisciplinary origins. Early theoretical influences include psychological anthropology, ethnopsychology, cultural anthropology, psychoanalytic anthropology, and folk healing. The interest in the *other* arrived in the mental-health fields during the 1940s and 1960s. Anthropologists and psychoanalysts collaborated on studying the relationship between culture and psyche. Proponents of these movements applied psychoanalytic analyses to social and cultural phenomena. Some scholars examined cross-cultural mental health, some studied the effects of oppression on ethnic minorities' mental health, and still others questioned the universal application of psychoanalytic concepts such as the oedipal complex.

Members of the cultural school of psychoanalysis argued that culture shapes behavior because individuals are contextualized and embedded in social interactions that varied across cultural contexts and historical periods (Seeley, 2000). Although the anthropological psychoanalytic orientations enriched the cultural and behavioral discourse, they failed to develop cultural theories that could be applied to psychotherapy (Seeley, 2000).

Psychological and psychiatric anthropologists studied the effects of culture on mental health and gave birth to transcultural psychiatry. Similar to *culturalism*—the psychotherapeutic use of culture-specific folk healing—transcultural psychiatry and psychology advocated for the use of community and indigenous resources (clergy, teachers, folk healers, and other ethnic minority individuals) for mental-health treatment.

The minority-empowerment movements furthered the development of multicultural psychotherapies. These movements examined the power and oppression dynamics between dominant group members and minorities. Known as *identity politics*, women's rights, black power, Chicano or brown power, and gay lesbian and bisexual movements highlighted the civil rights and needs of marginalized groups. Adherents of these movements raised consciousness and worked toward empowering marginalized groups in order to redress social and political inequities.

The desire to understand the effects of oppression on mental health led some clinicians to examine the psychology of colonization. Frantz Fanon (1967) articulated the principles of the psychology of colonization in terms of the economic and emotional dependence of the colonized on the colonizer. He used the concepts of imperialism, dominance, and exploitation to examine the relationship between the colonizer and the colonized. The dynamics of colonization echoed in the United States as the first president of color of the American Psychological Association, Kenneth B. Clark, identified the condition of Americans of color as similar to being colonized (Comas-Diaz, 2007).

A major influence on multicultural psychotherapies is the *education for the oppressed* model. Paulo Freire (1973) identified dominant models of education as instruments of oppression that reinforce and maintain the status quo and social inequities. He coined the term *conscientizacion* or critical consciousness as a process of personal and social liberation. Education for the oppressed teaches individuals to become aware of their circumstances and change them through a dialectical conversation with their world. Because oppression robs its victims of their critical thinking, the development of *conscientizacion* involves asking critical questions such as "What? Why? How? For whom? Against whom? By whom? In favor of whom? In favor of what? To what end?" (Freire & Macedo, 2000). Answering these questions helps clients examine "what matters" and uncovers clients' existential reasons for being, as well as purpose, and position in life. Critical consciousness helps oppressed individuals to author their own reality.

Reevaluation counseling (RC) is another influence in the emergence of multicultural psychotherapies. RC is an empowering co-counseling approach in which two or more individuals take turns listening to each other without interruption in order to recover from the effects of racism, classism, sexism, and other types of oppression (Roby, 1998). Harvey Jackins developed RC based on his belief that everyone has tremendous intellectual and loving potential but that these qualities have become blocked as a result of accumulated distress. Recovery involves a natural discharge process through which the "counselor" encourages the "client" to discharge emotions (catharsis). Afterward, the "client" becomes the "counselor" and listens to the client. RC proponents are committed to ending racism at the individual, collective, and societal levels. For more information, visit www.rc. org.

The struggle against colonization and oppression challenged women's subservient position. As daughters of empowerment movements, feminist therapists embraced diversity as a foundation for practice. Such an empowerment position influenced the development of multicultural psychotherapies. Feminist clinicians believe dominant psychotherapists act as agents of the status quo; in contrast, feminist psychotherapy attempts to empower all people, women as well as men, and promote equality at individual, interpersonal, institutional, national, and international levels (Brown, 2010). Feminist therapy and multicultural therapies equally influence each other. For instance, women of color challenged feminist therapists to become culturally sensitive. As a result, cultural feminist therapy and the feminist therapy of women of color were born. Although cultural feminist therapists use the empathic relationship to increase women's subjectivity, interdependence, connection to others, and other female values (Worell & Remer, 2003), feminist therapists for women of color address the interaction between racism, sexism, classism, heterosexism, ethnocentrism, ableism, and other forms of oppressions.

Ethnic Family Therapy

Like feminist therapy, family therapy has benefited from an interaction with multiculturalism. With its history of recognizing ethnicity and culture in its theory and practice (McGoldrick, Giordano, & Gracia-Preto, 2005), family therapy witnessed the emergence of ethnic family therapy. Ethnic family therapists attempt to (1) know their own culture, (2) avoid ethnocentric attitudes and behaviors, (3) achieve an insider status, (4) use intermediaries, and (5) have selective disclosure. An illustration of ethnic family therapy is Boyd-Franklin's (2003) multisystemic approach in *Black Families in Therapy*. Just as family therapy uses genograms to show the relationships between family members (McGoldrick, Gerson, & Shellenberger, 1999), ethnic family therapists use *cultural genograms* (Hardy & Laszloffy, 1995). Cultural genograms are discussed in more detail later in this McGoldrick chapter.

Several professional and academic organizations have supported the development of multicultural psychotherapies. For example, the American Psychological Association has a recent history of examining the needs of minority populations. Several of its societies—such as the Society of the Psychology of Women, the Society for the Psychological Study of Ethnic Minority Psychology, and the Society for the Psychological Study of Gay, Lesbian, Bisexual and Transgender Issues—are examples. In particular, the Society for the Psychological Study of Ethnic Minority Psychology has promoted the need for multiculturalism in all aspects of psychology, especially in professional psychology. The society's official journal, *Cultural Diversity and Ethnic Minority Psychology*, is an important vehicle for dissemination of scholarly and professional work on multicultural psychology (Comas-Diaz, 2009). Other APA dissemination multicultural psychological outlets include the *Asian American Journal of Psychology* and the *Journal of Latina/o Psychology*.

Counseling psychologists demonstrated a commitment to multicultural issues and have recognized the importance of multiculturalism in publications such as the

Journal of Multicultural Counseling and Development. Feminist psychologists find an outlet for their writing in journals such as *Psychology of Women Quarterly*, the official journal of the American Psychological Association Society of the Psychology of Women. In addition, the Association of Women in Psychology publishes its official journal, *Women & Therapy*.

The ethnic minority psychological associations—the Asian American Psychological Association, the Association of Black Psychologists, the National Latina(o) Psychological Association, and the Society of Indian Psychologists—have been powerful advocates for the mental-health needs of people of color. The Council of National Psychological Associations for the Advancement of Ethnic Minority Issues is a coalition composed of the APA Society for the Psychological Study of Ethnic Minority Issues, the Asian American Psychological Association, the Association of Black Psychologists, the National Latina(o) Psychological Association, and the Society of Indian Psychologists. This group advocates for the delivery of effective psychological services to people of color. In addition, the Society for the Study of Culture and Psychiatry is an interdisciplinary and international society devoted to furthering research, clinical care, and education in cultural *aspects* of mental health and illness (www.psychiatryandculture.org/cms/).

Current Status

The collectivistic concept of unity through diversity achieved prominence during the 21st century. Multiculturalism promotes empowerment, change, and a transformative dialogue on oppression and privilege. Indeed, multicultural psychotherapists advocate for social justice action (Comas-Diaz, 2012b; Ratts, D'Andrea, & Arredondo, 2004).

The creation of the American Psychological Association Office of Ethnic Minority Affairs advanced the role of multiculturalism in psychological theory and practice. This office provided a forum for ethnic minority psychologists to voice their concerns about the lack of cultural relevance in psychological practice. Afterward, the establishment of the American Psychological Association's Society for the Psychological Study of Ethnic Minority Issues helped cement the position of multicultural psychotherapies. Currently, multicultural psychotherapists practice following three models: (1) a cultural adaptation of dominant psychotherapy, (2) ethnic psychotherapies, and (3) holistic approaches. Psychotherapists frequently combine these frameworks.

Psychotherapy can be culturally adapted through the development of generic cross-cultural skills or through the incorporation of culture specific skills (Lo & Fung, 2003). The generic term *cultural competence* refers to knowledge and skills required to work effectively in any cross-cultural clinical encounter. Psychotherapists working within the culture-specific skills level assimilate ethnic dimensions into mainstream psychotherapy. As an example of culture specificity, Bernal, Bonilla, and Bellido (1995) recommended the inclusion of eight cultural dimensions—language, persons, metaphors, content, concepts, goals, method, and context—into mainstream psychotherapy. Within this framework, therapists use culturally appropriate *language* to fit client's worldview and life circumstances. The dimension of *persons* refers to the therapeutic relationship. *Metaphors* relate to concepts shared by members of a cultural group. The dimension of *content* refers to a therapist's cultural knowledge (e.g., Does the client feel understood by the therapist?). *Concepts* examine whether the treatment concepts are culturally consonant with the client's context. The dimension of *goals* examines whether clinical objectives are congruent with clients' adaptive cultural values. *Methods* pertain to the cultural adaptation and validation of methods and instruments. Finally, Bernal and his associates defined *context* as clients' environment, including history and sociopolitical circumstances.

In another example of culture specificity, Ricardo Muñoz (Muñoz & Mendelson, 2005) suggested culturally adapting CBT through (1) involving culturally diverse people in the development of interventions, (2) including collectivistic values, (3) attending to religion or spirituality, (4) paying attention to the relevance of acculturation, and (5) acknowledging the effects of oppression on mental health. Notwithstanding CBT's evidence-based foundation, there is a dearth of empirical studies on the cultural validity of empirically supported treatments (Hall, 2001). Consequently, multicultural practitioners identified the need for culture-specific psychotherapy with an evidence base to address the day-to-day realities of people of color. As a response, the American Psychological Association's presidential task force included in its definition of evidence-based practice in psychology the integration of patients' characteristics, culture, and preferences with clinical expertise and research (APA, 2006).

Pamela Hays (2008) provided an example of a successful incorporation of cultural elements into therapy, highlighting cultural complexities in the conceptualization of identity. Her ADDRESSING framework recognizes the interacting cultural influences of Age, Developmental and acquired Disabilities, Religion, Ethnicity, Socioeconomic status, Sexual orientation, Indigenous heritage, National origin, and Gender. Another culturally adapted psychotherapy, culturally sensitive psychotherapy (CSP), targets specific ethnocultural groups so that one group may benefit more from a specific intervention than from interventions designed for another (Hall, 2001). Furthermore, ethnocultural psychotherapy integrates cultural variables in treatment through the examination of worldviews, cultural transitions, relationships, and context (Comas-Diaz & Jacobsen, 2004).

Notwithstanding psychotherapy's cultural adaptation, several multiculturalists advocated for the use of ethnic psychotherapies in order to reaffirm their ethnocultural roots. As ethnic psychotherapies provide continuity, they may help clients repair their fractured identities. Ethnic and indigenous psychotherapies appeal to culturally diverse individuals because they are grounded in a cultural context and thus are responsive to clients' life experiences. They offer a culturally relevant framework that validates racial and ethnic meanings. Moreover, ethnic psychotherapies are based on a philosophical spiritual foundation that promotes connective, ancestral, and sacred affiliations in healing. As a result, they impart hope to sufferers, particularly when dominant psychotherapy approaches fail. Ethnic psychotherapies empower at both individual and collective levels. Some of the ethnic psychotherapies include folk healing, network therapy, narratives, the psychology of liberation, and holistic approaches based on Eastern philosophical traditions.

A historical antecedent of multicultural psychotherapies, folk healing is form of indigenous psychotherapy. Folk healing reestablishes clients' sense of cultural belonging and historical continuity, promotes self-healing, and nurtures a balance between the sufferer, family, community, and cosmos (Comas-Diaz, 2006). Folk healers use mechanisms similar to those used by mainstream psychotherapists; the main difference revolves around folk healers' spiritual belief systems. In other words, folk healers foster empowerment, encourage liberation, and promote spiritual development. APA multicultural guideline number 5 encourages psychologists to strive to learn about non-Western healing traditions that could be appropriately integrated into psychotherapy. When appropriate, this guideline encourages psychologists to acknowledge and enlist the assistance of recognized helpers (community leaders, change agents) and traditional healers in treatment.

Following these notions, Carolyn Attneave developed network therapy as an extended family treatment and group intervention (Speck & Attneave, 1973). Based on a Native American healing approach, network therapy re-creates the entire social context of a clan's network in order to activate and mobilize a person's family, kin, and relationships in the healing process. Network therapy is a community-based form of healing.

Another communal ethnic psychotherapy is the psychology of liberation. Based on the Latin American theology of liberation, the psychotherapy of liberation emerged as a response to sociopolitical oppression. Its architect—Ignacio Martín-Baro (in Blanco, 1998)—was both a psychologist and a priest. Likewise, psychology of liberation resonates with African American psychology based on black liberation theology and Africanist traditions. Such a spiritual basis affirms ethno-racial-cultural strengths through indigenous traditions and practices. Liberation practitioners attempt to work with people in context through strategies that enhance awareness of oppression and of the ideologies and structural inequality that have kept them subjugated and oppressed. Similar to Paulo Freire's critical consciousness, liberation therapists collaborate with the oppressed in developing critical analysis and engaging in transformative actions.

Ethnic psychotherapists frequently use narratives as a form of treatment. Therefore, stories are context-rich communications full of cultural nuances and meanings. Indeed, telling a story is a collectivistic way of relating. A reaction to Latin American political oppression, *testimonio* chronicles traumatic experiences and how these have affected the individual, family, and community (Cienfuegos & Monelli, 1982). Another healing narrative, *cuento* therapy, has been empirically proven to be an effective treatment for Puerto Rican children (Costantino, Malgady, & Rogler, 1997). Furthermore, *dichos* (sayings) are a form of flash psychotherapy that consists of Spanish proverbs or idiomatic expressions that capture folk wisdom (Comas-Díaz, 2006).

PERSONALITY

Theory of Personality

Multicultural psychotherapists recognize the development of identity within several contexts. As mind inhabits the body, personality develops within multiple contexts. Multicultural clinicians acknowledge multiple perspectives, hence they adhere to diverse theories of personality and follow theories that are consistent with their preferred theoretical orientation. However, multicultural psychotherapies' unique contribution to the theory of personality is the formulation of cultural identity development theories.

Cultural Identity Development

Following Gehrie's (1979) assertion, multicultural psychotherapists view the self as an internal representation of culture. For instance, being a member of an oppressed minority group influences identity development. The identify formation of people of color involves both personal identity and cultural-racial-ethnic group identity. Minority identity developmental theories illuminate the worldviews of people of color. The minority identity development theories offer a lens for understanding how individuals process and perceive the world. Indeed, the ethnic and racial identity stage affects beliefs, emotions, behaviors, attitudes, expectations, and interpersonal style. As a result, these stages influence how individuals present to treatment and even how they select their psychotherapist.

The diverse models of minority identity development propose that members of racial and ethnic minority groups initially value the dominant group and devalue their own group, then move to value their own group while devaluing the dominant group, and then, in a final stage, integrate appreciation for both groups (Atkinson, Morten, & Sue, 1998). More specifically, minority identity development stages include:

1. conformity—individuals internalize racism and choose values, lifestyles, and role models from the dominant group;
2. dissonance—individuals begin to question and suspect the dominant group's cultural values;
3. resistance-immersion—individuals endorse minority-held views and reject the dominant culture's values;
4. introspection—individuals establish their racial ethnic identity without following all cultural norms, beginning to question how certain values fit with their personal identity; and
5. synergistic—individuals experience a sense of self-fulfillment toward their racial-ethnic-cultural identity without having to categorically accept their minority group's values.

Moreover, a key milestone in the racial identity development of people of color is overcoming internalized racism and becoming critically conscientized.

Racial identity development potentially interacts with client and therapist ethnic match. Consider the case of Jose, a bilingual, bicultural teacher. Jose's racial ethnic identity placed him at the dissonance stage (characterized by suspicion of whites). When referred to a mental-health center, Jose refused to see a European American therapist. He asked to see a counselor who "spoke his language and understood" his culture. When Dr. Delgado was assigned to see Jose, the therapist said, "I'm sorry, I don't speak Spanish." Jose answered, "That's okay, I just didn't want to see a white therapist." Jose's case illustrates the relevance of understanding racial identity developmental stages.

Racial identity development models extend to members of the dominant society. A white American identity developmental theory suggests that European Americans develop a specific cultural identity because of their status as members of the dominant majority group. According to Janet Helms (1990), white American cultural racial identity occurs in specific stages:

1. contact—individuals are aware of minorities but do not perceive themselves as racial beings;
2. disintegration—they acknowledge prejudice and discrimination;
3. reintegration—they engage in blaming the victim and in reverse discrimination;
4. pseudoindependence—they become interested in understanding cultural differences; and
5. autonomy—they learn about cultural differences and accept, respect, and appreciate both minority and majority group members.

Similarly, identity developmental stages have been proposed for biracial individuals (Poston, 1990). These are (1) personal identity, (2) choice of group categorization, (3) enmeshment or denial, (4) appreciation, and (5) integration.

Multicultural psychotherapies also contributed to the formulation of gays' and lesbians' minority identity development. Gay and lesbian identity developmental stages include:

1. confusion—individuals question their sexual orientation;
2. comparison—individuals accept the possibility that they may belong to a sexual minority;
3. tolerance—recognition that one is gay or lesbian;

4. acceptance—individuals increase contacts with other gays and lesbians;

5. pride—people prefer to be gay or lesbian; and

6. synthesis—people find peace with their own sexual orientation and reach out to supportive heterosexuals (Cass, 2002).

Feminist identity developmental theory also emerged from the minority identity developmental models. The feminist identity development theory articulates the premise that women struggle and continuously work through their reactions to the prejudice and discrimination they encounter to achieve a positive feminist identity. According to Downing and Roush (1985), feminist identity develops as (1) passive acceptance, (2) revelation, (3) embeddedness or emanation, (4) synthesis, and (5) active commitment.

Variety of Concepts

Multicultural psychotherapists aim to empower clients by fostering their cultural identity development. To promote this goal, psychotherapists reinforce clients' strengths rather than focus on deficits. In this fashion, multicultural psychotherapists promote *cultural resilience*—a set of strengths, values, and practices that enhances the coping mechanisms and adaptive reactions of clients of color to trauma and oppression (Elsass, 1992).

Within this framework, multicultural psychotherapists encourage clients of color to develop *cultural consciousness*, a process that helps clients increase their psychocultural awareness. In other words, psychotherapists assist clients of color to rescue their ethnocultural legacies in order to reauthor their history. Likewise, psychotherapists aim to develop *multicultural consciousness* during and beyond the clinical hour. Multicultural consciousness refers to therapists' internalization and incorporation of cultural competence into their everyday activities and into every aspect of their behavior (Comas-Díaz, 2012).

Equally important, multicultural consciousness fosters the development of *cultural intelligence*, which is the understanding of the impact of culture on individuals' behavior. Cultural intelligence requires inductive and analogical reasoning because individuals need these forms of thinking to approach and understand a new context without being constrained by previous experiences and preconceived ideas (Early & Ang, 2003). Multicultural psychotherapists aspire to promote cultural intelligence among their clients as well as among themselves.

PSYCHOTHERAPY

Theory of Psychotherapy

Multicultural psychotherapists do not subscribe to a unifying theory of psychotherapy; instead, they endorse multiple perspectives. Such a pluralistic framework functions as a metatheory from which clinicians use concepts, strategies, and interventions from diverse therapeutic orientations to conceptualize, critically examine, and empirically evaluate their multiple therapeutic processes (Cooper & McLeod, 2007). Therefore, a multicultural metatheory recognizes that all helping traditions are culturally embedded (Ivey, Ivey, & Simek-Morgan, 1997). Such culture-centered metatheory addresses clients' meaning making and co-construction of reality (Valsiner & Rosa, 2007). However, at the center of their theoretical approach, multicultural psychotherapists attempt to answer the question, "How can a therapist understand the life of a culturally different client?" Multiculturalists view the cultivation of the therapeutic alliance as a crucial aspect in healing and critically important to understanding clients. For this reason, the therapeutic alliance guides the multicultural psychotherapy process.

Cultural Self-Awareness

Multicultural therapeutic encounters are full of conscious or unconscious messages about the client's and the therapist's feelings and attitudes about their cultural backgrounds. Indeed, the perception of cultural differences evokes feelings of being excluded, compared, and relatively powerless (Pinderhughes, 1989). To address these issues, multicultural psychotherapists engage in cultural self-awareness. They initiate the self-awareness by identifying the dominant culture's values in which they communicate and practice. Psychotherapists can explore these issues through the following questions (adapted from Pinderhughes, 1989):

- What is my cultural heritage?
- What was the culture of my parents and ancestors?
- With what cultural group(s) do I identify?
- What is the cultural meaning of my name?
- What is my worldview?
- What aspects of my worldview (values, beliefs, opinions, and attitudes) do I hold that are congruent with the dominant culture's worldview? Which are incongruent?
- How did I decide to become a psychotherapist? How was I professionally socialized? What professional socialization do I maintain? What do I believe to be the relationship between culture and psychotherapy/counseling?
- What abilities, expectations, and limitations do I have that might influence my relations with culturally diverse individuals?

    Other potential questions include:

- How do my clients answer some of the questions above?
- Are there differences between my answers and those of my culturally diverse clients?
- How do I feel about these differences?
- How do I feel about the similarities?

    To further their cultural self-awareness, psychotherapists can use Bennett's (2004) multicultural sensitivity development model. Bennett divided multicultural sensitivity development into ethnocentric and ethnorelative stages. The ethnocentric stages include the following.

1. Denial: Individuals deny the existence of cultural differences and avoid personal contact with culturally diverse people.
2. Defense: Individuals recognize other cultures but denigrate them.
3. Minimization: Individuals view their own culture as universal, and although they recognize cultural differences, they minimize them, believing that other cultures are just like theirs.

    The ethnorelative stages of developing multicultural sensitivity include the following.

1. Acceptance: Individuals recognize and value cultural differences without judging them.
2. Adaptation: Individuals develop multicultural skills; in other words, they learn to shift perspectives and move in and out of alternative worldviews.
3. Integration: Individuals' sense of self expands to include diverse worldviews.

    The development of multicultural sensitivity facilitates appreciation of diverse worldviews and the emergence of a positive therapeutic alliance. Indeed, a successful therapeutic relationship rests on the recognition of the self in the other.

Process of Psychotherapy

The Therapeutic Relationship

Most psychotherapists recognize that a positive alliance increases psychotherapy's effectiveness. Moreover, research has repeatedly demonstrated the importance of the therapeutic relationship as a curative factor. However, the development of a therapeutic alliance requires cultural congruence between clients' and therapists' worldviews. When both therapist and client share worldviews, the development of a positive alliance is enhanced. Conversely, different worldviews may obstruct the development of the therapeutic alliance, and they may require adjustments. For example, Kakar (1985) modified his psychoanalytic approach when working with East Indians by being active and didactic. In addition, he emphasized feeling and expressing pity, interest, and warmth.

Culture affects how clients perceive therapists. For example, cultural attitudes toward authority and healing figures shape clients' expectations about their therapists. If Eastern collectivistic clients perceive therapists as wise teachers, then they will adopt the role of students. The ideal therapist role varies from culture to culture. Hence, psychotherapists need to understand culturally diverse expectations. For example, therapists who have an egalitarian and nondirective style may not work well with clients who prefer hierarchical and directive relationships and specific instructions about what to do to change (Koss-Chioino & Vargas, 1992).

Similarly, Atkinson, Thompson, and Grant (1993) identified eight intersecting therapist roles that depend on clients' acculturation to the mainstream society. They asserted that low acculturated clients expect therapists to behave as *adviser*, *advocate*, or *facilitator of indigenous support systems*. As an illustration, the use of modeling, selective self-disclosure, and didactic strategies seems culturally relevant for low-acculturated immigrant clients. More-acculturated clients may expect their clinician to act as a consultant, change agent, counselor, or psychotherapist.

However, in reality, culturally diverse clients have complex expectations of their therapists. Besides acculturation, clients' expectations are shaped by interpersonal needs, developmental stages, ethnic identity, spirituality, and numerous other factors. Even though clients' expectations range from a collaborative to a hierarchical therapeutic style, these expectations are not mutually exclusive. For instance, regardless of clients' level of acculturation, psychotherapists tend to respond according to their clients' needs. In other words, therapists move from one role to another or simultaneously engage in several helping roles. Along these lines, an empirical investigation found that although clients of color expected to get relief from their problems, they also expected to work in therapy to overcome their contribution to their distress (Comas-Diaz, Geller, Melgoza, & Baker, 1982). Even though they expected their therapist to be active, give advice, teach, and guide them, they also believed that psychotherapists would help them to grow emotionally in a process that at times would be painful. Concisely put, clients of color exhibited psychological mindedness and viewed psychotherapy as a process to work though their issues.

Cultural Empathy

Clients of color expect psychotherapists to demonstrate cultural credibility. *Credibility* refers to the client's perception of the psychotherapist as a trustworthy and effective helper. For example, many American Indians expect psychotherapists to exemplify empathy, genuineness, availability, respect, warmth, congruence, and connectedness. Certainly, a therapist's credibility and trust foster a positive therapeutic alliance. To achieve this goal, multicultural psychotherapists aim to develop empathy for the "other." Empathy is an interpersonal concept referring to a clinician's capacity to attend to the emotional experience of clients. In dominant psychotherapy, empathy has somatic, cognitive, and affective components. The somatic aspect of empathy refers to nonverbal communication and body language. Therapists develop cognitive empathy for culturally diverse clients by becoming empathic witnesses. As empathic witnesses, psychotherapists study clients' culture and reaffirm the clients' experience and reality. Empathy's affective component involves emotional connectedness, a capacity to take in and contain the feelings of the client. Succinctly put, affective empathy is similar to the subjective experience of *being* like the other. Therapists who can only empathize at a cognitive level keep their identity separate from their client's. This "separation" hinders the therapist's development of affective empathy for culturally different clients. Such empathic failure is associated with the difficulty of being "like the other." Indeed, the development of affective empathy is critical in multicultural psychotherapy because we tend to empathize with people who remind us of ourselves; conversely, we have difficulty empathizing with those who are culturally different from us.

Besides cognitive and affective empathy, therapists need to develop cultural empathy. Cultural empathy is a learned ability to obtain an understanding of the experience of culturally diverse individuals informed by cultural knowledge and interpretation (Ridley & Lingle, 1996). Therefore, cultural empathy promotes therapists' cultural responsiveness through the integration of perceptual, cognitive, affective, and communication skills. Cultural empathy involves a process using a cultural framework as a guide for understanding the client and recognizing cultural differences between self and other (Ridley & Lingle, 1996). Interestingly, research has suggested that practitioners reduce their stereotypic and ethnocentric attitudes if they are able to take the perspective of others (Galinsky & Moskowitz, 2000). Thus, cultural empathy entails an attunement to the other—a combined cultural, cognitive, emotional, affective, and behavioral connection to the culturally different person. In short, cultural empathy is the ability to place yourself in the other's culture. As such, it facilitates the recognition of self in the culturally diverse other. Multicultural psychotherapists develop cultural empathy by engaging in self-reflection, unpacking their invisible knapsack, exploring their own worldview, challenging ethnocentrism, developing openness and respect for cultural differences, and understanding power dynamics.

Ethnocultural Transference and Countertransference

The therapeutic relationship is a fertile ground for the projection of conscious and unconscious feelings, and every therapeutic encounter promulgates the projection of conscious or unconscious messages about the client's and the therapist's cultures. The examination of *transference* (clients' projections of feelings from previous relationships onto their therapists) and *countertransference* (therapists' reactions to clients' transference) helps to manage these processes. Although the examination of transference reactions can be an important part of psychotherapy, most dominant psychotherapists ignore transferential cultural issues. Instead, they adhere to the universalistic perspective that endorses a culture-blind and race-neutral position of human relations (Pinderhughes, 1989). Simply put, many clinicians ignore ethnic, cultural, and racial aspects of transference and countertransference.

Multicultural psychotherapists examine transferential reactions through the initiation of a dialogue on cultural differences and similarities. During this dialogue, among others aims, they seek to:

1. suspend preconceptions about clients' race and ethnicity contexts;
2. recognize that clients may be quite different form other members of their racial or ethnic group;

3. consider how racial or ethnic differences between therapist and client may affect psychotherapy;

4. acknowledge that power, privilege, oppression, and racism might affect their interactions with clients; and

5. err on the side of discussion, particularly when in doubt about the role of race and ethnicity in treatment (Cardemil & Battle, 2003).

Moreover, multicultural psychotherapists specifically ask clients questions such as, "How do you feel about my being from a different culture from yours?" and "How do you feel about our being from similar cultures?" This line of questioning fosters a discussion of ethnocultural transference and countertransference.

Ethnocultural transference and countertransference play a significant role in the therapeutic relationship because providers and clients tend to bring their imprinting of ethnic, cultural, and racial experiences into psychotherapy. Ethnocultural reactions can provide a blueprint for the relationship between self and others.

Comas-Díaz and Jacobsen (1991) described several types of ethnocultural transference and countertransference within intra- and interethnic dyads. Some of the interethnic transferential reactions include:

1. overcompliance and friendliness (observed when there is a societal power differential in the client–therapist dyad);

2. denial (when the client avoids disclosing issues pertinent to ethnicity or culture);

3. mistrust, suspiciousness, and hostility ("What are this therapist's real motivations for working with me?"); and

4. ambivalence (clients in an interethnic psychotherapy may struggle with negative feelings toward their therapist while simultaneously developing an attachment to him or her).

Intraethnic transference may transform a client's image of the therapist into one of several predictable roles:

1. the omniscient or omnipotent therapist—fantasy of the reunion with the perfect parent as promoted by the ethnic similarity;

2. the traitor—client exhibits resentment and envy at therapist's successes, which is equated with betrayal of his or her ethnoculture;

3. the autoracist—client does not want to work with a therapist of his or her own ethnocultural group because of projection of strong negative feelings onto the ethnoculturally similar therapist; and

4. the ambivalent—clients may feel at once comfortable with their shared ethnocultural background while at the same time fearing too much psychological closeness.

Some interethnic dyad countertransferential reactions include:

1. denial of cultural differences—we are all the same;

2. the clinical anthropologist's syndrome—excessive curiosity about clients' ethnocultural backgrounds at the expense of their psychological needs;

3. guilt—about societal and political realities that dictate a lower status for people of color;

4. pity—a derivative of guilt or an expression of political impotence within the therapeutic hour;

5. aggression; and

6. ambivalence—toward the client's culture, which may originate from ambivalence toward a therapist's own ethnoculture.

Within the intraethnic dyad, some of the countertransferential manifestations include:

1. overidentification;

2. an us-and-them mentality—shared victimization because of racial discrimination may contribute to therapist ascribing a client's problems as being solely the result of membership in a minority group;

3. distancing;

4. survivor's guilt—therapists may have the personal experience of escaping the harsh socioeconomic circumstances of low-income ethnic minorities, leaving family and friends in the process, and generating guilt—feelings that can impede professional growth and may lead to denying clients' psychological problems;

5. cultural myopia—inability to see clearly because of ethnocultural factors that obscure therapy;

6. ambivalence—working through the therapist's own ethnocultural ambivalence; and

7. anger—being too ethnoculturally close to a client may uncover painful and unresolved intrapsychic issues.

Identifying the cultural parameters of transference and countertransference is central in multicultural psychotherapy. For example, the gendered ethnicity—the gender and ethnicity interaction—can evoke strong countertransference as well as transference. Indeed, multicultural psychotherapists recognize that ethnic, cultural, gender, and racial factors (as well as their intersectionality) often lead to a more rapid unfolding of core problems in psychotherapy.

Mechanisms of Psychotherapy

Multicultural psychotherapists use whatever tools and techniques they learned in graduate school and those endorsed by their theoretical orientations and professional organizations. However, these techniques are not applied automatically and thoughtlessly. These therapists also think carefully and hard about using psychotherapeutic mechanisms that are congruent with their clients' worldviews. For instance, many individualistic group members prefer a verbal therapy that works through and promotes change by *externalizing*, or moving from the unconscious to the conscious. Conversely, a significant number of collectivistic members require a holistic healing approach that acknowledges nonverbal communication and promotes change by *internalizing*, or moving from the conscious to the unconscious (Tamura & Lau, 1992). Therefore, many multicultural psychotherapists integrate holism into their practices. Most of these practices are based on non-Western philosophical and spiritual traditions. In addition to verbal therapy, many clients of color require a mind, body, and spirit approach. For example, Cane (2000) successfully used mind, body, and spirit self-healing practices complemented with a liberation method.

Also known as *contemplative* practices (see Chapter 12), holistic approaches such as meditation, yoga, breathwork, creative visualization, and indigenous healing are gaining popularity among mainstream psychotherapists. With their holistic emphasis, many multicultural psychotherapists promote spiritual development. Spirituality—a sense of connection to self, others, community, history, and context—is an important aspect in the lives of many people of color. Spirituality provides a worldview, a way of life, and a meaning-making process. Within this context, multicultural psychotherapists help individuals overcome adversity and find meaning in their existence. Many people of color require liberation approaches in order to recover from historical and contemporary cultural and racial trauma.

Multicultural psychotherapists foster creativity as part of their holistic approach, and they encourage clients to use art, folklore, ethnic practices, and other creative cultural forms. The therapeutic use of creativity enhances resilience and *cultural consciousness*—the affirmation, redemption, and celebration of one's ethnicity and culture (Comas-Diaz, 2007). For example, many psychotherapists use clients' oral traditions in healing because people of color frequently answer questions by telling a story. This communication style is consistent with an inferential reasoning based on contextual, interpersonal, and historical factors. In other words, telling a story is a creative way of constructing reality in both linear and nonlinear ways, and the patient's narrative combines both analytical and gestalt elements. Asking clients "What happened to you?" offers a cultural holding environment in which the therapist can become an emphatic witness. It is not surprising that storytelling has been found to be effective in cross-cultural psychotherapy (Semmler & Williams, 2000).

Moreover, because of their experiences of disconnection and trauma, people of color use creativity to cope with past trauma and create meaning and purpose in their lives. Examples of such resilient creativity include flamenco music (originated by gypsy or Romaney people), spoken word (New York Puerto Rican and African American urban spoken poetry), memoirs and narratives of people of color, and other narrative performances. For example, Southeast Indian novelist Chitra Banerjee Divakaruni began to write creatively after immigrating to the United States and confronting her first racist incident (personal communication, May 1, 2002).

Using photos for storytelling enhances self-esteem among visible people of color (Falicov, 1998) and addresses issues of skin color and race. Many oppressed people of color have used creativity as a means of resistance, recovery, redemption, and reformulation.

It is clear that creative activities promote healing. Indeed, songs, chants, music, and dance induce emotional states in patients that affect the way the immune system responds to illness (Lyon, 1993). Holistic healers understand this process very well. They use metaphors to help their clients manipulate sensory, emotional, and cognitive information to alter their perceptions of illness. For example, empirical studies revealed that folk healers who encouraged their patients to publicly perform their dreams in poetry, song, and dance were significantly more effective in healing as opposed to therapists who encouraged their patients to talk about their dreams in private (Joralemon, 1986).

There is an intimate relationship between multiculturalism and creativity, and research has demonstrated that exposure to diverse cultures enhances creativity. To illustrate, Leung, Maddux, Galinsky, and Chiu (2008) empirically showed that the relationship between multicultural experiences and creativity is stronger when people are open to new experiences and when the creative context emphasizes flexibility. In summary, multicultural psychotherapists employ holistic approaches in addition to more traditional psychotherapy mechanisms used in mainstream healing approaches. Out of this amalgamation, with its specific emphasis on cultural strengths, healing emerges.

Ethnopsychopharmacology

All clients come to therapy expecting amelioration of symptoms and some relief from their distress. Medications such as antidepressants are often the quickest way to offer at least temporary relief from pain. Consequently, psychotherapists need to work in tandem with physicians, prescribing psychologists, advanced practice nurses, and other health-care providers to help patients access the medications they need.

Regrettably, ethnocentrism has resulted in culturally diverse clients' mistrust of psychopharmacology. This problem is compounded by the fact that different racial and ethnic minority groups may respond differently to medication than European American individuals (Rey, 2006). Notwithstanding the empirical evidence of the relevance of ethnicity in assessing likely pharmacological response to psychotropic medications (Ruiz, 2000), ignorance of the ways in which different ethnic groups respond to different medications has contributed to misdiagnosis and mistreatment. Ethnopsychopharmacology is the field that specializes in the relationship between ethnicity and responses to medications. For example, African Americans with affective disorders are often misdiagnosed and thus mistreated with antipsychotic medications (Lawson, 2000; Strickland, Ranganeth, & Lin, 1991). Similarly, because of the fact that many health-care providers do not understand or appreciate the different metabolic rates associated with different ethnic groups, many Asians and Latinos are treated inappropriately with psychotropic medications (Ruiz, 2000). Consequently, many people of color have deepened their mistrust of mental-health establishments, especially toward the prescription of psychotropic medications. These individuals fear, sometimes correctly, that psychotherapists' ignorance of ethnic variations in drug metabolization reflects cultural unawareness, incompetence, or indifference.

The field of ethnopsychopharmacology emerged out of the need to address the specific mental-health needs of culturally diverse people. Ethnopsychopharmacologists take special care in assessing potential gender and ethnic interactions when prescribing medications. In addition, they are knowledgeable about the interface of multiculturalism and psychopharmacology (Rey, 2006). For example, it is common for Latinos to share medications with family members and significant others. This practice reflects the cultural value of familism, where family interdependence naturally and predictably results in the sharing of resources. They also may self-medicate and combine medications with herbal remedies. Therefore, multicultural psychotherapists are alert to the need to educate clients about the dangers of self-medication, sharing medications with relatives, using medications obtained over the counter from outside the United States, and combining herbal remedies with psychotropic medications. Besides exploring the biological characteristics that affect response to medications, multicultural clinicians examine their clients' lifestyles. For example, the diets of some people of color contain foods (i.e., Mexican Americans' consumption of cheese) that are incompatible with certain kinds of psychotropic medications (e.g., MAOIs), but this problem can't be assessed unless the clinician knows something about the dietary habits of his or her client. In addition, multicultural psychotherapists collaborate with psychopharmacologists who are knowledgeable about ethnicity medication interactions.

APPLICATIONS

Who Can We Help?

To paraphrase Murray and Kluckhohn (1953), every multicultural therapist is "like all other therapists, like some other therapists, and like no other therapists." In other words, multiculturalists share similarities with all therapists (by virtue of being therapists), with some therapists (by belonging to a particular theoretical orientation), and with no other therapist (because of their unique personal and cultural experiences). Multicultural clinicians engage in diverse therapy formats, including individual, family, and group. In addition, some use community interventions such as network therapy. This section presents specific examples of clinical interventions prevalent in multicultural psychotherapies.

Multicultural psychotherapies apply to everyone because they emphasize a person-in-context model. As such, multicultural practitioners attempt to use culturally appropriate assessment and treatment modalities. However, multicultural psychotherapies are particularly helpful when individuals present to treatment with identity issues, relationship problems, cultural adaptation, ethnic and racial stressors, and conflicts of diverse nature.

Treatment

A multicultural assessment is a process-oriented tool that leads to culturally appropriate treatment. Some examples of multicultural assessment include the explanatory model of distress, cultural formulation, the use of a cultural genogram, and ethnocultural assessment.

Explanatory Model of Distress

Clients' worldviews and life experiences affect how they present their problems to their psychotherapists, the meaning they attribute to their distress, their help-seeking behavior, their level of social support, and their perseverance in treatment (Anderson, 1995). The explanatory model is a culture-centered assessment based on an anthropological method developed to address these issues. In other words, an explanatory model elicits clients' perspectives of their illness, experience, and healing (Kleinman, 1980). Multicultural psychotherapists use the explanatory model to unfold clients' treatment expectations by asking the following questions (Kleinman, 1980):

> What do you call your problem (illness)?
> What do you think your problem (illness) does?
> What do you think the natural course of your illness is?
> What do you fear?
> Why do you think this illness or problem has occurred?
> How do you think the distress should be treated?
> How do want me to help you?
> Who do you turn to for help?
> Who should be involved in decision making?

Cultural Formulation and Analysis

The cultural formulation is a clinical tool for assessment and treatment included in the fourth edition of the American Psychiatric Association's (2000) *Diagnostic and Statistical Manual* (DSM-IV). The cultural formulation is a process-oriented approach that places diagnosis in a cultural context. Although the cultural formulation is a medical model that emphasizes pathology, its application increases psychotherapists' cultural awareness. The cultural formulation examines:

1. individual's cultural identity,
2. cultural explanations for individual illnesses,
3. cultural factors related to the psychosocial environment and levels of functioning,
4. cultural elements of the therapist–client relationship, and
5. overall cultural assessment for diagnosis and treatment (APA, 2000).

The cultural formulation facilitates a cultural analysis. Like the explanatory model of distress, the cultural analysis uncovers the cultural knowledge people use to organize their behaviors and interpret their experiences (Spradley, 1990). Lo and Fung (2003) recommended a cultural analysis based on an object relation treatment model, emphasizing the importance of self and relationships with others and with the world. The domains of the cultural analysis include self, relations, and treatment. According to Lo and Fung, the self-domain captures cultural influences on the psychological aspects of the self that may be relevant in psychotherapy (i.e., affect, cognition, behavior, body, and self-concept, plus individual goals and motivations). The relations domain relates to cultural influence on clients' relationships with family, groups, others, society, possessions, environment, spirituality, and time. The treatment domain accentuates therapy elements influenced by culture such as communication (both verbal and nonverbal), problem-solution models, and the therapeutic relationship.

Cultural Genogram

Psychotherapists use genograms to enhance their cultural self-awareness. A family therapy tool, genograms diagram a genealogical tree that highlights dynamics from a nuclear to an extended family perspective (McGoldrick et al., 1999). Genograms are particularly useful when psychotherapists compare their genealogy to their clients' and examine similarities as well as differences. Many psychotherapists complete their own genogram during personal therapy or professional training. You can see how to complete a genogram at www.genopro.com/genogram_rules/default.htm.

Although the genogram is a well-known family therapy tool, few psychotherapists complete their cultural genograms, even when working with multicultural clients. Hardy and Laszloffy (1995) developed the cultural genogram as a tool to emphasize the role of culture and collective contexts in the lives of individuals and their families. Cultural genograms diagram the genealogical, developmental, historical, political, economical, sociological, ethnic, spiritual and religious, and racial influences in people's lives. The cultural genogram places individuals within their communal contexts.

Clinicians begin a cultural genogram with three or more generations of ancestors. If appropriate and if the information is unavailable, they invite clients to use their imaginations to summon up family information. To aid in this process, clients bring family photos to therapy sessions. This approach is useful when discussing racial differences and other types of physical characteristics. In preparing the cultural genogram, Hardly and Lazloffy recommended the use of color to designate different ethnic groups and mixed colors to identity mixed race individuals. Likewise, clients can use their creativity—drawing, painting, sculpting, and so on—to prepare their cultural genogram. Cultural genograms share the symbols used in family genograms such as squares to designate males and circles for females, in addition to symbols specific to cultural genograms (Comas-Diaz, 2012).

The following factors can be used in completing a cultural genogram (adapted from Comas-Diaz & Ramos Grenier, 1998; Hardy Lazloffy, 1995):

- Individual and family culture(s)
- Meaning of race:
  - identity and identification; and
  - significance of skin color, body type, hair texture, phenotype.
- Meaning of ethnicity:
  - national origin, collective history, wars, conflicts with other ethnic groups;
  - languages spoken by client, family of origin, and current family; and
  - ethnocultural heritage.
- Sexual orientation:
  - interaction of gender, ethnicity, race, class, and sexual orientation.
- Family:
  - intact, blended, single parent, nuclear, extended, multigenerational, and so forth; and
  - cultural meanings of family roles.

- Adoption and foster parenting:
  - family of origin and multigenerational history;
  - assessment of non–blood-related extended family members;
  - family life-cycle development and stages;
  - family structure (nuclear, extended, traditional, intact, reconstituted); and
  - gender and family roles.
- Social class:
  - educational level;
  - financial history (e.g., Great Depression, culture of poverty, change in socioeconomic class); and
  - occupation and avocation.
- Marriage:
  - common-law, civil law, religious, commitment ceremonies, same-sex unions, and so on;
  - gender roles; and
  - gender-specific trauma.
- Relations (intimate, friends, comrades or padres, sister friends, etc.):
  - intraethnic and interethnic.
- Migration:
  - history of (im)migration and generations from (im)migrations; and
  - patterns, reasons for migration.
- Refugee experience
- Refugee trauma
- Acculturation:
  - assimilation, separation, marginalization, and integration.
- Stress:
  - types of stress,
  - acculturative stress,
  - life stressors,
  - ecological stress (e.g., inner-city living), and
  - stress management.
- Spirituality and faith:
  - spiritual assessment and
  - use of contemplative practices.
- History and politics
- Trauma:
  - political torture and repression;
  - history of slavery, colonization, holocaust, genocide, wars; and
  - history of human trafficking.
- Sexual and gender trauma:
  - rape, incest, molestation, and harassment.
- Meaning of differences:
  - individual, family, group, and community.

Multicultural psychotherapists frequently complement their use of cultural genograms with community genograms (Rigazio-DiGillio, Ivey, Grady, & Kunkler- Peck, 2005) and spiritual genograms (Hodge, 2000). In addition, they use ecomaps to examine clients' relationships and connections to multiple systems such as significant others, neighborhoods, service providers, and social support systems (Hartman, 1995). When working with clients with a history of immigration, multicultural psychotherapists use a culturagram to map their cultural translocations (Congress, 2002).

Finally, multicultural assessments can be complemented with a *power-differential analysis*. Such analysis requires going beyond the power differential inherent in the psychotherapist–client dyad. It should include an analysis of the client's cultural group's social status compared with the practitioner's. This comparison entails the identification and challenge of internalized privilege and oppression

Ethnocultural Assessment

A multicultural tool for both evaluation and treatment, the ethnocultural assessment explores diverse areas in the development of cultural identity. The domains of ethnocultural assessment include heritage, journey, self-adjustment, and relationships (Comas-Diaz & Jacobsen, 2004). In exploring heritage, therapists examine clients' ethnocultural ancestry (including parents' genealogy), history, genetics, and sociopolitical contexts. Of particular relevance is the examination of cultural trauma. Exploring journey entails examining the family, clan, and group story. In addition, they explore their clients' history of immigration and other significant transitions. Moreover, they explore the posttransition analysis, giving special attention to clients' intellectual and emotional interpretation of their journey. Therapists examine clients' individual adaptation separate from their family during the self-adjustment phase. Clients' coping styles, including cultural resilience, are assessed in this domain. In the relationships domain, therapists explore clients' significant affiliations, including the therapeutic relationship.

Evidence

Multicultural psychotherapists combine cultural knowledge with clinical skills and ecological understanding. Instead of endorsing cultural reductionism, they argue for research on the effectiveness of multicultural approaches to psychotherapy—that is, they advocate for research findings that are applicable to the lives of culturally diverse individuals and communities. Multicultural psychotherapies' evidence base is a reality-based perspective, one that moves from the "couch to the bench" and from the "clinic to the laboratory." Such an approach reflects the need for psychotherapy research to be culturally relevant and accountable to ethnic communities.

Some early psychotherapy research focused on ethnic similarities between psychotherapists and clients. Empirical findings suggested that clients working with psychotherapists of similar ethnic backgrounds and languages tended to remain in treatment longer than those whose therapists were not ethnically or linguistically similar. However, ethnic and linguistic match does not necessarily translate into mutual cultural identification (Hall, 2001) nor is it necessarily desirable for some clients. A review of the research on therapist–client ethnic matching revealed inconclusive results and low validity for ethnic matching (Karlsson, 2005). Nonetheless, research has indicated that clients of color in similar race dyads participate more in their care than do those in racially dissimilar dyads (Cooper-Patrick et al., 1999). In contrast, an empirical study on the effects of ethnic matching on treatment satisfaction among migrant patients showed that these clients did not view ethnic matching as important, and they considered clinical competence, compassion, and sharing their worldview as far more important factors (Knipscheer & Kleber, 2004). In toto, however, the available research suggests that culturally competent therapists enhance their clients' satisfaction with treatment.

Much more research is needed on multicultural psychotherapies. Some of the questions that need to be answered include the following:

What kinds of treatments work best with which kind of clients?

What is the connection between a psychotherapist's cultural competence and his or her treatment outcomes?

What is spirituality's effect on psychotherapy effectiveness?

What are the effects of cultural resilience on physical and mental health? How does language (e.g., bilingualism, being a polyglot) influence psychotherapy process?

How do creativity and multicultural experiences affect mental health?

What are the gender, ethnobiological, and neurohomonal factors that influence clients' responses to psychotropic medications?

What are the cultural and ethical contexts of therapists' self-disclosure?

The empirical exploration of these questions and others can reveal the effectiveness of multicultural therapy.

Psychotherapy in a Multicultural World

The inclusion of a section in each chapter of *Current Psychotherapies* on multicultural psychotherapy—and, of more significance, the addition of an entire chapter devoted to the topic in the two most recent editions—underscores the growing importance of multicultural issues for all psychotherapists. Students who are reading this chapter are encouraged to go back and reread the multicultural sections of all of the other psychotherapy specific chapters and evaluate these sections, these chapters, and these therapies vis-à-vis what they have learned from reading the current chapter. To facilitate this process, students can examine the clinical insights provided by the application of multicultural psychotherapies in the following case illustration.

CASE EXAMPLE

Grace:	I don't know why I'm here.
Dr. Martin:	You are wondering why you are in therapy.
Grace:	Don't paraphrase me. I hate it when shrinks do that.
Dr. Martin:	It sounds like you have been in therapy before.
Grace:	Yes, and I despised it.
Dr. Martin:	What did you despise?
Grace:	I was never understood.
Dr. Martin:	Help me understand you.
Grace:	It's simple: Just listen to me, look at me. What do you see?
Dr. Martin:	An attractive young woman who needs help and doesn't know why she is here.
Grace:	Now you are getting somewhere. Anything else?
Dr. Martin:	How do you see yourself?
Grace:	What do you mean?
Dr. Martin:	Let's start with where do you come from? Family, ethnic, racial, cultural background.
Grace:	You are the first shrink who asked me that. Hum . . . Although I look white, I'm mixed race.

Background

Grace was the daughter of an African American man and a white European American woman. She grew up in an upper-middle-class family; her father worked as a clinic administrator and her mother as a high school teacher. Both parents grew up Catholic and sent Grace to Catholic school. She excelled at academics until her senior year when she experienced a traumatic loss. A drunk driver killed her boyfriend, Adolph, who was on his way home after leaving his 17th birthday party.

"I created a macabre dance," Grace said as she described her birthday gift to Adolph—a choreographed birthday dance. Dr. Martin noticed that Grace did not cry while relating the tragedy.

After the accident, Grace's grades plummeted. She saw three different therapists, all of whom she fired.

Grace's developmental history was unremarkable. Her health history indicated episodic sleep paralysis during times of severe stress. Based on her sleep laboratory study, Grace received medication (Tofranil 25 mg) to control her symptoms. However, she stopped treatment because of side effects from the medication. "I have a sleep paralysis episode every year on Adolph's birthday," Grace said. On completion of the explanatory model of distress, Grace told Dr. Martin, "This is the first time I feel a therapist listened to me." Dr. Martin cemented the emerging therapeutic alliance by teaching Grace relaxation techniques. Grace expressed some relief from her anxiety symptoms.

Assessment

Grace's responses to the explanatory model of distress revealed a fear of being cursed. Immediately after her birth, Grace's father lost his job. The "curse" continued until two years later when her parents had a second child. "My sister Mary brought joy and luck," Grace said. "My parents won the lottery and used the money to pay for my father's graduate studies." "What did your parents think about your 'curse'?" Dr. Martin asked Grace. "My mother denied it, but Dad has always been distant from me." As further evidence of her "curse," Grace connected her "macabre dance" with Adolph's death.

When asked about her views on her problem, Grace responded, "I'm a 25 year old woman looking for myself."

Cultural Genogram

Dr. Martin invited Grace to complete a cultural genogram. Grace began to gather information by talking with her relatives. She traced her maternal family to Germany back three generations. Dr. Martin asked her to bring photos of her relatives to therapy sessions. In response, Grace compiled a photo album and complemented it with drawings. She chose a pink color to identify her maternal ancestors and assigned lavender to her paternal side of the family. At this time, Grace did not choose a color to identify herself in the cultural genogram.

Grace had a dream about a town in Germany during the completion of her cultural genogram. She conducted research and discovered that part of her maternal family was from an area that Germany annexed from Denmark. She found a great aunt of German-Danish ancestry and began communicating with her by Internet. Fortunately, her great aunt spoke enough English to communicate with Grace.

Grace became a genealogy fan and researched her paternal ancestry. She discovered that her father was a descendant of the free people of color in New Orleans. As the term implies, free people of color were not enslaved during the United States slavery period. Most of the free people of color were of mixed race and had similar rights to whites—that is, they owned property, were educated, and participated in diverse occupations and professions. This legacy filled Grace with excitement and pride. "I'm the product of contradictions." The exploration of Grace's contrasts led to the examination of her cultural identity development. At the beginning of treatment, Grace appeared to be at the biracial identity appreciation stage. Her words during the first session with Dr. Martin, "Although I look white, I'm mixed race," denoted positive regard for her mixed race identity. It is interesting that Grace's genealogy work signaled her movement toward an integrative stage where biracial identity began to coalesce. Grace selected a gold color to self-identify at the completion of her cultural genogram.

Treatment

Dr. Martin worked on Grace's complicated bereavement during the beginning stages of treatment. However, before deepening the treatment, Dr. Martin—a European American middle-aged married woman—engaged in cultural self-assessment. The process revealed an English and Italian ethnocultural heritage. Both maternal and paternal great-grandparents had been immigrants. Dr. Martin compared her ethnocultural heritage with Grace's. Like her client, she felt proud of being a product of the union of two ethnicities. Also like her client, Dr. Martin had received a Catholic school education. Another connection between them was the loss of a significant person during adolescence; Dr. Martin's best friend died after an accident during her senior year in high school. These similarities seemed to facilitate Dr. Martin's development of empathy. Nonetheless, the therapist acknowledged not knowing was like to be a mixed-race woman.

Grief work helped Grace accept Adolph's death. Her anxiety symptoms decreased. However, Adolph's next birthday and death anniversary found Grace with another episode of sleep paralysis. Grace described it to Dr. Martin. "It's like someone is sitting on my chest and I can't move. Grandma says that when this happens, a witch is riding you."

Dr. Martin researched the topic of sleep paralysis and found that the condition is prevalent among some African Americans who suffer from anxiety (Paradis & Freidman, 2005). After reviewing the literature, Dr. Martin suggested that Grace consult her grandmother about the "riding witch." Grace, who was named after her paternal grandmother, reported that her grandmother believed Adolph to be the cause of her sleep affliction. When Dr. Martin asked her what she thought about this explanation, Grace replied that relationships don't end with death. Indeed, some people of color believe that relationships between significant others continue after death.

Dr. Martin used grief counseling to treat Grace's complicated bereavement. Although Grace was able to sleep better, she continued to experience sleep paralysis. Dr. Martin interpreted Grace's symptoms as survivor's guilt and treated Grace with cognitive-behavioral techniques. After several months of treatment, Dr. Martin began to feel frustrated and angry toward Grace. She examined her countertransference and realized that she was comparing her own grief (around her friend's death) with Grace's experience of losing Adolph. Dr. Martin consulted a colleague and worked through her own bereavement. Afterward, Dr. Martin suggested a guided-imagery exercise to Grace. She asked Grace to remember the last time she saw Adolph. Grace used the relaxation techniques she learned in therapy to help her visualization.

"Adolph just turned into my father," Grace said during the exercise. "Was Adolph black?" asked Dr. Martin. "Yes," Grace answered.

Dr. Martin realized that she had an ethnocultural countertransference involving a cultural denial. She had assumed that Adolph was white. The realization that Adolph was African American helped her better understand Grace's circumstances around his death. Dr. Martin interpreted Grace's reaction to Adolph's death as a repetition of a pattern in which Grace felt abandoned by significant others (like her father's reaction to her "curse"). Dr. Martin worked with Grace on this dynamic interpretation. She suggested another holistic guided visualization. In this exercise, Dr. Martin asked Grace to relax deeply and imagine a safe and serene place. Grace saw herself choreographing a new dance. While she danced, Grace envisioned herself getting healed. She named the piece the Dance of Life.

Grace did not experience sleep paralysis during Adolph's next birthday and death anniversary. She examined her relationships with significant others during the rest of psychotherapy. Grace improved her relationship with her father, and for the first time she felt close to her sister Mary. Her grandmother died during the last phase of therapy. Grace experienced sadness but completed her bereavement. Afterward, Grace formed an advocacy group to raise community consciousness about drunk driving. Grace stayed in therapy for two and a half years. On her last therapy session, she told Dr. Martin, " I found myself. " She took a tissue from the Kleenex box. "I finally own my name. No longer a curse, I'm a Grace to my family, community, and to myself."

SUMMARY

The United States' population is becoming more culturally, racially, and ethnically diverse. The election of the first president of color of the United State is a sign of such diversity. Multiculturalism emerged as a product of sociopolitical and civil rights movements. Multicultural theories of psychotherapy came to light out of the concerns of people of color, and they were later expanded to embrace diversity regarding gender, sexual orientation, class, religion spirituality, age, ability, and disability.

Originally considered a transforming force in psychology, multiculturalism is at the vanguard of psychotherapy. To illustrate, multicultural theories constitute a shift in psychological paradigm. They provide conceptual and practical methods designed to enhance all types of clinical interventions. Multicultural psychotherapies facilitate adaptation and growth because they address the management of diverse and complex environments. With their emphasis on context, multicultural theories enhance our ability to cope with change and thus foster transformation and evolution.

Multicultural psychotherapies promote the development of cultural competence as a lifelong process. Fostering flexibility, they facilitate the incorporation of pluralistic and holistic approaches into practice. Multicultural theories accommodate the current resurgence of ancient healing traditions and promote their integration into mainstream psychotherapy.

As every human encounter is multicultural in nature, multicultural psychotherapies are relevant to all individuals. They offer tools for the effective management of differences, similarities, and power disparities. Finally, multicultural theories facilitate our adjustment to the globalization of our society. They offer a compass for the multicultural journey on which all of us embark.

Counseling CourseMate Website:

See this text's Counseling CourseMate website at www.cengagebrain.com for learning tools such as chapter quizzing, videos, glossary flashcards, and more.

ANNOTATED BIBLIOGRAPHY

Bernal, G., & Domenech Rodriguez, M. (Eds.) (2012). *Cultural adaptations: Tools for evidence-based practice with diverse populations*. Washington, DC: American Psychological Association.
This edited book promotes culturally adapted evidence-based practice as empirically viable approaches for treating ethnic minorities.

Comas-Díaz, L. (2012). *Multicultural care: A clinician's guide to cultural competence*. Washington, DC: American Psychological Association.
This clinically applicable text is grounded in scholarship and research. It presents complex clinical material and multicultural strategies in accessible ways.

Fadiman, A. (1997). *The spirit catches you and you fall down: A Hmong child, her American doctors and the collision of two cultures*. New York: Noonday Press (Farrar, Straus & Giroux).
This true story of cultural misunderstanding within the healing profession illustrates the utility of the explanatory model of distress.

Gerstein, L. H., Hepper, P. P., Ægisdóttir, S., Leong, S-M. A., & Norsworthy, K. (Eds.). (2009). *International handbook of cross-cultural counseling: Cultural assumptions and practices worldwide*. Thousand Oaks, CA: Sage.
This is an excellent resource for psychotherapists who work with international and cross-cultural clients.

Hoffman, E. (1989). *Lost in translation: A life in a new language*. New York: Penguin Books.
In this superb memoir, an immigrant woman struggles with cultural change and eventually becomes a psychotherapist.

Pinderhughes, E. (1989). *Understanding race, ethnicity, and power: The key to efficacy in clinical practice*. New York: The Free Press.
This classic text articulates the relationship between race, ethnicity, and power in clinical work.

Ridley, C. R. (1995). *Overcoming unintentional racism in counseling and therapy: A practitioner's guide to intentional intervention*, Thousand Oaks: Sage.
An eye opener, this book offers practical guidelines for clinicians to overcome prejudice and racism.

Web resources

www.apa.org/pi/oema/guide.html
American Psychological Association Guidelines for Providers of Psychological Services to Ethnic, Linguistic, and Culturally Diverse Populations

www.genopro.com/genogram_rules/default.htm
Psychological Treatment of Ethnic Minority Populations (Council of National Psychological Associations, 2003)

www.apa.org/pi/oema/resources/brochures/treatment-minority.pdf

CASE READING

Comas-Díaz, L. (2006). Latino healing: The integration of ethnic psychology into psychotherapy. *Psychotherapy: Theory, Research, Practice, Training, 46*(4), 463–453.

One of these cases is reprinted in D. Wedding & R. J. Corsini (Eds.) (2013). *Case studies in psychotherapy*. Belmont, CA: Cengage.

This article illustrates the integration of ethnic psychotherapy into mainstream psychotherapy and includes examples of Latino ethnic psychology such as *cuento, dichos*, and spirituality.

REFERENCES

Allport, G. W. (1954). *The nature of prejudice*. Cambridge, MA: Addison-Wesley.

Altman, N. (1995). *The analyst in the inner city: Race, class and culture through a psychoanalytic lens*. New York: Analytic Press.

Altman, N. (2010). *The analyst in the inner city* (2nd ed.) New York: Routledge.

American Psychiatric Association. (2000). *Diagnostic and statistical manual of mental disorders* (4th ed., Text revision). Washington, DC: Author.

American Psychological Association. (1990). *Guidelines for providers of psychological services to ethnic, linguistic, and culturally diverse populations.* Washington, DC: Office of Ethnic Minority Affairs, American Psychological Association. Retrieved from www.apa.org/pi/oema/guide.html

American Psychological Association. (2003). Guidelines on multicultural education, training, research, practice, and organizational change. *American Psychologist, 58,* 377–402.

American Psychological Association. (2010). *Ethical principles of psychologists and code of conduct with the 2010 amendments*. Retrieved from www.apa.org/ethics/code/index.aspx

American Psychological Association, Presidential Task Force on Evidence-Based Practice (2006). Evidence-based practice in psychology. *American Psychologist, 6*(4), 271–285.

Anderson, N. (1995). Behavioral and sociological perspectives on ethnicity and health: Introduction to the special issue. *Health Psychology, 14,* 589–591.

Atkinson, D. R., Morten, G., & Sue, D. W. (1998). *Counseling American minorities: A cross cultural perspective* (5th edition). New York: McGraw-Hill.

Atkinson, D. R., Thompson, C. E., & Grant, S. K. (1993). A three-dimensional model for counseling racial/ethnic minorities. *Counseling Psychologist, 21*, 257–277.

Bennett, M. J. (2004). From ethnocentrism to ethnorelativism. In J. S. Wurzel (Ed.), *Toward multiculturalism: A reader in multicultural education* (pp. 62–77). Newton, MA: Intercultural Resource Corporation.

Bernal, G. Bonilla, J., & Bellido, C. (1995). Ecological validity and cultural sensitivity for outcome research: Issues for cultural adaptation and development of psychosocial treatments with Hispanics. *Journal of Abnormal Child Psychology, 23*(1), 67–82.

Betancourt, J. R., Green, A. R., Carrillo, J. E., & Ananch-Firempong, O. (2003, July–August). Defining cultural competence: A practical framework for addressing racial/ethnic disparities in health and health care. *Public Health Reports, 118*, 293–302.

Blanco, A. (1998). *Psicología de la liberación de Ignacio Martín-Baró*. Madrid: Editorial Trotta.

Boyd-Franklin, N. (2003). *Black families in therapy: Understanding the African American experience* (2nd ed.). New York: Guilford.

Brown, L. S. (1997). The private practice of subversion: Psychology as Tikkun Olam. *American Psychologist, 52*, 449–462.

Brown, L. S. (2010). *Feminist therapy*. Theories of Psychotherapy Series. Washington, DC: American Psychological Association.

Cane, P. (2000). *Trauma, healing and transformation: Awakening a new heart with body mind spirit practices*. Watsonville, CA: Capacitar.

Cardemil, E. V., & Battle, C. L. (2003). Guess who's coming to therapy? Getting comfortable with conversations about race and ethnicity in psychotherapy. *Professional Psychology: Research and Practice, 34*, 278–286.

CIEBP. (2008, March 13–14). Culturally Informed Evidence Based Practice: Translating Research and Policy for the Real World. Conference sponsored by the National Institute of Mental Health (NIMH), Bethesda, MD.

Cienfuegos, A. J., & Monelli, C. (1983). The testimony of political repression as a therapeutic instrument. *American Journal of Orthopsychiatry, 53*, 43–51.

Comas-Díaz, L. (2006). Latino healing: The integration of ethnic psychology into psychotherapy. *Psychotherapy Theory, Research, Practice, & Training, 43*(4), 436–453.

Comas-Díaz, L. (2007). Ethnopolitical psychology: Healing and transformation. In E. Aldarondo (Ed.), *Promoting social justice in mental health practice*. Hillsdale, NJ: Lawrence Erlbaum Associates.

Comas-Díaz, L. (2008). Spirita: Reclaiming womanist sacredness in feminism. *Psychology of Women Quarterly, 32*, 13–21.

Comas-Díaz, L. (2009). Changing psychology: History and legacy of the Society for the Psychological Study of Ethnic Minority Issues. *Cultural Diversity and Ethnic Minority Psychology, 15*(4), 400–408.

Comas-Díaz, L. (2012a). *Multicultural care: A clinician's guide to cultural competence*. Washington, DC: American Psychological Association.

Comas-Díaz, L. (2012b). Psychotherapy as a healing practice, scientific endeavor, and social justice action. *Psychotherapy, 49*(4), 473–474.

Comas-Díaz, L., Geller, J., Melgoza, B., & Baker, R. (1982, August). *Ethnic minority patients' expectations of treatment and of their therapists*. Presentation made at the American Psychological Association Annual Meeting.

Comas-Díaz, L., & Jacobsen, F. M. (1991). Ethnocultural transference and countertransference in the therapeutic dyad. *American Journal of Orthopsychiatry, 61*(3), 392–402.

Comas-Díaz, L., & Jacobsen, F. M. (2004). Ethnocultural psychotherapy. In E. Craighead & C. Nemeroff (Eds.), *The Corsini encyclopedia of psychology and behavioral science* (pp. 338–339). New York: Wiley.

Comas-Díaz, L., & Ramos Grenier, J. (1998). Migration and acculturation. In J. Sandoval, C. L. Frisby, K. F. Geisinger, J. D. Scheuneman, & J. Ramos-Grenier (Eds.), *Test interpretations and diversity: Achieving equity in assessment* (pp. 213–239). Washington, DC: American Psychological Association.

Congress, E. (2002). Using culturagrams with culturally diverse families. In A. Roberts & G. Greene (Eds.), *Social desk reference* (pp. 57–61). New York: Oxford.

Cooper, M., & McLeod, J. (2007). A pluralistic framework for counselling and psychotherapy: Implications for research. *Counselling and Psychotherapy Research, 7*(3), 135–143.

Cooper-Patrick, L., Gallo, J., Gonzales, J. J., Vu, H. T., Powe, N. E., Nelson, C., & Ford, D. (1999). Race, gender and partnership in the patient–physician relationship. *Journal of the American Medical Association, 282*, 583–589.

Costantino, G., Malgady, R., & Rogler, L. (1986). Cuento therapy: A culturally sensitive modality for Puerto Rican children. *Journal of Consulting and Clinical Psychology, 54*, 639–645.

Cross, T. Bazron, B., Dennis, K., & Issacs, M. (1989). *Towards a culturally competent system of care: A monograph on effective services for minority children who are severely emotionally disturbed* (pp. 13–17). Washington, DC: CASPP Technical Assistance Center, Georgetown University Child Development Center.

Diala, C., Muntaner, C., Walrath, C., Nickerson, K., LaVeist, T., & Leaf, P. (2000). Racial differences in attitudes toward professional mental health care in the use of services. *American Journal of Orthopsychiatry, 70*(4), 455–456.

Dovidio, J. F., & Gaertner, S. L. (1986). *Prejudice, discrimination, and racism*. San Diego: Academic Press.

Dovidio, J. F., & Gaertner, S. L. (1998). On the nature of contemporary prejudice: The causes, consequences and challenges of aversive racism. In J. L. Eberhardt & S. T. Fiske (Eds.), *Confronting racism: The problem and the response* (pp. 3–32). Thousand Oaks, CA: Sage.

Downing, N., & Roush, K. (1985). From passive acceptance to active commitment: A model of feminist identity development for women. *The Counseling Psychologist, 13*(4), 695–709. doi: 10. 1177/0011000085134013.

Duran, E. (2006). *Healing the soul wound: Counseling with American Indians and other native people.* New York: Teachers College Press.

Early, C., & Ang, S. (2003). *Cultural intelligence: Individual interactions across cultures.* Stanford, CA: Stanford University Press.

Elsass, P. (1992). *Strategies for survival: The psychology of cultural resilience in ethnic minorities.* New York: New York University Press.

Essed, P. (1991). *Everyday racism: Reports from women in two cultures.* New York: Hunter House.

Falicov, C. J. (1998). *Latino families in therapy: A guide to multicultural practice.* New York: Guilford.

Fanon, F. (1967). *Black skin, White masks.* New York: Grove Press.

Freire, P. (1973*). Education for critical consciousness.* New York: Seabury.

Freire, P., & Macedo, D. (2000). *The Paulo Freire reader.* New York: Continuum.

Gehrie, M. J. (1979). Culture as an internal representation. *Psychiatry, 42,* 165–170.

Hall, G. C. N. (2001). Psychotherapy research with ethnic minorities: Empirical, ethical, and conceptual issues. *Journal of Consulting and Clinical Psychology, 69,* 502–510.

Hardy, K. V., & Laszloffy, T. (1995). The cultural genogram: Key to training culturally competent family therapists. *Journal of Marital and Family Therapy, 21*(3), 227–237.

Hartman, A. (1995). Diagrammatic assessment of family relations. *Families in Society, 76*(2), 111–122.

Hays, P. (2008). *Addressing cultural complexities in practice: Assessment, diagnosis and therapy.* (Second edition). Washington, DC: American Psychological Association.

Helms, J. E. (1990). *Black and white racial identity: Theory, research and practice.* Westport, CT: Greenwood.

Howard-Hamilton, M. F., Phelps, R. E., & Torres, V. (1998). *Meeting the needs of all students and staff members: The challenge of diversity. New directions for student services.* San Francisco: Jossey-Bass.

Ivey, A., Ivey, M., & Simek-Morgan, L. (1997). *Counseling and psychotherapy: A multicultural perspective.* Boston: Allyn & Bacon.

Joralemon, D. (1986). The performing patient in ritual healing. *Social Science and Medicine, 23,* 841–845.

Kakar, S. (1985). Psychoanalysis and non-Western cultures. *International Review of Psychoanalysis, 12,* 441–448.

Karlsson, R. (2005). Ethnic matching between therapist and patient in psychotherapy: An overview of findings, together with methodological and conceptual issues. *Cultural Diversity and Ethnic Minority Psychology, 11*(2), 113–129.

Kleinman, A. (1980). *Patients and healers in the context of culture: An exploration of the borderland between anthropology, medicine, and psychiatry.* Berkeley: University of California Press.

Knipscheer, J. W., & Kleber, R. J. (2004). A need for ethnic similarity in the therapist-patient interaction? Mediterranean migrants in Dutch mental health care. *Journal of Clinical Psychology, 60*(6), 543–554.

Koss-Chioino, J. D., & Vargas, L. (1992). Through the cultural looking glass: A model for understanding culturally responsive psychotherapies. In L. A. Vargas & J. D. Koss-Chioino, *Working with culture: Psychotherapeutic interventions with ethnic minority, children and adolescents* (pp. 1–22). San Francisco: Jossey Bass.

Galinsky, A. D., & Moskowitz, G. B. (2000). Perspective-taking: Decreasing stereotype expression, stereotype accessibility, and in-group favoritism. *Journal of Personality & Social Psychology, 78,* 708–724.

Gehrie, M. J. (1979). Culture as an internal representation. *Psychiatry, 42,* 165–170.

Gergen, K. J., & Gergen, M. M. (1997). Toward a cultural constructionist psychology. *Theory and Psychology, 7,* 31–36.

Lawson, W. B. (2000). Issues in pharmacotherapy for African Americans In P. Ruiz (Ed.), *Ethnicity and psychopharmacology* (pp. 37–47). Washington, DC: American Psychiatric Press.

Leininger, M. (1978). Changing foci in American nursing education: Primary and transcultural nursing care. *Journal of Advanced Nursing, 3*(2), 155–166.

Leung, A. K., Maddux, W., Galinsky, A., Chiu, C. (2008). Multicultural experience enhances creativity: The when and how. *American Psychologist, 63*(3), 169–181.

Lo, H-T., & Fung, K. P. (2003). Culturally competent psychotherapy. *Canadian Journal of Psychiatry, 48*(3), 161–170.

Lyon, M. (1993). Psychoneuroimmunology: The problem of the situatedness of illness and the conceptualization of healing. *Culture Medicine and Psychiatry, 17,* 77–97.

McIntosh, P. (1988). *White privilege and male privilege: A personal account of coming to see correspondences through work in women's studies.* Available from the Wellesley College Center for Research on Women, Wellesley, MA 02181.

McGoldrick, M., Gerson, R., & Shellenberger, S. (1999). *Genograms: Assessment and intervention.* New York: W.W. Norton.

McGoldrick, M., Giordano, J., & Garcia-Preto, N. (Eds.). (2005). *Ethnicity and family therapy* (3rd ed.). New York: Guilford.

Miranda, J., Bernal, G., Lau, A., Kohn, L., Hwang, W.-C., & La Framboise. T. (2005). State of the science on psychosocial interventions for ethnic minorities. *Annual Review of Clinical Psychology, 1,* 113–142.

Morales, E., & Norcross, J. C. (2010). Evidence based practices with ethnic minorities: Strange bedfellows no more. *Journal of Clinical Psychology, 66*(8), 1–9.

Muñoz, R. F., & Mendelson, T. (2005). Toward evidence-based interventions for diverse populations: The San Francisco General Hospital prevention and treatment manuals. *Journal of Clinical and Consulting Psychology, 73*(5), 790–799.

Murray, H. A., & Kluckhohn, C. (1953). *Personality in nature, society, and culture.* Cambridge, MA: Harvard University Press.

Norcross, J. C., Hedges, M., & Prochaska, J. O. (2002). The face of 2010: A delphi poll on the future of psychotherapy. *Professional Psychology, Research, & Practice, 33,* 316–322.

Paradis, C., & Freidman, S. (2005). Sleep paralysis in African Americans with panic disorder. *Transcultural Psychiatry, 42*(1), 123–134.

Pierce, C. M. (1995). Stress analogs of racism and sexism: Terrorism, torture, and disaster. In C. V. Willie, P. P. Reiker, & B. S. Brown (Eds.), *Mental health, racism, and sexism* (pp. 277–293). Pittsburgh: University of Pittsburgh Press.

Pinderhughes, E. (1989). *Understanding race, ethnicity, and power: The key to efficacy in clinical practice.* New York: The Free Press.

Poston, W. C. (1990, November–December). The biracial identity development model: A needed addition. *Journal of Counseling and Development, 69*(2), 152–155.

Ratts, M., D'Andrea, M., & Arredondo, P. (2004, July). Social justice counseling: "Fifth force" in field. *Counseling Today, 47*, 28–30.

Rey, J. (2006, December 1). The interface of multiculturalism and psychopharmacology. *Journal of Pharmacy Practice, 19*(6), 379–385.

Ridley, C., & Lingle, D. W. (1996). Cultural empathy in multicultural counseling: A multidimensional process model. In P. B. Pedersen, J. G. Draguns, W. J. Lonner, & J. E. Trimble (Eds.), *Counseling across cultures* (4th ed., pp. 21–46). Thousand Oaks, CA: Sage.

Rigazio-DiGilio, S. A., Ivey, A. E., Grady, L. T., & Kunkler-Peck, K. P. (2005). *Community genograms: Using individual, family, and cultural narratives with clients.* New York: Teachers College, Columbia University.

Rhode, D. L., & Williams, J. C. (2007). Legal perspectives on employment discrimination. In F. J. Crosby, M. S. Stockdale, & S. A. Ropp (Eds.), *Sex discrimination in the workplace* (pp. 235–270). Malden, MA: Blackwell.

Roby, P. (1998, January). Creating a just world: Leadership for the twenty-first century. *Social Problems, 45*(1), 1–20.

Ruiz, P. (Ed.). (2000). *Ethnicity and psychopharmacology.* Washington, DC: American Psychiatric Press.

Seeley, K. M. (2000). *Cultural psychotherapy: Working with culture in the clinical encounter.* Northvale, NJ: Jason Aronson.

Semmler, P. L., & Williams, C. B. (2000). Narrative therapy: A storied context for multicultural counseling. *Journal of Multicultural Counseling and Development, 28*, 51–62.

Speck, R. V., & Attneave, C. L. (1973). *Family networks.* New York: Parthenon Books.

Spradley, J. P. (1990). *Participant observation.* New York: Holt, Rinehart & Winston.

Strickland, T. L., Ranganeth, V., & Lin, K.-M. (1991). Psychopharmacologic considerations in the treatment of black American populations. *Psychopharmacology Bulletin, 27*, 441–448.

Sue, D. W., & Sue, D. (2008). *Counseling the culturally diverse: Theory and practice* (5th ed.). New York: Wiley.

Sue, D. W., Bingham, R. P., Porche-Burke, L., & Vasquez, M. (1999). The diversification of psychology: A multicultural revolution. *American Psychologist, 54*(12), 1061–1069.

Sue, D., Capodilupo, C. M., Torino, G. C., Bucceri, J. M., Holder, A. M., Nadal, K. L., & Esquilin, M. (2007). Racial microagressions in everyday life: Implications for clinical practice. *American Psychologist, 62*(4), 271–286.

Tamura, T., & Lau, A. (1992). Connectedness versus separateness: Applicability of family therapy to Japanese families. *Family Process, 31*, 319–340.

Triandis, H. (1995). *Individualism and collectivism.* Boulder, CO: Westview.

Valsiner, J., & Rosa, A. (2007). Contemporary socio-cultural research: Uniting culture, society, and psychology. In J. Valsiner & A. Rosa (Eds.), *The Cambridge handbook of sociocultural psychology* (pp. 1–20), Cambridge, UK: Cambridge University Press.

Varma, V. K. (1988). Culture personality and psychotherapy. *International Journal of Social Psychiatry, 43*(2), 142–149.

Whaley, A. (1998). Racism in the provision of mental health services: A social–cognitive analysis. *American Journal of Orthopsychiatry, 68*, 47–57.

Whaley, A. L., & Davis, K. E. (2007). Cultural competence and evidence-based practice in mental health services: A complementary perspective. *American Psychologist, 62*(6), 563–574.

Worell, J., & Remer, P. (2003). *Feminist perspectives in therapy* (2nd ed.). New York: Wiley.

Wu, E., & Martinez, M. (2006, October). *Taking cultural competence from theory to action.* The Commonwealth Fund Publication No. 964. Retrieved from www.cmwf.org

Young, M. I. (1990). *Justice and the politics of difference.* Princeton, NJ: Princeton University Press.

16 | CONTEMPORARY CHALLENGES AND CONTROVERSIES

Kenneth S. Pope and Danny Wedding

The other chapters in this book show psychotherapy's fascinating diversity. Therapists from diverse disciplines—psychology, psychiatry, social work, and counseling, to name just a few—apply different principles from different perspectives in working with people who come to them for help.

Yet for all the diversity, every therapist who shows up for work in a private office, clinic, community center, hospital, or elsewhere faces an array of contemporary challenges and controversies. This chapter takes a look at 11 of them:

1. the mental-health workforce;
2. physicians, medications, and psychotherapy;
3. the *Diagnostic and Statistical Manual* (DSM);
4. empirically supported therapies;
5. phones, computers, and the Internet;
6. therapists' sexual involvement with patients, nonsexual physical touch, and sexual feelings;
7. nonsexual multiple relationships and boundary issues;
8. accessibility and people with disabilities;

9. the American Psychological Association, the law, and the individual's ethical responsibility;

10. detainee interrogations; and

11. cultures.

THE MENTAL-HEALTH WORKFORCE

You and your partner have just moved to a new state. After a week, your partner tells you, "I've been feeling a little depressed and anxious since we moved. It's not one of those things I can pull myself out of. I think I need some help. We don't know anyone here, so there's no one we trust to ask for a recommendation, but I've looked in the phone book and here are the people who are available: a counselor, a life coach, a marriage and family therapist, a psychiatrist, a psychologist, and a social worker. The phone book doesn't give anything more than the title. Which do you think I should choose?" How do you respond?

Mental-health services are delivered by numerous health professionals, including psychologists, social workers, psychiatrists, licensed professional counselors, rehabilitation counselors, pastoral counselors, substance-abuse counselors, and general practice physicians and nurses. Whatever their professional identification, the majority of these individuals practice *technical eclecticism* (described in Chapter 14) and use a variety of methods, many of which are described in *Current Psychotherapies.*

Because of this diversity of service personnel, defining the mental-health workforce with any precision presents complex challenges, especially in light of the fact that many therapists work part-time and many identify with more than one mental-health profession (for example, a therapist may be both a social worker *and* a marriage and family therapist).

The best available data on the mental-health workforce in the United States are found in biennial monographs published by the U.S. Substance Abuse and Mental Health Services Administration (SAMHSA) titled *Mental Health, United States.* The administration's most recent biannual publication (SAMHSA, 2012) documents the need for mental-health services (e.g., 34,000 deaths in the United States annually from suicide), the falling percent of health-care expenditures devoted to mental health, the rapid increase in national and per capita spending on psychotropic medications, and the shortages of mental-health providers in almost every state (e.g., Idaho is the state with the most dramatic shortage of mental-health professionals—31.6%; West Virginia is the state with the highest percentage of its residents living in counties with a marked shortage of prescribing professionals—85%).

The SAMHSA estimates for clinically trained mental health personnel by discipline are presented in Table 16.1. According to the table, there are 31 psychologists in the United States for every 100,000 people. This number may be far less than the proportion of psychologists in many other countries. For example, "The number of practicing psychologists in Argentina has been surging, to 196 per 100,000 people last year, according to a study by Modesto Alonso, a psychologist and researcher, from 145 per 100,000 people in 2008" (Romero, 2012).

Despite the clear need for more mental-health services in the United States, the American Psychiatric Association (2012) reports that the number of psychiatrists is declining, noting "the number of U.S. medical students choosing psychiatry as a specialty has been declining for the past six years," and "about half of currently practicing psychiatrists are over the age of 55 and many will soon start retiring" (American Psychiatric Association, 2012).

In contrast, the numbers of nonphysician mental-health providers have continued to grow over the past decade. As early as 2000, some writers expressed concern about

TABLE 16.1 **Number and Rate of Mental-Health Personnel by Discipline, United States**

Discipline	Number	Rate per 100,000 Population
Social Work	244,900	82
Counseling	128,886	54
Psychology	92,227	31
Marriage and Family Therapy	48,666	16
Psychiatry	43,120	14
Advanced Practice Psychiatric Nursing	9,764	3

Source: (SAMHSA, 2012)

market saturation (e.g., Robiner & Crew, 2000). These concerns have been fueled by the growth and success of the professional school movement in psychology, the development of the doctor of psychology (PsyD) degree, the proliferation of online and for-profit universities offering degrees in mental-health fields, and the internship crisis in clinical and counseling psychology.

Psychologists, social workers, and other nonmedical personnel have drawn closer to achieving the status of physicians, especially in the areas of insurance reimbursement, participation in federal health programs, and admission to psychoanalytic training. In many states, psychologists have gained hospital admitting privileges, and some states have enacted laws requiring hospitals that offer psychology services to allow psychologists to directly admit their patients.

The accreditation standards of the Joint Commission on Accreditation of Health-care Organizations (JCAHO) influence the hiring practices and staffing decisions made by administrators of hospitals, community mental-health centers, and other settings where psychotherapy services are delivered. Confronted with fiscal limitations and budget constraints, these administrators recognize that although a variety of professions are licensed to provide psychotherapy, the base salary that therapists expect may differ significantly, depending on the profession.

Nearly all states classify psychotherapy as a legitimate part of medical practice without restricting its use to psychiatrists. However, psychiatrists now devote most of their time to medication management, and far fewer psychiatrists are being trained to provide psychotherapy to their patients (Luhrmann, 2000; Moran, 2009). This trend results in part from the fact that approximately half of new psychiatrists licensed in the United States are international medical graduates (IMGs), and these physicians are more likely to be trained in biological psychiatry.

In 2013, psychologists, social workers, psychiatric nurse practitioners, and marriage and family therapists were required to be licensed or certified in all 50 states; likewise, professional counselors and substance-abuse counselors must be licensed or certified in many states.

Licensing is more meaningful than certification because licensure restricts the practice of a profession, whereas certification restricts the use of a profession's name. These distinctions are difficult to apply to psychotherapy because it is virtually impossible to restrict the practice of a profession that includes such a varied range of activities. States may regulate certain professional activities, however. Psychological testing may be restricted to psychologists, for example, and the authority to prescribe medication may be granted only to physicians, dentists, and other health-care practitioners such as advanced practice nurses, nurse practitioners, physicians' assistants, optometrists, and podiatrists.

Regulatory authority is usually invested in a state board appointed by the governor and composed of professionals and members of the public. Frequently, state boards will use reciprocity to license professionals who hold a license to practice in other states.

It is difficult to decide who should have the right to practice psychotherapy because there are few unambiguous and universally accepted practice guidelines to define what is appropriate professional care for patients with mental and emotional disorders. A psychoanalyst and a behavior therapist may provide dramatically different treatment for a patient with an anxiety disorder, for example. Yet both will claim—and genuinely believe—that their mode of treatment is appropriate.

PHYSICIANS, MEDICATIONS, AND PSYCHOTHERAPY

You are a psychologist practicing in a small town. You and a psychiatrist, who is also in solo practice, provide the town's only mental-health services. Over the years, you have noticed that whenever one of your therapy patients needs to be evaluated for medications and you refer him or her to the psychiatrist, the patient soon stops seeing you. It's one of those small towns where there are few secrets, so you discover that the psychiatrist encourages your patients to discontinue seeing you so that they can consolidate their care and receive both medication and psychotherapy from the same person, even though many of them are subsequently treated only with medication. Rosa Gonzales, for example, had been seeing you in connection with her work-related depression. Her employer was exploitive, abusive, and disrespectful. She'd been working on developing the confidence and courage to change jobs. However, once she went to the psychiatrist for a medication consult, she stopped coming to therapy. When you happen to see her in the grocery store several months later, she looks at the floor and comments, "The medications made me feel better and the job doesn't seem so bad now." What are your reactions to your experiences with the psychiatrist? And how do you think you'd respond to your former patient's comment?

No therapist works in isolation. All therapists must cope with frequently changing rules about the allocation and delivery of clinical services. The patterns reflecting which people receive—and which people fail to receive—clinical services, in what forms, for what problems, and from whom constantly evolve. Therapists must decide how they want to respond to these shifting patterns and what role, if any they want to play in changing them.

What are the major trends? Many studies document that treatment consisting solely of psychotherapy is becoming less common. Wang et al. (2006), for example, found that a

> mental-health-specialty-only profile, representing possible use of psychotherapy alone, had been the most popular profile in the NCS [National Comorbidity Survey] but declined significantly in the past decade. This finding is consistent with a significant decrease in psychotherapy visits during the 1990s. . . . It could reflect new restrictions on the number of psychotherapy sessions, increased patient cost sharing, and reduced provider reimbursements for psychotherapy visits imposed by many third-party payers. . . . It could also reflect changes in the popularity of therapeutic modalities, particularly patients' growing preferences for psychotropic medications. (p. 1195)

In a 2010 article, "National Trends in Psychotherapy," Olfson and Marcus described how the role of psychotherapy had shifted:

> Despite impressive progress by academic researchers in demonstrating the efficacy of several specific forms of psychotherapy for some of the most common psychiatric disorders (35–41), a decreasing proportion of mental health outpatients receive psychotherapy, and those who do are receiving fewer visits. Over the course of a

decade that witnessed substantial growth in outpatient medical expenditures, spending on outpatient mental health care underwent little change, and spending on psychotherapy significantly declined. During the same period, a large and growing number of mental health outpatients received psychotropic medications without psychotherapy. These changes have helped to redefine outpatient mental health care in America. (p. 1462)

Those findings echo an earlier study by Olfson, Marcus, Druss, Elinson, Tanielian, and Pincus (2002) who found that

[s]ignificant growth occurred in the number of Americans who received treatment for depression during the past decade, and at the same time the treatments they received underwent a profound transformation. Antidepressant medications became established as a mainstay, psychotherapy sessions became less common and fewer among those receiving treatment, and physicians assumed a more prominent role. (pp. 206–207)

Some people have questioned the general value of psychotherapy as a meaningful way of addressing society's needs. For example, in 2011, Alan Kazdin, a Yale psychology professor and the 2008 president of the American Psychological Association (APA), argued in a provocative *Time* magazine interview that 70% of people with mental and emotional problems don't receive needed treatment, in part because the most common approaches to treatment (e.g., many of the kinds of therapy discussed in this book) simply weren't adequate to address the pressing health needs of the general public.

The research data not only trace a trend that deemphasized psychotherapy but also suggest that people seeking help for problems such as depression are turning more to physicians and less to psychologists. Olfson, Marcus, Druss, Elinson, Tanielian and Pincus (2002) reported that

there was a significant increase in the proportion of patients whose treatment of depression involved visits to a physician. . . . By 1997, more than 8 (87.3%) of 10 patients who received outpatient treatment of depression were treated by a physician, compared with 68.9% in 1987. Conversely, the percentage who received treatment from psychologists declined (29.8% vs. 19.1%). Treatment of depression by social workers remained little changed and relatively uncommon. (p. 206)

Interestingly, this shift to seeking help from physicians, particularly primary care physicians, involves obtaining not only medications but also psychotherapy from those primary care physicians. Wang and his colleagues note that

[t]he general medical-only profile experienced the largest growth over the past decade and is now the most common profile. This increased use of general medical providers without specialists may be because primary care physicians now act as "gatekeepers" for nearly one-half of patients. . . . The development and heavy promotion of new antidepressants and other psychotropic medications with improved safety profiles have further spurred care of mental disorders exclusively in general medical settings. . . . There has also been a growing tendency for some primary care physicians to deliver psychotherapies themselves. (Wang et al., 2006, p. 1194)

Although some mental-health practitioners may be concerned about competition with physicians, there is a growing national trend toward collaborative practice and integrated care (Curtis & Christian, 2012). This model involves co-location of mental-health practitioners with physicians and nurses, joint training, and shared continuing education opportunities. The model facilitates respect between different professional groups and supports the "curbside consults" and "hallway hand-offs" that are critical to continuity of care.

Several studies also suggest a shift away from longer-term psychotherapies. As early as 2002, Olfson, Marcus, Druss, and Pincus noted the heavy focus on brief treatment and a significant decline in the average number of psychotherapy sessions.

In some cases, the focus on medication may mean that patients receive little monitoring or other help of any kind. A study of 84,514 adult and pediatric patients found that "during the first 4 weeks of treatment with antidepressants, only 55. 0% of the patients saw a health-care provider for any purpose, and only 17. 7% saw a provider for mental health care" (Stettin, Yao, Verbrugge, & Aubert, 2006, p. 453). Four years later, Olfson and Marcus (2010) documented a decade-long trend of the "increasing proportion of mental-health outpatients received psychotropic medication without psychotherapy" (p. 1456).

The increased use of medications to treat psychological disorders was one factor that led psychologists to seek prescription privileges. The issue soon erupted into controversy, with thoughtful arguments made on each side. Would prescription privileges enable psychologists to provide a more comprehensive array of clinical services to clients? Would psychologists' ability to prescribe enable them to provide services in geographic areas of critical need that lacked psychiatrists? Would psychologists betray their professional identity and values, shifting toward a medical model in which medication is often an initial intervention? If psychologists were not going to add a year or two to their doctoral training, what part of their current curriculum and training would have to be abandoned to make room for training in psychopharmacology?

As this chapter is written, only New Mexico, Louisiana, and the U.S. Territory of Guam have laws providing limited prescription authority to psychologists with special training, and almost 1,700 psychologists have completed level 3 clinical pharmacotherapy training (Robert McGrath, personal communication, June 10, 2012). McGrath notes, "Technically, since 1993 Indiana also has had a law 'providing limited prescription privileges to psychologists with special training.' However, the Indiana law is limited to individuals participating in a 'federal government sponsored training or treatment program'" (personal communication, June 10, 2012).

The prescriptive authority movement has not progressed as rapidly as early proponents had hoped, in part because of a handful of psychologists who feel strongly about the issue and who travel to testify *against* any state legislation that would allow psychologists to prescribe. In addition, organized medicine has adamantly opposed allowing psychologists to prescribe, and state medical societies have been successful in having bills that authorize this enhanced scope of practice for psychologists overturned by the governors of states such as Oregon and Hawaii. This issue remains a hotly debated topic within the profession of psychology.

THE *DIAGNOSTIC AND STATISTICAL MANUAL* AND THE *INTERNATIONAL CLASSIFICATION OF DISEASES*

You have been seeing a couple contemplating divorce, and you are proud of the progress the couple has made in only three short sessions. There are still significant problems in the marriage, however, and the wife remains very angry about a brief affair her husband had with a co-worker at a professional meeting in Hawaii. However, at the end of the third session, the husband asks to see you alone and says "Look, Doc. My insurance company won't pay for marital counseling, but they do pay for the treatment of mental illness. We still have a long way to go, but one of us needs a diagnosis. It can be anxiety, depression, pretty much anything—but without a diagnosis, there's no more treatment, and with treatment, there's no more marriage. Can you help me out here?" How would you respond?

As we write this chapter, the American Psychiatric Association has scheduled the publication of the fifth edition of the *Diagnostic and Statistical Manual* (DSM-5) for May 2013, but criticism and controversy surround the project. For example, the British Psychological Society's (2011) critique of the DSM-5 draft stated:

> The Society is concerned that clients and the general public are negatively affected by the continued and continuous medicalisation of their natural and normal responses to their experiences; responses which undoubtedly have distressing consequences which demand helping responses, but which do not reflect illnesses so much as normal individual variation. . . . The criteria are not value-free, but rather reflect current normative social expectations. . . . Diagnostic systems such as these therefore fall short of the criteria for legitimate medical diagnoses. . . . We are also concerned that systems such as this are based on identifying problems as located within individuals. This misses the relational context of problems and the undeniable social causation of many such problems.

Financial conflicts of interest have served as another focus of concern:

> "The ties between the D. S. M. panel members and the pharmaceutical industry are so extensive that there is the real risk of corrupting the public health mission of the manual," said Dr. Lisa Cosgrove, a fellow at the Edmond J. Safra Center for Ethics at Harvard, who published a study in March that said two-thirds of the manual's advisory task force members reported ties to the pharmaceutical industry or other financial conflicts of interest. (Urbina, 2012, p. A11)

Similarly, Spence (2012), in an article "The Psychiatric Oligarch Who Medicalise Normality" in the *British Medical Journal* (BMJ), wrote, "75% of the authors of the new, fifth edition of the DSM report conflicts of interest. . . . It is yet more industrial mass production psychiatry to serve the drug industry, for which mental ill health is the profit nirvana of lifelong multiple medications. . . . [The] DSM-5 . . . is riddled with conflicts of interest; its definitions are soft, nonspecific, and seem counterintuitive." (Spence is also critical of the tendency to pathologize those experiences and situations that we all experience as a normal part of life. He notes, "the U.S. Centers for Disease Control and Prevention (CDC) report that a staggering 25% of people in the United States have a 'mental illness.' This is so large a figure that there can be only one conclusion: psychiatry is medicalising normality.")

In a thoughtful article in the *New England Journal of Medicine*, McHugh and Slavney (2012) explored the ways in which the DSM works against understanding either the patient or the disorder:

> Its emphasis on manifestations persuaded psychiatrists to replace the thorough "bottom-up" method of diagnosis, which was based on a detailed life history, painstaking examination of mental status, and corroboration from third-party informants, with the cursory "top-down" method that relied on symptom checklists. Checklist diagnoses cost less in time and money but fail woefully to correspond with diagnoses derived from comprehensive assessments . . . . Identifying a disorder by its symptoms does not translate into understanding it.

"More Psychiatrists Attack Plans for DSM-5," an article appearing in the BMJ, reported University of East London clinical psychologist Mark Rapley's analysis:

> "The APA insists that psychiatry is a science," he said, before posing some barbed questions. "Why, I wonder, does the Royal College of Physicians not seek Web site comments from the public on the diagnosis of breast cancer. . . . When, oh, when will the Geological Society finally solicit 'views from the general public' on the appropriateness of diagnosing granite as an igneous rock?" Responding to his own

questions he went on: "Real sciences do not decide on the existence and nature of the phenomena they are dealing with via a show of hands with a vested interest and pharmaceutical industry sponsorship." (Watts, 2012)

Most international health-care providers use a diagnostic and coding system developed by the World Health Organization (WHO) titled the *International Classification of Diseases* (ICD). The 10th edition of the ICD is currently being field-tested, and we hope it will be widely adopted in the United States. It is clearly inefficient and confusing to have a separate and unique taxonomy for mental and emotional disorders, and this duel system of classification makes international epidemiological research difficult if not impossible. In an October 2009 article in the *APA Monitor*, WHO psychologist Geoffrey Reed noted four major distinctions between these two diagnostic systems:

1. The ICD is produced by a global health agency with a constitutional public health mission, while the DSM is produced by a single national professional association.

2. WHO's primary focus for the mental and behavioral disorders classification is to help countries to reduce the disease burden of mental disorders. ICD's development is global, multidisciplinary and multilingual; the primary constituency of the DSM is U.S. psychiatrists.

3. The ICD is approved by the World Health Assembly, composed of the health ministers of all 193 WHO member countries; the DSM is approved by the assembly of the American Psychiatric Association.

4. The ICD is distributed as broadly as possible at a very low cost, with substantial discounts to low-income countries, and available free on the Internet; the DSM generates a very substantial portion of the American Psychiatric Association's revenue, not only from sales of the book itself, but also from related products and copyright permissions for books and scientific articles.

EMPIRICALLY SUPPORTED THERAPIES

It is your first week as executive director of a community mental-health clinic. The clinic offers individual therapy, group therapy, and family therapy, as well as a suicide hotline and a walk-in crisis clinic. At the end of the week, the board of directors informs you that because it wants to be sure money is spent wisely and effectively, it has adopted a new policy for you to implement: The clinic will offer only services that have been empirically supported through well-designed scientific research. If research has not demonstrated that an intervention is both safe and effective, then it is prohibited. Would you agree with this policy? If required to implement it, what steps would you take?

The push to put therapy on sound scientific footing led to the concept of *empirically supported treatments* (ESTs). Proponents of ESTs believed that each form of therapy needs to be tested in carefully controlled experimental research. The results would show which therapies actually worked and which, though well intended, did nothing to help the patient or, worse, were harmful.

Eager to stop wasting money on worthless interventions, managed care companies and other third-party payment sources rushed to embrace the concept. ESTs held the promise of allowing insurance companies to restrict payments to those therapies that well-designed experiments had demonstrated to be the most effective and efficient.

The concept of empirically supported therapy, appealing to so many in theory, has turned out to be difficult and controversial to put into practice, and many practitioners have resisted training in empirically supported therapies for both theoretical and practical reasons (Stewart, Chambless, & Baron, 2012). Drew Westen and Rebekah Bradley (2005) note that

> evidence-based practice is a construct (i.e., an idea, abstraction, or theoretical entity) and thus must be operationalized (i.e., turned into some concrete form that comes to define it). The way it is operationalized is not incidental to whether its net effects turn out to be positive, negative, or mixed. (p. 226; see also Westen, Novotny, & Thompson-Brenner, 2004)

One challenge is that a therapy cannot be described simply as "effective" any more than a psychological test can be described simply as "valid" or "reliable." The validity and reliability of psychological tests do not exist in the abstract. They must be established for a specific purpose (e.g., identifying malingering), for a specific setting (e.g., forensic), and for a specific population (e.g., adults who can read and write English at a seventh-grade or more advanced level). Gordon Paul acknowledged this complexity in 1967 when many were searching for therapies that were "effective." Paul wrote that both therapists and researchers must confront the question "What treatment, by whom, is most effective for this individual with that specific problem, and under which set of circumstances?" (p. 111).

David Barlow reviewed research showing the importance of these complex sets of variables. He notes, for example, that studies show "that therapist variables such as experience contribute to successful outcome. . . . But this research on therapist variables occurs in the context of considering, first and foremost, the presenting pathology of the patient" (2004, p. 874). He concludes that

> there are three overriding principles in evaluating the robustness of [psychotherapies]. . . . First, it is important to match the psychological intervention to the psychological or physical disorder or problem. . . . Second, it is important to match the treatment to patient and therapist characteristics. . . . Finally, the evaluation of treatments must be considered in the context of the actual settings in which the treatments are provided. (p. 874)

Another challenge is that it is difficult to define with precision exactly what variables are significant in a specific situation. Imagine, for example, that a series of experiments had evaluated the effectiveness and efficiency of different treatments for a specific psychological syndrome, perhaps one of those found in DSM. As Robert Sternberg (2006) points out,

> [if] every client was a textbook-pure case of a particular syndrome, then it might be possible to comfortably generalize the results of many and even most . . . [random assignment studies] . . . to clinical settings. [But] the degree of fidelity is, at best, variable. . . . [E]cological validity is a matter of degree, and as the universe of therapy situations to which one wishes to generalize expands, one has to be increasingly cautious in interpreting the results of RAS designs. Will the treatment work in other cultures? Will it work for people with co-morbid diagnoses? Will it work for people on a particular combination of drugs? How will it work for people who are highly resistant to psychotherapy? In the end, one must ask just how general the results of any given study or set of studies can be. (p. 269)

The daunting complexity of the research needed to investigate a particular psychological therapy adequately stands in stark contrast with the sheer number of available therapies. Kazdin (2008b; see also 2008a), for example, notes that there are more than 550 psychological interventions for children and adolescents, but only a relatively small minority have been subjected to research.

Trying to determine whether a set of studies can be validly generalized to other individuals, other cultures, and other situations is difficult enough, but Kazdin (2006) takes the challenge to a deeper level: In light of the kinds of measures used in most therapy research, do we have logical, empirical, or other scientific proof that the individuals in the research studies themselves are being helped? A fundamental scientific and clinical question, according to Kazdin, "is whether our findings 'generalize' to patient functioning. Stated more empirically, what exactly is the evidence that EBTs [evidence-based therapies] help patients? I believe it is possible to delineate an EBT . . . that improves the life of no one" (p. 46). Furthermore, he states,

> In most therapy studies, measures are not linked to specific referents in everyday life and are arbitrary metrics. Fancy data transformations, creation of new metrics, and statistical razzle-dazzle can be very useful (and worked with my dissertation committee, even if only for the first hour of my six-hour root-canal-like oral defense). However, these statistical strategies do not alter the arbitrariness of the metric, and in the case of psychotherapy research, they say little to nothing about whether patients have changed in ways that make a difference. (p. 46)

Carol Goodheart (2006) identified a challenge on yet another level:

> Psychotherapy is first and foremost a human endeavor. It is messy. It is not solely a scientific endeavor, nor can it be reduced meaningfully to a technical mechanistic enterprise. . . . Psychotherapy is a fluid, mutual, interactive process. Each participant shapes and is shaped by the other. They are masters of tact and timing, of when to push and when to be patient. They know the spectrum of disruptions that can occur in a working alliance and are versatile and empathetic in their reparative responses. They are creative in finding paths to understanding, in matching an intervention to a need. (pp. 42–42)

Despite such challenges, the APA 2005 Presidential Task Force on Evidence-Based Practice emphasized the value of evidence-based practice, defining it as

> the integration of the best available research with clinical expertise in the context of patient characteristics, culture, and preferences. . . . Many strategies for working with patients have emerged and been refined through the kinds of trial and error and clinical hypothesis generation and testing that constitute the most scientific aspect of clinical practice. Yet clinical hypothesis testing has its limits, hence the need to integrate clinical expertise with the best available research. (p. 282)

Despite the enthusiasm among some, controversies remain. Goodheart and Kazdin (2006), for example, in their introduction to the APA-published book *Evidence-Based Psychotherapy: Where Practice and Research Meet,* wrote:

> It is not clear whether the EBP movement is good for clients. . . . There is agreement on the interest and priority of improving client care. There is disagreement on the extent to which conclusions from research ought to be applied to and constrain clinical practice and the extent to which practitioners can genuinely identify client needs and apply the best or more appropriate combination of treatments based on that evaluation. (pp. 7–8)

In a thoughtful article, "Braking the Bandwagon: Scrutinizing the Science and Politics of Empirically Supported Therapies," Hagemoser (2009) discusses the ways in which "political variables may be contributing to the expansion of EST and the resulting restriction of practitioner autonomy" and "the perils of equating the EST paradigm with the scientist-practitioner ideal" (p. 601).

The debate about evidence-based practice is not limited to the mental-health professions; the absence of clear guidelines characterizes much of medical practice. The United States government has attempted to deal with this lack of uniform standards by establishing the Agency for Healthcare Research and Quality (AHRQ). This agency and several professional organizations have developed explicit treatment guidelines for behavioral problems such as depression and anxiety, but the use of practice guidelines in mental-health remains controversial. Proponents of practice guidelines argue that they bring much-needed standardization to a field that has suffered greatly from extensive but unnecessary variance in practice (largely as the result of a lack of standardized training in the mental-health professions). Critics of the guidelines, on the other hand, argue that every clinical case is unique and adamantly reject any attempt to apply standardized treatment protocols, algorithms, or "cookbooks." Moreover, Terrence Shaneyfelt and Robert Centor (2009) argue that "too many current guidelines have become marketing and opinion-based pieces, delivering directive rather than assistive statements" and that "Most current articles called 'guidelines' are actually expert consensus reports" (p. 868). They wrote:

> The overreliance on expert opinion in guidelines is problematic. All guideline committees begin with implicit biases and values, which affects the recommendations they make. However, bias may occur subconsciously and, therefore, go unrecognized. Converting data into recommendations requires subjective judgments; the value structure of the panel members molds those judgments. (p. 868)

In a similar vein, John Kraemer and Laurence Gostin (2009) caution against the "politization of professional practice guidelines."

Anyone interested in reviewing the large number of existing guidelines for treating behavioral disorders can visit the *AHRQ Guideline Clearinghouse* (www.guidelines.gov).

The other chapters in this book illustrate the great diversity of approaches to psychotherapy. In light of that diversity, and the diversity of human nature itself, perhaps it should not be surprising that there is no general agreement about the definition, methodology, or value of evidence-based psychotherapy. Diverse views and a lack of general agreement among therapists about basic definitions, methodology, and the like have deep historical roots. APA president Carl Rogers set in motion an organized effort to define psychotherapy when he appointed David Shakow to chair a special committee. The APA convention of 1947 adopted the Shakow committee report, which led to the Boulder Conference in 1949. The Boulder Conference recorder summarized the result of this massive effort to define psychotherapy in a memorable passage: Psychotherapy is "an undefined technique which is applied to unspecified problems with a nonpredictable outcome. For this technique we recommend rigorous training" (Lehner, 1952, p. 547).

PHONES, COMPUTERS, AND THE INTERNET

You have established a busy practice, and you schedule eight 1-hour sessions each day. You use your computer both for billing and for record keeping, and all of your client files are maintained on your office computer. You also use e-mail extensively as a way to follow up and check on your patients. Because so much of your work depends on access to your computer, it is especially frustrating when your hard drive crashes, and you realize that you have not backed up your files in months. When you frantically call a local computer repair company, you are told that your data can probably be recovered but a technician will need access to your computer for an entire day. You can bring your computer into the shop for repair, or the technician can visit your clinic to do the work on-site. A colleague is on vacation, and you will be able to use her office to see your patients, so you tell the computer repair company to send somebody out the next day. What ethical dilemmas does this vignette present? Is it reasonable to expect a therapist to cancel eight patients in order to simply sit and watch someone work on her computer for eight hours? Is it sufficient to simply "check in" on the technician between patients?

Scenario One

The digital age makes it possible for psychotherapy to occur without therapist and patient ever meeting face-to-face or even being in the same country. Consider the following scenario.

Someone seeking therapy begins the search on the Internet, examining a number of therapists' Web sites. One site offers just what the prospective patient is looking for. The site provides a list of available times for initial sessions, one of which is convenient. The prospective patient reads a series of passages describing the nature and ground rules of the therapy, the exceptions to confidentiality, the responsibilities of both therapist and patient, and so on. After reading each passage, the individual indicates "agree" or "disagree" as part of the informed-consent process.

Once the basics are covered, the soon-to-be patient answers a series of open-ended questions about personal history, demographics, health status, the reasons for seeking therapy, and so on. The therapist offers an initial session at half price—therapist and prospective patient will get to know a little about each other and decide whether they both want to work together. The prospective patient must pay the fee in advance, by credit card, to reserve the time for the initial session.

Therapist and patient meet on the Internet using Skype or a similar communication platform once a week for 45-minute sessions for a total of 12 weeks. They focus on the patient's depression, which they trace to the patient's unsatisfying career. They discuss the barriers—both internal and external—that have kept the patient from finding a new line of work. When the patient decides it is time to end the therapy after 3 months, the depression is no longer constant and debilitating. The patient has started to implement a plan to change careers.

Scenario Two

The therapist and patient in this scenario live more than 300 miles from each other. They communicate only by computer. The words of both therapist and patient appear on their computer monitors.

The patient in this scenario is particularly appreciative of this mode of therapy. Not only was she able to find a therapist whose skills and personal approach were what she was looking for—the kind of therapist who was simply not available in her own small, remote community—but this patient is in the advanced stages of a neuromuscular disease that makes it very difficult for her to leave home. No longer able to speak, she communicates with others via assistive technology on her computer that enables her to control the computer using a "sip and puff" switch. Her words are displayed on a monitor.

Technologies enabling therapist and client to work together without meeting each other face-to-face, without living in the same state or even in the same country, and without either of them leaving home have brought many benefits. Patients, especially those living in small or remote communities, are more likely to find a therapist with particular qualities, values, approaches, skills, or experience. Therapists specializing in a very rare disorder can reach patients with this disorder living across a wide range of states, provinces, and other locales. Many patients—for example, those in the final stages of terminal diseases, those whose physical conditions limit their mobility, and those with highly contagious diseases—can choose among a great variety of therapeutic approaches, even though any attempted travel outside their home is arduous, painful, risky, and perhaps impossible. Some patients whose fears, anxieties, or conditions (such as agoraphobia) might discourage them from trying more traditional modes of therapy may find that therapy by computer or telephone seems safe as an initial intervention. Therapists whose physical condition makes it impractical for them to travel to and from a job site or to spend extended time in an office can work from home, hospital, or hospice.

Scenario Three

These forms of long-distance therapy have also brought challenges and controversy. For example, imagine a scenario in which a therapist begins work traditionally, working with the client in an office setting. However, the company for which the client works transfers the client to another state. Both client and therapist believe that it would be in the client's interest to continue working with the same therapist rather than starting over in the new state with a new therapist. Therapist and client continue to work for the next 2 years, holding sessions by phone and computer. However, the client becomes profoundly depressed and confesses to the therapist that he has been sexually abusing children in his new neighborhood. Then the client becomes acutely suicidal and takes his life. The client's family subsequently sues the therapist for malpractice.

During the extended litigation, the following issues arise.

- Was the therapist practicing without a license in the state to which the client had moved? If a therapist and patient are in different jurisdictions during therapy sessions, then is the therapist required to maintain appropriate licensing status in both jurisdictions? If a therapist lives in Missouri and is licensed only in Missouri, then what authority, if any, does the state licensing board in Missouri have over the therapist's work via telephone or Internet with a client living in Illinois? What authority, if any, does the licensing board in Illinois have to regulate the work of the therapist who lives in Missouri? Does it make any difference if the patient and therapist live only minutes apart but on different sides of the Mississippi River?

- What are the standards of care regarding basic competence when therapy is conducted by telephone or Internet? What education, training, or supervised experience in telephone therapy or Internet therapy establishes that therapists are not working outside their areas of competence?

- Do the laws regarding privacy, confidentiality, privilege, mandatory reporting (of child abuse or elder abuse, for example), and duty to protect third parties that prevail in the state where the therapist lives apply, or do such laws of the state in which the client lives apply, or do both sets of laws apply? What happens if the laws in the therapist's state conflict with the laws in the client's state? For example, what if the laws in one state require that certain information be kept confidential, whereas the laws of the other state require that the information be reported?

- What information about telephone therapy or Internet therapy must a therapist be sure that a client understands and consents to as part of the process of informed consent and informed refusal?

- Under what conditions is telephone therapy or Internet therapy covered—or not covered—under different professional liability policies?

Formal guidelines relevant to therapy provided by telephone or Internet, as well as discussion of the other topics included in this chapter, can be found on the Web page "Ethics Codes & Practice Guidelines for Assessment, Therapy, Counseling, & Forensic Practice" (http://kspope.com/ethcodes/index.php), which provides links to more than 100 formal sets of guidelines and codes, and on the Web page "Telepsychology, Telehealth, & Internet-Based Therapy" (http://kspope.com/telepsychology.php).

Digital technology has created changes and challenges for therapists in another area of practice: the storage and transmission of records. Even though the widely hailed "paperless office" has not come to pass for most therapists, many therapists use computers to handle clinical data. Some may use computers to administer, score, or interpret psychological tests and other assessment instruments. Many use computers for recording information about their clients and notes on psychotherapy sessions. Spreadsheets and specialized software handle billing, track accounts receivable, and provide documentation to insurance companies and other third-party payment sources.

How can therapists make sure that this confidential information is restricted to those authorized to see it? It may seem a reasonably easy challenge, but therapists and patients have been stunned by instances in which supposedly secure information fell into the wrong hands. The following are some of the things that can happen.

- A desktop or laptop computer containing confidential patient information is stolen from an office.

- A car is vandalized, and a laptop stored in the trunk is stolen.

- Someone hacks into a computer that is connected to the Internet and steals the information stored on the computer's hard drive.

- A virus, worm, Trojan, or other malware infects a computer and sends confidential files to a hacker, uploads confidential files to a Web site where anyone can read them, and sends confidential files to everyone listed in the computer's address book. This includes all the Internet discussion groups to which the therapist belongs and all addresses in the computer's memory.

- A hacker makes subtle and undetected changes in a therapist's files (such as adding numbers randomly to billing records or changing the dates in the records of therapy sessions).

- Someone sits down at an unattended computer that is not password protected or whose password is easy to find (in the desk drawer, under the keyboard, or on a Post-it note nearby) or easy to guess (the person's name, the word *password*) and reads, downloads, or transmits confidential data to unauthorized sources.

- Someone reads a monitor—and obtains confidential information—by standing near the monitor sitting next to a laptop user in an airport, on a flight, or in some other public setting.

- A therapist and client discuss extremely sensitive information, unaware that because one of them is using a cordless phone, the conversation can be overheard by someone using a cordless phone close by.

- A therapist e-mails a message containing confidential information to a colleague who is authorized to have it, but it is accidentally sent to the wrong e-mail address.

- A therapist e-mails a message containing confidential information to a colleague who is authorized to have it, but the recipient shares his or her computer with someone else who opens the e-mail message.

- A therapist faxes confidential information, but the recipient's fax machine is shared with others.

- A therapist keeps clinical and financial records on a computer, unaware that spyware has been installed on the computer.

- A therapist faxes confidential information but, by mistake, punches in the wrong fax number.

- A therapist sells a computer, forgetting that confidential information, thought to be "erased" from the hard drive, is still recoverable because a more thorough form of "scrubbing" the hard drive was not used.

Computers and other electronic devices for storing information and communicating with others offer obvious benefits. However, the mental-health community has been slow to recognize their potential pitfalls and the need for creativity and care in their use. Therapists have extensive education, training, and supervised experience in working with people. For most of us in this field, however, working with computers and other digital devices is not our strong suit. When we use digital devices to handle the most sensitive and private information about our clients, we must remember to live up to an ancient precept: First, do no harm.

Therapists—and all students learning to be therapists—should also realize that most clients will Google their therapist's name either before or immediately after the first session. This can be particularly problematic when a therapist's Facebook page or a similar social networking site (e.g., a dating service) contains highly personal information that one would not want to have shared with one's clients. Admissions committees for professional training programs are currently grappling with the issue of whether or not highly personal information (e.g., nude photos) obtained from an Internet search is appropriate data to be shared with other members of the committee and used in making decisions about admission to professional training programs.

THERAPISTS' SEXUAL INVOLVEMENT WITH PATIENTS, NONSEXUAL PHYSICAL TOUCH, AND SEXUAL FEELINGS

You are a therapist in a mental-health center seeing your last client of the day. She is dressed in a short skirt and T-shirt, and she has for several sessions hinted at some secret that she is too embarrassed to talk about. You find her very attractive and enjoy spending time with her. She begins by saying that she had an intense dream that may have given her the courage to work on her secret in therapy. She tells you the dream in detail. It is an erotic dream, and you find yourself becoming intensely aroused. She says that all the graphic sexual activity in the dream is related to her secret, which is that she has always been ashamed that her breasts were so small and that she had wanted to ask you if you thought so. She then raises her T-shirt so her breasts are exposed. What do you think you would do if you were this therapist? What, if anything, would you tell your supervisor about it? What, if anything, would you write in the client's chart? If you imagine the same scenario adapted to a male patient who is concerned about the size of his penis and suddenly pulls down his pants, are your responses to these questions different in any way?

Sex is the focus of one of the most ancient rules of working with patients, is a cause of discomfort and confusion for many therapists, and is a contemporary challenge for the profession.

Therapist–Patient Sexual Involvement

No circumstances or rationale justify sexual involvement with a patient. This basic rule has ancient roots. Annette Brodsky's (1989) research led to her discovery that the prohibition is older than the Hippocratic oath, which included it. In fact, she found that this prohibition was set forth centuries earlier in the Nigerian Code of the Healing Arts.

The prohibition continues to be fundamental to the profession for many reasons, including the issue of harm to patients. In the landmark 1976 case of *Roy v. Hartogs,* for example, New York Supreme Court Presiding Justice Markowitz wrote, "Thus from [Freud] to the modern practitioner we have common agreement of the harmful effects of sensual intimacies between patient and therapist" (*Roy v. Hartogs,* 1976, p. 590).

Studies of the effects of therapist–patient sexual involvement have looked at both patients who never returned to therapy and those who worked with a subsequent therapist; have compared those who engaged in sex with a therapist with matched groups of those who engaged in sex with a nontherapist physician and of those who did not engage in sex with a health-care professional; and have evaluated the effects of sexual involvement between patients and therapists using an array of measures including standardized psychological tests, clinical interview by subsequent therapists and by independent clinicians, behavioral observation, and self-report (Pope, 1994).

The effects of therapist–patient sexual involvement on clients often seem to cluster into 10 very general areas: (1) ambivalence, (2) guilt, (3) emptiness and isolation, (4) sexual confusion, (5) impaired ability to trust, (6) confused roles and boundaries, (7) emotional liability, (8) suppressed rage, (9) increased suicidal risk, and (10) cognitive dysfunction, frequently in the areas of concentration and memory and often involving flashbacks, intrusive thoughts, unbidden images, and nightmares (Pope, 1988, 1994; Pope & Vasquez, 2011).

In light of the harm associated with sexual boundary violations, almost half the states have determined that the civil legislation and case law prohibiting sex with patients were insufficient and have added criminal penalties that can be applied in some situations.

Despite the harm that therapist–patient sexual involvement can cause to patients, despite the long-standing professional prohibition, and despite civil and even criminal penalties, a small minority of therapists sexually exploit their patients. A study of the combined data from the first eight national, anonymous self-report surveys that appeared in peer-reviewed journals found that 4.4% of the 5,148 therapists surveyed reported having engaged in sex with at least one patient (Pope & Vasquez, 2011).

Statistical analysis found no significant differences among the three professions surveyed in these studies: Social workers, psychiatrists, and psychologists report becoming sexually involved with their patients at roughly the same rates.

These studies do, however, reveal significant gender differences. Male therapists reported engaging in sex with their patients at much higher rates (6.8%) than did female therapists (1.6%). By far the most common pairing is a male therapist with a female patient, accounting for about 88% to 95% of the instances of therapist–patient sex in large-scale peer-reviewed studies that report gender data.

Gender is a significant factor in a variety of other sexual dual or multiple relationships and boundary issues (e.g., supervisor–supervisee, professor–student)—even when the base rates of gender in each role are taken into account—and in other nonsexual dual or multiple relationship situations. For example, Pope and Vasquez (2011) reviewed studies showing that in both psychology training situations and in psychotherapy, a much greater proportion of men than women engage in sex in the professional roles of teacher, supervisor, administrator, therapist. A much greater percentage of women than men, however, engage in sex in the roles of student or therapy client with their teacher, supervisor, administrator, or therapist.

Therapists usually become sexually involved with their patients through a variety of common scenarios. Pope and Bouhoutsos (1986, p. 4) presented 10 of the scenarios that seem to occur most often (see Table 16.2).

Nonsexual Physical Touch

It is important to distinguish therapist–patient sexual involvement from two very different phenomena. First, nonsexual physical touch is clearly different from sexual involvement. Pope, Sonne, and Holroyd (1993) documented the ways in which nonsexual physical touch within therapy had acquired a "guilt by association" with sexual touch. Their review of the research and other professional literature found no harm from nonsexual touch per se, although context, culture, and meaning should always be considered

TABLE 16.2   **Ten Common Scenarios**

Scenario	Description
Role trading	Therapist becomes the "patient," and the wants and needs of the therapist become the focus.
Sex therapy	Therapist fraudulently presents therapist–patient sex as valid treatment for sexual or related difficulties.
As if . . .	Therapist treats positive transference as if it were not the result of the therapeutic situation.
Svengali	Therapist creates and exploits the dependence of the patient.
Drugs	Therapist uses cocaine, alcohol, or other drugs as part of the seduction.
Rape	Therapist uses physical force, threats, or intimidation.
True love	Therapist uses rationalizations that attempt to discount the clinical or professional nature of the professional relationship and its duties.
It just got out of hand	Therapist fails to treat the emotional closeness that develops in therapy with sufficient attention, care, and respect.
Time-out	Therapist fails to acknowledge and take account of the fact that the therapeutic relationship does not cease to exist between scheduled sessions and outside the therapist's office.
Hold me	Therapist exploits patient's desire for nonerotic physical contact and patient's possible confusion between erotic and nonerotic contact.

© Cengage Learning

before touching a patient. When consistent with the patient's clinical needs and the therapist's approach, nonsexual touch can be comforting, reassuring, grounding, caring, and an important part of the healing process. When discordant with clinical needs, context, competence, or consent, even the most well-intentioned nonsexual physical contact may be experienced as aggressive, frightening, intimidating, demeaning, arrogant, unwanted, insensitive, threatening, or intrusive.

Sexual Attraction to Patients

Like nonsexual touch, sexual feelings about patients seem to have acquired a guilt by association with therapist–patient sex. National studies indicate that *simply experiencing sexual attraction to a client*—without acting on it and without necessarily even feeling tempted to act on it—makes a majority of both social workers and psychologists feel guilty, anxious, and confused (see Pope & Vasquez, 2011). Although a large majority of therapists report feeling sexually attracted to one or more clients, and most also report discomfort with the feelings, these studies also suggest that adequate training in this area is relatively rare. A majority reported no training in the area, and only around 10% of social workers and psychologists reported adequate training in their graduate programs and internships.

Pope, Sonne, and Greene (2006) discuss the seemingly taboo nature of sexual feelings about clients as reflecting one of several basic myths about therapists that interfere with training and effective therapy. The myth is that *good* therapists (those who don't sexually exploit their patients) never have sexual feelings about their patients, don't become sexually aroused during therapy sessions, don't vicariously enjoy the (sometimes) guilty pleasures of their patients' sexual experiences, don't have sexual fantasies or dreams about their patients. (p. 28)

Because of the widespread discomfort with sexual feelings about clients and the inadequacy of training in this area, it is not surprising that many professional books do not focus on this topic.

In light of the multitude of books in the areas of human sexuality, sexual dynamics, sex therapies, unethical therapist–patient sexual contact, management of the therapist's or patient's sexual behaviors, and so on, it is curious that sexual attraction to patients per se has not served as the primary focus of a wide range of texts. The professor, supervisor, or librarian seeking books that turn their *primary* attention to exploring the therapist's *feelings* in this regard would be hard pressed to assemble a selection from which to choose an appropriate course text. If someone unfamiliar with psychotherapy were to judge the prevalence and significance of therapists' sexual feelings on the basis of the books that focus exclusively on that topic, he or she might conclude that the phenomenon is neither widespread nor important (Pope, Sonne, & Holroyd, 1993, p. 23).

There may be a circular process at work here: The discomfort about sexual feelings may have fostered a relative absence of books and a lack of adequate training in this area. The relative dearth of books and training may have, in turn, led to further discomfort with the topic.

NONSEXUAL MULTIPLE RELATIONSHIPS AND BOUNDARY ISSUES

You are a social worker providing weekly psychotherapy sessions to an extremely rich and successful CEO, Ms. Chin. Your client is struggling with how to implement her decision to acquire a medium-sized company. When she makes the public announcement that she is buying the company, should she immediately announce the planned layoffs at the new company or should she take time to try to cushion the blow? It is about this time that you decide to buy some stock in her company. Ms. Chin is so appreciative of your help in sorting through her difficult issues that she asks you if you will attend a special event at her home, a celebration of her installation as the new president of the company. You accept the invitation and, during the all-day celebration, wind up playing tennis with her and some of her friends in the business community, leading to new referrals to your practice and to a weekly tennis game on the courts of her estate.

As your practice and the value of your stock holdings grow, you reflect on your choices. Your buying the stock harmed no one, did not disclose confidential information, was not based on illegally obtained information, and, as you think about it, was something you had planned to do all along, even before you heard that Ms. Chen's investment group would be buying a new company. Your weekly visits to Ms. Chen's estate allow you to see her in another setting and interacting with other people—and this provides invaluable information that helps you understand and treat your client. The visits enable you to bond with your client more deeply and in more varied ways, strengthening your working relationship with her and giving you a better basis for your therapy. It is all very proper, and everyone benefits. As you imagine yourself as the therapist in this vignette, do you have any second thoughts?

Sound judgments about nonsexual boundaries always depend on context.

Nonsexual boundary crossings can enrich therapy, serve the treatment plan, and strengthen the therapist–client working relationship. They can also undermine the therapy, sever the therapist–patient alliance, and cause immediate or long-term harm to the client. Choices about whether to cross a boundary confront us daily, are often subtle and complex, and can sometimes influence whether therapy progresses, stalls, or ends. (Pope & Keith-Spiegel, 2008, p. 638)

In the 1980s and the early and mid-1990s, the full, often daunting complexity of boundary issues made itself known to the profession through clinical experimentation, research, articles challenging virtually every aspect of the status quo, and open discussion from diverse points of view. A vigorous, wide-ranging, and healthy controversy over therapists' nonsexual multiple relationships and other boundary excursions blossomed. Was it good practice for a therapist to enter into dual professional roles with a client, serving both as a client's therapist and as that client's employer? What about multiple social roles? Is it helpful, hurtful, or completely irrelevant for a therapist to provide therapy to a close friend, spouse, or stepchild? Are there any potential benefits or risks to social outings with a client (meeting for dinner, going to a movie, playing golf, or heading off for a weekend of sightseeing), so long as there is no sexual or romantic involvement? Are financial relationships (say, the therapist borrowing a large sum from a client to buy a new house or car, or inviting a client to invest in the therapist's new business venture) compatible with the therapeutic relationship? What about lending a client money to help pay the rent or buy food and medications, or driving a patient home after a session because she doesn't have a car and can't afford cab fare? Under what circumstances should a therapist accept bartered services or products as payment for therapy sessions?

The 15 years or so from the early 1980s to the mid-1990s saw these and other questions about multiple relationships and boundaries discussed—and often argued—from virtually every point of view, every discipline, and every theoretical orientation. In 1981, for example, Samuel Roll and Leverett Millen presented "A Guide to Violating an Injunction in Psychotherapy: On Seeing Acquaintances as Patients." In her 1988 article on "Dual Role Relationships," ethicist Karen Kitchener provided systematic guidance to readers on the kinds of "counselor–client relationships that are likely to lead to harm and those that are not likely to be harmful" (p. 217). Similarly, in the 1985 edition of their widely used textbook *Ethics in Psychology: Professional Standards and Cases,* Patricia Keith-Spiegel and Gerald Koocher discussed ways in which boundary crossings may be unavoidable in good clinical practice and presented ways to think through the ethical implications of specific dual relationships or other boundary issues. Patruksa Clarkson, who wrote "In Recognition of Dual Relationships," discussed the "mythical, single relationship" and noted that "it is impossible for most psychotherapists to avoid all situations in which conflicting interests or multiple roles might exist" (1994, p. 32).

Vincent Rinella and Alvin Gerstein argued that "the underlying moral and ethical rationale for prohibiting dual relationships . . . is no longer tenable" (1994, p. 225). Similarly, Robert Ryder and Jeri Hepworth (1990) set forth thoughtful arguments that the AAMFT ethics code should not prohibit dual relationships. Jeanne Adleman and Susan Barrett (1990) took a fresh and creative look, from a feminist perspective, at how to make careful decisions about dual relationships and boundary issues. Laura Brown (1989; see also 1994) examined the implications of boundary decisions from another perspective in "Beyond Thou Shalt Not: Thinking about Ethics in the Lesbian Therapy Community." Ellen Bader (1994) urged that the focus on the duality of roles be replaced by an examination of whether each instance did or did not involve exploitation.

Research Leading to a Call for a Change in the APA Ethics Code

The first ethics code of the American Psychological Association was empirically based. APA members responded to a survey asking them what ethical dilemmas they encountered in their day-to-day work. A replication of that survey, performed 50 years after the original, led to a call for a change in the APA ethics code regarding dual relationships.

The second most often reported ethical dilemma that psychologists reported was in the area of blurred, dual, or conflictual relationships. These responses from such a wide range of psychologists led investigators Pope and Vetter (1992) to include in their report a call for changes to the APA ethics code in the areas of dual relationships, multiple relationships, and boundary issues so that the ethics code would, for example,

1. define dual relationships more carefully and specify clearly conditions under which they might be therapeutically indicated or acceptable;

2. address clearly and realistically the situations of those who practice in small towns, rural communities, remote locales, and similar contexts (emphasizing that neither the current code in place at the time nor the draft revision under consideration at that time fully acknowledged or adequately addressed such contexts); and

3. distinguish between dual relationships and accidental or incidental extratherapeutic contacts (e.g., running into a patient at the grocery market or unexpectedly seeing a client at a party) . . . [in order] to address realistically the awkward entanglements into which even the most careful therapist can fall.

The following section from the *American Psychologist* report of the study presents the relevant findings, examples, specific suggestions for changes, and reasoning.

Blurred, Dual, or Conflictual Relationships

The second most frequently described incidents involved maintaining clear, reasonable, and therapeutic boundaries around the professional relationship with a client. In some cases, respondents were troubled by such instances as serving as both "therapist and supervisor for hours for [patient/supervisee's] MFCC [marriage, family, and child counselor] license" or when "an agency hires one of its own clients." In other cases, respondents found dual relationships to be useful "to provide role modeling, nurturing and a giving quality to therapy." One respondent, for example, believed that providing therapy to couples with whom he has social relationships and who are members of his small church makes sense because he is "able to see how these people interact in group context." In still other cases, respondents reported that it was sometimes difficult to know what constitutes a dual relationship or conflict of interest; for example, "I have employees/supervisees who were former clients and wonder if this is a dual relationship." Another . . . respondent felt a conflict between his own romantic attraction to a patient's mother and responsibilities to the child who had developed a positive relationship with him:

> I was conducting therapy with a child and soon became aware that there was a mutual attraction between myself and the child's mother. The strategies I had used and my rapport with the child had been positive. Nonetheless, I felt it necessary to refer to avoid a dual relationship (at the cost of the gains that had been made).

Taken as a whole, the incidents suggest, first, that the ethical principles need to define dual relationships more carefully and to note with clarity if and when they are ever therapeutically indicated or acceptable. For example, a statement such as "Minimal or remote relationships are unlikely to violate this standard" ("Draft," 1991, p. 32) may be too vague and ambiguous to be helpful. A psychologist's relationship to a very casual acquaintance whom she or he meets for lunch a few times a year, to an accountant who only does very routine work in filling out her or his tax forms once a year (all such business being conducted by mail), to her or his employer's husband (who has no involvement in the business and with whom the psychologist never socializes), and to a travel agent (who books perhaps one or two flights a year for the psychologist) may constitute relatively minimal or remote relationships. However, will a formal code's assurance that minimal or remote relationships are unlikely to violate the standard provide a clear, practical, valid, and useful basis for ethical deliberation to the psychologist who serves as therapist to all four individuals? Research and the professional literature focusing on nonsexual dual relationships underscores the importance and implications of decisions to enter into or refrain from such activities (e.g., Borys & Pope, 1989; Ethics Committee, 1988; Keith-Spiegel & Koocher, 1985; Pope & Vasquez, 2011 Stromberg et al., 1988).

Second, the principles must address clearly and realistically the situations of those who practice in small towns, rural communities, and other remote locales. Neither the current code nor the current draft revision explicitly acknowledges and adequately addresses such geographic contexts. Forty-one of the dual-relationship incidents involved such locales. Many respondents implicitly or explicitly complained that the principles seem to ignore the special conditions in small, self-contained communities. For example,

> I live and maintain a . . . private practice in a rural area. I am also a member of a spiritual community based here. There are very few other therapists in the immediate vicinity who work with transformational, holistic, and feminist principles in the context of good clinical training that "conventional" people can also feel confidence in. Clients often come to me because they know me already, because they are not satisfied with the other services available, or because they want to work with someone who understands their spiritual practice and can incorporate its principles and practices into the process of transformation, healing, and change. The stricture against dual relationships helps me to maintain a high degree of sensitivity to the ethics (and potentials for abuse or confusion) of such situations, but doesn't give me any help in working with the actual circumstances of my practice. I hope revised principles will address these concerns!

Third, the principles need to distinguish between dual relationships and accidental or incidental extra therapeutic contacts (e.g., running into a patient at the grocery market or unexpectedly seeing a client at a party) and to address realistically the awkward entanglements into which even the most careful therapist can fall. For example, a therapist sought to file a formal complaint against some very noisy tenants of a neighboring house. When he did so, he was surprised to discover "that his patient was the owner–landlord."

It is worth emphasizing that the complexity of both therapy itself and specifically of boundary issues can never obscure, erode, or minimize the clinician's inescapable responsibility to maintain boundaries that protect and serve the patient's safety and the goals of therapy. As Robert Simon and Daniel Shuman (2007) wrote,

> [it] is always the therapist's responsibility to maintain appropriate boundaries, no matter how difficult or boundary testing the patient may be. . . . The conduct of psychotherapy is an impossible task because there are no perfect therapists and no perfect therapies. Knowing one's boundaries, however, makes the impossible task easier. (p. 212; see also Appelbaum & Gutheil, 2007; Gutheil & Brodsky, 2008)

On Not Overlooking How Difficult This Topic Tends to Be for Us

In closing this section, it's worth noting what a vexing challenge this area is for mental-health practitioners. Part of the problem is the difficulty of psychotherapy itself. We can never go on automatic pilot, never let the formal standards and guidelines do our thinking for us, and never let the general principles obscure the uniqueness of every therapeutic encounter.

> Awareness of the ethics codes is crucial to competence in the area of ethics, but the formal standards are not a substitute for an active, deliberative, and creative approach to fulfilling our ethical responsibilities. They prompt, guide, and inform our ethical consideration; they do not preclude or serve as a substitute for it. There is no way that the codes and principles can be effectively followed or applied in a rote, thoughtless manner. Each new client, whatever his or her similarities to previous clients, is a unique individual. Each situation also is unique and is likely to change significantly over time. The explicit codes and principles may designate many possible approaches as clearly unethical. They may identify with greater or lesser degrees of clarity the types of ethical concerns that are likely to be especially significant, but they cannot tell us how these concerns will manifest themselves in a particular clinical situation. They may set forth essential tasks that we must fulfill, but they cannot tell us how we can accomplish these tasks with a unique client facing unique problems. . . . There is no legitimate way to avoid these struggles. (Pope & Vasquez, 2011)

But another part of the difficulty is the topic itself, how often we jump to conclusions, rely on stereotypes, or fail to consider carefully what is actually occurring rather than what seems to be happening. Former APA president Gerry Koocher (2006) provides a vivid example of how others tend to react when he tells them about crossing time boundaries (i.e., letting a session run far beyond its schedule), financial boundaries (i.e., not charging), and other boundaries with one of his clients.

> On occasion I tell my students and professional audiences that I once spent an entire psychotherapy session holding hands with a 26-year-old woman together in a quiet darkened room. That disclosure usually elicits more than a few gasps and grimaces. When I add that I could not bring myself to end the session after 50 minutes and stayed with the young woman holding hands for another half hour, and when I add the fact that I never billed for the extra time, eyes roll.
>
> Then, I explain that the young woman had cystic fibrosis with severe pulmonary disease and panic-inducing air hunger. She had to struggle through three breaths on an oxygen line before she could speak a sentence. I had come into her room, sat down by her bedside, and asked how I might help her. She grabbed my hand and said, "Don't let go." When the time came for another appointment, I called a nurse to take my place. By this point in my story most listeners, who had felt critical of or offended by the "hand holding," have moved from an assumption of

sexualized impropriety to one of empathy and compassion. The real message of the anecdote, however, lies in the fact that I never learned this behavior in a classroom. No description of such an intervention exists in any treatment manual or tome on empirically based psychotherapy. (p. xxii)

Setting appropriate boundaries and limits presents vexing dilemmas for all therapists. Consider the following situations and discuss how you would respond:

- Several of your clients ask to follow you on Twitter and to be listed as a friend on Facebook.

- A longtime client dies, and her sister asks you to say a few words at your client's funeral.

- Your client, a travel agent, offers you a free upgrade to first class when you are only paying for an economy-class seat.

- A patient you have seen for many years commits suicide, and the patient's sister— a trial attorney who has been paying the bills for therapy for many years—asks to have a private session to "get closure on David's death."

- A client reveals that she is in fact "Maria," a woman you have been flirting with on an Internet dating site for the past two months.

- A state trooper—who also happens to be one of your clients—stops you for speeding but tells you he is only going to give you a warning ticket because you've helped him so much in therapy.

ACCESSIBILITY AND PEOPLE WITH DISABILITIES

You are a therapist with a thriving practice in a large city. You see clients in a large suite atop a high-rise office building with a magnificent view of the city. There is a new client who will be showing up that evening for an initial session. The office building closes and locks its doors at 5 p.m. each day, but both heating in winter and air conditioning in summer remain on until 10 p.m., and at the top of the front steps is a call-box system allowing people outside to call the phone in any of the offices to ask to be buzzed in. The new client never shows up at your office. It is only the next day that you learn that the client is blind. Finding the front door locked, he was unable to locate a way to enter the building. There were no instructions in Braille or any other indications of how to gain access to the building that would be perceived by someone who was blind or had any form of severely impaired vision. As you consider this situation, the phone rings. It is someone whose initial appointment is scheduled to begin five minutes from now. She is calling with her cell phone. She is outside your building but does not know how to enter. She uses a wheelchair for mobility and is unable to use the front steps that lead up to your building's front door. What are your feelings as you imagine yourself the therapist in this vignette? What do you think you would say to these two people? What, if anything, do you wish you had done differently?

This vignette illustrates two of the many ways in which psychotherapists and their offices may be blocked off from people with disabilities. These physical barriers may shut out many people. As psychologist Martha Banks noted,

[a]pproximately one-fifth of U.S. citizens have disabilities. The percentage is slightly higher among women and girls (21.3%) than among men and boys (19.8%). Among women, Native American women and African American women have the highest percentages of disabilities. . . . As a result of limited access to funds, more than one-third of women with work disabilities and more than 40% of those with severe work disabilities are living in poverty. . . . (2003, p. xxiii)

Individual therapists and the profession as a whole face the challenge of identifying the barriers that screen out people with disabilities or make it unnecessarily difficult for them to become therapists or to find appropriate therapeutic services. Think back to the classrooms, lecture halls, and therapy offices you have seen. Would a person using a wheelchair or walker find reasonable access to those places? Would a person who is blind or has severe visual impairment experience unnecessary hardships in navigating those buildings? For additional information and strategies to identify and address issues of physical access, see Pope (2005), Chapter 4, in *How to Survive and Thrive as a Therapist: Information, Ideas, and Resources for Psychologists* (Pope & Vasquez, 2005), and the the Web site "Accessibility & Disability Information & Resources in Psychology Training & Practice" at http://kpope.com.

In addition to the challenge of identifying and addressing physical barriers is the challenge of providing adequate training. A survey of American Psychological Association members by Irene Leigh and her colleagues found reports of problems resulting from lack of adequate training.

> "A deaf woman [was] diagnosed as having schizophrenia by a mental health agency because she flailed her arms around; she was signing." Another respondent indicated that a child with hearing impairment had been misdiagnosed with mental retardation. With regard to test interpretation, a respondent reported that a provider administered a short version of the Minnesota Multiphasic Personality Inventory and did not take into consideration how disability might affect some responses such as "I have difficulty standing or walking." Other examples . . . included providers not using an interpreter and provider refusal to treat persons with disabilities. (Leigh, Powers, Vash, & Nettles, 2004)

Similarly, in "Impact of Professional Training on Case Conceptualization of Clients with a Disability," Nancy Kemp and Brent Mallinckrodt (1996) reported the results of their study:

> Therapists gave different priorities to treatment themes depending on whether the client had a disability and whether they, the therapists, had received any training in disability issues. Untrained therapists were more likely to focus on extraneous issues and less likely to focus on appropriate themes for a sexual abuse survivor with a disability. (p. 378)

Among the findings were that "even a small amount of training on issues of disability may be associated with significantly less bias in case conceptualization and treatment planning" (Kemp & Mallinckrodt, 1996, p. 383).

Unfortunately, studies of how therapists are trained suggest that we have a long way to go in meeting these challenges. In "ADA Accommodation of Therapists with Disabilities in Clinical Training," Hendrika Kemp and her colleagues noted that

> Despite the obvious need . . . disability is not a standard part of clinical training. . . . We found that of the 618 internship sites recently listed on the APPIC web-site, only 81 listed a disabilities rotation. . . . The picture is even bleaker when we examine how training sites accommodate clinicians with disabilities. (Kemp, Chen, Erickson, & Friesen, 2003)

Finally, flaws in our training programs may affect students with disabilities. Taube and Olkin (2011), for example, state that

> [t]here are three broad areas in which trainees with disabilities might encounter discrimination in rehabilitation, clinical, and counseling psychology training programs. The first area relates to structural barriers to access, such as not having books on tape or in Braille, failure to provide handouts online and in advance, failure to provide sign language interpreters, and failure to have wheelchair-accessible facilities. . . .

The second area relates to policies and procedures for completing graduate programs. These may include, for example, a refusal to allow trainees with disabilities to engage in part-time training or to permit extra time on assignments. . . . The third area relates to less tangible discriminatory barriers such as how a trainee is treated by instructors and peers, whether the trainee is seen as a viable candidate for clinical placements, whether the trainee is steered away from disability topics, and whether disability is included in diversity training. . . . However, psychologists are subject to the same prejudices about disability as are others [and] . . . . it is in this third area that trainees with disabilities (as well as trainees from other traditionally marginalized groups) may be most subject to discrimination and least protected by law. (p. 329)

THE AMERICAN PSYCHOLOGICAL ASSOCIATION, THE LAW, AND INDIVIDUAL ETHICAL RESPONSIBILITY

In collaboration with the local police chief, you establish a creative program in which you provide therapy to any police officer who requests it. Although all officers signed confidentiality waivers when joining the force, the chief tells you that he and the department will keep hands off and that you and your clients can consider your work confidential. A little more than a year later, Internal Affairs visits your office and tells you to open your files on several police officers as part of a high-profile investigation. You call the chief, who apologizes profusely but says it is out of his hands and you'll have to rely on the signed waivers. You turn over the files. Several officers file ethics complaints. You point out that you were forced to follow the law and, because you had no other legal option, you committed no ethical violation. Should the APA Ethics Committee accept your defense?

One of the most closely watched series of trials in history focused on the question of whether following the law relieves one of ethical responsibility. The Nuremberg Trials after World War II evaluated the Nazi defense of "just following the law" or "just following orders." The verdicts reaffirmed that individual ethical responsibility existed beyond the dictates of law, and this became known as the Nuremberg Ethic. In short, the Nuremberg Trials established that an individual who decided to violate a fundamental ethical responsibility could not escape ethical accountability by trying to place all responsibility and agency on laws, orders, or regulations.

Whatever their setting or specialty, clinicians can feel that laws or regulations are at odds with the legitimate needs of their clients or with their own conscience and most deeply help values. What does the individual clinician do when facing such dilemmas? To illustrate such a dilemma in which people of good faith can differ on the right course of action, we've chosen a high-profile controversy involving the psychology profession. It is important to keep in mind that the kinds of issues that follow appear in countless forms in our work, regardless of our profession, locale, or clientele.

Less than a year after the horrendous attacks of September 11, 2001, on the United States, the American Psychological Association broke with other major health and behavioral science organizations and took a stance directly opposing the Nuremberg Ethic. On August 21, 2002, APA adopted an ethics code that, for the first time in its long history, stated that when encountering an irreconcilable conflict between their "ethical responsibilities" and the state's authority, "psychologists may adhere to the requirements of the law, regulations, or other governing legal authority" (Section 1. 02).

An earlier draft had mandated that psychologists' decisions in such cases must be "in keeping with basic principles of human rights." However, APA decided to remove that restriction from the code's enforceable section and to mention it only in the code's introduction, where it would be aspirational rather than required and enforceable.

APA's long history, stretching back more than a century, had included arguments that it would be in psychologists' interests to allow the law, regulations, and other governing legal authority to shield them from violating ethical standards. Before 9/11, various ethics code drafts had ventured opposition to the Nuremberg Ethic and the controversy about how to handle ethical–legal conflicts served as a focus of journal articles. In the 1980s, for example, a survey of psychologists' beliefs and behaviors when confronting such conflicts appeared in the *American Psychologist* with the title "When Laws and Values Conflict: A Dilemma for Psychologists" (Pope & Bajt, 1988). However, before the 9/11 attacks, APA had never approved any draft code that opposed the Nuremberg Ethics.

Occurring less than a year after and in the context of both the 9/11 attack on the United States and the U.S. military's launch of Operation Enduring Freedom in Afghanistan in response to that attack, the APA Council of Representatives voted to let psychologists set aside basic ethical responsibilities if they conflicted irreconcilably with laws, regulations, and other forms of governing legal authority. These legal orders included military orders clearly communicated to the profession, policy makers, and the public. This was a profound shift in values.

The U.S. military supported this shift and emphasized APA's new enforceable ethical standard in its own formal policy for psychologists (U.S. Department of the Army, 2006, p. 152). Citing APA's new ethical standard, the army policy stated: "A process for maintaining adherence to the Code when it conflicts with applicable law, regulation, and policy is outlined below" (p. 154). The policy stated that after consultation and attempts to resolve the conflict, "If the issue continues to elude resolution, adhere to law, regulations, and policy in a responsible manner."

Although the military—as well as many APA members and others—tended to support this historic change in APA's ethics code, there was also widespread criticism. The editor of the *British Medical Journal*, for example, wrote: "So deeply ingrained is [the Nuremberg] ethic in health care that it's surprising, even shocking, to find that the same code isn't shared by psychologists, at least in the United States" (Godless, 2009).

Writing in the British Psychological Society's *The Psychologist*, Burton and Kagan (2007), stated,

> Most concerning of all, the APA allows its members the "Nuremberg defence" that "I was only following orders.". . . The implication is that psychologists are permitted to assist in torture and abuse if they can claim that they first tried to resolve the conflict between their ethical responsibility and the law, regulations or government legal authority. Otherwise they can invoke the Nuremberg defence. (p. 485)

Other health associations continued to speak out against the notion that governmental authority can serve as a valid defense when violating basic ethical responsibilities. Less than a year after APA adopted an ethics code that opposed the Nuremberg Ethic, for example, the World Medical Association's president issued a public reminder:

> At Nuremberg in 1947, accused physicians tried to defend themselves with the excuse that they were only following the law and commands from their superiors. . . the court announced that a physician could not deviate from his ethical obligations even if legislation demands otherwise. (World Medical Association, 2003)

Adopting a formal ethics code that opposed the Nuremberg Ethic, the American Psychological Association continued to support, teach, and promote it as official ethical policy for eight years. APA did not reverse its stance against the Nuremberg Ethic until 2010.

DETAINEE INTERROGATIONS

Scenario One

You are a therapist in independent practice. Several government officials arrive at your office to explain that one of your clients has been placed in a high-security center for questioning. The Department of Homeland Security has reason to believe that your client has knowledge of a terrorist network planning a massive attack. An interrogation team hopes to obtain enough information from your client, who has so far refused to discuss the topic, in time to prevent the attack. Emphasizing that lives are at stake and there is not a moment to waste, the officials ask for your client's evaluation and treatment records so that they can be faxed immediately to the interrogation team. They ask you to accompany them to the holding center so that the interrogation team can consult with you about the strategies most likely to gain the client's trust and persuade him to cooperate. They also ask you to talk with your client because he trusts you. When you hesitate, they stress that the attack may be only a matter of hours away, that surely you would not want to be the one person who could have prevented the attack and whose delay or refusal to help resulted in widespread death and destruction.

What ethical issues does this scenario raise? What reasons would you give for cooperating fully, cooperating in some ways but not in others, or refusing to cooperate with the government officials?

Scenario Two

You are a military psychologist transferred to a detention center holding those suspected of being enemy combatants, unlawful combatants, and others who pose a threat to national security. You are ordered to use interviews and other appropriate methods to prepare psychological profiles of several detainees so that they may be interrogated effectively.

What ethical issues, if any, does this scenario present? Would you have concerns about any aspects of your participation?

In the aftermath of the 9/11 attacks on the United States, the United States began interrogating detainees in Abu Ghraib prison in Iraq, the detention center at Bagram Airfield in Afghanistan, and Camps Delta, Iguana, and X-Ray at Guantanamo Bay Naval Base. The American Psychological Association took the position that psychologists should play a key role in detainee interrogations because the interrogations were inherently a psychological process requiring psychological expertise. The "Statement of the American Psychological Association on Psychology and Interrogations Submitted to the United States Senate Select Committee on Intelligence" stated:

> Conducting an interrogation is inherently a psychological endeavor. . . . Psychology is central to this process because an understanding of an individual's belief systems, desires, motivations, culture and religion likely will be essential in assessing how best to form a connection and facilitate educing accurate, reliable and actionable intelligence. Psychologists have expertise in human behavior, motivations and relationships. . . . Psychologists have valuable contributions to make toward . . . protecting our nation's security through interrogation processes. (APA, 2007)

Psychologists' special expertise sets them apart, according to the American Psychological Association, from psychiatrists and other physicians. The Director of the APA Ethics Office wrote: "This difference, which stems from psychologists' unique competencies, represents an important distinction between what role psychologists and physicians may take in interrogations" (Behnke, 2006, p. 66).

The American Psychological Association's emphasis on its unique competencies in interrogation and the value of its contributions to the interrogations led the Pentagon to adopt a new policy in 2006 that focused solely on psychologists, rather than including psychiatrists, for help in developing strategies for interrogating detainees.

Assurances by the APA and its representatives that "psychologists knew not to participate in activities that harmed detainees" was part of a central theme of the organization that psychologists would keep interrogations safe and ethical.

In 2007, for example, the president of the American Psychological Association wrote, "The Association's position is rooted in our belief that having psychologists consult with interrogation teams makes an important contribution toward keeping interrogations safe and ethical."

The 2007 APA president emphasized that psychologists' involvement makes an important contribution toward keeping interrogations safe and ethical (Brehm, 2007). The following statement from the APA Ethics Office appearing in *Psychology Today* emphasized what psychologists' participation would achieve in *all* interrogations: "The ability to spot conditions that make abuse more likely uniquely prepares psychologists for this task. Adding a trained professional ensures that all interrogations are conducted in a safe, legal, ethical, and effective manner that protects the individual and helps to elicit information that will prevent future acts of violence" (Hutson, 2008).

APA's assurances that psychologists' involvement would ensure that *all* interrogations would be safe, legal, ethical, and effective were controversial and deserve careful consideration. What evidence did APA have to support such sweepingly absolute statements? Were APA's public statements supported by the facts?

It is worth noting that some reports suggested that the effects of psychologists' involvement were not all positive. Eban (2007; see also Goodman, 2007), for example, documented ways in which "psychologists weren't merely complicit in America's aggressive new interrogation regime. Psychologists, working in secrecy, had actually designed the tactics and trained interrogators in them. . . ." According to the Associated Press, "Military psychologists were enlisted to help develop more aggressive interrogation methods, including snarling dogs, forced nudity and long periods of standing, against terrorism suspects, according to a Senate investigation." Mayer (2008) reported, "[General] Dunlavey soon drafted military psychologists to play direct roles in breaking detainees down. The psychologists were both treating the detainees clinically and advising interrogators on how to manipulate them and exploit their phobias. . . ." After publishing a series of investigative reports, the *Boston Globe* stated, "From the moment U.S. military and civilian officials began detaining and interrogating Guantanamo Bay prisoners with methods that the Red Cross has called tantamount to torture, they have had the assistance of psychologists" ("Psychologists and Torture," 2008).

The sharp disagreements over interpretations of the effects of psychologists' participation in detainee interrogations are exemplified by the contrasting reactions to a set of government documents obtained by the American Civil Liberties Union (ACLU). The ACLU released the documents under the heading "Newly Unredacted Report Confirms Psychologists Supported Illegal Interrogations in Iraq and Afghanistan." The ACLU disagreed with the view that the director of the APA Ethics Office had expressed:

> We do not, however, agree with your conclusion that documents recently obtained by the ACLU through its Freedom of Information Act Litigation demonstrate that the APA's "policy of engagement served the intended purpose." . . . Rather, we are deeply concerned by the fact that, viewed in context, these documents warrant the opposite conclusion. (Romero, 2008)

APA's approach attracted sharp criticism. The editor of *British Medical Journal* wrote that APA's approach was shocking (Goddlee, 2009). Professor of Medicine and Bioethics Steven Miles wrote: "The American Psychological Association was unique among U.S. health professional associations in providing policy cover for abusive interrogations" (2009). Amnesty International et al. (2009) sent an open letter to APA describing necessary steps to acknowledge and confront "the terrible stain on . . . American psychology." For a more comprehensive review of APA's policy documents and public statements in this area, see Pope (2011).

This controversy provides a rich opportunity to engage in critical thinking about policies, public assurances, and evidence. Here are a few examples of questions that may be useful in thinking through complex issues:

What evidence does an individual psychologist or a psychological association need before providing assurances to the public that a particular approach or intervention is safe and effective?

What hazards are there in making absolute assurances about all cases?

What costs, if any, are there when an individual organization makes public assurances that are not supported by the evidence?

CULTURES

You are a marriage and family counselor who works in a large mental-health clinic. One client immigrated to the United States from another country and has learned enough English to communicate adequately during therapy. During the fourth session, the client says, "As you know, I come from another culture and I was wondering: Do you think that your own culture and the culture of this clinic have any effects on me and my therapy? For example, I notice that all the therapists and administrators in this clinic seem to be of the same race, while the people who clean the building and take care of the grounds all seem to be of a different race. Why do you think that is and do you think it has any effects on what happens between us in my therapy?"

How do you think you would respond to the client? What are your thoughts about how a therapist's culture and a mental-health organization's culture might affect individual clients and the therapeutic process? How would you design a research study to explore the possible effects of culture on therapy, therapists, and clients? What hypotheses would you advance? When you imagined this situation, what country did you imagine the client emigrated from? What race was the client? The therapist? The cleaning staff? Why did these particular images come to mind?

The United States is a diverse nation enriched by the presence of many different cultures. However, cultural differences between therapist and client can sometimes pose significant challenges to everyone involved. One of the most obvious challenges occurs when the cultures speak different languages.

Even when therapist and patient both speak the same language (Spanish or Chinese, for example), each language may have many dialects that can prevent clear communication. And furthermore, "variations in language barriers experienced by immigrant groups are often reflective of differences in the local migration histories and socio-economic status of these groups" (Kretsedemas, 2005, p. 109).

In addition to language challenges are the challenges imposed when the research studies that inform our understanding overlook potentially significant cultural and other group differences. For example, Beverly Greene (1997) notes,

> A preponderance of the empirical research on or with lesbians and gay men has been conducted with overwhelmingly white, middle-class respondents. . . . Similarly, research on members of ethnic minority groups rarely acknowledges differences in sexual orientation among group members. Hence there has been little exploration of the complex interaction between sexual orientation and ethnic identity development, nor have the realistic social tasks and stressors that are a component of gay and lesbian identity formation in conjunction with ethnic identity formation been taken into

account. Discussion of the vicissitudes of racism and ethnic identity in intra- and in-terracial couples of the same gender and their effects on these couples' relationships has also been neglected in the narrow focus on heterosexual relationships found in the literature on ethnic minority clients. There has been an equally narrow focus on predominantly white couples in the gay and lesbian literature. (pp. 216–217)

Research that does take into account cultural complexity suggests that culture may sometimes play a significant role in the development of psychological disorders. Jeanne Miranda (2006) wrote,

Rates of depression and substance abuse disorders are low among Mexican Americans born in Mexico . . . and immigrant Mexican American women have a lifetime rate of depression of 8%, similar to the rates of nonimmigrant Mexicans. . . . However, after 13 years in the United States, rates of depression for those women who immigrated to the United States rise precipitously. U.S.-born women of Mexican heritage experience lifetime rates of depression similar to those of the White population in the United States, nearly twice the rate of immigrants. These findings are mirrored in other indicators of health. . . . Despite high rates of poverty, Mexican American immigrant women have low rates of physical and mental health problems. . . . Chinese American immigrant women have a lifetime rate of major depression near 7%, approximately half that of White women. . . . These results suggest that some aspects of culture protect against depression. (pp. 115–116)

Shankar Vedantam (2005) provides other examples of how culture and other group differences may influence mental health:

- Patients with schizophrenia, a disease characterized by hallucinations and disorganized thinking, recover sooner and function better in poor countries with strong extended family ties than in the United States as two long-running studies by the World Health Organization have shown.

- People of Mexican descent born in the United States have twice the risk of disorders such as depression and anxiety, and four times the risk of drug abuse, compared with recent immigrants from Mexico. This finding is part of a growing body of literature that indicates that the newly arrived are more resilient to mental disorders, and that assimilation is associated with higher rates of psychiatric diagnoses.

- Black and Hispanic patients are more than three times as likely to be diagnosed with schizophrenia as white patients—even though studies indicate that the rate of the disorder is the same in all groups.

- White women in the United States are three times as likely to commit suicide as black and Hispanic women—a difference that experts attribute in part to the relative strengths of different social networks.

- A host of small studies suggest that the effects of psychiatric drugs vary widely across different ethnic groups. There are even differences in the effect with dummy pills.

Remember that even though any names and descriptions we might use to identify cultures, groups, and similar characteristics relevant to a client may help us understand the client's words, experiences, and behavior, they are *not* a substitute for learning directly from and about this unique individual. Individual differences within a group may overwhelm between-group differences, and an individual within a group may not reflect group characteristics. Any attempt to view, describe, or understand a person as the sum of a fixed set of descriptors oversimplifies in ways that are misleading. The descriptors themselves may not be as clear as some of the research seems to assume. As Connie Chan (1997) puts it,

Although identity is a fluid concept in psychological and sociological terms, we tend to speak of identities in fixed terms. In particular, those aspects of identity that characterize observable physical characteristics, such as race or gender, are perceived as unchanging ascribed identities. Examples of these would include identifications such as *Chinese woman,* or *Korean American woman,* or even broader terms such as *woman of color,* which are ways of grouping together individuals who are not of the hegemonic "white" race in the United States. We base these constructions of identity upon physical appearance and an individual's declaration of identity. However, even these seemingly clear distinctions are not definitive. For example, I, as a woman of Asian racial background, may declare myself a woman of color because I see myself as belonging to a group of ethnic/racial minorities. However, my (biological) sister could insist that she is not a woman of color because she does not feel an affiliation with our group goals, even though she is a person of Chinese ancestry. Does her nonaffiliation take her out of the group of people of color? Or does she remain in regardless of her own self-identification because of her obvious physical characteristics? Generally, in the context of identities based upon racial and physical characteristics, ascribed identities will, rightly or wrongly, continue to be attributed to individuals by others. It is left up to individuals themselves to assert their identities and demonstrate to others that they are or are *not* what they might appear to be upon first notice. (pp. 240–241)

It is also crucial that therapists be aware not only of the client's culture but also of the therapist's own culture and how it influences the therapist's values, frameworks, theoretical orientation, understanding, and decisions. An exceptional book, *The Spirit Catches You and You Fall Down: A Hmong Child, Her American Doctors, and the Collision of Two Cultures* (Fadiman, 1997) documents in vivid detail the efforts of health-care professionals at a California hospital and a refugee family from Laos to help a Hmong child whom the health-care professionals had determined was experiencing epileptic seizures. Despite the great expertise and dedication of the girl's physicians, the failure to take culture into account had disastrous consequences. Medical anthropologist Arthur Kleinman is quoted in the book:

> As powerful an influence as the culture of the Hmong patient and her family is on this case, the culture of biomedicine is equally powerful. If you can't see that your own culture has its own set of interests, emotions, and biases, how can you expect to deal successfully with someone else's culture? (p. 261)

Kleinman addresses the effects of culture, such as the culture of biomedicine, in more detail in an article (2004) in the *New England Journal of Medicine:*

> The culture of biomedicine is also responsible for some of the uncertainty surrounding depression. Symptoms that represent a depressive disorder for the practitioner (say, sadness and hopelessness in a patient dying from cancer) may not denote a medical problem to the patient, his or her family, or their clergy, for whom depression may be a sign of the moral experience of suffering. What is seen by a particular social network as a normal emotional response—say, grief lasting for years—may count as a depressive disorder for the psychiatrist, since the *Diagnostic and Statistical Manual of Mental Disorders* . . . defines normal bereavement as lasting for two months. In this area, the professional culture, driven by the political economy of the pharmaceutical industry, may represent the leading edge of a worldwide shift in norms.
>
> Yet many people with clinical depression—at least 50 percent among immigrants and minority groups in the United States—still receive neither a diagnosis nor treatment from a biomedical practitioner. Lack of access to appropriate services is a major reason for this failure, but cultural causes of misdiagnosis also

contribute. Culture confounds diagnosis and management by influencing not only the experience of depression, but also the seeking of help, patient–practitioner communication, and professional practice. Culture also affects the interaction of risk factors with social supports and protective psychological factors that contribute to depression in the first place. Culture may even turn out to create distinctive environments for gene expression and physiological reaction, resulting in a local biology of depression: research already shows that persons from various ethnic backgrounds metabolize antidepressant drugs in distinct ways. (pp. 951–952)

Melba Vasquez (2007) provides an evidence-based analysis of the ways in which cultural differences can affect the therapeutic alliance specifically and therapy more generally. Lillian Comas-Díaz explores the relationship between culture and psychotherapy more fully in Chapter 15 of this book.

The same question arises here as with the other challenges and controversies noted in this chapter: Are we addressing these issues adequately in our training programs? Research conducted by Nancy Hansen and her colleagues (2006) suggests that we may need to pay more attention to issues of culture in our graduate programs, practica is, internships, and other educational settings to develop competencies in this area and the ability to follow through. Hansen and colleagues' "Do We Practice What We Preach?" provides the results of a survey that found that "Overall and for 86% of the individual items, participants did not practice what they preached" (p. 66) in terms of what they endorsed as the need for multicultural competencies. Hansen and her colleagues concluded that psychotherapists need to recognize their vulnerability to not following through with what they know to be competent practice, and they need, in advance, to problem solve creative solutions. It would be helpful to identify your personal barriers in this regard: Are you anxious about raising certain issues with racially or ethnically different clients? Are you uncertain about how best to intervene? Do you fear you will "get in over your head" exploring these issues? What will it take to work through (or around) these barriers to become more racially and ethnically responsive in your psychotherapy work? (Hansen et al., 2006, p. 72)

Taking seriously the reality that *every* therapist is influenced by culture and *every* client is influenced by culture saves us from the misleading stereotype that multicultural counseling is something you need to know about only if you happen to find yourself working with someone from a different country, say, or someone of a different ethnicity who speaks a different language. As Pedersen, Draguns, Lonner, and Trimble (1989, p. 1) remind us in *Counseling Across Cultures:* "Multicultural counseling is not an exotic topic that applies to remote regions, but is the heart and core of good counseling with any client."

ANNOTATED BIBLIOGRAPHY

Pope, K. S., & Vasquez, M. J. T. (2011). *Ethics in psychotherapy and counseling: A practical guide* (4th ed.). Hoboken, NJ: Wiley.

This book provides an expanded discussion and in-depth analysis of almost all of the issues discussed in this chapter.

WEB RESOURCES

PsycCRITIQUES blog (http://psyccritiquesblog. apa.org/) *PsycCRITIQUES: Contemporary Psychology—APA Review of Books* is a weekly online journal that reviews books and films relevant to the science and practice of psychology. Many of the issues and topics covered in this chapter are also debated in response to provocative probes on the journal's blog.

REFERENCES

Adleman, J., & Barrett, S. E. (1990). Overlapping relationships: Importance of the feminist ethical perspective. In H. Lermamn & N. Portman (Eds.), *Feminist ethics in psychotherapy* (pp. 87–91). New York: Springer.

American Psychiatric Association. (2012, March). Fewer medical school seniors electing psychiatry as a specialty. Retrieved from http://bit.ly/KOBNrj

American Psychological Association, Presidential Task Force on Evidence-Based Practice. (2005). Evidenced-based practice in psychology. *American Psychologist, 61,* 271–285. Retrieved from www.apa.org/practice/resources/evidence/evidence-based-report.pdf

American Psychological Association. (2007, September 21). Statement of the American Psychological Association on Psychology and Interrogations submitted to the United States Senate Select Committee on Intelligence. Retrieved from www.apa.org/ethics/statement092107.html

Amnesty International, Physicians for Human Rights, and 11 other organizations. (2009, June 29). Open letter in response to the American Psychological Association Board. Retrieved from http://bit.ly/Y2bFj

Appelbaum, P. S., & Gutheil, T. G. (2007). *Clinical handbook of psychiatry and the law* (4th ed.). New York: Lippincott Williams & Wilkins.

Bader, E. (1994). Dual relationships: Legal and ethical trends. *Transactional Analysis Journal, 24*(1), 64–66.

Banks, M. E. (2003). Preface. In M. E. Banks & E. Kaschak (Eds.), *Women with visible and invisible disabilities: Multiple intersections, multiple issues, multiple therapists* (pp. xxi–xxxix). New York: Haworth Press.

Barlow, D. H. (2004). Psychological treatments. *American Psychologist, 59*(9), 869–878.

Behnke, S. (2006). Ethics and interrogations: Comparing and contrasting the American Psychological, American Medical and American Psychiatric Association positions. *Monitor on Psychology, 37*(7), 66.

Borys, D. S., & Pope, K. S. (1989). Dual relationships between therapist and client: A national study of psychologists, psychiatrists, and social workers. *Professional Psychology: Research and Practice, 20,* 283–293. Available at http://kspope.com

Brehm, S. (2007, January 9). American Psychological Association news release of letter from the APA president to the editor of *The Washington Monthly.* Retrieved from www.apa.org/releases/washingtonmonthly.pdf

British Psychological Society. (2011). *Response to the American Psychiatric Association: DSM-5 Development.* London: Author. Retrieved from http://bit.ly/KenPopeBPSDSMCritique

Brodsky, A. M. (1989). Sex between patient and therapist: Psychology's data and response. In G. O. Gabbard (Ed.), *Sexual exploitation in professional relationships* (pp. 15–25). Washington, DC: American Psychiatric Press.

Brown, L. S. (1989). Beyond thou shalt not: Thinking about ethics in the Lesbian therapy community. *Women and Therapy, 8,* 13–25.

Brown, L. S. (1994). *Subversive dialogues.* New York: Basic Books.

Burton, M., & Kagan, C. (2007). Psychologists and torture: More than a question of interrogation. *The Psychologist, 20,* 484–487.

Caplan, P. J. (2012, April 27). Psychiatry's bible, the DSM, is doing more harm than good. *Washington Post.* Retrieved from http://wapo.st/KenPopeDSMAsCausingHarm

Chan, C. S. (1997). Don't ask, don't tell, don't know: The formation of a homosexual identity and sexual expression among Asian American lesbians. In B. Greene (Ed.), *Ethnic and cultural diversity among lesbians and gay men* (pp. 240–248). Thousand Oaks, CA: Sage.

Clarkson, P. (1994). In recognition of dual relationships. *Transactional Analysis Journal, 24*(1), 32–38.

Curtis, R., & Christian, E. (2012). (Eds.). *Integrated care: Applying theory to practice.* New York: Routledge.

Eban, K. (2007, July 17). Rorschach and awe. *Vanity Fair.* Retrieved from http://tinyurl.com/2zkg9p

Fadiman, A. (1997). *The spirit catches you and you fall down: A Hmong child, her American doctors, and the collision of two cultures.* New York: Farrar, Straus and Giroux.

Flores, G. (2006). Language barriers to health care in the United States. *New England Journal of Medicine, 355*(3), 229–231.

Godlee, F. (2009, May 16). Rules of conscience. *British Medical Journal, 338,* 7704. Retrieved from www.bmj.com/content/338/bmj. b1972. short

Goodheart, C. D. (2006). Evidence, endeavor, and expertise in psychological practice. In C. D. Goodheart, A. E. Kazdin, & R. J. Sternberg (Eds.), *Evidence-based psychotherapy: Where practice and research meet* (pp. 37–61). Washington, DC: American Psychological Association.

Goodheart, C. D., & Kazdin, A. E. (2006). Introduction. In C. D. Goodheart, A. E. Kazdin, & R. J. Sternberg (Eds.), *Evidence-based psychotherapy: Where practice and research meet* (pp. 3–10). Washington, DC: American Psychological Association.

Goodman, A. (2007, June 8). Psychologists implicated in torture. *Seattle Post-Intelligencer.* Retrieved from http://seattlepi. nwsource.com/opinion/318745_amy07.html

Greene, B. G. (Ed.). (1997). *Ethnic and cultural diversity among lesbians and gay men.* Thousand Oaks, CA: Sage.

Gutheil, T. G., & Brodsky, A. (2008). *Preventing boundary violations in clinical practice.* New York: Guilford.

Hansen, N. D., Randazzo, K. V., Schwartz, A., Marshall, M., Kalis, D., Frazier, R., Burke, C., Kershner-Rice, K., & Norvig, G. (2006). Do we practice what we preach? An exploratory survey of multicultural psychotherapy competencies. *Professional Psychology: Research and Practice, 37*(1), 66–74.

Hagemoser, S. D. (2009). Braking the bandwagon: Scrutinizing the science and politics of empirically supported therapies. *Journal of Psychology: Interdisciplinary and Applied, 143*(6), 601–614.

Kazdin, A. E. (2006). Arbitrary metrics: Implications for identifying evidence-based treatments. *American Psychologist, 61*(1), 42–49.

Kazdin, A. E. (2008a). Evidence-based treatments and delivery of psychological services: Shifting our emphases to increase impact. *Psychological Services, 5*(3), 201–215.

Kazdin, A. E. (2008b). Evidence-based treatment and practice: New opportunities to bridge clinical research and practice, enhance the knowledge base, and improve patient care. *American Psychologist, 63*(3), 146–159.

Keith-Spiegel, P., & Koocher, G. P. (1985). *Ethics in psychology: Professional standards and cases.* New York: Crown/Random House.

Kemp, H. V., Chen, J. S., Erickson, G. N., & Friesen, N. L. (2003). ADA accommodation of therapists with disabilities in clinical training. *Women & Therapy, 26*(1–2), 155–168.

Kemp, N. T., & Mallinckrodt, B. (1996). Impact of professional training on case conceptualization of clients with a disability. *Professional Psychology: Research and Practice, 27*(4), 378–385.

Kitchener, K. S. (1988). Dual role relationships: What makes them so problematic? *Journal of Counseling & Development, 67*(4), 217–221.

Kleinman, A. (2004). Culture and depression. *New England Journal of Medicine, 351*(10), 951–953.

Koocher, G. P. (2006). Foreword to the second edition: Things my teachers never mentioned. In K. S. Pope, J. L. Sonne, & B. Greene, *What therapists don't talk about and why: Understanding taboos that hurt us and our clients* (2nd ed., pp. xxi–xxiv). Washington, DC: American Psychological Association.

Kraemer, J. D., & Gostin, L. O. (2009). Science, politics, and values: The politicization of professional practice guidelines. *Journal of the American Medical Association, 301*(6), 665–667.

Kretsedemas, P. (2005). Language barriers & perceptions of bias. *Journal of Sociology & Social Welfare, 32*(4), 109–123.

Lehner, G. F. J. (1952). Defining psychotherapy. *American Psychologist, 7,* 547.

Leigh, I. W., Powers, L., Vash, C., & Nettles, R. (2004). Survey of psychological services to clients with disabilities: The need for awareness. *Rehabilitation Psychology, 49*(1), 48–54.

Lewis, A. (2006, June 7). Psychologists preferred for detainees. *New York Times.* Retrieved from http://tinyurl.com/2gfjdz

Luhrmann, T. M. (2000). *Of two minds: The growing disorder in American psychiatry.* New York: Knopf.

Mayer, J. (2008). *The dark side.* New York: Doubleday.

McHugh, P. R., & Slavney, P. R. (2012). Mental illness—comprehensive evaluation or checklist? *New England Journal of Medicine, 366*(20), 1853–1855. Retrieved from www.nejm.org/doi/full/10. 1056/NEJMp1202555

Miles, S. H. (2009b, May 1). Psychologists and torture [Letter to the Editor published online]. *British Medical Journal.* Retrieved from http://bmj.com

Miranda, J. (2006). Improving services and outreach for women with depression. In C. M. Mazure & G. P. Keita (Eds.), *Understanding depression in women: Applying empirical research to practice and policy* (pp. 113–135). Washington, DC: American Psychological Association.

Moran, M. (2009). Psychiatrists lament decline of key treatment modality. *Psychiatric News, 44*(13), 8. Retrieved from http://pn. psychiatryonline.org/cgi/content/full/44/13/8

Olfson, M, & Marcus, S. C. (2010). National trends in outpatient psychotherapy. *American Journal of Psychiatry, 167*(12), 1456–1463.

Olfson, M., Marcus, S. C., Druss, B., Elinson, L., Tanielian, T., & Pincus, H. A. (2002). National trends in the outpatient treatment of depression. *Journal of the American Medical Association, 287*(2), 203–209.

Olfson, M., Marcus, S. C., Druss, B., & Pincus, H. A. (2002). National trends in the use of outpatient psychotherapy. *American Journal of Psychiatry, 159*(11), 1914–1920.

Paul, G. L. (1967). Strategy of outcome research in psychotherapy. *Journal of Consulting Psychology, 31*(2), 109–118.

Pedersen, P. D., Draguns, J. G., Lonner, W. J., & Trimble, E. J. (1989). Introduction and overview. In P. D. Pedersen, J. G. Draguns, W. J. Lonner, & E. J. Trimble (Eds.), *Counseling across cultures* (3rd ed., pp. 1–2). Honolulu: University of Hawaii Press.

Pope, K. S. (1988). How clients are harmed by sexual contact with mental health professionals. *Journal of Counseling and Development, 67,* 222–226.

Pope, K. S. (1994). *Sexual involvement with therapists: Patient assessment, subsequent therapy, forensics.* Washington, DC: American Psychological Association.

Pope, K. S. (2005). Disability and accessibility in psychology: Three major barriers. *Ethics & Behavior, 15*(2), 103–106. Available at http://kspope.com

Pope, K. S. (2011). Are the American Psychological Association's detainee interrogation policies ethical and effective? Key claims, documents, and results. *Zeitschrift für Psychologie/Journal of Psychology, 219*(3), 150–158. Available at http://kspope.com/apa/detainee.php

Pope, K. S., & Bajt, T. R. (1988). When laws and values conflict: A dilemma for psychologists. *American Psychologist, 43,* 828.

Pope, K. S., & Bouhoutsos, J. C. (1986). *Sexual intimacies between therapists and patients.* New York: Praeger/Greenwood.

Pope, K. S., & Keith-Spiegel, P. (2008). A practical approach to boundaries in psychotherapy: Making decisions, bypassing blunders, and mending fences. *Journal of Clinical Psychology: In Session, 64*(5), 638–652.

Pope, K. S., Sonne, J. L., & Greene, B. (2006). *What therapists don't talk about and why: Understanding taboos that hurt us and our clients.* Washington, DC: American Psychological Association.

Pope, K. S., Sonne, J. L., & Holroyd, J. (1993). *Sexual feelings in psychotherapy: Explorations for therapists and therapists-in-training.* Washington, DC: American Psychological Association.

Pope, K. S., & Vasquez, M. J. T. (1998). *Ethics in psychotherapy and counseling.* San Francisco: Jossey-Bass.

Pope, K. S., & Vasquez, M. J. T. (2005). *How to survive and thrive as a therapist: Information, ideas, and resources for psychologists in practice*. Washington, DC: American Psychological Association.

Pope, K. S., & Vasquez, M. J. T. (2011). *Ethics in psychotherapy and counseling: A practical guide* (4th ed.). New York: Wiley.

Pope, K. S., & Vetter, V. A. (1992). Ethical dilemmas encountered by members of the American Psychological Association: A national survey. *American Psychologist, 47,* 397–411. Available at http://kspope.com

Psychologists and torture. [Editorial]. (2008, August 30). *Boston Globe*. Retrieved from http://tinyurl.com/5qhtf2

Reed, G. (2009). What is the difference between the ICD and DSM? *Monitor on Psychology, 40*(9), 63.

Rinella, V. J., & Gerstein, A. I. (1994). The development of dual relationships: Power and professional responsibility. *International Journal of Law and Psychiatry, 17*(3), 225–237.

Robiner, W. N., & Crew, D. P. (2000). Rightsizing the workforce of psychologists in health care: Trends from licensing boards, training programs, and managed care. *Professional Psychology: Research and Practice, 31,* 245–263.

Roll, S., & Millen, L. (1981). A guide to violating an injunction in psychotherapy: On seeing acquaintances as patients. *Psychotherapy: Theory, Research & Practice, 18*(2), 179–187.

Romero, A. D. (2008, June 18). Letter from the American Civil Liberties Executive Director to Dr. Stephen Behnke, Director, Ethics Office, American Psychological Association. Retrieved from http://tinyurl.com/6o5grc

Romero, S. (2012). Do Argentines need therapy? Pull up a couch. *The New York Times*. Retrieved from http://nyti.ms/OiIpLG

Roy v. Hartogs. (1976). 381 N.Y. S. 2d 587; 85 Misc. 2d 891.

Ryder, R., & Hepworth, J. (1990). AAMFT ethical code: "Dual relationships." *Journal of Marital & Family Therapy, 16*(2), 127–132.

Shaneyfelt, T. M., & Centor, R. M. (2009). Reassessment of clinical practice guidelines. *Journal of the American Medical Association, 301*(8), 868–869.

Simon, R. I., & Shuman, D. W. (2007). *Clinician's manual of psychiatry and law*. Washington, DC: American Psychiatric Press.

Spence, D. (2012). The psychiatric oligarchs who medicalise normality. *British Medical Journal, 344,* e3135. Retrieved from www.bmj.com/content/344/bmj. e3135

Sternberg, R. J. (2006). Evidence-based practice: Gold standard, gold plated, or fool's gold? In C. D. Goodheart, A. E. Kazdin, & R. J. Sternberg (Eds.), *Evidence-based psychotherapy: Where practice and research meet* (pp. 261–271). Washington, DC: American Psychological Association.

Stettin, G. D., Yao, J., Verbrugge, R. R., & Aubert, R. E. (2006, August). Frequency of follow-up care for adult and pediatric patients during initiation of antidepressant therapy. *American Journal of Managed Care, 12,* 453–461.

Stewart, R. E., Chambless, D. L., & Baron, J. (2012). Theoretical and practical barriers to practitioners' willingness to seek training in empirically supported treatments. *Journal of Clinical Psychology, 68*(1), 8–23.

Stromberg, C. D., Haggarty, D. J., Leibenluft, R. F., McMillian, M. H., Mishkin, B., Rubin, B. L., & Trilling, H. R. (1988). *The psychologist's legal handbook*. Washington, DC: Council for the National Register of Health Service Providers in Psychology.

Substance Abuse and Mental Health Services Administration. (2012). *Mental health, United States, 2010*. HHS Publication No. (SMA) 12-4681. Rockville, MD: Author.

Taube, D. O., & Olkin, R. (2011). When is differential treatment discriminatory? Legal, ethical, and professional considerations for psychology trainees with disabilities. *Rehabilitation Psychology, 56*(4), 329–339.

Urbina, I. (2012, May 12). Addiction diagnoses may rise under guideline changes. *The New York Times*, p. A11.

U.S. Department of the Army. (2006). *Behavioral science consultation policy* (OTSG/MEDCOM Policy Memo 06–029, October 20). Washington, DC: Author.

Vasquez, M. J. T. (2007). Cultural difference and the therapeutic alliance: An evidence-based analysis. *American Psychologist, 62*(8), 878–885.

Vedantam, S. (2005, June 26). Patients' diversity is often discounted: Alternatives to mainstream medical treatment call for recognizing ethnic, social differences. *Washington Post*, p. A1.

Wang, P. S., Demler, O., Olfson, M., Pincus, H. A., Wells, K. B., & Kessler, R. C. (2006). Changing profiles of service sectors used for mental health care in the United States. *American Journal of Psychiatry, 163*(8), 1187–1198.

Watts, G. (2012, May 11). More psychiatrists attack plans for DSM-5. *British Medical Journal, 344,* e3357. doi:10.1136/bmj.e3357

Westen, D., & Bradley, R. (2005). Empirically supported complexity: Rethinking evidence-based practice in psychotherapy. *Current Directions in Psychological Science, 14,* 266–271.

Westen, D., Novotny, C. M., & Thompson-Brenner, H. (2004). The empirical status of empirically supported psychotherapies: Assumptions, findings, and reporting in controlled clinical trials. *Psychological Bulletin, 130,* 631–663.

World Medical Association. (2003, June 23). Physicians under threat, warns WMA president, Press release. Retrieved from http://bit.ly/bXfPFM

GLOSSARY

The following abbreviations are used to indicate primary associations: (AD) Adlerian Psychotherapy; (BT) Behavior Therapy; (CC) Client-Centered Therapy; (CN) Contemplative Psychotherapy; (CT) Cognitive Therapy; (EX) Existential Therapy; (FT) Family Therapy; (GT) Gestalt Therapy; (INT) Integrative Therapy; (IP) Interpersonal Psychotherapy; (MC) Multicultural Psychotherapy; (PPT) Positive Psychotherapy; (PA) Psychodynamic Psychotherapy; (REBT) Rational Emotive Behavior Therapy.

Acceptance and Commitment Therapy (BT) A form of behavior therapy developed by Steven Hayes that focuses on experiential avoidance and cognitive fusion as key determinants of psychopathology and commitment as one component of therapeutic success.

Activity Scheduling (CT, BT) Setting up routine activity in order to offset inertia.

Actualizing Tendency (CC) An innate human predisposition toward growth and fulfilling one's potential.

Agape Unconditional love for humanity (literally, "love between friends").

Aggression (GT) The basic biological movement of energy extending out from the organism to the environment. Aggression is required for assimilation, love, assertion, creativity, hunger, humor, discrimination, warmth, and so on.

Agoraphobia A fear of situations in which escape might be difficult or help unavailable in the event of experiencing a panic attack or panic symptoms. Commonly feared situations include enclosed places, being alone, crowded places, and travel.

Aha! (GT) Awareness of a situation in which a number of separate elements come together to form a meaningful whole; sudden insight into the solution to a problem or the structure of a situation.

Albert Ellis Institute (REBT) An organization founded by Albert Ellis in 1959. There was considerable controversy in psychotherapy circles in 2005 when the institute removed Albert Ellis from its board.

Albert Ellis Foundation (REBT) An organization established in 2006 to support the work and legacy of Albert Ellis.

Anorectic A person engaging in self-starving behavior.

Antisuggestion (AD) *See* Paradoxical Intervention.

Aphasia An organic speech deficit involving difficulty understanding or using language.

Applied Behavior Analysis (BT) A form of behavior therapy, closely tied to Skinner's philosophy of radical behaviorism, that stresses observable behavior rather than private events and uses single-subject experimental design to determine the relationship between behavior and its antecedents and consequences.

Arbitrary Inference (CT) Drawing conclusions without supporting evidence or despite evidence to the contrary.

Armamentarium The complete range of psychotherapeutic methods and techniques used by a therapist.

Assertiveness Training (BT, REBT) A treatment procedure designed to teach clients to openly and effectively express feelings and needs.

Assimilation (GT) The process of breaking something into component parts so that these parts can be accepted and made part of the person, rejected, or modified into suitable form.

Attachment Theory (FT, IP) A theory developed by John Bowlby, who proposed that all humans have an innate tendency to develop strong affectional bonds and that threats to these bonds resulted in psychopathology.

Authentic Mode (EX) A way of being described by Heidegger in which one understands and appreciates the fragility of being while acknowledging responsibility for one's own life. Also referred to as the *Ontological Mode*.

Automatic Thought (CT) A personal notion or idea triggered by particular stimuli that lead to an emotional response.

Autonomy A personality dimension based on the need to be independent and self-determining and to attain one's goals.

Auxiliary A person who aids a therapist or client in enacting a particular scene.

Aversive Racism (MC) A theory proposed by Gaertner and Dovidio that maintains that whites can sincerely endorse egalitarian values while at the same time being racist and harboring unacknowledged negative attitudes toward racial or ethnic out-groups.

Awfulizing (REBT) Seeing something inconvenient or obnoxious as awful, horrible, or terrible.

Basic Encounter (CC) One member of a group responding with empathy to another member being genuine and real.

Basic Mistake (AD) Myth used to organize and shape one's life. Examples include overgeneralizations, a desperate need for security, misperceptions of life's demands, denial of one's worth, and faulty values.

Behavioral Experiment (CT, REBT) Testing distorted beliefs or fears scientifically in a real-life situation (e.g., having a shy person initiate a conversation to see what actually happens).

Behavioral Medicine (BT) Applying learning theory techniques to prevent or treat physical problems (e.g., pain reduction, weight loss).

Behavioral Rehearsal (CT, BT) Practicing an emotionally charged event and one's response to it before its actual occurrence.

Belonging (AD, BT) An innate need, drive, and source of human behavior. It leads people to seek relationship and involvement with other human beings.

Boundary (FT) A barrier between parts of a system, as in a family in which rules establish who may participate and in what manner.

Broaden-and-Build Hypothesis (PPT) Barbara Fredrickson's theory, which postulates that positive emotions broaden an individual's momentary thought–action repertoire, building an individual's enduring personal resources, which have an undoing effect on negative emotions.

Catastrophizing (REBT, CT) Exaggerating the consequences of an unfortunate event.

Catharsis The expression and discharge of repressed emotions; sometimes used as a synonym for *abreaction.*

Character Strengths (PPT) Manifested through feelings, thoughts, actions, or reactions, character strengths are ubiquitous traits that are morally valued in their own right and not necessarily tied to tangible outcomes. Character strengths contribute to fulfillment and life satisfaction.

Circular Causality (FT) The feedback model of a network of interacting loops that views any causal event as the effect of a previous cause as in family interactions.

Circular Questioning (FT) An interviewing technique directed at eliciting differences in perceptions about events or relationships from different family members, especially regarding those points in the family life cycle when significant coalition shifts occur.

Classical Conditioning (BT) A form of learning in which existing responses are attached to new stimuli by pairing those stimuli with those that naturally elicit the response; also referred to as *respondent conditioning.*

Classification of Strengths and Virtues (PPT) The first and most comprehensive classification of 24 core human character strengths that are subsumed under 6 virtues. Edited by Peterson and Seligman (2004), this volume is also referred as the *un-DSM* or the "Manual of Sanities."

Closed System (FT) A self-contained system that has impermeable boundaries and thus is resistant to new information and change.

Cognitive Behavior Therapy (BT) An extension of behavior therapy that treats thoughts and cognition as behaviors amenable to behavioral procedures. Cognitive behavior therapy is most closely associated with the work of Aaron Beck, Albert Ellis, and Donald Meichenbaum.

Cognitive Distortion (CT, REBT) Pervasive and systematic errors in reasoning.

Cognitive Restructuring (AD, BT, REBT) An active attempt to alter maladaptive thought patterns and replace them with more adaptive cognitions.

Cognitive Shift (CT, REBT) A systematic and biased interpretation of life experiences.

Cognitive Triad (CT) Negative views of the self, the world, and the future that characterize depression.

Cognitive Vulnerability (CT) Individual ways of thinking that predispose one to particular psychological distress.

Collaborative Empiricism (CT) A strategy of seeing the patient as a scientist capable of objective interpretation.

Common Factors Approach (INT) An approach that seeks to determine and apply the core ingredients different therapies share, predicated on the assumption that commonalities across therapies account for more of the variance in therapeutic success than do unique factors. Common factors include the therapeutic alliance, catharsis, acquisition of new behaviors, and positive expectations.

Complex (AP) An energy-filled cluster of emotions and ideas circling a specific subject. A complex has an archetypal core but expresses aspects of the personal unconscious. Jung's discovery and explanation of the complex lent validity to Freud's belief in the personal unconscious.

Compromise Formation (PA) A theoretical proposition emerging from the ego psychology tradition that stipulates that all experience and action is the result of a compromise between an underlying instinctually derived wish and a defense against it.

Conditional Assumption (CT) An erroneous "if–then" interpretation of events that leads to an erroneous conclusion (e.g., "*If* one person dislikes me, *then* I am not likable").

Confluence(GT) A state in which the contact boundary becomes so thin, flexible, and permeable that the distinction between self and environment is lost. In confluence, one does not experience self and others as distinct. The beliefs, attitudes, and feelings of self and others become merged. Confluence can be healthy or unhealthy.

Congruence (CC) State of being integrated and whole in which the person's actual experiencing matches his or her concept of self. Congruence is an aspect of psychological adjustment. *See also* Genuineness.

Conscientization (MC) An educational concept, also known as *critical consciousness,* that was developed by Paulo Freire. Conscientization involves learning to perceive the social, political, and economic contradictions associated with oppression.

Consensus Trance (CN) View of the normal waking state of mind as dreamlike, lacking clear awareness.

Conjoint Session (FT) Psychotherapy in which two or more patients are treated together.

Constructivism (FT) The view that emphasizes the subjective ways in which each individual creates a perception of reality.

Contact (GT) Basic unit of relationship involving an experience of the boundary between "me" and "not me"; feeling a connection with the "not me" while maintaining a separation from it.

Containment (PA) A model of development and therapeutic change originating in the work of Wilfred Bion that stipulates that the therapist's ability to process the client's difficult or "intolerable" affective experience in a nondefensive fashion, and to help him or her make sense of it, is an important therapeutic mechanism.

Convenient Fiction A philosophy of science phase signifying concepts that are imaginary and unreal but may be helpful in conceptualization.

Conviction Conclusion based on personal experience and perceptions, usually biased because each person's perspective is unique.

Core Conditions (CC) According to Carl Rogers, the core conditions for growth in therapy are congruence, unconditional positive regard, and empathy. Other theorists such as Albert Ellis have argued that these three conditions are neither necessary nor sufficient for therapeutic growth.

Counterconditioning (BT) Replacing a particular behavior by conditioning a new response incompatible with the maladaptive behavior. Counterconditioning is one of the explanations for the effectiveness of systematic desensitization.

Countertransference (PA, AP) Traditionally defined as the activation of unconscious wishes and fantasies on the part of the therapist toward the patient. It can either be elicited by and indicative of the patient's projections or come from the therapist's tendency to respond to patients as though they were significant others in the life, history, or fantasy of the therapist. Many contemporary psychoanalytic theorists conceptualize countertransference as the totality of the therapist's feelings and other spontaneous responses emerging in the context of the relationship with the client. *See also* Transference.

Courage (AD) Willingness to take risks without being sure of the consequences; necessary for effective living.

Cultural Competency (MC) The set of knowledge, behaviors, attitudes, skills, and policies that enable a practitioner to work effectively in a multicultural situation. Cultural competence requires congruent behaviors, attitudes, and policies that reflect an understanding of how cultural and sociopolitical influences shape individuals' worldviews and related health behaviors.

Cultural Genogram (MC) A therapeutic tool that emphasizes the role of culture and context in the lives of individuals and their families.

Cybernetic Epistemology (FT) A framework for conceptualizing and analyzing what is being observed in terms of the flow of information through a system.

Cybernetic System (FT) The study of methods of feedback control within a system.

Decatastrophizing (CT, REBT) A "what-if" technique designed to explore actual rather than feared events and consequences.

Decentering (CT) Moving the supposed focus of attention away from oneself.

Deconstructionism A theory of literary criticism that challenges many of the prevailing assumptions of psychotherapy. Therapists influenced by deconstructionism attempt to "deconstruct" the ideological biases and traditional assumptions that shape the practice of psychotherapy. Like postmodernism, deconstructionism rejects all claims of ultimate truth.

Defense (PA) Method mobilized by the ego in response to its danger signal of anxiety as protection from inner and outer threat. Examples include repression, denial, and projection.

Deflection (GT) A means of blunting the impact of contact and awareness by not giving or receiving feelings or thoughts directly. Vagueness, verbosity, and understatement are forms of deflection.

Dehypnosis (CN) Awakening from the usual consensus trance state of mind—for example, by recognizing thoughts as thoughts rather than identifying with them.

Demandingness (REBT) The belief of some clients that they must get what they want in life—and it is a terrible tragedy if this does not occur.

Dementia Praecox An obsolete term for schizophrenia.

Dereflection (CN) Directing one's attention away from the self.

Determinism The assumption that every mental event is causally tied to earlier psychological experience.

Dialectical Behavior Therapy (BT) A therapy developed by Marsha Linehan for use with patients with borderline personality disorder. DBT balances the need to change with acceptance of the way things are; this is the central dialectic of psychotherapy. Mindfulness is a central component of DBT.

Dialogue (EXT, GT) Genuine, equal, and honest communication between two people; the "I–Thou" relationship.

Dichotomous Thinking (CT, REBT) Categorizing experiences or people in black-and-white or extreme terms only (e.g., all good vs. all bad) with no middle ground.

Dichotomy (GT) A split in which a field is experienced as comprising competing and unrelated forces that cannot be meaningfully integrated into a whole.

Differentiation of Self (FT) Psychological separation by a family member, increasing resistance to being overwhelmed by the emotional reactivity of the family.

Discriminative Stimulus (BT) A stimulus signifying that reinforcement will (or will not) occur.

Disengaged Family (FT) A family whose members are psychologically isolated from one another because of overly rigid boundaries between the participants.

Disorientation Inability to correctly identify time and place (e.g., dates and locations).

Dissociation (PA) A partial or complete disruption of the normal integration of a person's conscious or psychological functioning resulting from anxiety or trauma.

Disturbances at the Boundary (GT) A disturbance in the ongoing movement between connection and withdrawal. Blocking connection results in *isolation*; blocking withdrawal results in *confluence*.

Double The auxiliary role that involves playing the protagonist's inner self or what the protagonist might be feeling or thinking but not expressing outwardly. *See also* Auxiliary.

Double Bind (FT) Conflict created in a person who receives contradictory messages in an important relationship but is forbidden to leave or escape from the relationship or to comment on the discrepancy.

Drama Therapy Use of theater techniques to gain self-awareness or increase self-expression in groups.

Dramaturgical Metaphor Framing situations as if they were like scenes in a play, which helps to include and more effectively describe vividly the range of psychosocial phenomena that are difficult to describe in more prosaic or abstract terms.

Dyadic (FT) Pertaining to a relationship between two persons.

Dynamic Strengths Assessment (PPT) An assessment approach in which signature strengths are a composite of self-identified strengths, strengths identified by a family member and a close friend, and a self-report measure. Clients also identify their desired strengths and highlight under- and overuse of strengths.

Dynamics (PA) Interactions, usually conflicted, between one's basic drives or id and the ego's defenses. *See also* Psychodynamics.

Dysarthria Speech deficit involving difficulty with the mechanical production of language.

Early Recollection (AD) Salient memory of a single incident from childhood; used as a projective technique by Adlerian therapists.

Eclecticism The practice of drawing from multiple and diverse sources in formulating client problems and devising treatment plans. Multimodal therapists are technical eclectics (e.g., they employ multiple methods without necessarily endorsing the theoretical positions from which they were derived).

Effectiveness Study Less well-controlled studies that do not typically use treatment manuals or specific training for the therapists involved in the study. Effectiveness research tends to be conducted in community settings under conditions that approximate day-to-day clinical practice. *Contrast with* Efficacy Study.

Efficacy Study A controlled study that typically uses random assignment of patients to treatments, treatment manuals, carefully trained therapists, and rigorous assessment of outcome by impartial evaluators. This is the type of research typically conducted in universities. *Contrast with* Effectiveness Study.

Ego (PA) The central controlling core of the personality mediating between the *id* (primitive, instinctive needs) and the *superego* (civilized, moralistic elements of the mind). *See also* Id, Superego.

Eigenwelt (EX) One level of the way each individual relates to the world. *Eigenwelt* literally means "own world" and refers to the way each of us relates to self.

Elegant Solution (REBT) Solution that helps clients make a profound philosophical change that goes beyond mere symptom removal.

EllisREBT (REBT) An organization founded in 2012 dedicated to continuing the work and legacy of Albert Ellis through the worldwide teaching, writing and perpetuation of the distinct Ellis approach.

Emotive Techniques (REBT) Therapy techniques that are vigorous, vivid, and dramatic.

Empathic Understanding (CC) The ability to absorb the expressed meanings of the client as if the therapist were seeing the world as the client sees it; and to feel along with the client his or her pain or joy.

Empathy (CC) Accurately and deeply feeling someone else's expressed emotions, concerns, or situation.

Empirically Supported Treatments Therapies that have been shown to be effective in scientific studies that meet rigid criteria (e.g., randomized clinical trials). For a treatment to be empirically supported, patients receiving the treatment must have been shown to be better off than patients who receive no treatment, and outcomes must be at least equal to that obtained by alternative therapies that have been documented to be beneficial.

Empty Chair (GT) A chair whose inhabitant is imagined by a client with all of the client's projected attitudes. The imaginary occupant might be a significant person in the client's life, a figure from a dream, a part of the client's body or mind, or even the therapist. The chair is usually used along with role reversal, and the term *shuttling* is used to describe the client's moving back and forth between the chairs as the two parts engage in an encounter. *See also* Encounter, Role Reversal.

Enactment (PA) An interaction between client and therapist shaped by both partner's unconscious contributions. Exploring and working through enactments can be an important mechanism of change.

Encounter (GT) A dialogue between two persons, or two aspects of the same person, either in reality or with one part played by someone else.

Encounter Group A small number of people who meet (sometimes only once, sometimes on a weekly basis for a specified time) to truly know and accept themselves and others.

Enmeshed Family (FT) Family in which individual members are overly involved in each other's lives, making individual autonomy impossible.

Epistemology The study of the origin, nature, methods, and limits of knowledge.

Ethicality (CN) Moral or principled intentions and behavior.

Ethnocentrism (MC) The belief that one's worldview is inherently superior and desirable to others.

Evenly Suspended Attention (PA) An attentive, open, and receptive listening style in which the therapist attempts to listen to whatever the client says without allowing his or her preconceptions or expectations to shape what he or she attends to.

Existential Isolation (EX) Fundamental and inevitable separation of each individual from others and the world; it can be reduced but never completely eliminated.

Existentialism (EX) A philosophical movement that stresses the importance of actual existence, one's responsibility for and determination of one's own psychological existence, authenticity in human relations, the primacy of the here and now, and the use of experience in the search for knowledge.

Existential Neurosis (EX) Feelings of emptiness, worthlessness, despair, and anxiety resulting from inauthenticity, abdication of responsibility, failure to make choices, and a lack of direction or purpose in life.

Experiencing (CC) Sensing or awareness of self and the world, whether narrowly and rigidly or openly and flexibly. Experience is unique for each person.

Experiential Family Therapist (FT) A therapist who reveals him- or herself as a real person and uses that self in interacting with families.

Extinction (BT) In classical conditioning, the result of repeated presentation of a conditioned stimulus without the unconditioned stimulus and the resulting gradual diminution of the conditioned response. In operant conditioning, extinction (no response) occurs when reinforcement is withheld following performance of a previously reinforced response.

Facilitator An individual who aids a group in going the direction they choose and accomplishing their chosen goals without doing harm to any member.

Factors of Enlightenment (CN) In Buddhist psychology, seven mental qualities important for psychological well-being: They are mindfulness, effort, investigation, rapture, concentration, calm, and equanimity.

Family Constellation (AD) The number, sequencing, and characteristics of the members of a family. The family constellation is an important determinant of lifestyle.

Family Sculpting (FT, PD) A nonverbal technique to be used by individual family members for physically arranging other family members in space to represent the arranger's symbolic view of family relationships.

Feedback The process by which a system makes adjustments in itself; can be negative (reestablishing equilibrium) or positive (leading to change).

Field Theory (GT) A theory about the nature of reality and our relationship to reality in which our experiences are understood within a specific context. A field is composed of mutually interdependent elements, and changes in the field influence how a person experiences reality. No one can transcend embeddedness in a field, and therefore no one can have an objective perspective on reality.

First-Order Change (FT) Change within a system that does not alter the basic organization of the system itself.

Flourishing (PPT) A state characterized by positive emotions, a strong sense of personal meaning, good work, and positive relationships—helping clients achieve a state of flourishing requires far more than simply relieving the symptoms of psychological distress.

Flow (PPT) Mihaly Csikszentmihalyi's concept refers to a psychological state marked by, among other features, intense concentration, a lost sense of time, and being deeply engaged as "one" with the experience.

Formative Tendency (CC) An overall inclination toward greater order, complexity, and interrelatedness common to all nature, including human beings.

Free Association (PA) A basic technique of psychoanalysis in which analysands are asked to report, without structure or censure, whatever thoughts come to mind.

Full Life (PPT) The full life entails happiness and life satisfaction and is much more than the sum of components of well-being (PERMA). These components are neither exclusive nor exhaustive. In contrast, *an empty life* lacks these features, particularly engagement and meaning, and results in psychological problems.

Functionally Specific States (CN) States of consciousness in which particular abilities such as introspection are increased, and others are reduced.

Fundamental Negativity Bias (PPT) An evolutionary tendency that makes us more responsive to negative experiences than positive ones.

Fusion (EXT, FT) In existential therapy, the giving up of oneself to become part of another person or a group; a particular attempt to reduce one's sense of isolation. In family therapy, a blurring of boundaries between family members with the resultant loss of a separate sense of self by each member.

Future Projection Demonstration of what one sees going on in life at some specified time in the future.

Gemeinschaftsgefühl (AD) A combination of concern for others and appreciation of one's role in a larger social order; usually translated as "social interest."

Generalization (BT) The occurrence of behavior in situations that resemble but are different from the stimulus environment in which the behavior was learned.

Genital Stage (PA) The final stage in psychosexual development, also termed the *oedipal phase*, in which heterosexual relations are achieved. Its roots are formed at ages five to six, and it is said to be the basis for the mature personality.

Genogram (FT, MC) A schematic diagram of a family's relationship system used to trace recurring family patterns over generations.

Genuineness (CC) The characteristic of being real and true to oneself; lack of pretense, social facade, or refusal to allow certain aspects of one's self into awareness. *See* Congruence.

Gestalt (GT) A word with no literal English translation, referring to a perceptual whole or a unified configuration of experience.

Givens of Human Existence (EX) Psychiatrist Irvin Yalom defines these as death, freedom, isolation, and meaninglessness. The courage with which we meet the givens of human existence defines our life.

Golden Mean (PPT) An Aristotelian notion that in the context of Positive Psychology refers to the right combination of strengths applied to the right degree in the right situation.

Graded-Task Assignment (CT, BT) Starting with a simple activity and increasing the level of complexity or difficulty in a step-by-step fashion.

Hedonic Treadmill (PPT) A barrier to happiness that causes one to rapidly and inevitably adapt to good things by taking them for granted. As one accumulates more material possessions and accomplishments, for example, one's expectations also rise.

Hidden Agenda The actual goal of an interaction between people (as in a game), which is different from what superficially appears to be the goal.

Higher States (CN) States of consciousness containing normal mental capacities plus additional heightened ones.

Holism (AD) Studying individuals in their entirety, including how they proceed through life, rather than trying to separate out certain aspects or parts, such as studying the mind apart from the body.

Homeostasis A balanced and steady state of equilibrium.

Homework (REBT, BT) Specific activities to be done between therapy sessions.

Hot Cognition (CT) A powerful and highly meaningful idea that produces strong emotional reactions.

Hysteria An early term for conversion reaction, a disorder in which psychological disturbance takes a physical form (e.g., paralysis in the absence of organic disturbance). Many of Freud's theories grew out of his experience in treating hysterical patients.

Id (PA) The reservoir of the biological, instinctual drives with innate and developmental components. *See also* Ego, Superego.

Identified Patient (FT) The person who seeks treatment or for whom treatment is sought.

Inauthentic Mode (EX) Heidegger believed the inauthentic mode of being was characterized by mindless responding and a failure to take responsibility for becoming one's true self.

Inclusion (GT) Putting oneself as completely as possible into another's experience without judging or evaluating while still maintaining a separate sense of self.

Individual Psychology (AD) An approach to understanding human behavior that sees each person as a unique, whole entity who is constantly becoming rather than being and one whose development can only be understood within a social context.

Inferiority Complex (AD) An exaggeration of feelings of inadequacy and insecurity resulting in defensiveness and neurotic behavior. It is usually, but not always, abnormal.

Inferiority Feeling (AD) Seeing oneself as inadequate or incompetent in comparison with others, with one's ideal self, or with personal values; considered universal and normal. *Contrast with* Inferiority Complex.

Insight (PA) A mechanism of change that has always been considered important in psychoanalysis. Insight involves becoming aware of a feeling, wish, fantasy, thought, or memory that has previously been unconscious. Can also involve becoming aware of how one's previous experiences or current unconscious expectations shape one's perceptions and self-defeating patterns in the present.

Integration Organized and harmonious relationships among personality components.

Intensive Group (CC) A small number of people who come together for a brief but condensed period (e.g., a weekend) to engage in special interpersonal experiences that are designed to expand awareness of self and others.

Interlocking Pathologies (FT) Multiple forms of dysfunction within a family that are interdependent in the way they are expressed and maintained.

Interlocking Triangles (FT) Basic units of family relationships consisting of a series of three-person sets of interactions (e.g., father–mother–child; grandparent–parent–child).

Internal Frame of Reference (CC) A view or perception of both the world and self as seen by the individual, as distinguished from the viewpoint of an observer, psychotherapist, or other person.

Internal Objects (PA) Hypothetical psychic structures developed through a combination of real interactions with others, fantasies, and defensive processes.

International Positive Psychology Association (IPPA; www.ippa.org) (PPT) A membership organization that exists to promote the science of Positive Psychology. The IPPA has six divisions: basic research, clinical, coaching, education, health, and organizations.

Interpersonal Problem Areas (IP) Grief, interpersonal disputes, role transitions, and interpersonal deficits. These four problem areas trigger depressive episodes.

Interpretation (PA) The therapist's attempt to help make sense of the client's experience, articulate a hypothesis about the client's unconscious experience, or draw the client's attention toward unconscious self-defeating patterns.

Intrapsychic Within the mind or psyche of the individual.

Introject (FT) Internalized object from one's past that affects current relationships.

Introjection (GT) Accepting information or values from the outside without evaluation; not necessarily psychologically unhealthy.

Irrational Belief (REBT) Unreasonable conviction that produces emotional upset (for example, insisting that the world should or must be different from what it actually is).

Isolation (GT) A state in which the contact boundary is so thick, rigid, and impermeable that the psychological connection between self and environment is lost, and the person does not allow access from or to the outside. Isolation can be healthy or unhealthy. *Contrast with* Withdrawal.

Leaning Tower of Pisa Approach (FT) A variation of paradoxical intention in which a therapist intentionally makes a problem worse until it falls of its own weight and is thereby resolved.

Libido (PA) The basic driving force of personality in Freud's system; includes but is not restricted to sexual energy.

Lifestyle (AD) One's characteristic way of living and pursuing long-term goals.

Life Tasks (AD) The basic challenges and obligations of life: society, work, and sex. The additional tasks of spiritual growth and self-identity are included by Rudolf Dreikurs and Harold Mosak.

Linear Causality (FT) The view that one event causes the other, not vice versa.

Locus of Evaluation (CC) The place of a judgment's origin, its source; whether the appraisal of an experience comes more from within the individual (internal) or from outside sources (external).

Logotherapy (EX) A therapeutic approach developed by Viktor Frankl emphasizing value and meaning as prerequisites for mental health and personal growth.

Lucid Dreaming (CN) A sleep state in which people know they are dreaming.

Magnification (CT) Exaggerating something's significance.

Manual-Based Treatments (BT) The use of standardized, manual-based treatments is advocated by most proponents of evidence-based treatment because manuals increase the likelihood of treatment fidelity. Critics of manualized treatment argue that the use of manuals represents a Procrustean approach that ignores individual differences in patients and problems.

Marital Schism (FT) A disturbed family arrangement characterized by disharmony, undermining of the spouse, and frequent threats of divorce. *See also* Marital Skew.

Marital Skew (FT) A disturbed family arrangement in which one person dominates to an extreme degree and in which the marriage is maintained through the distortion of reality. *See also* Marital Schism.

Masters in Applied Positive Psychology (PPT) This one-year program taught by luminaries in the field of Positive Psychology teaches advanced level theory, research, and application of Positive Psychology in various contexts.

Maya (CN) An illusory and encompassing distortion of one's perception and experience that is not recognized as such.

Mediational Stimulus–Response Model (BT) A behavioral model that posits internal events, such as thoughts and images, as links between perceiving a stimulus and making a response.

Medical Model (IP) An approach that is used to allow depressed individuals to adopt a sick role and understand that it is a treatable medical problem like diabetes.

Meditation (CN) Practices designed to train attention and bring various mental processes under greater voluntary control.

Microaggressions (MC) Psychological assaults that individuals receive on a regular basis solely because of their race, color, ethnicity, gender or culture.

Mindfulness (CN) Clear objective awareness of experience.

Minimization (CT) Making an event far less important than it actually is.

Mirror Person who imitates a client's behavior and demeanor so that the client can more clearly see him- or herself in action.

Mitwelt (EX) The way in which each individual relates to the world, socially and through being with others; the age we live in, our age, our own times, the present generation, our contemporaries.

Mode (CT) Network of cognitive, affective, motivational, and behavioral schema that composes personality and interprets ongoing situations.

Monadic (FT) Based on the characteristics or traits of a single person.

Monodrama (PD, GT) One client playing both parts in a scene by alternating between them.

Morita (CN) A Japanese therapy for treating anxiety by redirecting one's attention away from the self.

Multigenerational Transmission Process (FT) The passing on of psychological problems over generations as a result of immature persons marrying others with similar low levels of separateness from their families.

Multiple Psychotherapy (AD) A technique in which several therapists simultaneously treat a single patient.

Musturbation (REBT) A term coined by Albert Ellis to characterize the behavior of clients who are absolutistic and inflexible in their thinking, maintaining that they *must* not fail, *must* be exceptional, *must* be successful, and so on.

Mystification (FT) The deliberate distortion of another person's experience by misinterpreting or mislabeling it.

Naikan (CN) Japanese therapy using intensive reflection on past relationships to increase social and interpersonal contributions.

Narrative Therapy (FT) An approach to family therapy built on the belief that reality is constructed, organized and maintained through the stories we create. Associated with Australian therapist Michael White and others.

Negative Feedback (FT) The flow of output information back into a system to correct too great a deviation from normal and return the system to its steady state.

Negative Reinforcement (BT) Any behavior that increases the probability of a response by terminating or withdrawing an unpleasant stimulus. Negative reinforcement increases the likelihood of future occurrence of the behavior it follows.

Neurosis (PA) A term first used by Freud to include all but the most severe psychological syndromes; currently narrowly defined as an emotional disorder in which psychic functioning is relatively intact and contact with reality is sound.

Neurotic Anxiety (EX) A state of fear or apprehension out of proportion to an actual threat. Neurotic anxiety is destructive or paralyzing and cannot be used constructively. *Compare with* Normal Anxiety.

Nondirective Attitude (CC) Valuing the client's inherent capacity for and right to self-determination.

Normal Anxiety (EX) A sense of apprehension appropriate to a given threatening situation, which can be faced, dealt with, and used creatively. *Compare with* Neurotic Anxiety.

Object Relations Theory (PA, FT) The view that the basic human motive is the search for satisfying object (person) relationships. Associated with the writings of Melanie Klein, W. Ronald Fairbairn, and Donald Winnicott.

One-Person Psychology (PA) The perspective in classical psychoanalysis that assumes it is possible to understand the client's intrapsychic processes out of context of the therapist's ongoing contributions to the interaction.

Ontological (EX) Concerned with the science of being or existence.

Open System (FT) A system in which relatively permeable boundaries permit the exchange of information with its environment.

Operant Conditioning (BT) A type of learning in which responses are modified by their consequences. Reinforcement increases the likelihood of future occurrences of the reinforced response; punishment and extinction decrease the likelihood of future occurrences of the responses they follow.

Organ Inferiority (AD) Perceived or actual congenital defects in organ systems believed by Alfred Adler to result in compensatory striving to overcome these deficits.

Organismic Valuing Process (CC) Making individual judgments or assessments of the desirability of an action or choice on the basis of one's own sensory evidence and life experience.

Overgeneralization (CT, REBT) Constructing a general rule from isolated incidents and applying it too broadly.

Panacea A remedy for all diseases and difficulties; a cure-all.

Paradigm A set of assumptions limiting an area to be investigated scientifically and specifying the methods used to collect and interpret the forthcoming data.

Paradigm Shift A significant and widespread change in the concepts, values, perceptions, and practices that define a community or a structured activity (e.g., psychotherapy).

Paradoxical Intervention (FT) A therapeutic technique whereby the patient is directed to continue the symptomatic behavior. To comply is to admit voluntary control over the symptom; to rebel is to give up the symptom.

Paradoxical Theory of Change (GT) A theory of change that is based on a paradox: The more one tries to be who one is not, the more one stays the same; the more one tries to stay the same in a changing world, the more one changes relative to the world. When a person knows and accepts him- or herself, maximum growth can occur. When one rejects oneself—for example, by forcing oneself beyond one's support—growth is hindered by internal conflict.

Paraphilias Unusual or atypical sexual behaviors that are thought to have clinical relevance. The major paraphilias include exhibitionism, fetishism, frotteurism, pedophilia, sexual masochism, sexual sadism, transvestic fetishism, and voyeurism.

PERMA (PPT) Martin Seligman's theory postulates that well-being has five measurable elements (PERMA): **p**ositive emotion (of happiness and life satisfaction), **e**ngagement, **r**elationships, **m**eaning, and **a**ccomplishment.

Personalization (CT) Taking personal responsibility for negative events without supporting evidence of personal involvement.

Phenomenology (AD, EXT, GT) A method of exploration that primarily uses human experience as the source of data and attempts to include all human experience without bias (external observation, emotions, thoughts, and so on). Subjects are taught to distinguish between current experience and the biases brought to the situation. Phenomenology is the basic method of most existentialists.

Placebo In medicine, placebos are inert substances given to patients in place of bona fide medications. In psychotherapy, placebos are most often sham treatments used in research to control for the nonspecific effects of attention.

Pleasure Principle (PA) The basic human tendency to avoid pain and seek pleasure, especially salient in the first years of life. *Contrast with* Reality Principle.

Positive Cognitive Appraisal (PPT) An approach to unpack and reappraise bad and bitter memories by using four specific techniques: third-person perspective, inventory of positive and negative memories, diversion and distraction, and mindfulness.

Positive Feedback (FT) The flow of output information back into the system in order to amplify deviation from a steady state, thus leading to instability and change.

Positive Psychology Center (PPT) Located at the University of Pennsylvania, Philadelphia, with Martin Seligman as its director, the PPC is the leading institution promoting research, training, education, and the dissemination of Positive Psychology.

Positive Psychotherapy (PPT) A clinical Positive Psychology approach with the basic premise that psychopathology can be better understood and served if its symptoms and strengths are integrated and if strengths are used to overcome psychological distress.

Positive Psychotherapy Inventory (PPT) Based on Seligman's theory of well-being (PERMA), the PPI is an empirically validated, 25-item outcome measure of positive psychotherapy used to evaluate pre- to posttherapeutic changes in well-being.

Positive Reinforcement (BT) Any stimulus that follows a behavior and increases the likelihood of the occurrence of the behavior that it follows.

Postmodern Therapies (GT) Any approach to therapy that recognizes the validity and assumptions of multiple realities while rejecting the primacy of the worldview of the therapist. Postmodern therapies stress the importance of culture in determining reality and emphasize the influence of language and power relationships in shaping and defining psychopathology.

Primary Process Thinking (PA) Nonlogical thinking such as is found in dreams, creativity, and the operation of the unconscious. Freud believed primary process thinking characterized the operations of the Id. *Contrast with* Secondary Process Thinking.

Projection (PA, AP) Attributing to others unacceptable personal thoughts, feelings, or behaviors.

Projective Identification (PA) An interactional form of projection, used both normally and as a defense, through which one person places into another person his or her inner state and defenses.

Protagonist In psychodrama, the term used for the client whose situation is being explored, who is also usually the main player in the role-playing process.

Pseudohostility (FT) Superficial bickering that allows one to avoid dealing with deeper, more genuine, and more intimate feelings.

Pseudomutuality (FT) A facade of family harmony that gives the appearance of an open and satisfying relationship that does not truly exist.

Psychodrama A method of psychotherapy developed by J. L. Moreno in the mid-1930s in which clients role play their problems.

Psychodynamics (PA) A term similar to dynamics, which refers to mental interactions and conflict, usually formulated in terms of ego, id, and superego. *See also* Dynamics.

Psychodynamic Psychotherapy (PA) A general term for a variety of therapies that evolved from psychoanalysis. Dynamic psychotherapists generally see their clients once or twice each week, and the client is sitting up.

Psychological Masquerade Apparent psychological symptoms actually caused by physical or organic conditions.

Punishment (BT) An aversive event likely to terminate any behavior that it follows.

Randomized controlled trial (IP; BT; CT) A prospective experiment in which investigators randomly assign patients to one or more treatment groups; considered the gold standard method for evaluating evidence-based therapies. Most widely used in interpersonal psychotherapy, behavior therapy, and cognitive therapy. (Also known as *randomized clinical trial*.)

Rapture (CN) Delight in the awareness of experience.

Reality An individual's private world; more generally, a group of perceptions or "facts" with substantial consensus about their meaning.

Reality Principle (PA) The guiding principle of the ego, which permits postponement of gratification to meet the demands of the environment or secure greater pleasure at a later time. *Contrast with* Pleasure Principle.

Reattribution (CT) Assigning alternative causes to events; reinterpreting one's symptoms.

Redundancy Principle (FT) Repetitive behavioral sequences between participants, as within a family.

Reevaluation Counseling (MC) An empowering co-counseling approach in which two or more individuals take turns listening to each other without interruption in order to recover from the effects of racism, classism, sexism, and other types of oppression.

Reframing (FT, REBT) Relabeling behavior by putting it into a new, more positive perspective.

Reinforcement (BT) The presentation of a reward or the removal of an aversive stimulus following a response. Reinforcement always increases the future probability of the reinforced response.

Replay (PD, BT) A psychodramatic technique, often used in behavior therapy and other approaches, in which the client repeats a previous scene. It is often applied in the mastery of interpersonal skills.

Repression (PA) A major defense mechanism in which distressing thoughts are barred from conscious expression.

Relational Psychoanalysis (PA) An increasingly influential approach to psychoanalysis that consists of a synthesis of interpersonal psychoanalysis, object relations theory, self psychology, and feminist and postmodern theory. Important pioneers of the the relational tradition include Stephen Mitchell, Philip Bromberg, Emmanuel Ghent, Lewis Aron, Jessica Benjamin, and Adrienne Harris.

Resistance (PA, GT) In psychoanalysis, any obstacle, pathological or nonpathological, to the progress of an analysis or therapy, usually involving a modification of a ground rule of treatment and based on unconscious sources within both patient and analyst (i.e., interactionally

determined). In Gestalt therapy, the reluctance of people to know, show, or own aspects of themselves. Resistance can be healthy or unhealthy.

Respondent Conditioning (BT) *See* Classical Conditioning.

Retroflection (GT) A contact boundary disturbance in which a person self for the environment. One may do to one's self what they wish(ed) to do to another. Or one may do for one's self what they wish(ed) from another. Retroflection is the chief mechanism of isolation and is not necessarily unhealthy.

Role Playing Acting the part of oneself or someone else under therapeutic guidance. (Originally used in psychodrama, the term has now come to be used also as a way of problem exploration in many other therapies, as well as in education and business.)

Role Reversal In psychodrama, the dropping of the point of view of one's own role and taking on the attitudes and physical position and perspective of the other person in an interaction. A plays B, and B plays A. Or sometimes, if the actual other person isn't present, A takes the role of whoever he imagines B to be, using an empty chair, thus opening his mind to a deeper level of empathy. *See also* Empty Chair.

Rupture and Repair (PA) Ruptures are inevitable breakdowns in collaborative process or therapeutic impasses. The process of working through alliance ruptures or therapeutic impasses constructively is viewed as an important mechanism of change.

Samadhi (CN) Yogic state of consciousness marked by deep calm and concentration.

Scapegoating (FT) Casting a person in a role that unfairly exposes him or her to criticism, blame, or punishment.

Schema (CT) Strategy or way of thinking that comprises core beliefs and basic assumptions about how the world operates.

Secondary Process Thinking (PA) Linear, logical, and verbal thinking associated with the operations of the ego. *Contrast with* Primary Process Thinking.

Second-Order Change (FT) Fundamental change in a system's organization and function.

Selection Abstraction (CT) Basing a conclusion on a detail taken out of context and ignoring other information.

Self-Actualization A basic human drive toward growth, completeness, and fulfillment.

Self-Concept One's own definition of whom one is, including one's attributes, emotions, abilities, character, and faults.

Self-Instructional Training (BT) A technique, described most completely by Donald Meichenbaum, for replacing self-defeating thoughts with self-enhancing cognitions.

Self Psychology (PA) A psychoanalytic approach associated with the work and writings of Heinz Kohut. Self psychology stresses empathy, mirroring, and support for positive esteem.

Self-Regard (CC) That aspect of the self-concept that develops from the esteem or respect accorded to oneself.

Sensate Focus (BT) A series of exercises used in sex therapy designed to reintroduce clients to receiving and giving sensual pleasure.

Sharing The third phase of a psychodramatic enactment in which other group members in the audience and even auxiliaries share how that role playing may have touched on similar or related events in their own lives—in contrast to giving advice, interpretations, or analysis.

Sixty-five- (65)-percent barrier (PPT) Most treatments, including psychopharmacology and cognitive therapy, at best produce about a 65% response rate in alleviating symptoms. This number incorporates a placebo effect that ranges from 45% to 55%.

Social Interest (AD) The feeling of being part of a social whole; the need and willingness to contribute to the general social good. *See also* Gemeinschaftsgefühl.

Social Learning Theory (BT) A system that combines operant and classical conditioning with cognitive mediational processes (e.g., vicarious learning and symbolic activity) to account for the development, maintenance, and modification of behavior.

Sociometry A method in which groups give feedback about their interpersonal preferences (e.g., attraction or repulsion).

Sociotrophy (CT) A personality dimension characterized by dependency on interpersonal relationships and needs for closeness and nurturance.

Socratic Dialogue (CT, REBT) A series of questions designed to arrive at logical answers to and conclusions about a hypothesis.

Splitting (PA, GT) In psychoanalysis, a primitive defense through which persons are classified as all-good or all-bad individuals, making it impossible to have a full and balanced picture of other people. In Gestalt therapy, a situation in which a person splits off part of him- or herself as a polar opposite. The individual is aware of one pole and oblivious to the other. For example, an individual may split into competent and incompetent selves and vacillate between these roles. A split is one form of a dichotomy.

Spontaneity A frame of mind enabling one to address situations afresh, often with a significant measure of improvisation.

Stages of Change (INT) A model developed by Prochaska and DiClemente and used to match therapeutic approaches to a client's readiness to change. The model posits five stages: Precontemplation, contemplation, preparation, action, and maintenance. See Table 14.1 in Chapter 14.

Stimulus Control (BT) Arranging the environment in such a way that a given response is either more likely or less likely to occur (e.g., buying only one pack of cigarettes per day in order to decrease the likelihood of smoking).

Strategic Intervention Therapy (FT) An approach to family therapy employing specific strategies, plans, and tactics to force changes in behavior.

Strength-Based Assessment (PPT) Measurement of positive emotions, behaviors, competencies, strengths, and skills that facilitate personal and interpersonal well-being.

Structuralism (FT) An approach to family therapy, associated with Salvador Minuchin, that emphasizes the importance of the nuclear family and seeks to change pathological alliances and splits in the family.

Structuralist (FT) A therapist who emphasizes changing or realigning a family's organizational structure to improve its transactional patterns.

Structural Theory or Hypothesis (PA) Freud's second model of the mind. The model postulates three agencies of the mind—ego, superego, and id—each with conscious and unconscious components. *See also* Id, Ego, Superego.

Stuck-Togetherness (FT) A situation observed in schizophrenic families in which roles and boundaries are blurred and no family member has an identity distinct from the family.

Subjective Reasoning (CT) Believing that feelings are the same as, or equivalent to, facts.

Subsystem (FT) An organized component within an overall system such as a family.

Superego (PA) A structure of the mind, developed from innate tendencies and early parental interactions and identifications, that embraces moral and other standards and regulates psychic tensions, self-image, self-esteem, and drive discharge. *See also* Ego, Id.

Support (GT) To provide the psychological, physiological, social, or material aid needed to initiate, terminate, regulate, and maintain contact or withdrawal as needed by the person or the environment. People are self-supporting to the degree that they are the chief agents in initiating, terminating, regulating, and maintaining contact or withdrawal and do so based on self-identification. For example, knowing what one wants and being able to ask for it appropriately is self-supporting.

Surplus Reality Psychological experiences involving other than physical reality (e.g., spiritual events, a relationship with a significant deceased other).

Survival An innate need, drive, and source of human behavior. It leads human beings to seek health, nutrition, and protection from physical danger.

Symbiosis (FT) A relationship in which two people, often a mother and her child, become so intertwined that it is impossible to find a boundary between them.

Symbolization (CC) A process of allowing a life event or experience into one's consciousness or awareness and interpreting it in terms of the self-concept. Symbolization may be accurate and incorporate the fullness and intricacy of experiencing or it may be partial or distorted when experiencing threatens one's perceptions of self.

Syncretism (INT) A pejorative term referring to the uncritical and unsystematic combination of various therapeutic approaches.

Synthesis Making a whole from elements or parts; constructing the overall meaning of a situation from many different aspects of it.

System A complete unit made up of interconnected and interdependent parts operating in a stable way over time.

Systematic Desensitization (BT) A step-by-step procedure for replacing anxiety with relaxation while gradually increasing exposure to an anxiety-producing situation or object.

Systematic Eclecticism (INT) An approach advocated by Norcross and Beutler (Chapter 14) in which the various approaches to eclecticism (e.g., technical eclecticism, theoretical integration, common factors, and assimilative integration) are blended to meet the unique needs of each individual patient. Also referred to as *Systematic Treatment Selection* (STS).

Technical Eclecticism (INT) An integrative approach in which therapists use multiple procedures drawn from various therapeutic systems without particular concern about the theories from which they came.

Theoretical Integration (INT) The integration of two or more therapies with an emphasis on integrating the underlying theories associated with each therapeutic system.

Therapeutic Alliance The partnership between therapist and client that develops as the two work together to reach the goals of therapy.

Third-Party Payer Financial intermediary that controls payment to therapists. In therapy, third-party payers are usually insurance companies or government agencies.

Third Wave of Behavior Therapy (BT) The first wave of behavior therapy focused on modifying overt behavior. The second wave addressed cognitions (e.g., cognitive behavior therapy). The third wave addresses mindfulness and self-awareness and includes dialectical behavior therapy (DBT) and acceptance and commitment therapy (ACT).

Token Economy (BT) A program that provides people with short-term reinforcement for specific behaviors by allotting tokens (poker chips or points) that are accumulated and later exchanged for privileges or desired objects.

Topographic Theory (PA) Freud's first model of the mind in which access to awareness of contents and functions was the defining criterion. The model had interactional elements but was eventually replaced by Freud's structural model. *See also* Unconscious.

Trait Theory The belief in stable and enduring personality characteristics.

Transference (PA, AP) The therapy situation in which the patient responds to the therapist as though he or she were a significant figure in the patient's past, usually a parent. Many contemporary theorists emphasize that transference is usually (if not always) partially shaped by real characteristics of the therapist. *See also* Countertransference.

Triadic (FT) Pertaining to a relationship involving the interaction of three or more persons.

Trust (CC) Basic faith in oneself and others as being growth directed and positively oriented.

Two-Chair Technique (GT) An affective, experiential procedure in which the client engages in dialogue with another person (or with another part of the self) as symbolically represented by an empty chair. The client may assume different roles by switching from one chair to the other.

Two-Person Psychology (PA) The perspective common to many contemporary psychoanalytic models that assumes that both therapist and client are always contributing to everything that takes place in the therapeutic relationship.

Umwelt (EX) A way of relating to the world through its biological and physical aspects; one's relationship with nature and the surrounding world.

Unconditional Acceptance (REBT). A core philosophical emphasis in REBT that has three components: Unconditional Self Acceptance, Unconditional Other Acceptance, and Unconditional Life Acceptance.

Unconditional Positive Regard (CC) A nonpossessive caring and acceptance of the client as a human being, irrespective of the therapist's own values. One of Rogers's necessary and sufficient conditions for therapeutic change.

Unconscious (PA, AP) A division of the psyche; the repository of psychological material of which the individual is unaware.

Values in Action Institute (www.viacharacter.org) (PPT) This nonprofit organization advances both the science and practice of character strengths. More than 2 million people from more than 250 countries, in 17 languages, have completed its free online Values in Action—Inventory of Strengths, which measures strengths of character.

Vicarious Learning (BT) Learning through observation and imitation; a synonym for modeling.

Voluntary Simplicity (CN) Self-motivated choice to live more simply and to deemphasize material goods.

Well-being Therapy (PPT) Based on Carol Ryff's multi-dimensional model of psychological well-being, well-being therapy includes six dimensions: autonomy, personal growth, environmental mastery, purpose in life, positive relationships, and self-acceptance.

Warming-Up The process of becoming more spontaneous, often associated with a relaxation of self-consciousness, anxiety, a higher level of trust, and an increasing degree of involvement in the task at hand.

Warmth (CC) Positive and real feelings of acceptance toward another person.

Will to Power (AD) Individual striving for superiority and dominance in order to overcome feelings of inadequacy and inferiority.

Withdrawal (GT) Temporary withdrawing from contact while maintaining a permeable contact boundary. Withdrawal can be healthy or unhealthy. *Contrast with* Isolation.

Work (GT) The process of exploring by phenomenological focusing in order to increase awareness. One can work in any setting and focus on any theme (here and now contact, life problems, developmental themes, spiritual concerns, creativity and emotional expansion, dreams, belief systems, etc.).

Worldview (MC) Those ideas and beliefs, shaped by one's culture, that influence the way an individual interprets the world and interacts with it. Associated with the writings of Harry Triandis.

Yoga (CN) Disciplines dealing with ethics, lifestyle, body postures, breath control, intellectual study, and meditation.

Zeitgeist The spirit of the times; the prevailing cultural climate.

NAME INDEX

SUBJECT INDEX

A

Academy of Cognitive Therapy, 238, 254
Acceptance and commitment therapy
  (ACT), 60–61, 199, 216, 439
Acceptance-based behavioral therapies,
  199, 216
Accessibility, psychotherapy and, 591–593
Accomplishment, 479
Acting "as if," 59
Action, integrative therapy and, 511
Activity scheduling, 253
Actualizing tendency, 104, 115
Addiction, 428–429
ADDRESSING framework, 545
Adler, Alfred
  family therapy and, 379–380
  Freud and, 55, 62, 63–64
Adlerian psychotherapy
  applications, 79–84
  basic concepts, 55–59
  behavior therapy and, 195–196
  case example, 84–89
  concepts, 68–69
  family therapy and, 378–379
  history of, 62–65
  mechanisms of, 75–79
  other systems, 59–62
  process of, 72–75
  REBT and, 155
  theory of personality, 65–68
  theory of psychotherapy, 70–72
Adolescents, positive psychotherapy for,
  489–490
Agency, limits of, 42–43
Agency for Healthcare Research and
  Quality (AHRQ), 579
Aging, contemplative psychotherapies
  and, 443
Agoraphobia, cognitive model of, 242–243
Agreeableness, 200
AHRQ Guideline Clearinghouse, 579
Albert Ellis Institute, 159
All Out! (Ellis), 160
Altruism, 432
American Civil Liberties Union, detainee
  interrogation and, 596
American Psychiatric Association, 238,
  570
American Psychological Association
  (APA), 10, 65, 238, 536, 543
  detainee interrogation and, 595–597
  ethics code, 587–588
  Nuremberg Ethic and, 593–594
American Psychologist (journal), 505, 588,
  594
Analog observation, 208
Analytical psychology, 28
Ancillary services, 72
Annual Review of Behavior Therapy, 199
Anorexia nervosa, 244, 363

Antisocial personality disorder, 474
Antithetical modes of apperception, 60
Anxiety, 285, 315, 348–349, 473
Anxiety disorders, 206, 242
APA Monitor, 576
Applied behavior analysis, 198, 211
Applied Psychology: Health & Wellbeing,
  467
Arbitrary inference, 240
The Art of Loving (Fromm), 271, 282
Art therapy, 81
Asian American Journal of Psychology, 543
Assessment scales, 237
Assimilation, 311
Assimilative integration, 500, 501
Association for Behavioral and Cognitive
  Therapies (ABCT), 198, 238
Attachment avoidance, interpersonal psy-
  chotherapy for, 360
Attachment styles, 344, 348–349
Attachment theory, 32–33, 61, 344–345,
  348–349
Attention, development of, 450–451
Attention deficit hyperactivity disorder
  (ADHD), 439, 473
Authorship, 279
Automatic thoughts, 245, 251
Aversion, 429
Aversion therapy, 196
Aversive conditioning, 212
Aversive racism, 539
Avoidance, 348–349
Avoidant personality disorder, 475
Awakening experience, death as, 283–285
Awareness
  cultivating, 447–448
  enhanced, 436
  refining, 431
Awareness meditation, 427
Awareness of awareness, 316, 318
Awareness process, 301–302

B

Basic Adlerian Scales for Interpersonal
  Success (BASIS-A), 81, 83
Basic encounter, 129
Beck Depression Inventory (BDI-II), 491
Behavioral activation, for depression, 214
Behavioral approach test (BAT), 221
Behavioral assessment, 207–209
Behavioral change, in family therapy, 396
Behavioral family therapy, 196
Behavioral genetics, 8
Behavioral interviews, 208
Behavioral observation, 208
Behavioral rehearsal, 253
Behavioral techniques, 253–254
Behaviorism, 196
Behavior modification
  Gestalt therapy and, 303

REBT and, 156
Behavior therapy, 167–168
  basic concepts, 193–194
  cognitive therapy and, 234–235
  family therapy and, 379
  future directions in, 224–225
  other systems, 194–196
  treatment, 207–216
Behavior Therapy (journal), 198
Behaviour Research and Therapy, 198
Belief system, 151
Bell and pad, 197
Bias in psychological disorders, 241
Binge eating disorder, 363
Biological sciences, impact on
  psychotherapy, 6–8
Biomedicine, culture of, 599
Bipolar disorder, 362, 473
Birth order, 66–67, 83
Black Families in Therapy (Boyd-
  Franklin), 543
Body awareness, 323
Borderline personality disorder (BPD),
  349, 363, 474
Boundary(ies)
  disturbances at the, 311–312
  family therapy and, 376
  Gestalt therapy and, 309
Boundary issues, therapist-client, 586–591
Breathing, anxiety and, 315
Breathing retraining, 212
Breath meditation, 433
Brief therapy, REBT, 178
British Independents, 29
British Medical Journal, 575, 594, 596
Bulimia, 244, 363

C

Calm, contemplative psychotherapies and
  development of, 447
Cardiovascular system, contemplative
  psychotherapies for, 440
Carl Rogers Counsels a Black Client
  (Moodley, et al.), 124
Carl Rogers on Encounter Groups (Rogers),
  110
Carryover effects, 219
Causality, cognitive theory of, 240
Center for Cognitive Therapy, 238
Change processes, 516–517
Children
  contemplation for, 439
  positive psychotherapy for, 489–490
Children's Apperceptive Storytelling Test
  (CAST), 81
Circular causality, 327, 375
Circular questioning, 384, 395
Classical conditioning, 196, 200–201
Classical psychoanalysis, 29
Classroom teaching, 128–129